15 Maintenance communication in supervisor-subordinate work relationships, 250
Group leadership theories, 259

16 Role theory, 271

17 Team work. Building productive relationships, 286

18 Situational leadership theory, 304
Nurses' use and delegation of indirect care interventions, 306

19 Negotiating theories, 326
Conflict styles as indicators of behavioral patterns in interpersonal conflicts, 329

20 Role theory, 337
Predictors of absenteeism among hospital staff nurses, 338

22 Congruency between nurses' values and job requirements: A call for integrity, 381

24 Role theory, 404
Registered nurse role changes and satisfaction with unlicensed assistive personnel, 404
Professional identity: Values embedded in meaningful nursing practice, 410

25 Theory of types or bases of social power, 419
Culture of troubled work groups, 421

26 Mentoring in the career development of hospital staff nurses, 435

Leading and Managing in Nursing

Leading and Managing in Nursing

Second Edition

Patricia S. Yoder-Wise
RN, C, EdD, CNAA, FAAN
Texas Tech University Health Sciences Center
Lubbock, Texas, and Odessa, Texas

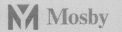

Mosby

A Harcourt Health Sciences Company

St. Louis   London   Philadelphia   Sydney   Toronto

Mosby

A Harcourt Health Sciences Company

Second Edition
Copyright © 1999 by Mosby, Inc.

Previous edition copyrighted 1995

Mosby, Inc.
11830 Westline Industrial Drive
St. Louis, Missouri 63146

Library of Congress Cataloging-in-Publication Data

Leading and managing in nursing / [edited by] Patricia S. Yoder-Wise.
  — 2nd ed.
     p.   cm.
  Includes bibliographical references and index.
  ISBN 1-55664-401-9
  1. Nursing services—Administration. 2. Leadership. I. Wise,
Pat S. Yoder
  [DNLM: 1. Nurse Administrators. 2. Leadership. 3. Personnel
Management.   WY 105L4325 1999]
RT89.L43 1999
362.1'73'068—dc21
DNLM/DLC

                                  98-11710

00   01   02 / 9   8   7   6   5   4   3

Contributors

Michael R. Bleich, RN, MPH, CNAA
Health Care Leadership and Systems Consultant
Lincoln, Nebraska

Carol Alvater Brooks, RN, DNSc, CNAA
Associate Professor
College of Nursing
Syracuse University
Syracuse, New York

Brenda Lewis Cleary, RN, CS, PhD, FAAN
Executive Director
North Carolina Center for Nursing
Raleigh, North Carolina

Karen A. Dadich, RN, MN
Associate Professor, Clinical Nursing
School of Nursing
Texas Tech University Health Sciences Center
Lubbock, Texas

Michael L. Evans, RN, PhD, FAHC, CNAA
Vice-President
Nursing and Patient Care Support Services
Presbyterian Hospital
Dallas, Texas

Jennifer Jackson Gray, RN, PhD
Assistant Professor
School of Nursing
The University of Texas at Arlington
Arlington, Texas

Ginny Wacker Guido, RN, MSN, JD
Professor and Chair
Department of Nursing
Eastern New Mexico University
Portales, New Mexico

Fran Hicks, RN, PhD
Professor
School of Nursing
University of Portland
Portland, Oregon

Joe Brannan Hurst, PhD, EdD
Professor
Education, Psychology, Research and Social Foundations
University of Toledo
Toledo, Ohio

Mary J. Keenan, RN, PhD
Associate Professor Emerita
School of Nursing
Medical College of Ohio
Toledo, Ohio

Karen Kelly, RN, EdD, CNAA
Director, Behavioral Healthcare/Social Services
St. Elizabeth's Hospital
Belleville, Illinois

Karren Kowalski, RN, PhD, FAAN
Director
Women's and Children's Services
Denver Metropolitan Service Area
Centura Health Care Systems
Denver, Colorado

Kerry A. Marrone, RN, MHA, CNA
Clinical Analyst
Veterans Memorial Medical Center
Meriden, Connecticut

Mary N. McAlindon, RN, EdD, CNAA
President
McAlindon Associates
Flint, Michigan

Kristi D. Menix, RN, MSN, CNAA
Associate Professor
School of Nursing
Texas Tech University Health Sciences Center
Lubbock, Texas

Dorothy A. Otto, RN, EdD
Associate Professor
University of Texas-Houston Health Science Center
School of Nursing
Houston, Texas

Amy Pettigrew, RN, DNS
Associate Professor
College of Nursing and Health
University of Cincinnati
Cincinnati, Ohio

Fay Carol Reed, RN, PhD
Director, Doctoral Program
College of Nursing and Health
University of Cincinnati
Cincinnati, Ohio

Cindy Whittig Roach, RN, DSN
Associate Professor
Co-Chair, Undergraduate Department
Beth-El College of Nursing and Health Sciences
Colorado Springs, Colorado

Linda Berger Spivack, RN, MSN
Director, Transition Planning
Veterans Memorial Medical Center
Meriden, Connecticut

Arlene P. Stein, RN, PhD
Former Clinical Manager
Surgical Unit
Memorial Hospital
Colorado Springs, Colorado

Darlene Steven, RN, MHSA, PhD
Associate Professor
School of Nursing
Lakehead University
Thunder Bay, Ontario, Canada

Ana M. Valadez, RN, EdD, CNAA, FAAN
Director, Undergraduate Program
Associate Professor, Roberts Practiceship
School of Nursing
Texas Tech University Health Sciences Center
Lubbock, Texas

Darla J. Vale, RN, DNSc, CCRN
Interim Chairperson
Department of Nursing
College of Mount St. Joseph
Cincinnati, Ohio

Rose Aguilar Welch, RN, EdD
Assistant Professor
Division of Nursing
California State University at Dominguez Hills
Carson, California

Deborah A. Wendt, RN, MS, CS
Assistant Professor
College of Mount St. Joseph
Cincinnati, Ohio

Donna Westmoreland, RN, PhD
Associate Professor
University of Nebraska Medical Center
College of Nursing
Omaha, Nebraska

This book is dedicated to the families who supported all of us who created it, to the faculty who use it to develop nursing's new leaders and managers, and to the learners who have the vision and insight to grasp today's reality and mold it into the future of dynamic nursing leadership.

Lead on... Adelanté!

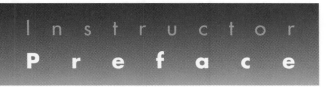
Leading and managing are two essential expectations of all professional nurses, and they are more important than ever in today's rapidly changing healthcare system. To lead and manage successfully, nurses must possess not only knowledge and skills but also a caring and compassionate attitude. After all, nursing management is about *people*.

Volumes of information on leadership and management principles can be found in the nursing, healthcare administration, business, and forecasting literature. The numerous journals in each of these fields offer research and opinion articles focused on improving leaders' and managers' abilities. The first edition of this text demonstrated that students, faculty, and registered nurses in practice found that a text that synthesized applicable knowledge and related it to contemporary practice was useful. Unlike clinical nursing texts, which offer exercises and assignments designed to provide opportunities for students to apply theory to practice, nursing leadership and management texts traditionally have offered limited opportunities of this kind. We changed that tradition by incorporating application exercises within the text and a skills workbook section for students.

This book results from our continued strong belief in the need for a text that focuses on the nursing leadership and management issues of today and tomorrow in a totally new way. We continue to find that we were not alone in this belief. Before the first edition, Mosby–Year Book, Inc., primarily through the efforts of Darlene Como, solicited faculty members' and administrators' ideas to find out what they thought professional nurses most needed to know about leading and managing, and what kind of text would best help them obtain the necessary knowledge and skills. Their comprehensive list of suggestions remains relevant in this edition.

CONCEPT AND PRACTICE COMBINED

Innovative in both content and presentation, *Leading and Managing in Nursing* merges theory, research, and practical application in key leadership and management areas. Our overriding concern remains in this edition to create a text that, while well grounded in theory and concept, presents the content in a way that is *real*. Wherever possible, we have used real-world examples from the continuum of today's healthcare settings to illustrate the concepts. Because each chapter contributor has focused on synthesizing his or her assigned content, you will find no lengthy quotations in these chapters. Instead, we have made every effort to make the content as engaging, inviting, and interesting as possible. Reflecting our view of the real world of nursing management today, the following themes pervade the text:

- The focus of healthcare is shifting from the hospital to the community.
- Healthcare clients and the healthcare work force are becoming increasingly culturally diverse.
- Today, virtually every professional nurse leads and manages regardless of his or her position.
- Consumer relationships play a central role in the delivery of nursing and healthcare.
- Communication, collaboration, team building, and other interpersonal skills form the foundation of effective nursing leadership and management.
- Change continues at a rapid pace in healthcare and society in general.

DIVERSITY OF PERSPECTIVES

The contributors have been recruited from diverse settings, roles, and geographical areas, enabling them to offer a broad perspective on the critical elements of nursing leadership and management roles. To help bridge the gap often found between nursing education and nursing practice, some contributors were recruited from academia; others, from practice settings. This blend not only contributes to the richness of this text, but also conveys a sense of oneness in nursing. The historical "gap" between education and service must become a sense of a continuum and not a chasm.

AUDIENCE

This book is designed for undergraduate students in nursing leadership and management courses, particularly those in BSN and BSN-completion courses. Today's students tend to be more visually oriented than past students. Thus we have incorporated illustrations, boxes, and a functional full-color design to stimulate their interest and maximize their learning. In addition, numerous examples and "A Manager's

Challenge" in each chapter remain to provide relevance to the real world of nursing.

ORGANIZATION

We have organized this text around issues that are key to the success of professional nurses in today's constantly changing healthcare environment:

Part I, Managing and Leading Presents basic concepts of managing and leading, with emphasis on their application to today's changing healthcare system. It includes coverage of legal and ethical issues, strategic planning, leading change in an evolving healthcare environment, and problem solving and decision making.

Part II, Managing the Organization Discusses healthcare organizations, cultural diversity in healthcare, various organizational structures, and collective action.

Part III, Managing Resources Explains the principles and practice of quality, risk, time, information, and financial management.

Part IV, Leading and Managing People Includes discussions on team building, staff development, communication, conflict management, and delegation.

Part V, Managing Consumer Care Focuses on consumer relationships, care delivery systems, and patient-related issues.

Part VI, Managing Personal Resources Offers career management and guidance via discussion of roles, power and politics, stress management, and career management.

Epilogue Provides tips and insights to prepare students for the future.

Workbook Section Included in the back of the text with exercises designed to meet individual and group learning needs.

Since repetition plays a crucial role in how well students learn and retain new content, some topics appear in more than one chapter and in more than one section. We have also made an effort to express a variety of different views on some topics, as is true in the real world of nursing.

DESIGN

A functional full-color design continues to distinguish this text. As described in later sections, the design is used to emphasize and identify the text's many teaching/learning strategies, which are featured to enhance learning. Full-color photographs provide visual reinforcement of concepts such as body language and the changes occurring in contemporary healthcare settings, while adding visual interest. Figures elucidate and graphically depict concepts and activities described in the text.

TEACHING/LEARNING STRATEGIES

The numerous teaching/learning strategies featured in this text are designed both to stimulate student interest and to provide constant reinforcement throughout the learning process. In addition, the visually appealing, full-color design itself serves a pedagogical purpose. Color is used consistently throughout the text to help the reader identify the various chapter elements described here:

CHAPTER OPENER ELEMENTS

The **introductory paragraph** briefly describes the purpose and scope of the chapter.

Objectives articulate the chapter's learning goals at the application level or higher.

Questions to Consider stimulate students to think about their personal viewpoint or experience with the topics and issues discussed in the chapter.

A Manager's Challenge presents a contemporary nurse manager's real-world concern related to the aspect of managing addressed in the chapter.

ELEMENTS WITHIN THE CHAPTERS

Glossary Terms appear in bold type in each chapter. They are also listed in the "Terms to Know" at the end of the chapter. Definitions appear in the Glossary at the end of the text.

Exercises stimulate students to think critically about how to apply chapter content to the work place and other "real world" situations. They provide experiential reinforcement of key leading and managing skills. Exercises are highlighted with an orange vertical rule and are numbered sequentially within each chapter to facilitate using them as assignments or activities.

Research and Literature Perspectives illustrate the relevance and applicability of current scholarship to practice. Perspectives always appear in orchid-color boxes with an "open book" logo.

Theory Boxes provide a brief description of relevant theory and key concepts. Application examples are included to illustrate the theory.

Boxes contain lists, tools such as forms and worksheets, and other information relevant to chapter content that students would find useful and interesting. Color boxes appear in each chapter.

END OF CHAPTER ELEMENTS

A Manager's Solution provides an effective method to handle the real-life situations set forth in A Manager's Challenge.

Chapter Checklists summarize key concepts from the chapter in both paragraph and itemized list form.

Tips offer practical guidelines for the student to follow before applying the information presented in each chapter.

Terms to Know are included as additional study/review aids.

References and Suggested Readings provide the student with a list of key sources for further reading on topics found in the chapter.

OTHER TEACHING/ LEARNING STRATEGIES

End-of-text Glossary contains a comprehensive list of definitions of all boldfaced terms used in the chapters.

COMPLETE TEACHING AND LEARNING PACKAGE

Together with *Leading and Managing in Nursing*, the workbook section, the Instructor's Resource Manual, and the accompanying video series comprise a complete teaching and learning package. Because students learn most successfully when information is presented in a variety of ways, the workbook section and video series are designed to give students the opportunity to reinforce their learning both experientially and visually.

INSTRUCTOR'S RESOURCE MANUAL with Transparency Masters and Test Bank prepared by Ginny Wacker Guido, RN, MSN, JD (also a contributor to the text), offers practical teaching suggestions and resources for presenting material in the text; making the most effective use of the workbook section and video series in conjunction with the text; and testing. The manual is divided into five distinct sections, including a chapter-by-chapter test bank containing a total of 260 multiple choice questions, with answer keys at the end of each set of chapter questions. Also 36 transparency masters of key illustrations from the text and other materials that instructors will find useful to present on overhead transparencies in the classroom are included.

MOSBY'S NURSING LEADERSHIP AND MANAGEMENT VIDEO SERIES Produced by David Wallace, PhD, Studio Three Productions, with Patricia Yoder-Wise, RN, C, EdD, CNAA, FAAN, as consultant, this series addresses the increasing demand for nursing graduates who can exercise leadership and management skills in today's varied healthcare settings. The series emphasizes the application of essential leadership and management principles to concrete practice situations. The video medium's ability to capture and convey both verbal nuance and body language with immediacy and clarity is particularly well-suited to a series illustrating interpersonal skills. Realistic case scenarios interspersed with narrative focus on key nursing leadership and management concepts and skills, while interviews demonstrate how real-life nurse managers successfully employ these concepts and skills in their practice. A survey of academic and staff development faculty was undertaken to identify the topics for which videos were most needed. The eight titles in the series are:

Video 1: Problem Solving and Decision Making: Critical Thinking in Action
Video 2: Dealing with Difficult People
Video 3: Effective Communication
Video 4: Managing Change
Video 5: Building Teams
Video 6: Delegating Effectively and Appropriately
Video 7: Managing Conflict
Video 8: Leadership

Each video is approximately 25 minutes long and is available either individually or as part of the set. An Instructor's Resource Booklet accompanies each.

Acknowledgments

We are indebted to our reviewers, whose insightful comments and suggestions were invaluable in helping revise this book. The end result of their efforts, as in any peer review process, is a stronger presentation. We are deeply grateful to the following people for their assistance:

Martha Butler, RN, PhD
Nursing Program Director
Southwestern College
Nursing Department
Winfield, Kansas

Mary L. Fisher, RN, PhD, CNAA
Associate Professor
Indiana University
Environments for Health, School of Nursing
Indianapolis, Indiana

Cecelia Gatson Grindel, RN, PhD
Assistant Professor
Northeastern University
College of Nursing
Boston, Massachusetts

Roselyn Holloway, RN, MSN
Lead Instructor, Nursing Management-Level III
Methodist Hospital
School of Nursing
Lubbock, Texas

Alice Nied, RN, MSN
Director of Nursing
Highland Community College
Nursing, Allied Health
Freeport, Illinois

Margaret B. Payne, RN, MNSc
Assistant Professor
William Carey College
School of Nursing
Hattiesburg, Mississippi

We also thank the numerous nurse educators and managers who participated in the surveys undertaken to plan the text and its ancillaries.

Special Acknowledgments

Many people helped to make this book a reality. First, I would like to acknowledge and thank the School of Nursing at Texas Tech University Health Sciences Center in Lubbock for allowing us to use its facilities in shooting many of the photographs that appear in this book. Special thanks to the Texas Nurses Association staff who consistently lead and role model.

Thanks to all who make Texas Tech University Health Sciences Center School of Nursing the special place it is.

All of the contributing authors to this book worked within very tight time frames to accomplish their work. To them I extend my deepest appreciation for being responsive, making the necessary revisions, and sounding eager to hear from me whenever I called. AT&T, Federal Express, fax, Kinko's, and email remain household words!

Special thanks go to our new editors, Yvonne Alexopoulos and Susan Epstein; to our developmental editors, Kimberly Netterville and Billi Carcheri, for answering questions, providing the "latest" version of whatever we were talking about, and doing all sorts of tasks that kept us on track; to Chuck Dresner (St. Louis) and Jim Childress (Lubbock) for their creative photography; to those who exceeded our wildest expectations of involvement (you know who you are); and to Robert Thomas Wise, my husband and best friend, for being such a great sounding board and consistent supporter.

One final note: no learner can remain stagnant. The context in which nurses manage and lead is constantly changing, sometimes for the better, sometimes for the worse. The key to success is to keep learning, keep caring, and maintain our passion for nursing. That, if nothing else, must be instilled in our leaders of tomorrow. **Lead on . . . Adelanté!**

Patricia S. Yoder-Wise, RN, C, EdD, CNAA, FAAN
Texas Tech University Health Sciences Center
Lubbock, Texas, and Odessa, Texas

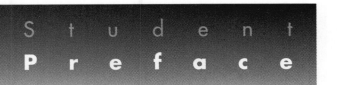

As a professional nurse in today's changing healthcare system, you will need strong leadership and management skills more than ever, regardless of your specific role. You will also need to be an independent, dependable follower. The second edition of *Leading and Managing in Nursing* not only provides the conceptual knowledge you will need but also offers practical strategies to help you hone the various skills so vital to your success as a leader and manager.

This book is divided into six parts that reflect the key issues in nursing leadership and management. Part I helps you gain insight into the concepts that underlie contemporary leading and managing practices. Parts II and III help you apply those concepts to the organization and its resources. Part IV focuses on managing the people who make up the nursing team, while Part V focuses on the healthcare consumer. Part VI offers information and practical strategies to help strengthen your ability to manage your professional and personal self. Because repetition is a key strategy in learning and retaining new information, you'll find many topics discussed in more than one chapter. And, as in the real world of nursing, you'll often find several different views expressed on a single topic.

To help you make the most of your learning experience, try the following strategy after you complete each chapter: Stop and think about what the chapter conveyed. What does it mean for you as a leader, follower, and manager? How does the chapter's content, and your interaction with it, relate to the other chapters you have already completed? How might you briefly synthesize the content for a non-nurse friend? Reading the chapter, restating its key points in your own words, and completing the text exercises and workbook activities will go far to help you make the content truly your own.

We think you'll find leading and managing to be an exciting, challenging field of study, and we've made every attempt to reflect that belief in the design and approach of this edition.

LEARNING AIDS

The second edition of *Leading and Managing in Nursing* incorporates some important tools to help you learn about leading and managing and apply your new knowledge to the real world. The next few pages graphically point out how to use these study aids to your best advantage.

The vivid full-color chapter opener **photographs** and other photographs throughout the text help convey each chapter's key message while providing a glimpse into the real world of leading and managing in nursing.

The **introductory paragraph** tells you what you can expect to find in the chapter. To help set the stage for your study of the chapter, read it first and then summarize in your own words what you expect to gain from the chapter.

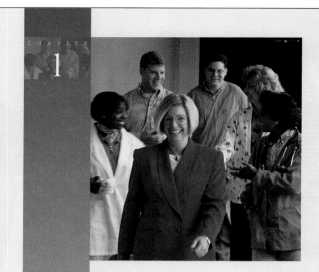

CHAPTER

1

Managing and Leading

Michael R. Bleich
RN, PhD.c, CNAA

This chapter explains the need to embrace leading and managing as an integral part of professional nursing practice, either at the bedside or in a management position. By examining leadership and management theories, personal attributes, and tasks, the student or nurse is able to reflect and assess leadership and management readiness to influence patient care and organizational outcomes.

Objectives

- Relate leading, managing, and following behaviors as important functions of professional nursing.
- Use leadership and management theories to guide self and others in managing patient care and human and material resources in various clinical settings.
- Develop personal attributes to promote self as an effective leader and follower.
- Apply nine essential tasks performed by leaders, managers, and executives to influence clinical practice outcomes.
- Assess and implement the use of follower strengths on a multidisciplinary team.

Questions to Consider

- Have you considered leading and managing as a part of professional nursing practice? How does effective followership promote successful leadership? What cultural and life experiences have influenced how you view leading, managing, and following?
- What leading and managing skills do you possess and practice in your current role? As you expand in personal and professional roles, what future expectations will you need to maintain your effectiveness?
- How can leadership and management theory guide your professional practice?

A Manager's Challenge

From the Director of Nursing of a Midwestern Healthcare System

As a Director of Nursing, it is my responsibility to ensure that effective clinical care is rendered to patients through the allocation of human and material resources. In my position, I cannot oversee the care given to each patient, but I do make use of management reports, consider staff and physician communications, and make selective rounds to observe the clinical practice environment. Using these management systems, I review and attend to critical problems that require immediate attention and examine the clinical outcomes for aggregate patient populations. This information helps me determine whether there are opportunities to improve or enhance the methods for delivering patient care, systems such as those for documentation, patient education, or discharge planning. With constrained or scarce human and material resources, one of my biggest challenges is getting adequate input from nurses and other bedside care providers so that systems can be enhanced to increase the value of care for patients. With high acuity and census, staff nurses do not have the time to redesign systems, or they are overwhelmed by the responsibility for suggesting changes in a turbulent work environment. Yet I need staff input and buy-in.

What do you think you would do if you were this manager?

INTRODUCTION

Too often, nurses think leading and managing responsibilities are reserved for nurses in management positions, or that being a follower means blindly observing the directions of others, such as following medical orders without question. What they fail to realize is that *all* professional nurses must display leadership behaviors when they are engaged in leading and managing activities at the bedside, in delegating assignments, or when serving in positions of formal authority over a clinical department or a cluster of services. Likewise, being an effective follower goes far beyond a display of passive actions without responsibility.

It takes effective leadership and followership behaviors to function optimally in clinical settings today. Furthermore, nurses are called on to be effective *both* as a leader and as a follower, shifting effortlessly between each role within moments of time, when necessary.

With many organizations designing, or even demanding, outcome-based, patient-centered healthcare systems, and with influential self-governed work teams and decentralized, "at-the-bedside" decision making, there are increased expectations and opportunities for professional nurses to influence patient care. Leadership and followership opportunities are available when nurses serve on shared governance committees, when they plan and execute a clinical

Each chapter opener includes these features:

The list of **Objectives** helps you focus on the key information you should be able to apply after having studied the chapter.

The **Questions to Consider** challenge you to think critically about issues in the chapter. You might want to write down your answers both before and after reading the chapter, and then compare them.

In **A Manager's Challenge,** practicing nurse managers offer their real-world views of a concern related to the chapter. Has a nurse manager you know had similar or dissimilar challenges?

Every chapter contains numbered **Exercises** that challenge you to think critically about concepts in the text and apply them to real-life situations.

Key Terms appear in boldface type throughout the chapter. (A list of all "Terms to Know" used in the chapter appears at the end of the chapter, and the Glossary at the end of the text contains a list of their definitions.)

The **boxes** in every chapter highlight key information such as lists and contain forms, worksheets, and self-assessments to help reinforce chapter content.

The **tables** that appear throughout the text provide convenient capsules of information for your reference.

---

8   Part one   **Managing and Leading: The Concepts**

the nurse and the patient. The leader/manager respects all opportunities for interaction with clients—patients or staff—and establishes goals based on this information.

Establishing **vision** is an important leadership concept. "Visioning" requires the leader to assess the current reality, determine what a desired state would be, and then manage the resultant tension between the two states in a positive manner. If the nurse manages the client positively, creative tension will result. Creative tension is positive tension that moves the client toward the desired goal. If the nurse fails to have a positive relationship with the client, or fails to recognize cues about the client's real circumstances, emotional tension results. Emotional tension drains the energy of the client and can cause even further distress. Visioning is an important function of leading and managing. Visioning goals gives purpose to all leadership activities.

Exercise 1-2

Develop a vision statement with a patient with whom you have a positive and knowing relationship. What is the patient's *current reality*, that is, what are the factors the client is facing as a result of disease, disability, lack of endurance, and so on? Ascertain with the client what his or her *future state* could be, such as adding your own professional knowledge and expertise to the client's perceptions. When you have finished your vision statement, ask the client, "If you could have your vision, would you take it?" Then ask the client to make an affirmation statement: "I choose to _____" (fill in the blank). A vision is then set for your collective intervention (Adapted from Fritz [1989]).

Affirming Values

Values are the inner forces that give us purpose and character. Organizations, through its members, have composite values that guide its purpose and character as expressed through its mission and philosophy. Leaders have values that influence decision making, priority setting, and the like, and clients (either patients or peers being influenced by the leader) have values that undergird their goals and are expressed through their behaviors. Values are deep-seated and are a persuasive force driving how we choose to act and respond to others.

The word *value* conjures up an image of something that has worth; our values have worth to us. A leader always seizes the opportunity to clarify and optimize the values that underlie the need to solve problems or create something new. This is because values are powerful forces that promote acceptance of change and achievement of a vision. In groups, awareness of the values that drive change helps those affected

> **Box 1-3**
>
> **Suggestions for Unlocking Individual and Group Motives**
>
> - Know your staff and patients and the factors that are influencing them to seek healthcare, work, and so on. Do your "homework" in a respectful and courteous manner.
> - Analyze individual and group responses to past rewards.
> - Ask for information from the group on how they would choose to celebrate work accomplishments.
> - Choose a variety of hygiene and motivator rewards to meet the variety of needs that may be present in a group.

relate to the importance of the change. Shared values build cohesiveness in a group. For example, the implementation of a new patient care delivery model will be enhanced if the persons affected by the change understand the guiding values, such as continuity of care, quality outcomes, and opportunities for demonstrating caring behaviors. If these values are known and important to the group, the change is more easily implemented and celebrated among all who share the values associated with it.

Motivating

When we let our values drive our actions, we make meaningful commitments to enacting our vision. Values become a source of motivation. **Motivation** is tapping into what we value, personally and professionally, and reinforcing those factors to achieve growth and movement toward our vision. Motivators are the reinforcers that keep positive actions alive. Examples of motivators include positively influencing patient outcomes, creating work efficiencies that improve teamwork, and the like.

Theories of motivation identify and describe the forces that motivate people. Examples of motivation theory are presented in the motivational theory box.

Motivating patients and staff as individuals is a challenging task. Leaders' recognize that often they do not have the luxury of working with individuals. The nurse leader taps into motivation of the patient and the patient's family and support system. Nurse managers often must lead whole groups of staff members toward a common vision. Leaders managing groups soon discover that various motivational strate-

---

38   Part one   **Managing and Leading: The Concepts**

Table 3-1	**ELEMENTS OF MALPRACTICE**
Elements	Example
Duty owed the patient 　Nature of the duty 　Existence of the duty	Failure to monitor a patient's response to treatment
Breach of the duty owed	Failure to communicate change in status to the primary healthcare provider
Foreseeability	Failure to ensure minimum standards are met
Causation	Failure to provide patient education
Injury	Patient falls
Damages	Fractured hip, concussion

nature of the duty. That a nurse owes a duty of care to a patient is usually not hard to establish. Often this is established merely by showing the valid employment of the nurse within the institution. The more difficult part is the nature of the duty, which involves standards of care that represent the minimum requirements that define acceptable practice. In the above scenario, the applicable standard of care is taken from the institution policy and procedure manual and concerns the standard of care owed the elderly patient regarding his or her safety. Standards of care are established by reviewing the institution's policy and procedure manual, the individual's job description, and the practitioner's education and skills, as well as pertinent standards as established by professional organizations, journal articles, and standing orders and protocols.

Several sources may be used to determine the applicable **standard of care.** The American Nurses' Association (ANA), as well as a cadre of specialty organizations, publishes standards for nursing practice. The overall framework of these standards is the nursing process. In 1988 the ANA published *Standards for Nurse Administrators,* a series of nine standards incorporating responsibilities of nurse administrators across all practice settings. Accreditation standards, especially those published yearly by the Joint Commission on Accreditation of Healthcare Organizations (JCAHO), also assist in establishing the acceptable standard of care for healthcare facilities. In addition, many states have healthcare standards that affect the individual institution and its employees.

The second element is breach of the duty of care owed the patient. Once the standard of care is established, the breach or falling below the standard of care is easy to show. However, the standard of care may differ depending on whether the injured party is trying to establish the standard of care or whether

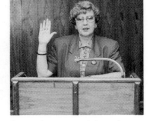

Nurses sometimes serve as expert witnesses whose testimony helps the judge and jury understand the applicable standards of nursing care.

the hospital's attorney is establishing an acceptable standard of care for the given circumstances. The injured party will attempt to show that the acceptable standard of care is much higher than the acceptable standard of care shown by the defendant hospital and staff. **Expert witnesses** give testimony in court to determine the applicable and acceptable standard of care on a case-by-case basis and to assist the judge and jury in understanding nursing standards of care. In the scenario involving Mrs. J., the injured party's expert witness would quote the institution policy manual, and the nurse's expert witness would note any viable exceptions to the stated policy.

A recent case example, *Sabol v. Richard Heights General Hospital* (1996), shows this distinction. In that

Most chapters contain at least one **Research** or **Literature Perspective** box that you can identify by the "open book" logo. These boxes summarize articles of interest and point out their relevance and applicability to practice. Check the journal that the article came from to find a list of indexing terms to help you locate additional and even more recent articles on the same topic.

Research Perspective

Boston, C., & Forman, H. (1994). A time to listen: Staff and manager views on education, practice, and management. Journal of Nursing Administration 24, 16-18.

A group of researchers from *The Nursing Spectrum* and the American Organization of Nurse Executives (AONE) surveyed 185 nurses eligible for middle management positions in healthcare to find out what would motivate them to apply for such a position. After learning that the nurses agreed unanimously that money alone was not enough, and that recruitment and retention of nurse middle managers were particular problems, the researchers asked the same group of nurses to participate in a series of focus groups to identify specific motivational and demotivational factors. The nurses chosen to participate were from major centers in the East, the Midwest and the South.

The researchers distributed a demographic assessment instrument and questionnaires to the nurses, who had been divided into three groups: middle managers, manager-eligible nurses, and relatively new graduates. Responses were very similar regardless of the area of the country the nurse was from. Nearly all nurses agreed that the prime motivational factors for recruiting and retaining nurse managers were individual empowerment, recognition, respect, true autonomy, and participation in decision making—essentially the same factors identified earlier by Maslow and Herzberg.

The middle managers' responses to the survey indicated that their sense of job satisfaction came from having the power to effect change, enjoying a sense of personal accomplishment grounded in their ability to influence and develop staff to provide consistent quality nursing care; receiving recognition from their parents, staff, colleagues in other disciplines, and upper management; and being afforded the dignity concomitant with their position. The most frequently noted difficulties were fiscal constraints, insufficient time to do everything, uncompensated time, and accountability without authority. The group identified key components of the middle management role as including both traditional and transformational concepts such as planning, directing, and controlling, motivating, facilitating, mentoring, problem solving, and advocating (for both staff and patients), and communicating effectively in all directions. All respondents agreed that good managers needed both strong fiscal skills and clinical competence.

Implications for Practice

Nurse executives at the organizational level can use the information gleaned from this survey to help ensure that the work environment is truly supportive for all nurses and that strategies essential for nurse manager effectiveness, such as empowerment, recognition, and compensation, are in place. AONE is also using the focus groups' results to plan educational strategies for its members.

Exercise 1-3

Recall a successful change that you experienced with other family, friends, or work peers. What values did you all share that made the change successful? How did you celebrate those values? Was change easier because of the values you shared? Now recall an unsuccessful change and compare the experience with the successful change. What made the two experiences different?

The freedom that leaders give staff to meet customer needs is best evidenced in the quality of decision making that surrounds meeting customer needs. Staff who are free to make decisions without fear of repercussion can have positive impact on the organization's capacity to carry out its mission. The astute leader also examines the quality of the staff's decision making in order to become politically involved in developing the organization's agenda for improvement. When leaders are politically astute, they seek forums to continuously advance ways to enhance services, systems, and products.

This chapter has addressed the importance of establishing a vision and applying leadership skills to achieve a desired state. Leaders do not influence organizational or client-centered change by just focusing on problem solving. If this were the case, leaders would be satisfied solving the same problems over and over. Leadership is about creating new systems and methods to accomplish the desired vision.

Achieving Workable Unity

Another challenge when leading and managing is to achieve workable unity and to avoid or diminish

Leadership Theories

THEORY/CONTRIBUTOR	KEY IDEA	APPLICATION TO PRACTICE
Trait Theories Trait theories were first studied from 1900 to 1950. These theories are sometimes referred to as the "Great Man" theory, from Aristotle's philosophy extolling the virtue of being "born" with leadership traits. Stogdill (1948) is usually credited as the pioneer in this school of thought.	Leaders have a certain set of physical and emotional characteristics that are crucial for inspiring others toward a common goal. Some theorists believe that traits are innate and cannot be learned; others believe that leadership traits can be developed in each individual.	Self-awareness of traits is useful in self-development (for instance, developing assertiveness) and in seeking behavior that matches traits (drive, motivation, integrity, confidence, cognitive ability, and task knowledge).
Style Theories Sometimes referred to as group and exchange theories of leadership, style theories were derived in the mid-1950s because of the limitations of trait theory. The key contributors to this renowned research were Shartle (1956), Stogdill (1963), and Likert (1961).	Style theories focus on what leaders do in relational and contextual terms. The achievement of satisfactory performance measures requires supervisors to pursue effective relationships with their subordinates, while comprehending the factors in the work environment that influence outcomes.	To understand "style," it is probably useful to obtain feedback from followers, superiors, and peers, such as through the Managerial Grid Instrument developed by Blake and Mouton (1985). Employee-centered leaders tend to be the leaders most able to achieve effective work environments and productivity.
Situational-Contingency Theories In the 1960s through the mid-1970s the situational-contingency theorists emerged. These theorists believed that leadership effectiveness depended on the relationship among (1) the leader's task at hand, (2) their interpersonal skills, and (3) the favorableness of the work situation. Examples of theory development with this expanded perspective include Fiedler's (1967) Contingency Model, the Vroom-Yetton (1973) Normative Decision-Making Model, and House-Mitchell's (1974) Path-Goal Theory.	Three factors are critical: (1) the degree of trust and respect between leaders and followers; (2) the task structure denoting the clarity of goals and the complexity of problems faced; and (3) the position power in terms of where the leader was able to reward followers and exert influence. Consequently, leaders were viewed as able to adapt their style according to the presenting situation. The Vroom-Yetton model was a problem-solving approach to leadership. Path-goal theory recognized two contingent variables: (1) the personal characteristics of followers and (2) environmental demands. Based on these factors, the leader sets forth clear expectations, eliminates obstacles to goal achievement, motivates and rewards staff, and increases opportunities for follower satisfaction based on effective job performance.	The most important implications for leaders is that these theories consider the challenge of a situation and encourage an adaptive leadership style to complement the issue being faced. In other words, nurses must assess each situation and determine appropriate action based on the people involved.

Most chapters contain a **Theory Box** to highlight and summarize pertinent theoretical concepts.

The numerous full-color **illustrations** visually reinforce key concepts.

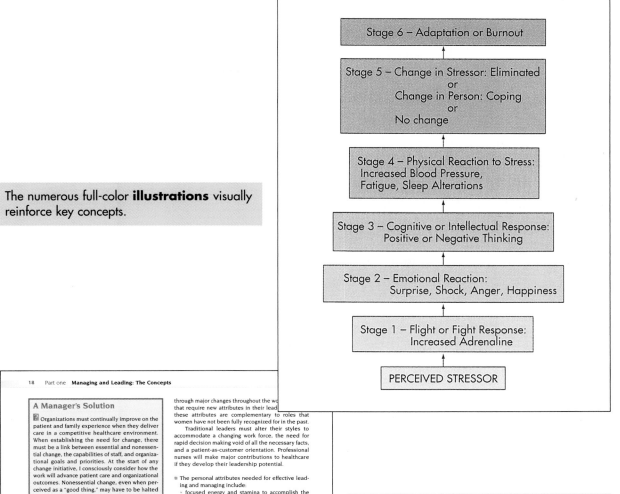

Each chapter ends with these features:

A Manager's Solution provides an effective method to handle the situations presented in A Manager's Challenge.

The **Chapter Checklist** provides a quick summary of key points in the chapter. To help you keep in mind the broad themes of the chapter, read it immediately *before* you start reading the chapter.

A Manager's Solution

Organizations must continually improve on the patient and family experience when they deliver care in a competitive healthcare environment. When establishing the need for change, there must be a link between essential and nonessential change, the capabilities of staff, and organizational goals and priorities. At the start of any change initiative, I consciously consider how the work will advance patient care and organizational outcomes. Nonessential change, even when perceived as a "good thing," may have to be halted in a turbulent work environment. Staff input is actively solicited. Through the use of practice councils, task forces, quality improvement teams, and career ladder change projects, staff must be represented despite acuity and census. This means added planning to ensure that staff participation is valued and that patient care is not compromised when staff attend to these added duties. Meetings must be led effectively to optimize staff input. Likewise, when an actual change is implemented, ample communication with staff is essential. What is being changed, what remains the same, and the benefits to be achieved from the change are communicated by myself *and* the staff who participated in the decision making. In this way, staff help "sell" the change to their peers by presenting their perspective on the changes taking place.

Would this approach be suitable for you? Why?

CHAPTER CHECKLIST

This chapter addresses the attributes and tasks of leadership and presents a case for active fellowship as significant functions for professional nurses to fulfill, whether in clinical or in management positions. Fulfilling leadership and followership roles requires understanding of self, commitment to the objectives of the organization and patient care, special skills and knowledge of organizations, human behavior, values, vision setting, problem solving and decision making, and the care of oneself. Organizations are going through major changes throughout the world that require new attributes in their leaders. Often, these attributes are complementary to roles that women have not been fully recognized for in the past.

Traditional leaders must alter their styles to accommodate a changing work force, the need for rapid decision making void of all the necessary facts, and a patient-as-customer orientation. Professional nurses will make major contributions to healthcare if they develop their leadership potential.

■ The personal attributes needed for effective leading and managing include:
- focused energy and stamina to accomplish the vision
- ability to make decisions in an intelligent manner
- willingness to use intuition, backed up with facts
- willingness to accept responsibility and to follow up
- sincerity in identifying the needs of others
- skill in dealing with people, for example, through coaching, communicating, or counseling
- comfortable standard/boundary setting
- flexibility in examining multiple options to accomplish the objective at hand
- trustworthiness, a good "steward of information"
- assertiveness in motivating others toward the objective at hand
- demonstrable competence and quick learning in the arena where change is desired

■ The tasks of leading and managing include:
- Envisioning goals
- Affirming values
- Motivating
- Managing
  - planning and priority setting
  - organizing and institution building
  - keeping the system functioning
  - setting agendas and making decisions
  - exercising political judgment
- Achieving workable unity
- Explaining
- Serving as symbol
- Representing the group
- Renewing

■ Traditional bureaucracies are changing because of the global changes in economy and healthcare. Organizations require new leadership skills and diversity in managing and leading.

■ The attributes of women are desirable for the new environments that are being created. Specifically,

The **Tips** offer guidelines to follow for each chapter before applying the information presented in the chapter.

The **Terms to Know** in every chapter includes all the key terms used in that chapter. You might find it helpful to review this list before reading the chapter and to look up in the Glossary any definitions that are unfamiliar.

---

56   Part one   Managing and Leading: The Concepts

- Nurse practice acts define the scope of acceptable practice for licensed registered nurses as well as licensed practical (vocational) nurses.
- Legal principles, if effectively integrated into all aspects of nursing management, minimize one's potential legal liability.
  - Malpractice is the failure of a person with professional education and skills to act in a reasonable and prudent manner.
  - Causes of malpractice for nurse managers include:
    - issues of delegation and supervision
    - duty to orient, educate, and evaluate
    - failure to warn
    - staffing issues
  - Liability may be classified as personal, vicarious, corporate, or strict product.
  - Protective and reporting laws ensure the safety or rights of specific groups of people.
  - Informed consent is the authorization by the patient or the patient's legal representative to do something to the patient.
  - Privacy and confidentiality rights protect the patient from unreasonable and unwanted interference and secure the privacy of the patient's medical record.
  - Federal and state governments have enacted a number of employment laws that nurses must understand and follow when dealing with managerial issues. These include:
    - Equal Pay Act of 1963
    - Civil Rights Act
    - Age Discrimination Act of 1967
    - Americans with Disabilities Act of 1990
    - Affirmative Action
    - Equal Employment Opportunity Laws
    - Occupational Safety and Health Act
    - Employment-at-Will and Wrongful Discharge
    - Collective Bargaining
- Ethical theories and principles relate to moral actions and value systems and apply both to patient situations and to management situations.
  - Ethical theories justify existing moral principles and are considered universally applicable.
  - Ethical theories include:
    - deontology
    - teleology
    - principlism
  - Ethical principles exert direct control over professional nursing practice and encompass basic premises from which rules are developed.
  - Ethical principles are:
    - autonomy

- beneficence
- nonmaleficence
- veracity
- justice
- paternalism
- fidelity
- respect for others
- The "MORAL" model is an easy acronym to remember in ethical decision making.
- Ethics committees aid in assisting nurses to implement solutions in everyday clinical practice.

TIPS ON LEGAL AND ETHICAL ISSUES

Before applying the information presented in the chapter, the following five tips are offered:

- Read the state nurse practice act carefully to fully comprehend the allowable scope of practice within the given state.
- Consult with risk management, the institutional attorney, or the legal department for a fuller understanding of how federal employment laws pertain to the individual nurse manager.
- Cultivate a group of professional consultants, either within the institution or outside the institution, who can assist with legal-ethical questions. Such a group or even one or two professional consultants may have great insight into issues as they arise and assist in preventing problems in the future.
- Discover who serves on the institutional ethics committee and develop friendships among selected members. Attend the meetings to see how ethical issues are addressed in the institution. Become an active part of the ethical rounds, if such exist in the institution.
- Think before you act. Remember it is always easier to hesitate, even briefly, so that the better approach can be implemented than to try to retract or amend something already done or already verbalized.

TERMS TO KNOW

apparent agency	emancipated minor
autonomy	ethics
beneficence	ethics committees
collective bargaining	expert witness
common law	failure to warn
confidentiality	fidelity
deontological theory	foreseeability

The **Glossary** at the end of the text lists alphabetically all the boldfaced terms from the chapters.

---

456   Glossary

Absenteeism The rate at which an individual misses work on an unplanned basis.

Acceptance The second phase of the change process when change is willingly used.

Accommodating An unassertive, cooperative approach to conflict in which the individual neglects personal needs, goals, and concerns in favor of satisfying those of others.

Accountability The expectation of explaining actions and results.

Acknowledgement Recognition that an employee is valued and respected for what he or she has to offer to the work place, team, or group; acknowledgements may be verbal or written, public or private.

Active listening Focusing completely on the speaker and listening without judgment to the essence of the conversation; an active listener should be able to repeat accurately at least 95% of the speaker's intended meaning.

Advocacy Multidimensional concept that refers to acting on or in behalf of another who is unable to act for himself or herself.

Agenda A written list of items to be covered in a meeting and the related materials that meeting participants should read beforehand or bring along. Types of agendas include structured agendas, timed agendas, and action agendas.

Apparent agency Doctrine whereby a principal becomes accountable for the actions of his or her agent; created when a person holds himself or herself out as acting in behalf of the principal; also known as *apparent authority.*

Assertions Statements about the truth of a matter; often these are only assumptions, postulations, or individual points of view that have little or no basis in fact or relevant evidence.

Associate nurse A licensed nurse in the primary nursing system who provides care to the patient according to the primary nurse's specification while the primary nurse is not working.

Autonomy Personal freedom and the right to choose what will happen to one's own person.

Average length of stay The number of patient days in a specific time period divided by the number of discharges in that same time period.

Avoiding An unassertive, uncooperative approach to conflict in which the avoider neither pursues his or her own needs, goals, and concerns nor helps others to do so.

Awareness The first phase of the change process when the need for change or innovation emerges.

Barrier A factor, internal or external to situation, that interferes with movement desirable outcome.

Beneficence Principle that states that the actions one takes should promote good.

Biomedical technology The use of machines and implantable devices to provide physiologic monitoring, diagnostic testing, drug administration, and therapeutic treatments in patient care.

Budget A detailed financial plan, stated in dollars, for carrying out the activities an organization wants to accomplish in a specific period of time.

Budgeting process An ongoing activity of planning and managing revenues and expenses in order to meet the goals of the organization.

Bureaucratic organization Characterized by formality, low autonomy, a hierarchy of authority, an environment of rules, division of labor, specialization, centralization, and control.

Burnout Disengagement from work characterized by emotional exhaustion, depersonalization, and decreased effectiveness.

Capital expenditure budget A plan for purchasing major capital items, such as equipment or a physical plant, with a useful life greater than 1 year and exceeding a minimum cost set by the organization.

Capitation A reimbursement method where healthcare providers are paid a per person per year (or per month) fee for providing specified services over a period of time.

Care delivery strategy A method nurses use to provide care to patients and clients.

CareMAP An abbreviation for a care multidisciplinary action plan, which combines a nursing care plan with a critical path. The purpose is to expedite patient care by improving expected outcome during a designated day.

Career Progressive achievement throughout a person's professional life.

Caring Behaviors and attitudes that denote special concern, interest, and/or feeling.

Case management A person-oriented service that reflects multidisciplinary cooperation and coordination.

Case management method A method of delivering patient care based on patient outcomes and cost containment. Components of case management are a case manager, critical paths, and unit-based managed care.

Case manager A baccalaureate or master's degree prepared clinical nurse who coordinates patient care from preadmission to and through discharge.

Chapter 4　**Strategic Planning, Goal Setting, and Marketing: Planning for the Future is the Key**　　15

◼ ACTIVITY 4-4

Planning is a critically important function. Without plans, we cannot sustain long-term initiatives. But planning must exist within a context of spontaneity, just as spontaneity must exist within a context of planning. To value one and eliminate the other will lead to system dysfunction!

1. List the benefits of planning.

2. List the problems associated with planning. Think about the problems that would occur if everything were planned and people were prohibited from taking any spontaneous action.

3. List the benefits associated with spontaneous action.

4. List the problems associated with spontaneous action. Think about the problems that would occur if no one in the organization did any planning.

Checking Your Thinking: See if your responses are similar to these benefits of planning:
- Enables allocation of resources
- Enables people to follow a common direction
- Provides a basis for performance measurement
- Enables long-term, proactive focus

Some problems of planning that is overdone and excludes spontaneity:
- Leads to organizational rigidity
- Impedes quick response to market changes
- Hinders individual creativity

Typical benefits of spontaneity:
- Allows for short-term flexibility
- Allows quick response to market changes
- Facilitates increased individual creativity

Some problems of spontaneity that is overdone and excludes planning:
- Impedes rational resource allocation
- Has no common direction
- Has no basis for performance measurement
- Has no basis for long-term focus

The **Workbook Section** is a built-in, perforated tool to help you self-assess and evaluate your learning and understanding of the content in the text.

◼ VIDEO SERIES

MOSBY'S NURSING LEADERSHIP AND MANAGEMENT VIDEO SERIES is an excellent tool to reinforce your learning of key leadership and management skills both visually and experientially. Using realistic case scenarios interspersed with narrative, each video demonstrates the application of interpersonal skills for leaders and managers. Whether you have personal access to these videos or view them only in class, you will find them especially helpful because of their ability to convey subtleties of communication such as verbal nuance and body language with immediacy and clarity. The eight titles in the series are:

Video 1: Problem Solving and Decision Making: Critical Thinking in Action
Video 2: Dealing with Difficult People
Video 3: Effective Communication
Video 4: Managing Change
Video 5: Building Teams
Video 6: Delegating Effectively and Appropriately
Video 7: Managing Conflict
Video 8: Leadership

Contents

PART one

MANAGING AND LEADING: THE CONCEPTS

1 **Managing and Leading,** 2
Michael R. Bleich, RN, MPH, CNAA

2 **Role Development,** 21
Ana M. Valadez, RN, EdD, CNAA, FAAN
Dorothy A. Otto, RN, EdD

3 **Legal and Ethical Issues,** 35
Ginny Wacker Guido, RN, JD, MSN

4 **Strategic Planning, Goal Setting, and Marketing,** 58
Darlene Steven, RN, MHSA, PhD

APPENDIX
Case Studies: The Strategic Plan of Action and the Strategic Marketing Planning Process, 68

5 **Leading Change,** 73
Kristi D. Menix, RN, EdD, CNAA

6 **Problem Solving and Decision Making,** 90
Rose Aguilar Welch, RN, MSN, EdD

PART two

MANAGING THE ORGANIZATION

7   **Healthcare Organizations,** 108
Carol Alvater Brooks, RN, DNSc, CNAA

8   **Cultural Diversity in Healthcare,** 123
Dorothy A. Otto, RN, EdD
Ana M. Valadez, RN, EdD, CNAA, FAAN

9   **Understanding and Designing Organizational Structures,** 137
Carol Alvater Brooks, RN, DNSc, CNAA

10   **Collective Action,** 151
Michael L. Evans, RN, PhD, CNAA
Fran Hicks, RN, PhD, FAAN

PART three

MANAGING RESOURCES

11 **Managing Quality and Risk,** 168
Deborah A. Wendt, RN, MS, CS
Darla J. Vale, RN, DNSc, CCRN

12 **Self-Management: Stress and Time,** 185
Fay Carol Reed, RN, PhD
Amy C. Pettigrew, RN, DNS

13 **Managing Information and Technology: Caring and Communicating With Computers,** 205
Mary N. McAlindon, RN, EdD, CNAA

14 **Managing Costs and Budgets,** 226
Donna Westmoreland, RN, PhD

PART four

LEADING AND MANAGING PEOPLE

15 **Communication and Partnership,** 246
Joe Brannan Hurst, PhD, EdD

16 **Selecting, Developing, and Evaluating Staff,** 265
Cindy Whittig Roach, RN, DSN

17 **Team Building,** 279
Karren Kowalski, RN, PhD, FAAN

18 **Delegation: An Art of Professional Practice,** 300
Patricia S. Yoder-Wise, RN, C, EdD, CNAA, FAAN

APPENDIX
The Best and the Worst of Delegation, 312

19 **Conflict: The Cutting Edge of Change,** 318
Joe Brannan Hurst, PhD, EdD
Mary J. Keenan, RN, PhD

20 **Managing Personal/Personnel Problems,** 335
Arlene P. Stein, RN, PhD
Cindy Whittig Roach, RN, DSN

PART five

MANAGING CONSUMER CARE

21 Consumer Relationships, 350
Brenda L. Cleary, RN, PhD, CS, FAAN

22 Care Delivery Strategies, 365
Karen A. Dadich, RN, MN

23 Patient Classification, Staffing, and Scheduling, 384
Linda Berger Spivack, RN, MSN
Kerry A. Marrone, RN, MHA, CNA

PART six

MANAGING
PERSONAL RESOURCES

24 **Role Transition**, 400
Jennifer Jackson Gray, RN, PhD

25 **Power, Politics, and Influence**, 415
Karen Kelly, RN, EdD, CNAA

26 **Career Management:
Putting Yourself in Charge**, 431
Patricia S. Yoder-Wise, RN, C, EdD, CNAA, FAAN

**APPENDIX
Marketing Yourself as a
Competent Professional**, 443

EPILOGUE **Thriving in the Future**, 451
Patricia S. Yoder-Wise, RN, C, EdD, CNAA, FAAN

Glossary, 454
Workbook Section, 465
Index, 555

Leading and Managing in Nursing

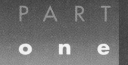

PART
one

Managing and Leading: The Concepts

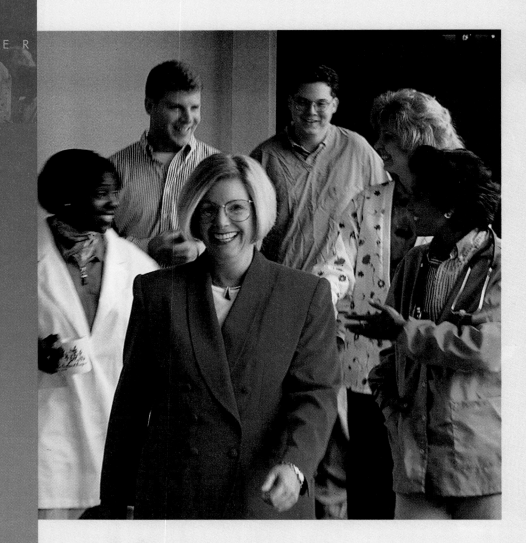

Managing and Leading

Michael R. Bleich
RN, MPH, CNAA

This chapter explains the need to embrace leading and managing as an integral part of professional nursing practice, either at the bedside or in a management position. By examining leadership and management theories, personal attributes, and tasks, the student or nurse is able to reflect and assess leadership and management readiness to influence patient care and organizational outcomes.

Objectives

- Relate leading, managing, and following behaviors as important functions of professional nursing.
- Use leadership and management theories to guide self and others in managing patient care and human and material resources in various clinical settings.
- Develop personal attributes to promote self as an effective leader and follower.
- Apply nine essential tasks performed by leaders, managers, and executives to influence clinical practice outcomes.
- Assess and implement the use of follower strengths on a multidisciplinary team.

Questions to Consider

- Have you considered leading and managing as a part of professional nursing practice? How does effective followership promote successful leadership? What cultural and life experiences have influenced how you view leading, managing, and following?
- What leading and managing skills do you possess and practice in your current role? As you expand in personal and professional roles, what future expectations will you need to maintain your effectiveness?
- How can leadership and management theory guide your professional practice?

A Manager's Challenge

From the Director of Nursing of a Midwestern Healthcare System

As a Director of Nursing, it is my responsibility to ensure that effective clinical care is rendered to patients through the allocation of human and material resources. In my position, I cannot oversee the care given to each patient, but I do make use of management reports, consider staff and physician communications, and make selective rounds to observe the clinical practice environment. Using these management systems, I review and attend to critical problems that require immediate attention and examine the clinical outcomes for aggregate patient populations. This information helps me determine whether there are opportunities to improve or enhance the methods for delivering patient care, systems such as those for documentation, patient education, or discharge planning. With constrained or scarce human and material resources, one of my biggest challenges is getting adequate input from nurses and other bedside care providers so that systems can be enhanced to increase the value of care for patients. With high acuity and census, staff nurses do not have the time to redesign systems, or they are overwhelmed by the responsibility for suggesting changes in a turbulent work environment. Yet I need staff input and buy-in.

What do you think you would do if you were this manager?

■ INTRODUCTION

Too often, nurses think leading and managing responsibilities are reserved for nurses in management positions, or that being a follower means blindly observing the directions of others, such as following medical orders without question. What they fail to realize is that *all* professional nurses must display leadership behaviors when they are engaged in leading and managing activities at the bedside, in delegating assignments, or when serving in positions of formal authority over a clinical department or a cluster of services. Likewise, being an effective follower goes far beyond a display of passive actions without responsibility.

It takes effective leadership and followership behaviors to function optimally in clinical settings today. Furthermore, nurses are called on to be effective *both* as a leader and as a follower, shifting effortlessly between each role within moments of time, when necessary.

With many organizations designing, or even demanding, outcome-based, patient-centered healthcare systems, and with influential self-governed work teams and decentralized, "at-the-bedside" decision making, there are increased expectations and opportunities for professional nurses to influence patient care. Leadership and followership opportunities are available when nurses serve on shared governance committees, when they plan and execute a clinical pathway, or when they lead an organizational quality improvement team. Still other opportunities are at the point of service, interacting with patients, family members, physicians, advanced practice nurses, and other healthcare team members to provide realistic, cost-effective, and patient-sensitive care.

With nurses playing the dual role of trying to complement patient and family care needs with organizational expectations for cost-effective care, the leadership-followership expectations are cofounded. In this chapter, **leadership** is defined as the use of personal traits to constructively and ethically influence patients, families, and staff through a *process* where clinical and organizational outcomes are achieved through collective efforts. The nurse as leader engages in relationship building to empower those being led toward a *vision* of optimal well-being and organizational achievement. **Followership** refers to those with whom the leader interacts. Followership is the healthy and assertive use of personal behaviors that contributes to patient, family, and healthcare team achievement leading toward clinical and organizational outcomes while practicing *acquiescence* in some tasks, such as direction setting, politicking, pacesetting, or planning, to the leader or others on the team. As defined, followership is *not* a passive process, but rather a set of behaviors that demonstrate collaboration, influence, and action *with* the leader.

It is important to realize that the attributes and behaviors of leaders are the complementary behaviors of followers. Finally, by virtue of organizational position, some nurses will be designated as managers. These nurses use their leadership skills and additional management skills to set organizational goals and objectives, manage human resources, provide performance feedback, and facilitate changes to meet patient care and organizational requirements.

PERSONAL ATTRIBUTES OF LEADERS/MANAGERS

Leading and managing require different skills from those associated with the technical aspects of nursing. Leading and managing require self-awareness of **personal motives**, those intangible driving factors that are influenced by our values and beliefs and that give meaning to our lives, both personally and professionally. Many nurses are motivated by the desire to help others, care for those who are unable to care for themselves, relieve social injustice, and the like. Still, the behaviors of nurses with these motives may vary greatly. One nurse who believes strongly in

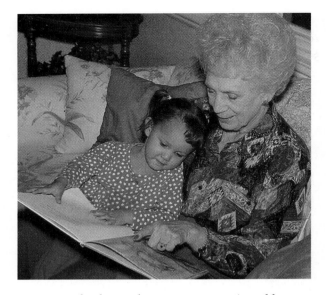

Many nurse leaders and managers are motivated by a strong desire to care for those who cannot care for themselves.

relieving social injustice may care for HIV/AIDS patients in an inner-city clinic, another may be an activist for social policy development, and another may engage in research. Being aware of one's motivations is not always an easy task; it is beyond the human condition to ever be totally self-aware. Leaders and managers must constantly seek self-awareness of their motives and values in order to inspire others.

Exercise 1-1

Imagine a clinical leader, manager, or teacher you admire and think of a specific situation in which this leader influenced positive change that affected you in some manner. Write down what you think the motivations were that made this leader want to facilitate change. Then describe the factors that made you feel drawn to work with this leader. Was it the leader's energy and stamina? His or her decision-making capabilities? Was it the leader's ability to make a decision without being paralyzed by too much data? Was it the leader's sincerity in dealing with people? Did the leader respect the confidence of those who shared information? Did you know where you stood at all times with the leader? Were you clear about the objective you were working toward? Was the leader competent in the issue being tackled? Did the leader act assertively? Did the leader have a plan for evaluating the impact of change? Share this assessment with the person you identified as the leader and get feedback on your observations.

Box 1-1
Attributes of Leader/Manager

- Uses focused energy and stamina to accomplish a vision
- Uses critical thinking skills in decision making
- Trusts personal intuition, then backs up intuition with facts
- Accepts responsibility willingly and follows up on the consequences of actions taken
- Identities the needs of others
- Deals with people skillfully: coaches, communicates, counsels
- Demonstrates ease in standard/boundary setting
- Examines multiple options to accomplish the objective at hand flexibly
- Is trustworthy; handles information from various sources with respect for the source
- Motivates others assertively toward the objective at hand
- Demonstrates competence or is capable of rapid learning in the arena where change is desired

The motives of the nurse influence the types of individuals who relate to that nurse as a leader and manager. These motives, coupled with other personal traits, shape the impact that the nurse as a leader/manager can have. Box 1-1 identifies some of the traits that attract other individuals to associate with a nurse leader.

DEVELOPMENT OF LEADERSHIP, MOTIVATION, AND MANAGEMENT THEORY

The development of leadership, motivation, and management theory rapidly evolved at the beginning of the twentieth century when industries flourished to achieve mass production. As large numbers of people migrated from rural communities to work together in these contained environments in urban settings, the factors that assured successful production were examined. Theory development began with an examination of the influence of *charismatic leaders* on the work force, followed by *motivational factors* that supported worker job satisfaction, and later, the *environmental determinants* that contributed to or deterred from achieving quotas.

Leadership theory emerged as the body of knowledge to explain the traits and behaviors of leaders perceived to successfully influence situations, people, and events toward organizational goal attainment. In the early years and continuing today, leadership theory was developed through the fields of sociology and psychology. The initial goal of leadership theory was to predict the qualities of leaders that would successfully influence others in meeting organizational outcomes.

Because leadership is an interactive process with others, several motivational theories were closely tied to leadership theory. The motivational theories explained how individuals derive and sustain behaviors to accomplish a goal, or how leaders and other environmental factors influence how workers maintain production. Motivational theories were developed primarily by the field of psychology.

Management theory constituted the body of knowledge that described how managers conduct activities to keep the organization operating in an effective manner. Management theory ranged from myriad topics such as how work is organized, planning accomplished, change managed, production quotas determined, and the like. Because of the diverse nature of activities that contribute to management theory development, representatives from a broad range of disciplines have contributed to its development, including managers, psychologists, sociologists, and anthropologists.

Leadership, motivational, and management theories overlap, although they are presented as distinctive. Each area of theory development continues to evolve, incorporating new learning about organizational culture, structure, and function; motivation, development, and learning; conflict management; team functioning; and other contemporary factors, such as globalization, diversity, and gender equity.

The theory boxes that follow are organized to provide an orientation to the major leadership and motivational theories and to introduce those concepts that apply in healthcare settings. Management theories, such as change theory, and other contemporary factors that are influencing leadership and motivation theory development are presented throughout this text. What should be evident from the theories presented is that the pattern of leadership research has been one of discarding, extending, and introducing ideas as the limitations of existing ideas were realized. There is a progression of different research orientations that has guided the development of leadership research.

Leadership Theories

THEORY/CONTRIBUTOR	KEY IDEA	APPLICATION TO PRACTICE
Trait Theories Trait theories were first studied from 1900 to 1950. These theories are sometimes referred to as the "Great Man" theory, from Aristotle's philosophy extolling the virtue of being "born" with leadership traits. Stogdill (1948) is usually credited as the pioneer in this school of thought.	Leaders have a certain set of physical and emotional characteristics that are crucial for inspiring others toward a common goal. Some theorists believe that traits are innate and cannot be learned; others believe that leadership traits can be developed in each individual.	Self-awareness of traits is useful in self-development (for instance, developing assertiveness) and in seeking employment that matches traits (drive, motivation, integrity, confidence, cognitive ability, and task knowledge).
Style Theories Sometimes referred to as group and exchange theories of leadership, style theories were derived in the mid-1950s because of the limitations of trait theory. The key contributors to this renowned research were Shartle (1956), Stogdill (1963), and Likert (1961).	Style theories focus on what leaders do in relational and contextual terms. The achievement of satisfactory performance measures requires supervisors to pursue effective relationships with their subordinates, while comprehending the factors in the work environment that influence outcomes.	To understand "style," it is probably useful to obtain feedback from followers, superiors, and peers, such as through the Managerial Grid Instrument developed by Blake and Mouton (1985). Employee-centered leaders tend to be the leaders most able to achieve effective work environments and productivity.
Situational-Contingency Theories In the 1960s through the mid-1970s the situational-contingency theorists emerged. These theorists believed that leadership effectiveness depended on the relationship among (1) the leader's task at hand, (2) their interpersonal skills, and (3) the favorableness of the work situation. Examples of theory development with this expanded perspective include Fiedler's (1967) Contingency Model, the Vroom-Yetton (1973) Normative Decision-Making Model, and House-Mitchell's (1974) Path-Goal Theory.	Three factors are critical: (1) the degree of trust and respect between leaders and followers; (2) the task structure denoting the clarity of goals and the complexity of problems faced; and (3) the position power in terms of where the leader was able to reward followers and exert influence. Consequently, leaders were viewed as able to adapt their style according to the presenting situation. The Vroom-Yetton model was a problem-solving approach to leadership. Path-goal theory recognized two contingent variables: (1) the personal characteristics of followers and (2) environmental demands. Based on these factors, the leader sets forth clear expectations, eliminates obstacles to goal achievements, motivates and rewards staff, and increases opportunities for follower satisfaction based on effective job performance.	The most important implications for leaders is that these theories consider the challenge of a situation and encourage an adaptive leadership style to complement the issue being faced. In other words, nurses must assess each situation and determine appropriate action based on the people involved.

Leadership Theories—cont'd

THEORY/CONTRIBUTOR	KEY IDEA	APPLICATION TO PRACTICE
Transactional/Transformational Theories		
These theory developments differ in that they describe the importance of dyadic relationships between leaders and followers. New concepts, such as empowerment, inspirations motivation, and social learning, are presented in these theories. While many theorists are currently exploring transformational theory development, Bass (1990), Bennis and Nanus (1985), and Tichy and Devanna (1986) are most frequently associated with its development through their qualitative studies.	Transformational leadership refers to a process whereby the leader attends to the needs and motives of followers, so that the interaction raises each to high levels of motivation and morality. The leader is a role model who inspires followers through displayed optimism, provides intellectual stimulation, and encourages follower creativity.	Transformed organizations are responsive to customer needs, are morally and ethically intact, promote employee development, and encourage self-management. Nurse leaders with transformational characteristics experiment with systems redesign, empower staff, create enthusiasm for practice, and promote scholarship of practice at the bedside.

TASKS OF LEADING AND MANAGING

The list of attributes of leaders and managers shown earlier provided some insight into the personal qualities that make leading and managing possible. But for individuals who have or are developing these attributes, opportunities to carry out leadership tasks will strengthen leadership and management functioning. Gardner (1990) describes the tasks of leadership in his book *On Leadership* (see Box 1-2).

Nurses as leaders and managers have daily opportunities to carry out these nine tasks, whether the focus is on patient care management or on unit/organizational management.

Envisioning Goals

Envisioning goals as a leader is not performed in isolation; it is the product of the relationship between the professional nurse and the patient or, in the case of a nurse manager, the manager and unit staff. The building of relationships is a product of time, circumstances, and the personal attributes of the nurse and the client. In a clinical emergency situation, where the patient is in crisis, the time factor may be reduced to moments before information is shared and a relationship established. The patient may not even realize who the attending nurse is, so long as the patient's perception of the nursing profession is positive and the individual providing care is perceived as some-

---

Box 1-2
Gardner's Tasks of Leadership

1. Envisioning goals
2. Affirming values
3. Motivating
4. Managing
   - planning and setting priorities
   - organizing and institution building
   - keeping the system functioning
   - setting agendas and making decisions
   - exercising political judgment
5. Achieving workable unity
6. Developing trust
7. Explaining
8. Serving as symbol
9. Representing the group
10. Renewing

From Gardner (1990).

---

one who can resolve the crisis. In other client-based situations, relationships are built over time, as the individual nurse or nurse manager proves to be competent and trustworthy, a good decision maker; able to prioritize the client's needs; and able to provide realistic options to solving problems. The point is this: effective goal development is contingent on trust, information, and mutual expectations between the nurse and the patient. The leader/manager respects all opportunities for interaction with clients—patients or staff—and establishes goals based on this information.

Establishing **vision** is an important leadership concept. "Visioning" requires the leader to assess the current reality, determine what a desired state would be, and then manage the resultant tension between the two states in a positive manner. If the nurse manages the client positively, creative tension will result. Creative tension is positive tension that moves the client toward the desired goal. If the nurse fails to have a positive relationship with the client, or fails to recognize cues about the client's real circumstances, emotional tension results. Emotional tension drains the energy of the client and can cause even further distress. Visioning is an important function of leading and managing. Visioning goals gives purpose to all leadership activities.

Exercise 1-2

Develop a vision statement with a patient with whom you have a positive and knowing relationship. What is the patient's *current reality,* that is, what are the factors the client is facing as a result of disease, disability, lack of endurance, and so on? Ascertain with the client what his or her *future state* could be, such as adding your own professional knowledge and expertise to the client's perceptions. When you have finished your vision statement, ask the client, "If you could have your vision, would you take it?" Then ask the client to make an affirmation statement: "I choose to _____" (fill in the blank). A vision is then set for your collective intervention (Adapted from Fritz [1989]).

Affirming Values

Values are the inner forces that give us purpose and character. Organizations, through its members, have composite values that guide its purpose and character as expressed through its mission and philosophy. Leaders have values that influence decision making, priority setting, and the like, and clients (either patients or peers being influenced by the leader) have values that undergird their goals and are expressed through their behaviors. Values are deep-seated and are a persuasive force driving how we choose to act and respond to others.

The word *value* conjures up an image of something that has worth; our values have worth to us. A leader always seizes the opportunity to clarify and optimize the values that underlie the need to solve problems or create something new. This is because values are powerful forces that promote acceptance of change and achievement of a vision. In groups, awareness of the values that drive change helps those affected

> ### Box 1-3
> ### Suggestions for Unlocking Individual and Group Motives
>
> - Know your staff and patients and the factors that are influencing them to seek healthcare, work, and so on. Do your "homework" in a respectful and courteous manner.
> - Analyze individual and group responses to past rewards.
> - Ask for information from the group on how they would choose to celebrate work accomplishments.
> - Choose a variety of hygiene and motivator rewards to meet the variety of needs that may be present in a group.

relate to the importance of the change. Shared values build cohesiveness in a group. For example, the implementation of a new patient care delivery model will be enhanced if the persons affected by the change understand the guiding values, such as continuity of care, quality outcomes, and opportunities for demonstrating caring behaviors. If these values are known and important to the group, the change is more easily implemented and celebrated among all who share the values associated with it.

Motivating

When we let our values drive our actions, we make meaningful commitments to enacting our vision. Values become a source of motivation. **Motivation** is tapping into what we value, personally and professionally, and reinforcing those factors to achieve growth and movement toward our vision. Motivators are the reinforcers that keep positive actions alive. Examples of motivators include positively influencing patient outcomes, creating work efficiencies that improve teamwork, and the like.

Theories of motivation identify and describe the forces that motivate people. Examples of motivation theory are presented in the motivational theory box.

Motivating patients and staff as individuals is a challenging task. Leaders' recognize that often they do not have the luxury of working with individuals. The nurse leader taps into motivation of the patient and the patient's family and support system. Nurse managers often must lead whole groups of staff members toward a common vision. Leaders managing groups soon discover that various motivational strate-

Motivational Theories

THEORY/CONTRIBUTOR	KEY IDEA	APPLICATION TO PRACTICE
Hierarchy of Needs Maslow is credited with developing a theory of motivation, first published in 1943.	People are motivated by a hierarchy of human needs, beginning with physiological needs, then progressing to safety, social, esteem, and self-actualizing needs. In this theory, when the need for food, water, air, and other life-sustaining elements is met, the human spirit reaches out to achieve affiliation with others, which promotes the development of self-esteem, competence, achievement, and creativity. Lower-level needs will always drive behavior before higher-level needs will be addressed.	When this theory is applied to staff, leaders must be aware that the need for safety and security will override the opportunity to be creative and inventive in promoting job change, for instance.
Two-Factor Theory Herzberg (1991) is credited with developing a two-factor theory of motivation, first published in 1968.	Hygiene factors, such as working conditions, salary, status, and security, motivate workers by meeting the safety and security needs and avoiding *job dissatisfaction*. **Motivator factors**, such as achievement, recognition, and the satisfaction of the work itself, promote job enrichment by creating *job satisfaction*.	Nurse managers need to use both hygiene and motivator factors to recruit and retain staff. Hygiene factors *do not* create job satisfaction; they simply *must* be in place for work to get accomplished. If not, these factors will only serve to *dissatisfy* staff. Transformational leaders use motivator factors liberally to inspire work performance.
Expectancy Theory Vroom (1964) is credited with developing the expectancy theory of motivation.	Felt needs of individuals cause their behavior. In the work setting, this motivated behavior is increased if a person perceives a positive relationship between effort and performance. Motivated behavior is further increased if there is a positive relationship between good performance and outcomes or rewards, particularly when these are valued.	Expectancy is the perceived probability of satisfying a particular need based on past experience. Therefore nurses in leadership roles need to provide specific feedback about positive performance.

Continued.

gies are necessary to move everyone toward the same vision. Box 1-3 provides suggestions for unlocking the motives of individuals and groups so that appropriate reward systems are in place to motivate behavior change. Chapter 16 in this text discusses motivation in more detail.

Managing

Ideally, managing is a subset of leading because leading reflects the importance of mutual relationships and vision setting between the leader and the clients. Managing is not void of relationship opportunities, but the tasks can be done in relative isolation of

Motivational Theories—cont'd

THEORY/CONTRIBUTOR	KEY IDEA	APPLICATION TO PRACTICE
OB Modification Luthans (1973) is credited with establishing the foundation for Organizational Behavior Modification, based on Skinner's work on operant conditioning.	OB mod is an operant approach to organizational behavior. OB Mod Performance Analysis follows a three step ABC Model: **A** (antecedent analysis of clear expectations and baseline data collection); **B** (behavioral analysis and determination); and **C** (consequence analysis, including reinforcement strategies).	The leader uses positive reinforcement to motivate followers to repeat constructive behaviors in the work place. Negative events that demotivate staff are negatively reinforced, so that the staff is motivated to avoid certain situations that cause discomfort. Extinction is the purposeful non-reinforcement (ignoring) of negative behaviors. Punishment is used sparingly because the results are unpredictable in supporting the desired behavioral outcome.

leading. The successful nursing leader today has both leadership and management skills.

Management skills require planning and priority setting. Once a vision has been established, planning requires the following (see also Chapter 4):

1. Deciding on a course of action.
2. Determining the chronology of events that must occur to achieve the vision.
3. Determining the talents and skills needed to accomplish the objective and assigning these tasks to individuals who can most effectively meet the needs.
4. Assessing the time requirements to accomplish the objectives and coordinate tasks around deadlines.
5. Considering the driving forces that will promote accomplishment of the objective. Driving forces are those political forces working in one's favor to promote transition to the established vision. The work that driving forces can achieve should be optimized.
6. Considering the restraining forces that will work against the desired accomplishments. Restraining forces are those political forces working *against* the desire to achieve the established vision. Decreasing these forces will help leaders achieve the vision. Political skills are used to develop alliances to assist in minimizing restraining forces.

7. Developing methods to stabilize the desired state once it is reached. Reinforcement is an important function of leadership.
8. Evaluating the attainment and maintenance of the desired state. Too often, leaders lose their effectiveness because they fail to recognize what they have accomplished. They must celebrate the accomplishment and reinforce the values and efforts that led to the success.

Other aspects of managing include using and promoting human resources to creatively develop new services or programs or extend existing services that help fulfill the mission and vision of the organization. By involving staff in service and program development, the leader promotes institution building through all levels of the organization.

Equally important is the leader's capacity to involve others in day-to-day problem solving. Keeping existing services and systems functioning is a challenging endeavor in healthcare organizations. Once a service or a system is designed, it may be taxed by the volume and/or acuity of patients who may use it. Realistically, not all patient needs can always be met with existing services or rigid systems. The leader empowers staff to respect, use, and adapt systems of care to meet the needs of customers. (Chapter 6 contains more on problem solving.)

Research Perspective

Boston, C., & Forman, H. (1994). A time to listen: Staff and manager views on education, practice, and management. Journal of Nursing Administration 24, 16-18.

A group of researchers from The Nursing Spectrum and the American Organization of Nurse Executives (AONE) surveyed 185 nurses eligible for middle management positions in healthcare to find out what would motivate them to apply for such a position. After learning that the nurses agreed unanimously that money alone was not enough, and that recruitment and retention of nurse middle managers were particular problems, the researchers asked the same group of nurses to participate in a series of focus groups to identify specific motivational and demotivational factors. The nurses chosen to participate were from major centers in the East, the Midwest and the South.

The researchers distributed a demographic assessment instrument and questionnaires to the nurses, who had been divided into three groups: middle managers, manager-eligible nurses, and relatively new graduates. Responses were very similar regardless of the area of the country the nurse was from. Nearly all nurses agreed that the prime motivational factors for recruiting and retaining nurse managers were individual empowerment, recognition, respect, true autonomy, and participation in decision making—essentially the same factors identified earlier by Maslow and Herzberg.

The middle managers' responses to the survey indicated that their sense of job satisfaction came from having the power to effect change, enjoying a sense of personal accomplishment grounded in their ability to influence and develop staff to provide consistent quality nursing care; receiving recognition from their parents, staff, colleagues in other disciplines, and upper management; and being afforded the dignity concomitant with their position. The most frequently noted difficulties were fiscal constraints, insufficient time to do everything, uncompensated time, and accountability without authority. The group identified key components of the middle management role as including both traditional and transformational concepts such as planning, directing, and controlling, motivating, facilitating, mentoring, problem solving, and advocating (for both staff and patients), and communicating effectively in all directions. All respondents agreed that good managers needed both strong fiscal skills and clinical competence.

Implications for Practice

Nurse executives at the organizational level can use the information gleaned from this survey to help ensure that the work environment is truly supportive for all nurses and that strategies essential for nurse manager effectiveness, such as empowerment, recognition, and compensation, are in place. AONE is also using the focus groups' results to plan educational strategies for its members.

Exercise 1-3

Recall a successful change that you experienced with other family, friends, or work peers. What values did you all share that made the change successful? How did you celebrate those values? Was change easier because of the values you shared? Now recall an unsuccessful change and compare the experience with the successful change. What made the two experiences different?

The freedom that leaders give staff to meet customer needs is best evidenced in the quality of decision making that surrounds meeting customer needs. Staff who are free to make decisions without fear of repercussion can have positive impact on the organization's capacity to carry out its mission. The astute leader also examines the quality of the staff's decision making in order to become politically involved in developing the organization's agenda for improvement. When leaders are politically astute, they seek forums to continuously advance ways to enhance services, systems, and products.

This chapter has addressed the importance of establishing a vision and applying leadership skills to achieve a desired state. Leaders do not influence organizational or client-centered change by just focusing on problem solving. If this were the case, leaders would be satisfied solving the same problems over and over. Leadership is about creating new systems and methods to accomplish the desired vision.

Achieving Workable Unity

Another challenge when leading and managing is to achieve workable unity and to avoid or diminish conflict so that the desired vision can be achieved. It is essential for leaders to acquire conflict-resolution skills.

When a dispute occurs, whether because of conflicting values or interests, it is useful to follow a defined set of principles for conflict resolution. Ury, Brett, and Goldberg (1988) describe a highly effective approach for restoring unity and movement toward the vision desired, as shown in Box 1-4. Chapter 19 in this text discusses conflict resolution in more detail.

Exercise 1-4

Examine the mechanisms available to you in your current capacity that are used for dispute resolution. How is the mechanism set up to accomplish the principles listed in Box 1-4? Has the system been used? What were the results? Were the disputants able to move on to achieve an outcome that was satisfactory to all parties? What role did the nurse leader or manager play in the resolution process?

Explaining

Leading and managing require a willingness to communicate and explain—again and again. The art of communication requires the leader to:

1. Know what information needs to be shared.
2. Know the parties who will receive the information. What will they "hear" in the process of the communication? Information must be presented that addresses the listener's self-interest.
3. Provide the opportunity for dialogue and feedback. Face-to-face communication is always preferable to written communication because of the immediacy of information feedback to the leader and the opportunity for clarification of information. Written feedback is useful for reinforcement of the message or to follow up on inquiries.
4. Know that it is possible to give too much information, which can temporarily paralyze the listener.
5. Be willing to repeat information in many different ways, at different times. The more diverse the group being addressed, the more important it is to avoid complex terms, concepts, or ideas. Information should be kept simple.
6. Always explain *why* something is being asked or is changing. The values behind the communication should be reinforced.
7. Acknowledge loss and provide the opportunity for honest communication about what

---

Box 1-4
Principles of Conflict Resolution

1. Put the focus on interests
   * examine the real issues of all parties
   * be expedient in responding to the issues
   * use negotiation procedures and processes such as ethics committees and other neutral sources
2. Build in "loop-backs" to negotiation
   * if resolution fails, allow for a "cooling off" period before reconvening
   * review the likely consequences of not proceeding with all parties, so that they understand the full consequences of failure to resolve the issue
3. Build in consultation *before* and feedback *after* the negotiations
   * build consensus and use political skills to facilitate communication before confrontation, if anticipated, occurs
   * work with staff or patients after the conflict to learn from the situation and to avoid a similar conflict in the future
   * provide a forum for open discussion
4. Provide the necessary motivation, skills, and resources
   * make sure that the parties involved in conflict are motivated to use procedures and resources that have been developed; this requires ease of access and a nonthreatening mechanism
   * ensure that those working in the dispute have skills in problem solving and dispute resolution
   * provide the necessary resources to those involved to offer support, information, and other technical assistance

Adapted from Ury, Brett, & Goldberg (1988).

---

will be missed, especially if change is involved.
8. Be sensitive to nonverbal communication. It may be necessary in complex situations to have someone reinterpret key points and provide feedback about the clarity of the message after the meeting. Leaders must use every opportunity for explaining as a vehicle to fine-tune communication skills. (See Chapter 15 for more on communication.)

Exercise 1-5

Examine a recent conversation in which you were in a leadership capacity. In one column, write down what you said. In the next column, write down the response you received. In a third column, write down what you were thinking but did *not* say. Analyze the conversation: Did you use language common to the listener? Did you share enough information to be clear, but not too much information, which could clutter the point of your communication? Were you honest in your communication? Did you allow time for feedback? Did you express main ideas in several different ways or summarize information for clarity? (Adapted from Chris Argyris as described in Senge [1990].)

Serving as Symbol

Every leader has the opportunity to speak for others. Nurses speak to physicians on behalf of patients; managers speak to other departments on behalf of their staff. Serving as a symbol means that unity, collective identity, and continuity of service are represented.

Representing the Group

While serving as a symbol of nursing, or of nursing management, there are many opportunities for leaders to represent the group. As mentioned in the introductory remarks to this chapter, progressive organizations today are creating more vehicles for employee participation. Many organizations are decentralizing decision making and removing layers of management. In an environment that is rapidly changing, the high technology and skill level associated with healthcare professionals, as well as the need for rapid organizational change, has created the need for collective decision making. Leaders should treat these newfound opportunities with respect and honestly try to represent the group with an attitude of openness and integrity. During these representative opportunities, leaders are called on to demonstrate an understanding of the organization's objectives and to contribute to its mission and purpose.

Whether on- or off-duty, leaders must be cognizant that their public image is always being viewed by others. As both a symbol of the organization and a representative of the professional discipline, the leader behaves in ways that uphold the dignity and quality of the organization and professional discipline.

Renewing

Leaders can generate energy within and among others. A true leader does not just expend the energy of the group or allow the group to lose its focus. In organizations and nursing practice, there is a constant need to find a balance between problem solving (energy expending) and vision setting (energy producing). When changes are made based on vision, they can be met with renewed spirit and purpose if the leader uses Gardner's nine tasks of leadership as a base. This chapter's "Literature Perspective" highlights the importance of vision setting.

Furthermore, leaders must take care of themselves—eat a balanced diet, get adequate sleep and exercise, and participate in other wellness-oriented activities—to maintain their perspective and the necessary energy level. Likewise, they must ensure that their constituents are given similar opportunities for renewal. Gardner (1990) states that, "The consideration leaders must never forget is that the key for renewal is the release of human energy and talent" (p. 136). This requires focused energy and personal well-being.

In Table 1-1 Gardner's leadership tasks are presented to provide a contrast between leaders who focus on the delivery of professional nursing and leaders who hold formal management positions representing the interests of the organization.

DIVERSITY IN LEADERSHIP, DIVERSITY IN ORGANIZATIONS

The healthcare industry is spiraling through unparalleled change, often away from the traditional industrial models that have reigned throughout the twentieth century. Today it is no longer acceptable for workers to understand only their single part in how the work of the organization is achieved; rather, they must understand how their work fits in with the whole system of care delivery. It is the responsibility of leadership to acquire this "whole system" knowledge, and then to impart and reinforce it to all staff. Healthcare organizations are being "retooled" to meet customer expectations and to achieve optimal clinical outcomes.

Traditional views of management and leadership are evolving in this chaotic environment (see "Literature Perspective," p. 16). Work forces are now characterized by workers who require more flexibility and balance in their work and personal lives; they want to know that what they do is being valued and is contributing toward a common goal, despite abbreviated work hours. Organizations are becoming known for their flexibility rather than their bureaucracy.

These changes create the opportunity for the emergence of a new type of nursing leader, both at

Table 1-1	CONTRASTING LEADING/MANAGING BEHAVIORS OF NURSES IN CLINICAL, MANAGEMENT, AND EXECUTIVE POSITIONS		
	Behaviors		
Gardner's Task	**Clinical Position**	**Management Position**	**Executive Position**
Envisioning goals	Visioning patient outcomes for single patients/families; assisting patients in formulating their vision of future well-being.	Visioning patient outcomes for aggregates of patient populations and creating a vision of how systems support patient care objectives; assisting staff in formulating their vision of enhanced clinical and organizational performance.	Visioning community health and organizational outcomes for aggregates of patient populations for which the organization can respond.
Affirming values	Assisting the patient/family to sort out and articulate personal values in relation to health problems and the impact of these problems on lifestyle adjustments.	Assisting the staff in interpreting organizational values and strengthening staff members' personal values to more closely align with those of the organization; interpreting values during organizational change.	Assisting other organizational leaders in the expression of community and organizational values; interpreting values to the community and staff.
Motivating	Relating to and inspiring patients/families to achieve their vision.	Relating to and inspiring staff to achieve the mission of the organization and the vision associated with organizational enhancement.	Relating to and inspiring management, staff, and community leaders to achieve desired levels of health and well-being, and appropriate use of clinical services.
Managing	Assisting the patient/family with planning, priority setting, and decision making; making sure that organizational systems work in the patients' behalf.	Assisting the staff with planning, priority setting, and decision making; making sure that systems work to enhance the staff's ability to meet patient care needs and the objectives of the organization.	Assisting other executives and corporate leaders with planning, priority setting, and decision making; ensuring that human and material resources are available to meet health needs.

the bedside and in formal management positions. While hospital leadership historically has been provided largely by men, women are assuming key organizational positions that add depth and diversity to management decision making. Research on the role of women in leadership positions supports the many personal characteristics that are desirable for organizations to succeed in the marketplace and in understanding the work force. Furthermore, in providing care to patients, nursing has historically been close to the true mission of the healthcare enterprise and is therefore in a strong position to recognize the impact that change can have on patient outcomes.

Helgeson (1990) described the characteristics of four women in top leadership and management positions:

Table 1-1	CONTRASTING LEADING/MANAGING BEHAVIORS OF NURSES IN CLINICAL, MANAGEMENT, AND EXECUTIVE POSITIONS—cont'd		
	Behaviors		
Gardner's Task	**Clinical Position**	**Management Position**	**Executive Position**
Achieving workable unity	Assisting patients/families to achieve optimal functioning to benefit the transition to enhanced health functions.	Assisting staff to achieve optimal functioning to benefit transition to enhanced organizational functions.	Assisting multidisciplinary leaders to achieve optimal functioning to benefit patient care delivery and collaborative care.
Explaining	Teaching and interpreting information to promote patient/family functioning and well-being.	Teaching and interpreting information to promote organizational functioning and enhanced services.	Teaching and interpreting organizational and community-based health information to promote organizational functioning and service development.
Serving as symbol	Representing the nursing profession and the values and beliefs of the organization to patients/ families and other community groups.	Representing the nursing unit service and the values and beliefs of the organization to staff, other departments, professional disciplines, and the community at large.	Representing the values and beliefs of the organization and patient care services to internal and external constituents.
Representing the group	Representing nursing and the unit in task forces, total quality initiatives, shared governance councils, and other groups.	Representing nursing and the organization on assigned boards, councils, committees, and task forces, both internal and external to the organization.	Representing the organization and patient care services on assigned boards, councils, committees, and task forces, both internal and external to the organization.
Renewing	Providing self-care to enhance the ability to care for staff, patients, families, and the organization served.	Providing self-care to enhance the ability to care for staff, patients, families, and the organization served.	Providing self-care to enhance the ability to care for patients, families, and the organization served.

1. Women worked at a steady pace, scheduling small breaks throughout the day to reduce the amount of "frantic" stress.
2. Women leaders were perceived as being more accessible. They did not view unscheduled tasks and encounters as interruptions and shared information with peers more readily.
3. Women were perceived as caring, involved, helpful, and responsible for their leading and managing functions.
4. Women were more likely to make time for functions not directly associated with their work. This enabled them to gain a broader perspective on the issues faced in the business environment.

Literature Perspective

Davidhizar, R. (1993). Leading with charisma: Journal of Advanced Nursing, *18, 675-679.*

Traditional approaches to management include the use of authority, control, competition, and logic through management behaviors that are autocratic, directive, and task oriented. Today, organizations are changing to focus on human needs, and *transformational leadership* is emerging as a modern management style to accommodate workers who value working in organizations that are personally fulfilling. Organizations with transformational leadership are characterized by mutuality and affiliation, acknowledging complexity and ambiguity, cooperating versus competing, emphasizing human relations, defining processes versus tasks, accepting feelings, promoting networking versus hierarchy building, and recognizing the value of intuition.

Charismatic leaders are required to guide organizations into transformational cultures. The effect of charismatic leaders is based on the leader's appeal to followers and the leader's ability to enter into the "psyche" of the followers in a manner that fosters the presence of loyalty or enthusiasm. "Charismatic effect" is created when there are a gifted leader, dependent followers, and situations for the leader to depict to followers.

To use charisma in leadership requires leaders to have positive self-regard/self-esteem, an orientation to people and a visible focus on the human needs of followers, a vision that gives individuals something to work for and be committed to, skill in promoting and selling the vision, and the ability to create structures and processes to attain the vision.

Implications for Practice

The organizational climate in healthcare is experiencing rapid change. Today's professional workers are characterized as individuals who relate more to their profession than to the organization that employs them; these attitudes are particularly prevalent given organizational mergers, department consolidation, and the addition of services extending beyond the traditional "walls" of the organization. These factors require charismatic leadership. Traditional leaders either will be reschooled in their approach to management or will find themselves replaced by others who are able to generate focus, enthusiasm, and energy in their staff. Hypervigilant supervision must be replaced by open communication, personal mentoring, and creative problem solving.

---

5. Women successfully maintained a complex network of relationships with people outside of their organizations. Again, this added a broader perspective on issues faced in the business environment.
6. Women focused on the ecology of leadership, reducing the likelihood of being caught in the here and now and focusing on future-oriented long-range planning.

As female nurses embark on the functions of leading and managing, they should do so recognizing that the characteristics that they bring to the healthcare setting are very much needed in this environment of change. Not only are these the characteristics of excellent clinical providers, but they are also characteristics consistent with excellent leadership in healthcare organizations.

In contrast to women, men tend to be socialized with values of distance and autonomy rather than connection and intimacy. Historically, society has expected men to use logic, analysis, and abstract thinking and to express their opinions (Belenky et al, 1986). Men who are in leadership positions must recognize that it may be difficult for women to merely "trust" this work of logic and fact-giving, particularly when their own experiences represent different truths. To capitalize fully on the potential of both genders, leaders must facilitate understanding of gender differences and, as mentioned earlier in this chapter, blend the use of intuition backed up by fact. Leaders must continue to grow in self-understanding so that they have the insight to appreciate the gifts of those they lead.

Box 1-5 lists typical masculine and feminine strengths women can develop to be effective in leadership and management positions.

Box 1-5

Typical Masculine and Feminine Strengths Related to Effective Androgynous Styles of Management

TYPICAL MASCULINE STRENGTHS WOMEN CAN DEVELOP	TYPICAL FEMININE STRENGTHS WOMEN CAN EXPAND
• Learn how to be powerful and forthright. • Become *entrepreneurial.* • Have a direct, visible impact on others, rather than just functioning behind the scenes. • State your own needs and refuse to back down, even if the immediate response is not acceptance. • Focus on a task and regard it as at least as important as the relationships with the people doing the task. • Build support systems with other women and share competence with them, rather than competing with them. • Build a sense of community among women instead of saying, "I pulled myself up by my bootstraps, so why can't you?" • Intellectualize and generalize from experience. • Behave "impersonally" rather than personalizing experience and denying another's reality because it is different. • Stop turning anger, blame, and pain inward. • Stop accepting feelings of suffering and victimization. • Take the option of being invulnerable to destructive feedback. • Stop being irritable, a "nag," and/or passive-resistant about resentments and anger. • Respond directly with "I" statements rather than with blaming "you" ones ("I'*m* not comfortable with that" rather than "*you* shouldn't do that"). • Become an effective problem solver by being analytical, systematic, and directive. • Change self-limiting behaviors, such as allowing interruptions or laughing after making a serious statement. • Become a risk-taker (calculating probabilities and making appropriate trade-offs).	• Be able to recognize, accept, and express feelings. • Respect feelings as a basic and essential part of life, as guides to authenticity and effectiveness, rather than as barriers to achievement. • Accept the vulnerability and imperfections of others. • Believe in the right to work for self-fulfillment as well as for money. • Believe in the value of nonwork roles as well as work identity. • Have the ability to fail at a task without feeling like a failure as a person. • Accept and express the need to be nurtured at all times. • Touch and be close to both men and women without necessarily experiencing or suggesting sexual connotations. • Be skillful at listening empathetically and actively without feeling responsible for solving others' problems. • Share feelings as the most meaningful part of one's contact with others, accepting the risk and vulnerability such sharing implies. • Be skillful at building support systems with other women, sharing competencies without competition, and sharing feelings and needs with sincerity. • Relate to experiences and people on a personal level rather than assuming that the only valid approach to life and interpersonal contact is an abstract, rational, or strictly objective one. • Accept the emotional, spontaneous, and irrational parts of the self.

Adapted from Sargent (1981). Cited in Carr-Ruffino (1993).

A Manager's Solution

🔲 Organizations must continually improve on the patient and family experience when they deliver care in a competitive healthcare environment. When establishing the need for change, there must be a link between essential and nonessential change, the capabilities of staff, and organizational goals and priorities. At the start of any change initiative, I consciously consider how the work will advance patient care and organizational outcomes. Nonessential change, even when perceived as a "good thing," may have to be halted in a turbulent work environment. Staff input is actively solicited. Through the use of practice councils, task forces, quality improvement teams, and career ladder change projects, staff must be represented despite acuity and census. This means added planning to ensure that staff participation is valued and that patient care is not compromised when staff attend to these added duties. Meetings must be led effectively to optimize staff input. Likewise, when an actual change is implemented, ample communication with staff is essential. What is being changed, what remains the same, and the benefits to be achieved from the change are communicated by myself *and* the staff who participated in the decision making. In this way, staff help "sell" the change to their peers by presenting their perspective on the changes taking place.

🔲 *Would this approach be suitable for you? Why?*

■ CHAPTER CHECKLIST

This chapter addresses the attributes and tasks of leadership and presents a case for active fellowship as significant functions for professional nurses to fulfill, whether in clinical or in management positions. Fulfilling leadership and followership roles requires understanding of self, commitment to the objectives of the organization and patient care, special skills and knowledge of organizations, human behavior, values, vision setting, problem solving and decision making, and the care of oneself. Organizations are going

through major changes throughout the world, changes that require new attributes in their leaders. Many of these attributes are complementary to roles that women have not been fully recognized for in the past.

Traditional leaders must alter their styles to accommodate a changing work force, the need for rapid decision making void of all the necessary facts, and a patient-as-customer orientation. Professional nurses will make major contributions to healthcare if they develop their leadership potential.

■ The personal attributes needed for effective leading and managing include:
  • focused energy and stamina to accomplish the vision
  • ability to make decisions in an intelligent manner
  • willingness to use intuition, backed up with facts
  • willingness to accept responsibility and to follow up
  • sincerity in identifying the needs of others
  • skill in dealing with people, for example, through coaching, communicating, or counseling
  • comfortable standard/boundary setting
  • flexibility in examining multiple options to accomplish the objective at hand
  • trustworthiness, a good "steward of information"
  • assertiveness in motivating others toward the objective at hand
  • demonstrable competence and quick learning in the arena where change is desired
■ The tasks of leading and managing include:
  • Envisioning goals
  • Affirming values
  • Motivating
  • Managing
    – planning and priority setting
    – organizing and institution building
    – keeping the system functioning
    – setting agendas and making decisions
    – exercising political judgment
  • Achieving workable unity
  • Explaining
  • Serving as symbol
  • Representing the group
  • Renewing
■ Traditional bureaucracies are changing because of the global changes in economy and healthcare. Organizations require new leadership skills and diversity in managing and leading.
■ The attributes of women are desirable for the new environments that are being created. Specifically,

women are suited for leadership positions because they:

- work at a steady pace, with less frantic stress
- do not view unscheduled tasks and encounters as interruptions and are more likely to share information
- are more likely to be perceived as caring, involved, helping, and being responsible
- are more likely to make time for functions not associated with their work and maintain a complex network of relationships that offer a broader perspective in problem solving in a business environment
- focus on the ecology of leadership, not losing sight of long-range objectives because of short-term pressures

TIPS FOR LEADING AND MANAGING

- When faced with a leadership opportunity or a management challenge, consider the source and nature of the issue. Does it involve a personal trait of the leader, the patient, the family, the physician, or other parties? If so, how can trait theory add perspective to the problem? To what degree does the issue pertain to the personal styles of the parties involved? Can awareness of style differences help resolve the issue? To what degree is the issue influenced by environmental factors? Would situational-contingency theory add richness to the problem-solving effort? Does the circumstance call for radical, charismatic change? Building on the work of the transformational theorists, what actions will be necessary to ensure outcomes?

- Never consider leadership the opposite of followership. Followership requires active presence and full engagement with the leader. Recognize that all leaders are followers in some situations, and the opposite is also true.

- Recall that in motivation theories at the organizational level, it is best to focus on positive reinforcement of behaviors, use extinction when you want to purposefully offer nonreinforcement of behaviors, and avoid negative reinforcement and/or punishment whenever possible.

- When solving conflict, put the focus on the interests, not the individuals involved. Give positive reinforcement to the disputing parties, whenever possible. Plan for the constructive and intentional use of communication feedback.

TERMS TO KNOW

followership	personal motives
leadership	values
management theory	vision
motivation	

REFERENCES

Bass, B.M. (1990). From transactional to transformational leadership: learning to share the vision. *Organizational Dynamics*, 18, 19-31.

Belenky, M.F., Clinchy, B.M., Goldberger, N.R., & Tarule, J.M. (1986). *Women's Ways of Knowing: The Development of Self, Voice, and Mind*. New York: Basic Books.

Bennis, W.G., & Nanus, B. (1985). *Leaders: The Strategies for Taking Charge*. New York: Harper & Row.

Blake, R.R. & Mouton, J.S. (1985). *The Managerial Grid III*, Houston, Gulf Publishing.

Boston, C., & Forman, H. (1994). A time to listen: Staff and manager views on education, practice, and management. *Journal of Nursing Administration*, 24, 16-18.

Carr-Ruffino, N. (1993). *The Promotable Woman*. Belmont, CA: Wadsworth.

Davidhizar, R. (1993). Leading with charisma. *Journal of Advanced Nursing*, 18, 675-679.

Fiedler, F.A. (1967). *A Theory of Leadership Effectiveness*. New York: McGraw-Hill.

Fritz, R. (1989). *The Path of Least Resistance: Learning to Become the Creative Force in Your Own Life*. New York: Fawcett Columbine.

Gardner, J.W. (1990). *On Leadership*. New York: Free Press.

Helgeson, S. (1990). *The Female Advantage: Women's Ways of Leadership*. New York: Bantam Doubleday.

Herzberg, F. (1991). One more time: How do you motivate employees? In Ward, M.J., & Price, S.A. *Issues in Nursing Administration: Selected Readings*. St. Louis: Mosby.

House, R.J., & Mitchell, T.R. (1974). Path-goal theory of leadership. *Journal of Contemporary Business*, Autumn, 81-97.

Likert, R. (1961). *New Patterns of Management*. New York: McGraw-Hill.

Luthans, F. (1973). *Organizational Behavior*. New York: McGraw-Hill Book Company.

Maslow, A. (1943). A theory of human motivation. *Psychological Review*, 50, 370-396.

Pugh, D.S., & Hickson, D.J. (1997). *Writers on Organizations*. 5th ed. Thousand Oaks, CA: Sage Publications.

Sargent, A.G. (1981). *The Androgenous Manager*. New York: Amacom.

Senge, P.M. (1990). The leader's new work: Building learning organizations. *Sloan Management Review*, 32(3), 7-22.

Shartle, C.L. (1956). *Executive Performance and Leadership*. Englewood Cliffs, NJ: Prentice-Hall.

Stogdill, R.M. (1948). Personal factors associated with leadership: A survey of the literature. *Journal of Psychology*, 25, 35-71.

Stogdill, R.M. (1963). *Manual for the Leader Behavior Description Questionnaire, form XII*. Columbus: The Ohio State University, Bureau of Business Research.

Tichy, N.M., & Devanna, M.A. (1986). *The Transformational Leader*. New York: John Wiley & Sons.

Ury, W., Brett, J., & Goldberg, S. (1988). *Getting Disputes Resolved: Designing Systems to Cut the Costs of Conflict*. San Francisco: Jossey-Bass.

Vroom, V.H. (1964). *Work and Motivation*. New York: John Wiley & Sons.

Vroom, V.H., & Yetton, P. (1973). *Leadership and Decision-Making*. Pittsburgh, PA: University of Pittsburgh Press.

■ SUGGESTED READINGS

Bass, B.M., & Avolio, B.J. (1994). *Improving Organizational Effectiveness Through Transformational Leadership*. Thousand Oaks, CA: Sage Publications.

Belenky, M.F., Clinchy, B.M., Goldberger, N.R., & Tarule, J.M. (1986). *Women's Ways of Knowing: The Development of Self, Voice, and Mind*. New York: Basic Books.

Bolman, L.G., & Deal, T.E. (1995). *Leading with Soul*. San Francisco: Jossey-Bass.

Bridges, W. (1991). *Managing Transitions: Making the Most of Change*. Reading, MA: Addison-Wesley.

Covey, S. (1991). *Principle-Centered Leadership*. New York: Summit.

DiRienzo, S.M. (1994). A challenge to nursing: Promoting followers as well as leaders. *Holistic Nursing Practice*, 9(1), 26-30.

Fisher, R., & Ury, W. (1991). *Getting to Yes: Negotiating Agreement Without Giving In*. New York: Penguin.

Holliday, M.E., & Parker, D.L. (1997). Florence Nightingale, feminism and nursing. *Journal of Advanced Nursing*, 26, 483-488.

Kohles, M.K., Baker, W.G., & Donaho, B.A. (1995). *Transformational Leadership: Renewing Fundamental Values and Achieving New Relationships in Health Care*. Chicago: American Hospital Publishing.

Leebov, W., & Scott, G. (1990). *Health Care Managers in Transition*. San Francisco: Jossey-Bass.

Luthans, F., & Kreitner, R. (1985). *Organizational Behavior Modification and Beyond*. Glenview, IL: Scott, Foresman.

Marriner-Tomey, A. (1993). *Transformational Leadership in Nursing*. St. Louis: Mosby.

McDaniel, R.R. (1997). Strategic leadership: A view from quantum and chaos theories. *Health Care Management Review*, 22(1), 21-37.

McGregor, D. (1960). *The Human Side of Enterprise*. New York: McGraw-Hill.

Northouse, P.G. (1997). *Leadership Theory and Practice*. Thousand Oaks, CA: Sage Publications.

Rainey, H.G., & Watson, S.A. (1996). Transformational leadership and middle management: Towards a role for mere mortals. *International Journal of Public Administration*, 19(6), 763-800.

Richardson, P., & Denton, D.K. (1996). Communicating change. *Human Resource Management*, 35(2), 203-216.

Van Wynen, E.A. (1997). Information processing styles: One size doesn't fit all. *Nurse Educator*, 22(5), 44-50.

Weeks, D. (1994). *The Eight Essential Steps to Conflict Resolution*. New York: G. Putney Sons.

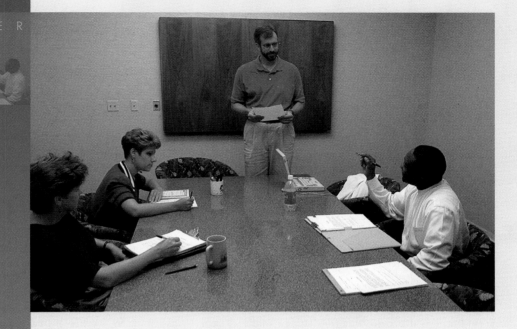

Role Development

Ana M. Valadez
RN, EdD,
  CNAA, FAAN

Dorothy A. Otto
RN, EdD

This chapter identifies key concepts related to the roles of nurse manager, leader, and follower. It describes basic manager functions; explains differences among leaders, managers, and followers; illustrates management principles that are inherent in the role of professional practice; and identifies descriptive competencies for the nurse manager, leader, and follower. Role development is crucial to forming the right questions to ask in a management or clinical situation, which help the practitioner both identify problems and anticipate needs. This chapter provides an overview for the further development of practical skills.

Objectives

- Analyze the relationship of the nurse manager, leader, and follower.
- Evaluate behaviors of professionalism of the nurse manager, leader, and follower.
- Analyze roles and functions of a nurse manager, leader, and follower.
- Evaluate management resource allocation/ distribution.
- Explain quality/outcomes of delivery systems.

Questions to Consider

- Why do you want to be a nurse manager or a nurse follower?
- What type of setting would you like to be in as a nurse manager or nurse follower?
- How do you manage current resources?
- Do you yearn for increased involvement in key decisions, changing systems, working with people, or improving client care?
- How will your clinical expertise be used in the setting?

A Manager's Challenge
From the Nurse Manager of a Post Anesthesia Care Unit at a Cancer Center in the Southwest

One of my major challenges is arranging for staff coverage for the night shift (11 PM to 7 AM). The pediatric acute care unit (PACU) is usually closed during this shift, and we do not know until late evening how many patients will remain in the unit or be transferred to the SICU. I have one registered nurse (RN) assigned to work nights and no ancillary staff is scheduled, except on call. A clerk is on call to work the night shift each week as an unlicensed assistant to the RN. If I have five patients remaining, my dilemma is, do I get an agency RN or another PACU staff nurse to report for the night shift?

What do you think you would do if you were this manager?

INTRODUCTION

The underpinnings of role theory began with management theory, a science that has undergone numerous changes in the last 10 decades. In the early 1990s the theory of scientific management was embraced, a theory based on the one best way to accomplish a task. Practice in the 1930s through the 1970s was dominated by participative, humanistic leadership theories. Situational and leadership theories, although introduced nearly a hundred years ago, did not gain recognition until the 1970s. Additionally, 1970s theorists recognized the influences of roles other than leadership roles on the leader and his or her followers. Covey's (1989) seven habits offer leaders a maturity continuum that culminates in interdependence and the "we can do" attitude. By combining their abilities, leaders and followers can achieve goals and collectively soar to higher achievement planes.

While changes in healthcare delivery no doubt are affecting the roles of nurse managers, the relevance of role theory remains a constant. Conway's (1978) definition, "**role theory** represents a collection of concepts and a variety of hypothetical formulations that predict how actors will perform in a given role, or under what circumstances certain types of behaviors can be expected" (p. 17), is still appropriate today.

Role theory is made up of two major theoretical perspectives: symbolic interaction and structural functional. Symbolic interaction focuses on individuals in reciprocal social interaction who actively construct and create their environment through a process of self-reflexive interaction. Problematic situations that demand new interpretations or new lines of action are the major foci of study. The structural functional perspective focuses on the bigger picture—society, social systems, the social structure—and on other pattern behaviors that develop over time. Social structures shape and determine individual behavior. Both of these perspectives have in common role, role behaviors, norms, sanctions, and status (Hardy & Hardy, 1988).

What is involved in management? What is the **role** of the nurse manager? Practicing **nurse managers** illustrate role perceptions. Some nurse managers would cite decision making and problem solving as major roles, for which maintaining objectivity is sometimes a special challenge.

Table 2-1	BASIC MANAGER FUNCTIONS AND NURSE MANAGER FUNCTIONS	
Basic Manager Function*		**Nurse Manager Function**
Establishes and communicates goals and objectives		Delineates objectives and goals for assigned area Communicates them effectively to staff members who will help attain goals
Organizes, analyzes, and divides work into tasks		Assesses and evaluates activities on assigned area Makes sound decisions about dividing up daily work activities for staff
Motivates and communicates		Stresses the importance of being a good team player Provides positive reinforcement
Analyzes, appraises, and interprets performance and measurements		Completes performance appraisals of individual staff members Communicates results to staff and management
Develops people including self		Addresses staff development continuously through mentoring and preceptorships Furthers self-development by attending educational programs and seeking specialty certification credentialing

*Drucker (1974).

An additional element is being a collaborator. Throughout educational programs, students have multiple opportunities to collaborate with other nurses. **Leaders** must also be involved in collaboration with other departments to enhance quality patient outcomes. Truly effective care is the result of efforts by the total healthcare team. Effective collaboration includes honesty, directness, and listening to other points of view.

Followers serve as leaders; however, most people are leaders in some situations and followers in others. A **follower** shares a common purpose with the leader, believes in the organization's goals, and desires success for both the leader and the organization.

Followership is imperative at this time. The leadership role cannot be set apart from the followership role. They have complementary and interdependent relationships and are influential only when interaction occurs (Corona, 1979).

Styles (1982) says that significant self-examination should be requisite for one who desires to become a nurse manager through the process of career development. A prerequisite for self-actualization is a bonding between the nurse and the community, for a nurse manager's clients and staff make up the community.

MANAGEMENT VERSUS LEADERSHIP ROLES

Management is a generic function that includes similar basic tasks in every discipline and in every society. However, before the nurse manager can be effective, she or he must be well grounded in nursing practice. Drucker (1974) identifies five basic functions for a manager:

- Establishes objectives and goals for each area and communicates them to the persons who are responsible for attaining them.
- Organizes and analyzes the activities, decisions, and relations needed and divides them into manageable tasks.
- Motivates and communicates with the people responsible for various jobs through teamwork.
- Analyzes, appraises, and interprets performance and communicates the meaning of measurement tools and their results to staff and superiors.
- Develops people, including self.

Table 2-1 shows how these basic management functions apply to the nurse manager.

A manager's development efforts focus on the individual. Their aim is to enable the person to develop his or her abilities and strengths to the fullest and to achieve excellence. According to Hershey and Blanchard (1977). "People differ not only in their ability to do, but also in their will to do or their motivation. . . . Commitment to a goal increases when people are involved in their own goal setting" (pp. 16, 25). Thus goals must be realistic before a person makes a real effort to achieve them. Goals should be set high enough, yet be attainable. Active participation, encouragement, and guidance from a director and from the organization are needed for the manager's developmental efforts to be fully productive. Nurse managers who are successful in motivating staff are often providing an environment that facilitates accomplishment of goals resulting in personal satisfactions.

Employees on all levels from lowest to highest must be given responsibility for the affairs of the institution and their community (Drucker, 1989). The manager's staff must be held responsible for setting goals for their own work and for managing themselves by objectives and self-control.

Shared governance, a concept that came into being in the 1980s, facilitates input from employees on the lower administrative level, such as staff nurses. It allows the staff nurse a greater voice in practice-related problems and emphasizes a pivotal decision-making role for the follower-caregiver.

The nurse manager must possess qualities similar to those of a good leader: knowledge, integrity, ambition, judgment, courage, stamina, enthusiasm, communication skills, planning, and administrative abilities. The arena of management versus leadership has been addressed by numerous authors, and while there are differences in points of view, there are some similarities between managers and leaders.

Managers address complex issues by planning, budgeting, and setting target goals. They meet their goals by organizing, staffing, controlling, and problem solving. By contrast, leaders set a direction, develop a vision, and communicate the new direction to the staff. Managers address complexity while leaders address change. Box 2-1 compares the characteristics of a leader with those of a manager and a follower.

Exercise 2-1

In a small group, discuss how clients pay for services of hospitals, clinics, hospices, or private provider offices. Hypothesize about what portion of those costs represents nursing care. How does a manager, or a follower, contribute to cost-effectiveness?

According to Drucker (1989), the most probable assumption today is the unique event, which cannot be predicted. However, unique events can be fore-seen and one can take advantage of them. Nurse managers can have strategies for the future that anticipate the area in which the greatest changes are likely to occur, strategies that enable the unit, department, or institution to take advantage of the unforeseeable. Strategic planning aims to exploit the new and different opportunities of tomorrow. The nurse manager can assist the staff to think strategically about what they are doing and what they should be doing for their clients, for example, in today's world of cost containment, examining what clients pay for the care they receive from the healthcare professionals.

Followers perform their roles at various levels from serving those for whom the organization exists to serving leaders and themselves. Leaders and followers enter into contractual agreements that facilitate both pursuing a common purpose within the context of their own value systems. For power to be balanced, leaders and followers must experience shared leadership. Being a follower does not connote a position of weakness; rather, it implies a condition that permits leadership not only to exist, but also to thrive and gain strength. Corona (1979) speaks to the lack of moral leadership and followership. The caring component long thought to be the "linchpin" for the nursing profession is being overlooked because of nursing's preoccupation with non–direct patient care tasks. Leaders and followers are asking for moral leadership when they ask for input in making nursing decisions. Followers, on the other hand, provide the "glue" for unity in the profession by debating leadership ideas and ultimately giving support to outcomes that offer both leader and follower a win-win situation. Corona provides a final thought on roles; that is, leader and follower roles cannot be seen as separate entities, but rather as synergistic and essential to each other.

Because the nursing profession is predominantly a woman's profession, it is important to acknowledge leadership styles attributed to women. Rosner (1990) reports that early women leaders tended to use commanding, controlling styles generally associated with men. Ames (1989) depicts the commanding, controlling, no-nonsense style of a male chief executive officer (CEO). Most of this leader's messages are not open for discussion, but rather are mandates for action. If outcomes do not meet expectations, the CEO does not hesitate to use punitive negative reinforcement. Rosner also reports that as women leaders became more comfortable with themselves they began to successfully use their own leadership style. This style often is called **transformational leadership.** Leadership of this type encourages followers to transform

Box 2-1		
Leader, Manager, and Follower Traits		
LEADER TRAITS	**MANAGER TRAITS**	**FOLLOWER TRAITS**
Values commitments, relationships with others, and esprit de corps in the organization.	Emphasizes organizing, coordinating, and controlling resources (for example, space, supplies, equipment, and people).	Perceives the needs of both the leader and other staff.
Provides a vision that can be communicated and has a long-term effect on the organization that moves it in new directions.	Attends to short-term objectives/goals.	Demonstrates cooperative and collaborative behaviors.
Communicates the rationale for changing paths; charts new paths that lead to progress.	Maximizes results from existing resources.	Exerts the power to communicate through various channels.
Endorses and thrives on taking risks that bring about change.	Interprets established policy, procedures, and mandates.	Remains fully accountable for actions while relinquishing some autonomy and conceding certain authority to the leader.
Demonstrates a positive feeling in the work and relates the importance of workers.	Moves cautiously; dislikes uncertainty.	Exhibits willingness to both lead and follow peers, as the situation warrants, allowing for competency-based leadership.
	Enforces policy mandates, contracts, etc. (acts as a gatekeeper).	Assumes responsibility to understand what risks are acceptable for the organization and what risks are unacceptable.

their own interests into group interests, with concern for a broader goal. Transformational leaders are interactive people who try diligently to make their interactions positive for everyone. They are not afraid to share their power to enhance their staff's self-worth.

Murphy and DeBack (1991) believe that the profession has a cadre of nursing leaders who are in influential positions and are providing the impetus for reshaping nursing practice to meet the challenges of the twenty-first century. They conducted research through in-depth interviews of 13 nurses considered to be leaders in this era of change. The data reveal many similar characteristics and competencies. Table 2-2 depicts these nurses' descriptive competencies.

Studies testing Kanter's theory of structural power in organizations (Sabiston & Laschinger, 1995) have addressed the empowerment of nurses in various positions ranging from high-level leadership to the staff nurse follower. A recent survey that tested Kanter's the-

ory with 101 staff nurses offered encouraging results (see the theory box on p. 26). All four hypotheses identified positive relationships: experiencing job-related empowerment led to a feeling of autonomy in their work situation; perceiving their job as flexible and having informal alliances led the nurses to believe they had access to job-related sources of empowerment; accessibility to the system's power sources and having job-related empowerment led to perceptions of autonomy and control over their work; and the more the staff nurses perceived their supervisor as being empowered, the more they felt empowered. This study is especially meaningful because followers, while they are extremely crucial to the organization, must be recognized more for their contributions to quality patient care. Finally, if the manager is perceived as empowered, their followers will reach out to attain higher levels of empowerment—a necessary element for job satisfaction and stability.

Table 2-2	NURSES' DESCRIPTIVE COMPETENCIES
Competencies	**Description**
Managing the dream	Sensing windows of opportunities; articulating the vision
Mastery of change	Providing life to the vision; taking risks; accepting error; managing change
Organizational design	Tailoring the organizational design to the vision; using pilot projects; retooling nurses to think differently
Anticipatory learning	Preparing futuristically, including preparing others; energizing the vision through learning with co-workers
Taking the initiative	Making things happen; beginning the idea and seeing it to completion; not allowing everyday distractions to blur their goals; using corporate strategies; presenting the "idea" for the organization, not for nursing

Kanter's Theory

THEORY/CONTRIBUTOR	KEY IDEA	APPLICATION TO PRACTICE
Power and Empowerment Kanter (1993) purports the tenets of power and empowerment in the work place.	The structure of an organization is a key factor in determining the worker's behavior. If the organization is viewed as empowering, its work force is likely to experience job satisfaction, commitment, and a sense of autonomy. If power is viewed in Kanter's context as the ability to get things done, then power can be viewed as a positive worker trait. Formal power allows worker flexibility, adaptability, creativity, and opportunities for recognition. Informal power is derived through association with significant others. Both sources of power facilitate job-related empowerment.	Managers, leaders, and followers, by virtue of the essential roles they play in the delivery of care, can use both sources of power and be an asset, not a liability. Empowerment can assist persons in all three roles to achieve optimum quality care outcomes by facilitating the access of resources.

Exercise 2-2

Select a nurse manager and a staff nurse follower in one of your clinical facilities. Observe them over a period of time (e.g., 4 to 8 hours). Compare and contrast the styles they exhibit. Is power shared or centralized? Are interactions positive or negative? How does your summation of this observation relate to managerial, leadership, and followership characteristics?

These leaders also exhibited other similarities. For example, their own leadership style denoted a commitment to decentralization, optimism, and a belief in the vision. They expected nothing but the best from the people around them, and they continuously maintained a telescopic view of the vision. Bennis (1992) describes leadership traits that are also found in the leaders in Murphy and DeBack's study. The traits include being expert articulators, admitting failures, and capitalizing on their strengths. They know the world they live in and what they want out of it. They are integrated selves, who are working on the new healthcare frontier and shaping the future for tomorrow's nurse leaders.

Nurse managers should use a leadership style that is comfortable for them and can bring about win-win situations. By ascribing to a particular leadership style a manager supports the belief that there is strength in diversity of leadership style. In the respect that they share common purposes with leaders, followers can strengthen the leadership style of managers. Followers, just like their leaders, believe and support the organizational goals and strive for organizational successes.

As Covey (1989) writes: "Our character, basically, is a composite of our habits. . . . Because they are consistent, often unconscious patterns, they constantly, daily, express our character and produce our effectiveness . . . or ineffectiveness" (p. 46). Nurse managers also must be credible clinicians in the areas they manage. A critical factor in being an excellent nurse manager is how to ensure optimal client outcomes, involve families/significant others in the plan of care, and allocate resources and technology in a fair and ethical manner. The nurse manager-clinician is confronted with complex and ambiguous client care situations. Sometimes decisions are made to meet one important client care need at the expense of another. Benner (1984) writes that not even expertise can rid the clinician of the uncertainty inherent in clinical practice. However, despite this uncertainty, some of the behaviors and qualities that enhance the nurse leader's effectiveness remain constant. Box 2-2 lists key abilities and skills that can assist the leaders and managers to meet the challenge.

Joiner and Corkrean (1986) refer to three types of skills needed by a nurse manager: technical, behavioral, and conceptual. However, the key to success in the nurse manager role includes linking three variables to these skills. These variables are motivation, ability, and role clarity. Figure 2-1 depicts these necessary elements for a successful nurse manager. Similarly, these elements are applicable to a nurse follower. The "Research Perspective" box on page 28 describes everyday nurse manager incidents that depict various roles inherent in a nurse manager position.

■ MANAGING HEALTHCARE SETTINGS

Current and emerging issues and the forces shaping them are the kinds of information that may be helpful for nurse managers to know in order to meet the challenges that arise in managing healthcare settings. Some of the current and emerging issues are the organization of health services, cost, quality, and ethics;

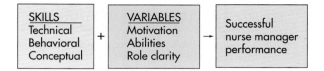

Figure 2-1   Skills and qualities of the successful nurse manager.

Box 2-2

Key Abilities and Skills for New Nurse Leaders/Managers

- Analyze nursing care requirements critically
- Influence others in their enactment of nursing
- Create a desire in others to continue self-development
- Synthesize data from multiple sources
- Develop staff, considering their abilities and the organization's needs
- Translate the organization's vision into work reality
- Make informed decisions readily
- Solve problems fairly and effectively using staff input
- Mentor, coach, acknowledge, empower, and challenge staff
- Communicate clearly and accurately
- Exhibit flexibility, creativity, commitment, enthusiasm, caring, and cultural sensitivity
- Demonstrate clinical competence
- Evaluate others and their work in light of standards
- Predict, control, and evaluate needed resources
- Have "long-short" vision (balance today's demands without losing sight of tomorrow's needs)
- Build teams and their commitment
- Choose a personal management style
- Assess, plan, implement, and evaluate
- Embrace change and quality
- Resolve "unending" disputes creatively
- Live a positive life
- Manage your career and facilitate others' careers
- Enjoy the work
- Value people
- Facilitate goal attainment
- Enrich the environment
- Maintain humor
- Have faith

Adapted from Marrelli (1993).

Research Perspective

Aroian, J.F., et al. (1997). Visions for a treasured resource: Part 1. Nurse manager role implementation. Journal of Nursing Administration, 27(3), 36-41.

This descriptive study used significant "everyday" nurse manager incidents to look at the roles inherent in the nurse manager position. Twenty-nine nurse managers at Beth Israel Hospital in Boston wrote and discussed salient incidents elicited through their managerial role. Using the Manager as Developer Model originated by Bradford and Cohen, data were interpreted through the phenomenological approach. Findings revealed that nurse managers often relied on traditional roles, such as being a hero—sole problem solver and conductor—using participative management and meetings to strengthen communication. Another role captured through the incident documentation was that of developer—involving the staff in all decisions affecting their unit. The study revealed that nurse managers differed in the way they implemented their role, and this was particularly evident when they addressed staffing issues of coaching and managing change. The length of experience as a nurse manager did not seem to make a significant difference in how the nurse manager implemented his or her various roles. By contrast, other factors, such as life experiences, did seem to influence and shape role performance.

Implications for Practice

Addressing the management roles that are elicited through the incident recordings can help employers in the development of their invaluable unit leaders. Additionally, capitalizing on the manager's life experiences may facilitate role implementation.

---

all are shaped significantly in some way by the forces of demand for greater fiscal and clinical accountability, technological growth and innovation, changing supply of labor, changing composition of the health industry and the population itself, and growing numbers of uninsured people (Crane, Hersh, & Shortell, 1992).

Exercise 2-3

Make a quick list that need not be all inclusive, but reflects a fairly accurate count of your "bag of skills" in each of the three categories: technical, behavioral, and conceptual. Describe yourself in terms of motivation. How can your skills assist in linking the three additional variables of motivation, ability, and role clarity in a position as a nurse manager? (For example, if you hold a high value for clinical expertise, then coordination of resources may be easier for you. Clinical expertise gives you insight about follow-up care of clients and delegation potential to selected staff.)

Healthcare settings are changing rapidly. They are an exciting, "full of opportunity" experience, yet there is flux in relation to where and how nurses will practice. Nurse managers may be redefining their role as case managers. The paradigm of client care is shifting from in-hospital settings to client-directed outpatient and community settings and from acute care disease treatment models to health promotion/disease prevention models.

Sigma Theta Tau International in *Nursing Leadership in the 21st Century*, ARISTA II, a think tank named for the Greek word denoting "the brightest" (1996, p. 4), emphasizes addressing the health needs of people in communities where they live and work. Effective healthcare programs identified within the context of the person's own environment and where community strengths and assets are clearly delineated will have the highest probability for success.

The Pew Health Professions Commission, in its report on *Reforming Health Care Workforce Regulation* (1995), addresses transformations in our healthcare systems that will impact the nurse manager's role and self-accountability. Managed care in a cost-conscious environment will place greater quality care demands on all healthcare providers. In addition, the Pew Health Commission report on *Critical Challenges: Revitalizing the Health Professions for the Twenty-First Century* (1995) envisions a healthcare system for the end of the century that has notable changes. Prevailing trends that encompass the new healthcare system delineate a more inclusive definition of health, diversified healthcare systems, a commitment toward improving health for entire populations, and shifting the focus from disease and treatment to prevention, education, and management of care. The professional nurse who manages care in this healthcare era will have to bring a new cadre of skills into his or her dynamic, rapidly changing managerial role.

High technology will continue to modify the nurse managers' roles. For example, because of the ability to perform more complex surgery through surgicenters, nurse managers will find themselves practicing with short-term or ambulatory care admissions. While there are no blueprints to help nurses practice in these new settings, old principles of management are not necessarily inapplicable.

With some modification, however, the basic principles of management still work. For instance, a key to successful management is interdependence. Covey (1989) makes a salient point when he addresses interdependence as a necessity to achieve life goals, whether family or organizational. A critical component of interdependence is collaboration, which uses the different strengths of each person. Collaboration requires one to be flexible and broadminded and to have a strong self-concept.

Roe (1997) addresses the use of collaboration and its importance particularly when people must work together for long periods of time and share in the accomplishment of the same objectives. As in compromise, the cornerstone of collaboration is mutual respect, and listening skills are crucial for successful collaborative ventures. In the healthcare arena, interdisciplinary collaboration should be the framework for effective client outcomes.

Organizations that lack shared values and consequently do not survive during stressful times are discussed by McCoy (1997). Conversely, organizations whose members share a strong work culture become effective survivors in turbulent times. McCoy challenges managers to reach decisions based on what they see and what variables they will allow to influence them.

Blanchard and O'Connor's book, *Managing by Values* (1997), provides a framework for stability, continuity, and growth in today's business world that is characterized by increasing change. Accordingly, the "Managing by Values" (MBV) process involves three phases: (1) clarification of mission/purpose and values; (2) communication of the mission and values; and (3) alignment of daily practices with the mission and values. Blanchard and O'Connor identify three core values as acts of life: achieving, connecting, and integrating. When was the last time that you defined or redefined your purpose in your personal and professional life? "Being values-aligned does not occur without changes in our daily habits, practices, and attitudes" (p. 144).

A way of demonstrating that employees are valued is by recognizing staff through the use of outstanding employee awards. The employees recognized have gone beyond the scope of their job to meet the needs of the patient, department, or institution. The award may reflect the institution's philosophy, beliefs, and mission as exemplified in one institution's "Quality Credo"—communication, competent performance, personal leadership, respect, and teamwork.

A significant new role for managers is emerging in the work place. *Facilitating* is a distinct role and not a subset of management skills. Weaver and Farrell (1997) write that leaders are concerned with doing the right thing, managers are concerned with doing things right, and facilitators are concerned with helping people do things. They consider active listening as the most important facilitation skill, a process by which one makes a conscious effort to understand someone else. Weaver and Farrell provide a simple listening self-assessment tool of 10 statements requiring a choice based on what you usually do, not on what you think a facilitator should do in a specific situation.

Exercise 2-4

You are about to embark on a management task force to address multifaceted issues of your client population. While you know these issues need to be addressed, an accrediting agency for your setting is due within the next few weeks, and this is requiring a lot of your time. What are your options for accomplishing the work you face as a manager? (For example, you know that delegation to your followers is included in your management role. You might then make use of the richness of interdependency and delegate the task force addressing the client issues to your expert clinician.)

MANAGING RESOURCES

The practice settings of tomorrow will no doubt continue to include in-hospital care; however, numerous innovative practice models operating from a community-based framework may also be found. Predictors of effective outcomes to ensure quality client care include rationed and multitiered distribution of healthcare services, such as health maintenance organizations (HMOs), Preferred Provider Organizations (PPOs), or independent private payment plans; very precise outcome-oriented quality assurance measures, such as critical pathways or care MAPs; and concerted efforts to control the spiraling health costs by increasing productivity and efficiency of healthcare providers. The nurse of the year 2005 may be a proprietor of a nurse-managed HMO. Other practice models, differentiated practice, shared governance, and restructured work environments make use of all levels of healthcare personnel.

The manager is responsible for managing all the resources designated to the unit of care. This includes all personnel, professional and nonprofessional, under the manager's span of control. The wise manager quickly determines that a unit must function economically and, in so doing, realizes that there are many opportunities to reshape how nursing is delivered. Budget and people have always been considered to be critical resources. However, as technology grows, informatics must be integrated with budget and people as a critical resource element. Basing practice on research findings, networking through the Internet with other nurse managers, sharing concerns/difficulties, and being willing to step outside of tradition can assist future managers in decisions about resource utilization.

Managed Care

Managed care, as the systematic integration and coordination of financing and delivering healthcare, is performed through healthcare plans. Such plans attempt to provide their constituents with prepaid access to high-quality care at relatively low cost. Nurse managers, as leaders or followers, must be knowledgeable about managed care and what their role performance evolves into, as definitions change. Grimaldi

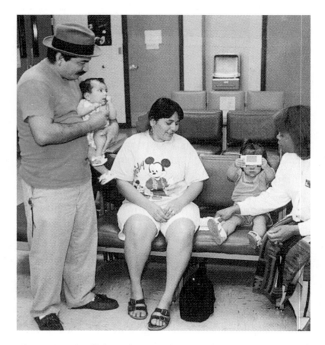

Client care is shifting from in-hospital settings to outpatient and community settings.

(1996) provides a glossary of managed care terms that facilitates such learning by the nurse manager.

Case Management

More and Mandell (1997) write that nurse case managers are catalysts and facilitators responsible for coordinating high-quality care in time-effective, cost-effective manner across the continuum of healthcare. They define **case management** as a "collaborative and multidisciplinary process" and a "24-hour phenomenon." Case management involves components of case selection, multidisciplinary assessment, collective planning, coordinating, negotiating, and evaluating and documenting the outcomes of client status in measures of cost and quality. Case managers are employed in acute care settings, rehabilitation facilities, subacute facilities, community-based programs, home care, and insurance companies. These managers must possess a broad range of personal, interpersonal, and management skills.

Informatics

Informatics is in a stage of constant change, and it highlights for nurse managers two roles that have prevailed: educator and research translator. Both of these roles have become easier to accomplish because informatics has given quick and ready access to current and retrospective clinical client data. The accessibility and use of the Internet and World Wide Web facilitate the education of staff, clients, and their families. Because of informatics, nurse managers have quick access to patient classification systems that denote acuity of care and to personnel hours that relate directly to client acuity. A manager must ensure that the staff's data input is accurate and demonstrate leadership in synthesizing how the data are used to deliver care.

Budgets

Budgetary allocations, whether they are related to the number of dollars available to manage a unit or in full-time equivalent employee formulas, may be the direct responsibility of nurse managers in the future. Budgets should be:

- outcome oriented
- understandable and based on informational data bases
- flexible, prompt, and contingency based on controllable factors
- fair and objective (Joiner & Corkrean, 1986).

Perhaps the most important aspect of a budget is the provision for a mechanism that allows some self-control, such as decision making at the point-of-service (POS), which does not require prior hierarchical approval and a rationale for budgetary spending.

Exercise 2-5

Visit a city health department or an adult day-care facility. What type of information system is used? Are both paper (hard copy) and computer sources used? What can you assume about the budget based on the physical appearance of the setting? Does any equipment appear dated? How do the employees (and perhaps volunteers) function? Do they seem motivated? Ask two or three to tell you, in a sentence or two, what the purpose (vision or mission) of the organization is. Can you readily identify the nurse manager? What does the manager do to manage the three critical resources? What is your impression of the follower as a complement to the nurse manager's role?

People and Work Place Violence

Human resources pose new challenges for nurse managers in today's society. One such challenge is violence in the work place. Lipscomb (1993) addresses violence in the work place as a recent addition to work place hazards facing healthcare workers. It is not only prevalent but also on the increase. Two issues complicate the existing research on violence: underreporting and the perception that assaults on healthcare workers are part of the job. Definitions of what is considered violence in the work place are open to many interpretations and biases.

The Institute of Medicine (1996) report on nursing staffs speaks to an increase in work place violence especially in inner-city emergency rooms and nursing homes. The committee that generated the report found that the safety of healthcare workers continues to be a growing concern and issue. Recommendations include (1) strongly urging healthcare organizations to address preventive assault strategies, (2) ensuring adequate security in high-risk areas, and (3) developing training programs that give the nursing staff effective tools to control violent clients. The policy statement from the Canadian Nurses' Association on interpersonal violence (March, 1996) speaks to the position of zero-based tolerance for violence on the health of individuals, families, groups, and societies, and it focuses on interpersonal violence, that is, violence in relationships, as well as violence from strangers or acquaintances. A strong tenet of this policy statement is in its stance that all registered nurses must articulate the message that everyone has the right to a violence-free life. The beginning or aspiring-to-be manager must be ever-vigilant to clues that indicate potential work place violence and take the necessary steps to ensure safety for his or her staff. One of the eight resolutions adopted by the Council of National Representatives, the governing body of the International Council of Nurses, in its June, 1997 proceedings, addressed the prevention of sexual violence against adults and children.

▐ QUALITY CARE

The shift from total quality management (TQM) programs toward a combination of quality processes that culminate in measurable outcomes of care is occurring rapidly. This paradigm requires the nurse man-ager to have a flexible, fluid outlook on quality care that may embrace more than one measurement process, with outcomes remaining the central focus.

Since 1994 the American Nurses Association (ANA) has been generating data for quality indicators that can be used in acute care settings. Quality indicators are measurements of care designed to reflect the effectiveness of nursing interventions related to a specific aspect of the patient's plan of care. Indicators may include measurable outcomes such as patient falls and urinary tract infections. At present, several state nurses' associations are conducting feasibility studies on these quality indicators. Preliminary results reflect favorable outcomes as to the value of the quality indicators when measuring outcomes of various aspects of care. The goal of the ANA is a redundant report card that can give healthcare organizations a measurement of quality of care in their organization. Their ultimate objective is to develop quality indicators for use in long-term and community-based client practice areas.

Influences that managed care has had on quality improvement programs are addressed by Katz and Green (1997). These authors propose a model for managed performance that addresses cost containment and performance levels expected by customers serviced. This model certainly shows effective applicability in a managed care environment, as do other quality indicators that continue to prevail in various settings. Jensen (1996) discusses the application of the Baldrige criteria, a self-evaluation tool that organizations can use to assess quality care effectiveness. Whatever tools, process, or model is used to evaluate the quality of care in an organization, the nurse manager must first and foremost address quality that meets customer expectations and yields measurable outcomes while controlling costs.

PROFESSIONALISM

Nurse managers must set examples of professionalism, which include academic preparation, roles and function, and increasing autonomy. The ANA's classic, Nursing: A Social Policy Statement (1995), provides significant ideals for all nurses, specifically, that nurses are guided by a humanistic philosophy that includes the highest regard for self-determination, independence, and choice in decision making, whether for personnel or for clients. A nurse manager's professional philosophy should also include the client's rights. These rights have traditionally identified such basic elements as human dignity, confidentiality, privacy, and informed consent. Additional basic rights now include self-determination through advance directives (living wills and durable power of attorney for healthcare) and the right to healthcare accessibility.

Exercise 2-6

Sue B., a young nurse on a surgical orthopedic unit, has been asked several times during her 8-hour shift for some medication for pain by one of her patients, Mr. Jones, who had foot surgery 3 days ago. Sue B.'s assessment of Mr. Jones leads her to believe that he is not having that much pain. Although he does have a p.o. medication order for pain, Sue independently decides to administer a placebo by subcutaneous injection and documents her medication intervention. Mr. Jones did not receive any relief from this subcutaneous medication. When Sue B. was relieved by the night nurse, Sue B. gave the nurse a report of her intervention concerning Mr. Jones' pain. The following morning, the night nurse reports Sue B.'s medication intervention to you, the nurse manager. You will have to address Sue's behavior. What will you do? What resources will you use to handle Sue B.'s behavior? How will you demonstrate professionalism?

Professionalism is all-encompassing; the way a manager interacts with personnel, other disciplines, and patients/clients and families reflects a professional philosophy. Professional nurses are ethically and legally accountable for the standards of practice as well as nursing actions delegated to others. Conveying high standards, holding others accountable, and shaping the future of nursing for a group of healthcare providers are inherent in the role of a manager.

Given the 1994 implementation of the North American Free Trade Agreement (NAFTA), aspects of the Canadian nurses' professional practice documents gain salient importance for United States nurses in practice settings. The College of Nurses of Ontario, a provincial organization analogous to a state's professional organization, has published various documents that will assist a registered nurse to practice within the province. For example, they include Guidelines for Professional Behaviour; A Decision Guide: Determining the Appropriate Category of Care Provider; The Regulated Health Professions Act: An Overview for Nursing (comparable to a state's nursing practice act); and Professional Standards for Registered Nurses and Registered Practical Nurses of Ontario. The Code of Ethics for the Canadian registered nurse addresses seven primary values that are congruent with the ANA's Code of Ethics. The values are intended to guide the nurse as to what is ethically and professionally acceptable. The values include health and well-being, choice, dignity, confidentiality, fairness, accountability, and practice environments conducive to safe, competent, and ethical care. One of the policy statements from the Canadian Nurses' Association (CNA) also speaks to a professional practice environment supported by nursing leadership that reflects quality, efficiency, and effective nursing services. When speaking of quality care, the CNA substantiates through empirical research a direct correlation between quality of nurses' work life and quality of client care. The CNA believes that nurses in general, as well as nurse managers, share the responsibility to create and foster work environments that promote quality patient care.

CHAPTER CHECKLIST

The role of the nurse manager is multifaceted and complex. Integrating clinical concerns with management functions, synthesizing leadership abilities with management requirements, and addressing human concerns while maintaining efficiency are the challenges facing a manager.

- There are five basic functions of a manager:
  - establishing and communicating goals and objectives
  - organizing and analyzing activities and decisions and dividing them into tasks
  - motivating and communicating with others
  - analyzing, appraising, and interpreting performance
  - developing people
- Differences exist between leaders, managers, and followers:
  - Leaders provide vision and bring about change.
  - Managers interpret and enforce policy, organize and coordinate resources, and act as gatekeepers for management.
  - Followers perceive leader and staff needs and share common purposes with leaders and managers.

A Manager's Solution

? I evaluate these factors in making my decision for nursing coverage:

1. Acuity level of patients: If the patient's condition is unstable, a transfer is made to the SICU; if the patient is in stable condition, keep him or her in the PACU. A major consideration is the patient who has had a craniotomy, who can be in stable condition by observation and then can suddenly deteriorate rapidly.
2. Competency of RN unit staff and RN agency staff: Can one or two RNs manage the patients or do I still need an unlicensed assistant? Cultural differences in the staff can be of concern.
3. Availability of needed staff: Who is available to help in an emergency? A physician? A nursing supervisor?
4. Safety of the patient and staff: This must be maintained. This challenge is not resolved without using my critical thinking skills as a nurse manager.

? *Would this be a suitable approach for you? Why?*

Nurse managers link technical, behavioral, and conceptual skills with the variables of motivation, abilities, and role clarity to form their own distinct style. Managing in today's healthcare settings involves working in a managed care environment that embraces case management and quality care. Nurse managers of today are on the cusp of a new healthcare era that offers them a multitude of patient care practice areas.

TIPS FOR IMPLEMENTING THE ROLE OF NURSE MANAGER

Aspects of the role of the nurse manager include being a leader as well as a follower. To implement the role, the nurse manager must profess to a:

■ Management philosophy that values people

■ Commitment to patient-focused quality care outcomes that address customer satisfaction
■ Desire to learn healthcare changes and their effect on his or her role and functions
■ Lifelong learning process for self and staff
■ Belief that all staff share in addressing and solving work place issues

TERMS TO KNOW

case management
follower
leader
managed care

nurse manager
role
role theory
transformational leadership

REFERENCES

American Nurses' Association (1980). *Nursing's Social Policy Statement*. Washington, D.C.: American Nurses Publishing.

Ames, C.B. (November-December 1989). Straight talk from the CEO. *Harvard Business Review*, 67, 132-138.

Arorian, J.F., Horvath, K.J., Secatore, J.A., Alpert, H., Costa, M.J., Powers, E., & Stengrevics, S.S. (March 1997). Vision for a treasured resource. Part I, Nurse manager role implementation. *Journal of Nursing Administration*, 27(3), 36-41.

Benner, P. (1984). *From Novice to Expert*. Menlo Park, CA: Addison-Wesley.

Bennis, W. (1992). *On Becoming a Leader*. Menlo Park, CA: Addison-Wesley.

Blanchard, K., & O'Connor, M. (1997). *Managing by Values*. San Francisco: Berrett-Koehler Publishers, Inc.

Canadian Nurses' Association. (March 1997). *Code of Ethics for Registered Nurses*. Ottawa, Ontario K2P 1E2: The Association.

Canadian Nurses' Association Policy Statements: *Interpersonal Violence* (March 1996); *Nursing Leadership* (November 1995); *The Quality of Nurses' Worklife* (November 1995). Ottawa, Ontario K2P 1E2: The Association.

College of Nurses of Ontario: *The Regulated Health Professionals Act: An Overview for Nursing* (April 1997); *A Decision Guide: Determining the Appropriate Category of Care Provider* (March 1997); *Professional Standards for Registered Nurses and Practical Nurses* (June 1996); *Guidelines for Professional Behaviour* (February 1995). Toronto, Ontario M5R 3P1: The College.

Conway, M.E. (1978). Theoretical approaches to the study of roles. Cited in Hardy, M.E., & Conway, M.E. (1978). *Role Theory: Perspectives for Health Professionals*. New York: Appleton-Century-Crofts.

Corona, D.F. (June 1979). Followership: The indispensable corollary to leadership. *Nursing Leadership*, 2(2), 5-8.

Covey, S.R. (1989). *The 7 Habits of Highly Effective People*. New York: Simon & Schuster.

Crane, S.C., Hersh, A.S., & Shortell, S.M. (1992). Challenges for Health Services Research in the 1990s. In Shortell, S.M., & Reinhart, U.E. *Improving Health Policy and Management: Nine Critical Research Issues for the 1990s*. Ann Arbor, MI: Health Administration Press.

Drucker, P.F. (1974). *Management Tasks, Responsibilities, and Practices*. New York: Harper & Row.

Drucker, P.F. (1989). *Managing in Turbulent Times*. New York: Harper & Row.

Grimaldi, P.L. (October 1996). A glossary of managed care terms. N*ursing Management, Special Supplement*, 5-7.

Hardy, M.E., & Hardy, W.L. (1988). Development of scientific knowledge. Cited in Hardy, M.E., & Conway, M.E. (1988). *Role Theory: Perspectives for Health Professionals*. 2nd ed. Norwalk, CT: Appleton & Lange.

Hershey, P., & Blanchard, K.H. (1977). *Management of Organizational Behavior*. 3rd ed. Englewood Cliffs, NJ: Prentice-Hall.

Institute of Medicine. (1996). *Nursing Staff in Hospitals and Nursing Homes: Is It Adequate?* Washington, D.C.: National Academy Press.

Jenson, L.A. (1996). Improving health care quality: Application of the Baldridge Process. *Journal of Nursing Administration*, 26(7/8), 51-54.

Joiner, C., & Corkrean, M. (1986). *Critical Incidents in Nursing Management*. Norwalk, CT: Appleton-Century-Crofts.

Kanter, R.M. (1993). *Men and Women of the Corporation*. 2nd ed. New York: Basic Books.

Katz, J.M., & Green, E. (1997). *Managing Quality: A Guide to System-wide Performance Management in Health Care*. St. Louis: Mosby.

Lipscomb, J. (1993). *Violence in the Health Care Industry: An Overview of the Problem with Policy Recommendations Regarding Research*. Presentation to the American Academy of Nursing.

Marrelli, T.M. (1993) *The Nurse Manager Survivor's Guide: Practical Answers to Everyday Problems*. St. Louis: Mosby.

McCoy, B.H. (May-June 1997). The parable of the Sadhu. *Harvard Business Review*, 75, 2-7 (Reprint 97307.)

More, P.K., & Mandell, S. (1997). *Nursing Case Management: An Evolving Practice*. New York: McGraw-Hill.

Murphy, M.M., & DeBack, V. (1991). Today's nursing leaders: Creating the vision. *Nursing Administration Quarterly*, 16(1), 71-80.

Pew Health Professions Commission (1995). *Critical Challenges: Revitalizing the Health Professions for the Twenty-first Century*. San Francisco: The Commission.

Pew Health Professions Commission (1995). *Reforming Health Care Workforce Regulation: Policy Considerations for the 21st Century*. San Francisco: The Commission.

Roe, S. (1997). Managing your work setting: Positive work relationships, conflict management, and negotiations.

Cited in Vestal, K.W. *Nursing Management: Concepts and Issues*. 2nd ed. Philadelphia: Lippincott.

Rosner, J.B. (November-December 1990). Ways women lead. *Harvard Business Review*, 68, 119-125.

Sabiston, J.A., & Laschinger, H.K. (1995). Staff nurse empowerment and perceived autonomy. *Journal of Nursing Administration*, 25(9), 42-50.

Sigma Theta Tau International (1996). *Nursing Leadership in the 21st Century: A Report of ARISTA II*. Indianapolis: Center Nursing Press.

Styles, M.M. (1982). *On Nursing Toward a New Endowment*. St. Louis: Mosby.

Weaver, R.G., & Farrell, J.D. (1997). *Managers as Facilitators*. San Francisco: Berrett-Koehler Publishers, Inc.

■ SUGGESTED READING

American Nurses Association (1995). Nursing's Social Policy Statement. Washington, D.C.: American Nurses Publishing, NP-107.

Bullough, B. (1978). Stratification. Cited in Hardy, M.E., & Conway, M.E. *Role Theory: Perspectives for Health Professionals*. New York: Appleton-Century-Crofts.

Carmel, H., & Hunter, M. (1989). Staff injuries from inpatient violence. *Hospital and Community Psychiatry*, 40(1), 41-46.

Donaho, B.A. (August 1996). *Strengthening Hospital Nursing: A Program to Improve Patient Care. Celebrating the Journal: A Final Report*. 1968 Peachtree Road, NW, Atlanta, GA 30309: Piedmont Hospital.

Ernst, D.H. (August 1995). The head nurse role in a rural hospital. *Nursing Management*, 26(8), 50, 52, 54-55.

Horn, S.D., Sharkey, P.D., Tracy, D.M., Horn, C.E., Blair, J., & Goodwin, F. (March 1996). Intended and unintended consequences of HMO cost-containment strategies: Results from the managed care outcomes project. *The American Journal of Managed Care*, 2(3), 253-264.

Huber, D. (1996). *Leadership and Nursing Care Management*. Philadelphia, PA: Saunders.

Marquis, B.L., & Huston, C.J. (1996). *Leadership Roles and Management Functions in Nursing: Theory and Application*. 2nd ed. Philadelphia: Lippincott.

Simons, G.F., Vazquez, C., & Harris, P.R. (1993). *Transcultural Leadership: Empowering the Diverse Workforce*. Houston: Gulf Publishing.

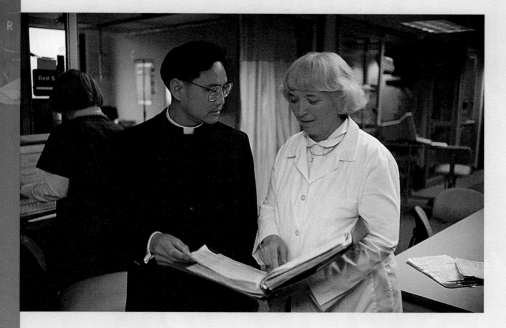

Legal and Ethical Issues

Ginny Wacker Guido
RN, JD, MSN

This chapter highlights and explains key legal and ethical issues as they pertain to managing and leading. It discusses malpractice, types of liability, and federal and state employment laws that pertain to legal and ethical issues. In addition to explaining basic ethical theories and principles, it also provides specific guidelines for avoiding legal liability. All of the issues as described are applicable to everyday professional practice.

Objectives

- Examine nurse practice acts, including the legal difference between licensed registered nurses and licensed practical (vocational) nurses.
- Apply various legal principles, including malpractice, privacy, confidentiality, reporting statutes, and doctrines that minimize one's liability to leading and managing roles in professional nursing.
- Analyze ethical theories and principles, including autonomy, beneficence, nonmaleficence, veracity, justice, paternalism, fidelity, and respect for others.
- Apply an ethical decision-making model to an ethical dilemma.
- Apply managers' rights and responsibilities from a legal and an ethical perspective to selected examples.
- Examine legal implications of resource availability versus service demand from a manager's perspective.
- Analyze key aspects of employment law and give examples of how these laws benefit professional nursing practice.
- Apply five guidelines that a nurse manager can implement to encourage a professional, satisfying work setting.

Questions to Consider

- What are the most common potential legal liabilities for nurse managers? How can they be avoided or minimized?
- How can nurse managers incorporate ethical principles in their everyday relationships with employees?
- What federal employment laws impact nurse managers' work settings?
- How do nurse managers determine which course of action to implement when a legal and/or ethical dilemma arises?

A Manager's Challenge

From the Director of Nurses at a Regional Medical Center in the Southwest

Recently, we were faced at our small hospital with the issue of either utilizing staff more effectively or closing the hospital. The rural hospital has 49 beds, an active emergency department, an obstetrical department, two operating rooms, a small special care unit with three monitored beds, and a general medical-surgical unit, serving both pediatric and adult patients. Not all units are fully utilized at all times, and it had become apparent that the numbers of staff were often greater than the numbers of patients being served. This caused us to face a true legal-ethical dilemma because the hospital serves a geographically large rural county and is critical to county residents' health care needs. Thus we wanted a solution that would meet the county's needs plus be cost-effective so that the hospital could remain open.

What do you think you would do if you were this manager?

▌ INTRODUCTION

The role of professional nursing has expanded rapidly within the past few years to include increased expertise, specialization, autonomy, and accountability, from both a legal and an ethical perspective. This expansion has forced new concerns among nurse managers and a heightened awareness of the interaction of legal and ethical principles. Areas of concern include professional nursing practice, legal issues, ethical principles, labor-management interactions, and employment. Each of these areas is individually addressed in this chapter.

▌ PROFESSIONAL NURSING PRACTICE

Nurse Practice Acts

The scope of nursing practice, those actions and duties that are allowable by a profession, is defined and guided individually by each state in the **nurse practice act** and by common law. **Common law** is "derived from principles rather than rules and regulations and consists of broad and comprehensive principles based on justice, reason, and common sense" (*Bishop v. United States*, 1971, p. 418). Common law principles govern most interactions affecting nursing; they are based on a traditional justice perspective rather than a caring relationship. The state nurse practice act is the single most important piece of legislation for nursing because the practice act affects all facets of nursing practice. Furthermore, the act is the **law** within the state and state boards of nursing cannot grant exceptions, waive the act's provisions, or expand practice outside the act's specific provisions.

Nurse practice acts and common law essentially define three categories of nurses: licensed practical or vocational nurses, licensed registered nurses, and advanced practice nurses. The acts, along with common law, set educational and examination requirements, provide for licensing by individuals who have met these requirements, and define the functions of each category of nurse, both in general and in specific terminology. The nurse practice act must be read to ascertain what actions are allowable for the three categories of nurses. Some states have separate acts for licensed registered nurses (RNs) and licensed practical/vocational nurses (LPNs/LVNs); if two acts exist, they must be reviewed at the same time to ensure that all allowable actions are included in one of the two acts and that there is no overlap between the acts. Some state acts do not have advanced nursing roles defined or delineated.

Each practice act also establishes a state board of nursing. The main purposes of the state boards of nursing are twofold. One purpose is to ensure enforcement of the act, serving to regulate those who come under its provisions and prevent those not addressed within the act from practicing nursing. The second purpose is to protect the public, ensuring that those who present themselves as nurses are licensed to practice within the state. The National Council of State Boards of Nursing (NCSBN) serves as a central clearinghouse, further ensuring that individual state actions against a nurse's license are recorded and enforced in all states in which the individual nurse holds licensure.

Since each state has its own nurse practice act and state courts hold jurisdiction on the common law of the state, all nurses are well advised to know and understand the provisions of the state's nurse practice act. This is especially true in the areas of diagnosis and treatment; states vary greatly on whether nurses can diagnose and treat or merely assess and evaluate. What may be an acceptable action in one state can be considered the practice of medicine in a bordering state.

Thus nurses must know applicable state law and use the nurse practice act for guidance and appropriate action. Nurse managers have this same basic responsibility to apply legal principles in their practice. They also have the responsibility for monitoring the practice of employees under their supervision and for ensuring that personnel maintain current and valid licensure.

Exercise 3-1

Read your state nurse practice act including rules and regulations that the state board of nursing has promulgated for the profession. You may need to read two acts if RNs and LPNs/LVNs come under different licensing boards. Does your state address advanced practice? How do the definitions of nursing vary for the RN, LPN/LVN, and advanced practice nurses? Using these definitions, formulate three lists showing which tasks or assignments you would delegate to each category of nurses, referencing the nurse practice act as needed.

Professional Malpractice

Malpractice concerns professional actions and is the failure of a person with professional education and skills to act in a reasonable and prudent manner. Issues of malpractice have become increasingly important to the nurse as nursing's authority, accountability, and autonomy have increased. There are essentially six elements that must be presented in a successful malpractice suit; all of these factors must be proven before the court will find liability against the nurse and/or institution. Table 3-1 outlines these elements.

To understand how the law applies each element of malpractice to specific court cases, the following scenario is offered. A nurse, employed by a state medical center, has been assigned to care for Mrs. J., a patient admitted for a right hip replacement. Mrs. J. is 69 years old, in relatively good health, and competent mentally. She is to have surgery tomorrow and requires assistance in ambulating to and from the bathroom. While caring for Mrs. J., the nurse fails to obtain the assistance of a second person when walking Mrs. J. to the bathroom, and the patient falls. Mrs. J. sustains a broken left hip and a mild concussion. She will be hospitalized for several additional days because she must undergo bilateral hip replacement and physical therapy. Additionally, she has spent 2 days in the Neurological Step-down Unit because of the concussion.

Elements of Malpractice

The first element is duty owed the patient and involves both the existence of the duty and the

Table 3-1	ELEMENTS OF MALPRACTICE	
Elements	**Example**

Duty owed the patient
  Nature of the duty
  Existence of the duty
	Failure to monitor a patient's response to treatment

Breach of the duty owed	Failure to communicate change in status to the primary healthcare provider
Foreseeability	Failure to ensure minimum standards are met
Causation	Failure to provide patient education
Injury	Patient falls
Damages	Fractured hip, concussion

nature of the duty. That a nurse owes a duty of care to a patient is usually not hard to establish. Often this is established merely by showing the valid employment of the nurse within the institution. The more difficult part is the nature of the duty, which involves standards of care that represent the minimum requirements that define acceptable practice. In the above scenario, the applicable standard of care is taken from the institution policy and procedure manual and concerns the standard of care owed the elderly patient regarding his or her safety. Standards of care are established by reviewing the institution's policy and procedure manual, the individual's job description, and the practitioner's education and skills, as well as pertinent standards as established by professional organizations, journal articles, and standing orders and protocols.

Several sources may be used to determine the applicable **standard of care.** The American Nurses' Association (ANA), as well as a cadre of specialty organizations, publishes standards for nursing practice. The overall framework of these standards is the nursing process. In 1988 the ANA published *Standards for Nurse Administrators*, a series of nine standards incorporating responsibilities of nurse administrators across all practice settings. Accreditation standards, especially those published yearly by the Joint Commission on Accreditation of Healthcare Organizations (JCAHO), also assist in establishing the acceptable standard of care for healthcare facilities. In addition, many states have healthcare standards that affect the individual institution and its employees.

The second element is breach of the duty of care owed the patient. Once the standard of care is established, the breach or falling below the standard of care is easy to show. However, the standard of care may differ depending on whether the injured party is trying to establish the standard of care or whether

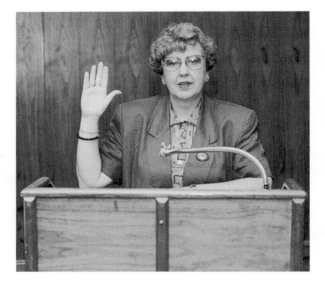

Nurses sometimes serve as expert witnesses whose testimony helps the judge and jury understand the applicable standards of nursing care.

the hospital's attorney is establishing an acceptable standard of care for the given circumstances. The injured party will attempt to show that the acceptable standard of care is much higher than the acceptable standard of care shown by the defendant hospital and staff. **Expert witnesses** give testimony in court to determine the applicable and acceptable standard of care on a case-by-case basis and to assist the judge and jury in understanding nursing standards of care. In the scenario involving Mrs. J., the injured party's expert witness would quote the institution policy manual, and the nurse's expert witness would note any viable exceptions to the stated policy.

A recent case example, *Sabol v. Richard Heights General Hospital* (1996), shows this distinction. In that case a patient was admitted to a general acute care hospital for treatment after attempting suicide by drug overdose. While in the acute care facility, the patient became increasingly paranoid and delusional. A nurse sat with the patient and tried to calm him. Restraints were not applied because the staff feared this would compound the situation by raising his level of paranoia and agitation. The patient got out of bed, knocked down the nurse who was in his room, fought his way past two nurses in the hallway, ran off the unit, and jumped from a third-story window, fracturing his arm and sustaining other relatively minor injuries.

Expert witnesses for the patient introduced standards of care pertinent to psychiatric patients, specifically those hospitalized in psychiatric facilities or in acute care hospitals with separate psychiatric units. The court ruled that the nurses in this general acute care situation were not negligent in this patient's care. The court stated that the nurses' actions were consistent with basic professional standards of practice for medical-surgical nurses in an acute care hospital. They did not have, nor were they expected to have, specialized psychiatric nursing training and would not be judged as if they did.

The third element, **foreseeability**, involves the concept that certain events may reasonably be expected to cause specific results. The nurse must have prior knowledge or information that failure to meet a standard of care may result in harm. The challenge is to show what was foreseeable given the facts of the case at the time of the occurrence, not when the case finally comes to court. In the given scenario, it was foreseeable that the patient could fall and harm herself if fewer than two people attempted to assist with ambulation.

The fourth element is causation, which means that the nurse's actions or lack of actions directly caused the patient's harm and not merely that the patient had some type of harm. There must be a direct relationship between the failure to meet the standard of care and the patient's injury.

The resultant injury, the fifth element, must be physical, not merely psychological or transient. In other words, there must be some physical harm incurred by the patient before malpractice will be found against the healthcare provider. In the given scenario, Mrs. J. came to harm as a direct result of ambulating to the bathroom, and she incurred both a broken hip and a concussion.

Finally, the injured party must be able to prove damages, the sixth element of malpractice. Damages are vital as malpractice is nonintentional and unintended. Thus the patient must show financial harm before the courts will allow a finding of **liability** against the defendant nurse and/or hospital. Mrs. J., in the given scenario, would be able to show additional hospital costs related to the second hip replacement surgery, physical therapy needs, and admission to the step-down unit.

As a nurse manager, one must know the applicable standards of care and ensure that all employees of the institution meet and/or exceed them. The standards must be reviewed periodically to ensure that the staff remain current and attuned to new technology and newer ways of performing tasks. If standards of care appear outdated or absent, the appropriate committee within the institution is notified so that timely revisions can be made. Finally, the nurse manager must ensure that all employees meet the standards of care by performing and/or reviewing all performance evaluations for evidence that standards of care are met, randomly reviewing patient charts for standards of care documentation, and inquiring of employees what constitutes standards of care and appropriate references for standards of care within the institution.

Exercise 3-2

Critically look at a policy and procedure manual at a community nursing service with which you are familiar. Are there policies that are outdated? Find out who is in charge of revising and writing policies and procedures for the agency. Take an outdated policy and revise it or use an issue that you determine should be included in the policy and procedure manual and write such a policy. Does your rewritten or new policy define standards of care? Where would you find criteria for ensuring that your policy and procedures fit a national standard?

LIABILITY: PERSONAL, VICARIOUS, AND CORPORATE

Personal liability defines each person's responsibility and accountability for individual actions or omissions. Even if others can be shown to be **liable** for a patient injury, each individual retains personal accountability for his or her own actions. The law sometimes allows other parties to be liable for certain causes of negligence. Known as **vicarious,** or substituted, **liability,** the doctrine of **respondeat superior** (let the master answer) makes employers accountable for the negligence of their employees. The rationale underlying the doctrine is that the employee would not have been in a position to have caused the wrongdoing unless hired by the employer and that the injured party will be allowed to suffer a double wrong merely because most employees are unable to pay damages for their wrongdoings. Nurse managers can best avoid these issues by ensuring that the staff they supervise know and follow hospital policy and procedure and deliver competent nursing care.

Often nurses believe that the doctrine of vicarious liability shields them from personal liability; the institution may be sued, but not the individual nurse or nurses. Patients injured because of substandard care have the right to sue both the institution and the nurse. In addition, the institution has the right under **indemnification** to sue the nurse for damages paid an injured patient. The principle of indemnification is applicable when the employer is held liable based solely on the actions of the staff member's **negligence** and the employer pays monetary damages because of the employee's negligent actions.

Corporate liability is a newer trend in the law and essentially holds that the institution has the responsibility and accountability for maintaining an environment that ensures quality healthcare delivery for consumers. Corporate liability issues include negligent hiring and firing issues, a duty to maintain safety in the physical environment, and maintenance of a qualified, competent, and adequate staff. Nurse managers play a key role in assisting the institution to avoid corporate liability. For example, the nurse manager is normally delegated the duty to ensure that the staff remains competent and qualified, that personnel within their supervision have current licensure, and that incompetent, illegal, or unethical practices are reported to the proper persons or agencies.

■ CAUSES OF MALPRACTICE FOR NURSE MANAGERS

Nurse managers are charged with maintaining a standard of competent nursing care within the institution. Several potential sources of liability for malpractice among nurse managers may be identified. Once identified, guidelines to prevent or avoid these pitfalls can then be developed.

Delegation and Supervision

The field of nursing management involves supervision of various personnel who directly provide nursing care to patients. The nurse manager remains personally liable for the reasonable exercise of delegation and supervision activities. The failure to delegate and supervise within acceptable standards of professional nursing practice may be seen as malpractice. Additionally, in a newer trend in the law, failure to delegate and supervise within acceptable standards may extend to direct corporate liability for the institution.

However, nurse managers are not liable merely because they have a supervisory function. The degree of knowledge concerning the skills and competencies of those one supervises is of paramount importance. The doctrine of "knew or should have known" becomes a legal standard in delegating tasks to the individuals one supervises. If it can be shown that the nurse manager delegated tasks appropriately and had no reason to believe that the assigned nurse was anything but competent to perform the task, then the nurse manager has no personal liability. But the converse is also true; if it can be shown that the nurse manager was aware of incompetencies in a given employee or that the assigned task was outside the employee's capabilities, then the nurse manager does become potentially liable for the subsequent injury to a patient.

Nurse managers have a duty to ensure that the staff members under their supervision are practicing in a competent manner. The nurse manager must be aware of the staff's knowledge, skills, and competencies and should know that they are maintaining their competencies. Knowingly allowing a staff member to function below the acceptable standard of care subjects both the nurse manager and the institution to potential liability. Some nurse practice acts also legislate fines and discipline for the nurse manager who assigns tasks or patient care loads that make a nursing assignment unsafe. Means of ensuring continuing competency include continuing education programs and assigning the staff member to work with a second staff member to improve technical skills.

Duty to Orient, Educate, and Evaluate

Most healthcare institutions have continuing education departments whose function is to orient nurses new to the institution and to supply inservice education addressing new equipment, procedures, and interventions. Nurse managers also have a duty to orient, educate, and evaluate. Nurse managers are responsible for the daily evaluation of whether nurses are performing competent care. The key to meeting this requirement is reasonableness. Nurse managers should ensure that they promptly respond to all allegations, whether by patients or staff, of incompetent or questionable nursing care. Nurse managers should thoroughly investigate, recommend alternatives for correcting the situation, and follow up on recommended alternatives and suggestions.

A recent North Carolina case, *Horton v. Carolina Medicorp, Inc.* (1996), shows the importance of monitoring those involved in patient care. In that case, a postoperative urological patient had not voided for 24 hours after the removal of a Foley catheter. By the time the patient was finally recatheterized, he had sustained severe bladder distention and dehiscence of the suture line in the bladder wall, which then required extensive additional surgery. In this case, there were obvious examples that those managed needed additional education and/or orientation as well as evaluation.

Failure to Warn

A newer area of potential liability for nurse managers is **failure to warn** potential employers of staff incompetencies or impairment. Information about suspected addictions, violent behavior, and incompetency is of vital importance to subsequent employers. If the institution has sufficient information and suspicion on which to discharge an employee or force a resignation, then subsequent employers should be advised of those issues.

One means of supplying this information is through the use of qualified privilege to certain communications. As a general rule, qualified privileged concerns communications made in good faith between persons or entities with a need to know. Most states now recognize this privilege and allow previous employers to give factual, objective information to subsequent employers (Trudeau, 1992).

Staffing Issues

Three different issues arise under the general term *staffing*. These include adequate numbers of staff members in a time of advancing patient acuity and limited resources, floating staff from one unit to another, and using temporary or "agency" staff to augment hospital staffing. Each area is addressed separately.

Accreditation standards, specifically those of the JCAHO and the Community Health Accreditation Program (CHAP), as well as other state and federal standards, mandate that healthcare institutions must provide adequate staffing with qualified personnel. This applies not only to numbers of staff, but also to the legal status of the staff. For instance, some areas of an institution must have greater percentages of RNs than LPNs/LVNs, such as critical care areas, postanesthesia care areas, and emergency centers, while other areas may have equal or lower percentages of RNs to LPNs/LVNs or nursing assistants, such as the general nursing areas and some long-term-care areas. Whether short-staffing or understaffing does exist in a given situation depends on a careful, objective analysis of the number of patients, the amount of care required by each patient, and the number and classification/type of staff (Fiesta, 1994). Courts will determine whether understanding did indeed exist on an individual case (Guido, 1997).

While the institution is ultimately accountable for staffing issues, nurse managers may also incur some potential liability as they directly oversee numbers of personnel assigned to a unit on a given shift. For such nurse manager liability to incur, it must be shown that the resultant patient injury was a direct result of the short-staffing and not due to the inappropriate or incompetent actions of an individual staff member, that is, it must be shown that sufficient numbers and competencies are available to meet nursing needs.

Exercise 3-3

Judy Jones, R.N., has worked in the emergency center for several years. She is currently advanced cardiac life support (ACLS) certified, as are the other emergency care nurses; the hospital policy requires ACLS certification for employment in critical care areas. A new hospital policy expressly forbids the intubation of patients by nurses; only physicians may intubate patients. A crisis occurred in the emergency center one evening and Judy Jones intubated (successfully) a patient in full cardiac arrest. What do you do about this issue?

Guidelines for nurse managers in "short-staffing" issues include alerting hospital administrators and upper-level managers of concerns. First, though, the nurse manager must have done whatever was under his or her control to have alleviated the circumstances, such as approving overtime for adequate coverage, reassigning personnel among those areas he or she supervises, and restricting new admissions to the area. Second, nurse managers have a legal duty to notify the chief operating officer, either directly or indirectly, when understaffing endangers patient welfare. One way of notifying the chief operating officer is through formal nursing channels, for example, by notifying the nurse manager's direct supervisor. Upper management must then decide how to alleviate the short-staffing, either on a short-term or on a long-term basis. Appropriate measures could be closing a certain unit or units, restricting elective surgeries, or hiring new staff members. Once the nurse manager can show that he or she acted appropriately, used sound judgment given the circumstances, and alerted his or her supervisors of the serious nature of the situation, then the institution becomes potentially liable for staffing issues.

Floating staff from unit to unit is the second issue that concerns overall staffing. Institutions have a duty to ensure that all areas of the institution are adequately staffed; thus units temporarily overstaffed because of either low patient census or a lower patient acuity ratio usually float staff to units less well staffed. Floating nurses to areas with which they have less familiarity and expertise can increase potential liability for the nurse manager, but to leave another area understaffed can also increase potential liability.

Before floating staff from one area to another, the nurse manager should consider staff expertise, patient care delivery systems, and patient care requirements. Nurses should be floated to units as comparable to their own unit as possible. This requires the nurse manager to match the nurse's home unit and float unit as much as is possible or to consider negotiating with another nurse manager to cross-float a nurse. For example, a manager might float a critical care nurse to an intermediate care unit and float an intermediate care unit nurse to a general unit. Or the manager might consider floating the general unit nurse to the postpartum unit and floating a postpartum nurse to labor and delivery. Open communications regarding staff limitations and concerns as well as creative solutions for staffing can alleviate some of the potential liability involved and create better morale among the floating nurses. A positive option is to cross-train nurses within the institution so that nurses are familiar with two or three areas and can competently float to areas in which they have been cross-trained.

A legal case shows that employees also have some responsibility in the area of cross-training. In *David W. Francis v. Memorial General Hospital* (1986), an intensive care nurse refused to float to an orthopedic unit because he felt that he was unqualified to act as a charge nurse on that unit. The hospital offered to orient him, but he declined and was subsequently terminated. The court sided with the employer, noting that the employee's unwillingness to be oriented or to even try working with hospital administration undermined his case.

The use of temporary or "agency" personnel has created increased liability concerns among nurse managers. Until recently, most jurisdictions held that such personnel were considered to be **independent contractors** and thus the institution was not liable for their actions, although their primary employment agency did retain potential liability. Today, courts have begun to hold the institution liable under the principle of **apparent agency.** Apparent authority or apparent agency refers to the doctrine whereby a principal becomes accountable for the actions of his or her agent. Apparent agency is created when a person (agent) holds himself or herself out as acting in behalf of the principal; in the instance of the agency nurse, the patient is unable to ascertain if the nurse works directly for the hospital (has a valid employment contract) or is working for a different employer. At law, lack of actual authority is no defense. This principle applies when it can be shown that the reasonable patient believed that the healthcare worker was an employee of the institution. If it appears to the reasonable patient that this worker is an employee of the institution, the law will consider the worker as an employee for the purposes of corporate and vicarious liability.

A recent case, though, seems to uphold the idea of independent contractor as the basis for liability. In *Hansen v. Caring Professionals, Inc.* (1997), the Appellate Court in Illinois held that a temporary nurse was an independent contractor and not an employee of the temporary nursing agency. The court cited the nurse's filing of a Form 1099, rather than a W-2 form, the payment of her own employment taxes, and the payment of her own workers' compensation coverage as proof of her independent employment status. The hospital, though, did have potential liability because it controlled which patients would be assigned to the agency nurse and directly supervised the agency nurse's clinical performance. Classification may be unimportant; what is important is that the hospital, and thus the nurse manager, may be sued for incompetent care when an agency nurse gives less than competent nursing care.

These trends in the law make it imperative that the nurse manager consider the temporary worker's skills, competencies, and knowledge when delegating tasks and supervising his or her actions. If there is reason to suspect that the temporary worker is incompetent, the nurse manager must convey this fact to the agency. The nurse manager must also either send the temporary worker home or reassign the worker to other duties and areas. Screening procedures, the same as those used with new institution employees, should also be performed with temporary workers.

Additional areas that nurse managers should stress when using agency or temporary personnel include ensuring that the temporary staff member is given a brief but thorough orientation to institution policies and procedures, is made aware of resource materials within the institution, and is made aware of documentation procedures. It is also advisable that nurse managers assign a resource person to the temporary staff member. This resource person serves in the role of mentor for the agency nurse and serves to prevent potential problems that could arise merely because the agency staff member does not know the institution routine or is unaware of where to turn for assistance. This resource person also serves as a mentor for critical decision making for the agency nurse.

STRICT PRODUCT LIABILITY

When patient injury occurs because of equipment, the issue becomes one of whether the patient was injured because of a defect in the equipment (product) or because of misusage or improper maintenance of the equipment. Nursing negligence associated with the improper use of equipment can arise in various ways. Nurses, once they learn the correct use of machinery, are expected to conform to manufacturer's recommendations. Two recent cases illustrate this point. In a 1991 Minnesota case a nurse disconnected the oxygen hose from a ventilator and reconnected it improperly, causing the patient to become hypoxic. Depositions in that case also showed that the same nurse had disconnected the ventilator alarms, so that the warning alarm did not sound when the oxygen was disconnected (*Mele v. St. Mary's Hospital of Rochester, Minnesota, and Mayo Foundations*, 1991). The second case involved a bed that malfunctioned, causing the patient who was recovering from back surgery to undergo a second surgical procedure. In investigating the complaint, the patient's attorney discovered that a previous patient had also complained about the bed and that nursing personnel had refused to change the bed or have the bed repaired (*Beltran v. Downey Community Hospital*, 1992).

Product liability cases usually involve the manufacturer of the equipment, the institution, and the staff using the equipment. Nurse managers can lessen potential liability by ensuring that equipment is used in the proper manner, that equipment is maintained properly, and that any storage of the equipment follows the written manufacturer's guidelines. These are most often ensured by holding frequent and mandatory inservice classes on new equipment or on a new use of previously used equipment, recording necessary maintenance procedures, and quickly in-

vestigating any concern or problem with equipment. Nurse managers may be found responsible along with staff members when equipment is misused or when maintenance procedures are not followed.

PROTECTIVE AND REPORTING LAWS

Protective and reporting laws ensure the safety or rights of specific classes of individuals. Most states have reporting laws for suspected child and elder abuse as well as laws for reporting certain categories of diseases and injuries. Examples of reporting laws include the reporting of venereal diseases, abuse of residents in nursing and convalescent homes, and organ donation. Nurse managers are frequently the individuals who are responsible for ensuring that the correct information is reported to the correct agencies, thus avoiding potential liability against the institution.

Many states now also have mandatory reporting of incompetent practice, especially through nurse practice acts, medical practice acts, and the National Practitioner Data Bank. Additionally, the National Council of State Boards of Nursing has developed an Electronic License Verification (ELVIS) system that monitors nurses' licensure status in all states and United States territories for discipline issues, competency ratings, and renewals. Frequently, reporting of incompetent practice is restricted to issues of chemical abuse, and special provisions prevail if the affected nurse voluntarily undergoes drug diversion or chemical dependency rehabilitation. Mandatory reporting of incompetent practitioners is a complex process, involving both legal and ethical concerns. Nurse managers must know what the law requires, when reporting is mandated, to whom the report must be sent, and what the individual institution expects of its nurse managers. When in doubt, the nurse manager should seek clarification from the state board of nursing and hospital administration.

INFORMED CONSENT

Informed consent is the authorization by the patient or the patient's legal representative to do something to the patient and is based on legal capacity, voluntary action, and comprehension. Legal capacity is usually the first requirement and is determined by age and competency. All states have a legal age for adult status defined by **statute;** competency involves the ability to understand the consequences of actions or the ability to handle personal affairs. In the instance that a minor or incompetent adult is involved, state statutes mandate who can serve as the patient's representative. In selected instances the following types of minors may be able to give valid informed consent: **emancipated minors**, minors for treatment related to substance abuse or communicable diseases, and pregnant minors. Voluntary action, the second requirement, means that the patient was not coerced by fraud, duress, or deceit into allowing the procedure or treatment.

Comprehension is the third requirement and the most difficult to ascertain. The law states that the patient must be given sufficient information, in terms he or she can reasonably be expected to comprehend, to make an informed choice. Information that must be included appears in Box 3-1.

Inherent in the doctrine of informed consent is the right of the patient to informed refusal. Patients must clearly understand the possible consequences of their refusal. In recent years, most states have enacted statutes to ensure that the competent adult has the right to refuse care and that the healthcare provider is protected should the adult validly refuse care.

Frequently, issues of informed consent among nurses concern the actual signing of the informed consent document, not the teaching and information that make up informed consent. Many nurses serve as witnesses to the signing of the informed consent document and are attesting only to the voluntary nature of the patient's signature. There is no duty on the part of the nurse to insist that the patient repeat what has been said or what he or she remembers. Should the patient ask questions that alert the nurse

to the inadequacy of true comprehension on the patient's part or express uncertainty while signing the document, the nurse has an obligation to inform the primary healthcare provider and appropriate persons that informed consent has not been obtained.

Exercise 3-4

A patient is admitted to your surgical center for minor surgery specifically for a breast biopsy under local anesthesia. The surgeon has previously informed the patient of the surgery risks, alternatives, desired outcomes, and possible complications. You give the surgery permit form to the patient for her signature. She readily states that she knows about the surgery and has no additional questions. She signs the form with no hesitation. Her husband, who is visiting with her, states he is worried because she will be awake during the procedure and he is afraid that something may be said to alarm her. What do you do at this point? Do you alert the surgeon that informed consent has not been obtained? Do you request that the surgeon revisit the patient and reinstruct her about the surgery? Or is there anything more that you should do as the patient has already signed the form?

■ PRIVACY AND CONFIDENTIALITY

Privacy is the patient's right to protection against unreasonable and unwarranted interference with the patient's solitude. This right extends to protection of personality as well as protection of one's right to be left alone. Within a medical context, the law recognizes the patient's right against (1) appropriation of the patient's name or picture for the institution's sole advantage, (2) intrusion by the institution on the patient's seclusion or affairs, (3) publication of facts that place the patient in a false light, and (4) public disclosure of private facts about the patient by the hospital or staff. **Confidentiality** is the right to privacy of the medical record.

Institutions can reduce potential liability in this area by allowing access to patient data, either written or oral, only to those with a "need to know." Persons with a need to know include physicians and nurses caring for the patient, technicians, unit clerks, therapists, social service workers, and patient advocates. Usually, this need to know extends to the house staff and consultants. Others wishing to access patient data must first ask the patient for permission to review a record. Administration of the institution can access the patient record for statistical analysis, staffing, and quality of care review.

The nurse manager is cautioned to ensure that staff members both understand and abide by rules

---

Box 3-1

Required Information for Informed Consent

- An explanation of the treatment/procedure to be performed and the expected results of the treatment/procedure
- Description of the risks involved
- Benefits that are likely to result because of the treatment/procedure
- Options to this course of action, including absence of treatment
- Name of the persons performing the procedure/treatment
- Statement that the patient may withdraw his/her consent at any time

regarding patient privacy and confidentiality. "Interesting" patients should not be discussed with others, and all information concerning patients should be given only in private and secluded areas. Individual managers may need to review the current means of giving reports to oncoming shifts and policies about telephone information. Many institutions have now added to the nursing care plan a reference for persons to whom the patient has allowed information to be given. If the caller identifies himself or herself as one of those listed persons, the nurse can give patient information without violating the patient's privacy rights. Patients are becoming more knowledgeable about their rights in these areas, and some have been willing to take offending staff members to court over such issues.

A concurrent issue in this area is the patient's right of access to his or her medical record. While the patient has a right of access, individual states mandate when this right attaches. Most states give the right of access only after the medical record is completed; thus the patient has the right to review the record after discharge. Some states do give the right of access while the patient is hospitalized, so individual state law governs individual nurses' actions. When supervising a patient's review of his or her record, the nurse manager should explain only the entries that the patient questions or about which the patient requests further clarification. The nurse manager then makes a note in the record after the session indicating that the patient has viewed the record and what questions were answered.

Patients also have a right to copies of the record, at their expense. The medical record belongs to the institution as a business record, and patients never have the right to retain the original record. This is also true in instances where a subpoena is obtained to secure an individual's medical record for court purposes. A hospital representative will verify that the copy is a "true and valid" copy of the original record.

An issue that is closely related to the medical record is that of incident reports or unusual occurrence reports. These reports are mandated by the JCAHO and serve to alert the institution concerning risk management and quality assurance within the setting. As such, incident reports are considered to be internal documents and thus not discoverable (open for review) by the injured party and/or attorneys representing the injured party. In most jurisdictions where this question has arisen, the courts have held that the incident report was discoverable and thus open to review by both sides of the suit.

It is therefore prudent for nurse managers to complete and to have staff members complete incident reports as though they will be open records. It is advisable to omit any language of guilt such as, "The patient would not have fallen if Jane Jones, R.N., had ensured that side rails were in their up and locked position." This document contains only pertinent observations and all care given the patient, such as x-rays for a potential broken bone, medication that was given, and consultants who were called to examine the patient. It is also advisable not to note the occurrence of the incident report in the official record because that incorporates the incident report "by reference" and there is no way to keep the report from being seen by the injured party and/or attorneys for the injured party.

POLICIES AND PROCEDURES

Risk management is a process that identifies, analyzes, and treats potential hazards within a given setting. The object of risk management is to identify potential hazards and to eliminate them before anyone is harmed or disabled. Written policies and procedures fall within the scope of risk management activities. Written policies and procedures are a requirement of JCAHO. These documents set standards of care for the institution and direct practice. They must be clearly stated, well delineated, and based on current practice. Nurse managers should review the policies and procedures frequently for compliancy and timeliness. If policies are absent or outdated, the nurse manager must request the appropriate person or committee to either initiate or update the policy.

Exercise 3-5

You are assigned some risk management activities in the nursing facility where you work. In investigating incident reports that were filed by your staff, you discover that this is the third patient this week who has fallen while attempting to get out of bed and sit in a chair. How would you handle this issue? Decide where you would start a more complete investigation of this issue. For example, is it a nursing facility-wide issue or one that is confined to one unit? What safety issues are you going to discuss with your staff and how are you going to discuss these issues? Design a unit inservice class for the staff concerning incident reports and safety of patients.

EMPLOYMENT LAWS

The federal and individual state governments have enacted laws regulating employment. To be effective and legally correct, nurse managers must be familiar with these laws and how individual laws affect the institution and labor relations. Many nurse managers have come to fear the legal system because of personal experience or the experiences of colleagues. Much of this concern, though, may be directly attributable to uncertainty with the law or partial knowledge of the law. By understanding and correctly following federal employment laws, nurse managers may actually lessen their potential liability because they have complied with both federal and state laws. Table 3-2 gives an overview of key federal employment laws.

Equal Employment Opportunity Laws

Several federal laws have been enacted to expand equal employment opportunities by prohibiting discrimination based on gender, age, race, religion, handicap, pregnancy, and national origin. These laws are enforced by the Equal Employment Opportunity Commission (EEOC). Additionally, states have enacted statutes that address employment opportunities, and the nurse manager should consider both when hiring and assigning nursing employees.

The most significant legislation affecting equal employment opportunities today is the amended 1964 Civil Rights Act (43 Fed. Reg. 1978). Section 703 (a) of Title VII makes it illegal for an employer "to refuse to hire, discharge an individual, or otherwise to discriminate against an individual, with respect to his compensation, terms, conditions, or privileges of employment because of the individual's race, color, religion, sex, or national origin." Title VII was also amended by the Equal Opportunities Act of 1972 so that it applies to private institutions with 15 or more employees, state and local governments, **labor unions,** and employment agencies.

In 1991 the Civil Rights Act was signed into law. This act further broadened the issue of sexual harassment in the work place and supersedes many of the sections of Title VII. Sections of the new legislation define sexual harassment, its elements, and the employer's responsibilities regarding harassment in the work place, especially prevention and corrective action. The Civil Rights Act is enforced by the EEOC as created in the 1964 act; its powers were broadened in the 1972 Equal Employment Opportunity Act. The primary activity of the EEOC is processing complaints

Table 3-2	SELECTED FEDERAL LABOR LEGISLATION	
Year	**Legislation**	**Purpose and Effect**
1935	Wagner Act; National Labor Act	Established many rights in unionizations; National Labor Relations Board (NLRB) established
1947	Taft-Hartley Act	Resulted in more equal balance of power between unions and management
1962	Executive Order 10988	Permitted public employees to join unions
1963	Equal Pay Act	Made it illegal to pay lower wages to employees based solely on gender
1964	Civil Rights Act	Protected against discrimination due to race, color, creed, national origin, etc.
1967	Age Discrimination Act	Made it illegal for employers to discriminate against older men and women
1974	Wagner Amendments	Allowed nonprofit organizations to join unions; opened unionization in nursing
1990	Americans with Disabilities Act	Barred discrimination against disabled individuals in the work place
1991	Civil Rights Act	Addressed specifically sexual harassment in the work place; overrode and modified previous legislation in this area
1993	Family and Medical Leave Act	Addressed needs for leave based on family and medical needs

Adapted from Marquis and Huston (1992).

of employment discrimination. There are three phases: investigation, conciliation, and litigation. Investigation focuses on determining whether or not Title VII has been violated by the employer. If the EEOC finds "probable cause," an attempt is made to reach an agreement or conciliation between the EEOC, the complainant, and the employer. If conciliation fails, the EEOC may file suit against the employer in federal court or issue to the complainant the right to sue for discrimination.

The EEOC also promulgated written rules and regulations that reflect its interpretation of the laws under its auspices, including those relating to staffing practices and sexual harassment in the work place. The EEOC defines sexual harassment broadly, and this has generally been upheld in the courts. Nurse managers must realize that it is the duty of employers (management) to prevent employees from sexually harassing other employees. The EEOC issues policies and practices for employers to implement both to sensitize employees to this problem and to prevent its occurrence; nurse managers should be aware of these policies and practices and seek guidance in implementing them if sexual harassment occurs in their units.

There are a number of bases on which employers may seek exceptions to Title VII. For example, it is lawful to make employment decisions on the basis of national origin, religion, and gender (never race or color) if such decisions are necessary for the normal operation of the business, though the courts have viewed this exception very narrowly. Promotions and layoffs based on bona fide seniority or merit systems are permissible (Herrero v. St. Louis University Hospital, 1997), as are exceptions based on business necessity.

Age Discrimination in Employment Act of 1967

This act made it illegal for employers, unions, and employment agencies to discriminate against older men and women. The law, in a 1986 amendment, prohibits discrimination against persons over the age of 40. The practical outcome of this act has been that mandatory retirement is no longer seen in the American work place.

As with Title VII, there are some exceptions to this act. Reasonable factors, other than age, may be used when terminations become necessary; such reasonable factors would be a performance evaluation system and some limited occupational qualifications, for example, the tedious physical demands of a specific job.

Americans with Disabilities Act of 1990

The Americans with Disabilities Act (ADA) of 1990 provides protection to persons with disabilities and is the most significant civil rights legislation since the Civil Rights Act of 1964. The purpose of the ADA is to provide a clear and comprehensive national mandate for the elimination of discrimination against disabled individuals and to provide clear, strong, consistent, enforceable standards addressing discrimination in the work place. The ADA is closely related to the Civil Rights Act and incorporates the antidiscrimination principles established in Section 504 of the Rehabilitation Act of 1973.

The act has five titles, and Table 3-3 shows the pertinent issues about each title. The ADA has jurisdiction over employers, private and public; employment agencies; labor organizations; and joint labor-management committees. It defines disability broadly: with respect to an individual a disability is (1) a physical or mental impairment that substantially limits one or more of the major life activities of such individual, (2) a record of such impairment, or (3) being regarded as having such an impairment [42 USC sec. 12102(2)]. The overall effect of the legislation is that

Table 3-3	AMERICANS WITH DISABILITIES ACT OF 1990
Title	**Provisions**
I	Employment: defines purpose of the act and who is qualified under the act as disabled
II	Public services: concerns services, programs, and activities of public entities as well as public transportation
III	Public accommodations and services operated by private entities: prohibits discrimination against disabled in areas of public accommodations, commercial facilities, and public transportation services
IV	Telecommunications: intended to make telephone services accessible to individuals with hearing or speech impairments
V	Miscellaneous provisions: certain insurance matters; incorporation of this act with other federal and state laws

Adapted from 42 USC sec. 12101 et seq.

persons with disabilities will not be excluded from job opportunities or adversely affected in any aspect of employment unless they are not qualified or are otherwise unable to perform the job. The ADA thus protects qualified and disabled individuals in regard to job application procedures, hiring, compensation, advancement, and all other employment matters.

Recent cases have assisted in defining disability eligibility. The court in *McIntosh v. Brookdale Hospital Medical Center* (1996) found that short-term conditions are not a disability under the ADA. In that case a nurse returned to work after a 1-month absence with her hypertension resolved and with no medical restrictions from her physician. "An impairment that prevents an individual from working for a period of one month, and that is not expected to recur in the foreseeable future, does not constitute a disability within the meaning of the Americans with Disabilities Act," stated the court.

A second case (*Howard v. North Mississippi Medical Center*, 1996) held that migraines and allergies are not disabilities under the ADA. In this case a home health aide was refused coverage under the act when her physician certified that she could not perform the duties of her employment because she could not call on patients in their homes, but needed a full-time position within the office or clinic. The court also noted that the employer had tried to accommodate her needs, but that the home health aide's skills were not sufficient for any of the open positions that currently existed. The court concluded that migraine headaches and allergies were not what the law was intended to include.

The act requires the employer or potential employer to make reasonable accommodations to employ the disabled. The law does not mandate that disabled individuals be hired before fully qualified, nondisabled persons; it does mandate that the disabled not be disqualified merely because of an easily accommodated disability.

This last point was well illustrated by the court in *Zamudio v. Patia* (1997). The court stated that the employer would be required to inform Ms. Zamudio when a position that she required as reasonable accommodation became available. She would be allowed to apply, but "as a disabled employee seeking reasonable accommodation she did not have to be given preference over other employees without disabilities who might have better qualifications or more seniority."

Nor will the court impose job restructuring on an employer if the person needing accommodation qualifies for other jobs not requiring such accommodation. In *Mauro v. Borgess Medical Center* (1995) the court refused to impose accommodation on the employer hospital merely because the affected employee desired to stay within a certain unit of the institution. In that case an operating surgical technician who was HIV positive was offered an equivalent position by the hospital in an area where there would be no patient contact. He refused the transfer, desiring accommodation within the operating arena, and was denied such accommodation by the Michigan court.

Also, the act specifically excludes from the definition homosexuality and bisexuality, sexual behavioral disorders, gambling, kleptomania, pyromania, and current use of illegal drugs [42 USC sec. 12211(a) and (b)(1)]. Moreover, employers may hold alcoholics to the same job qualifications and job performance standards as other employees even if the unsatisfactory behavior or performance is related to the alcoholism [42 USC sec. 12114 (c)(4)]. As with other federal employment laws, the nurse manager should have a thorough understanding of the law as it applies to the institution and his or her specific job description and should know whom to contact within the institution structure for clarification as needed.

Affirmative Action

The policy of affirmative action (AA) differs from the policy of equal employment opportunity (EEO). AA enhances employment opportunities of protected groups of people while EEO is concerned with utilizing employment practices that do not discriminate against or impair the employment opportunities of protected groups. Thus AA can be seen in conjunction with several federal employment laws; for example, in conjunction with the Vietnam Era Veterans' Readjustment Act of 1974, the AA requires that employers with government contracts take steps to enhance the employment opportunities of disabled veterans and other veterans of the Vietnam era.

Equal Pay Act of 1963

The Equal Pay Act makes it illegal to pay lower wages to employees of one gender when the jobs (1) require equal skill in experience, training, education, and ability; (2) require equal effort in mental or physical exertion; (3) are of equal responsibility and accountability; and (4) are performed under similar working conditions. Courts have held that unequal pay may be legal if it is based on seniority, merit, incentive systems, and a factor other than gender. The main cases filed under this law in the area of nursing have been by nonprofessionals.

Occupational Safety and Health Act

The Occupational Safety and Health Administration (OSHA) Act of 1970 was enacted to ensure that healthful and safe working conditions would exist in the work place. Among other provisions, the law requires isolation procedures, placarding areas containing ionizing radiation, proper grounding of electrical equipment, protective storage of flammable and combustible liquids, and the gloving of all personnel when handling bodily fluids. The statute provides that if no federal standard has been established, state statutes prevail. Nurse managers should know the relevant OSHA laws for the institution and his or her specific area. Frequent review of new additions to the law must also be undertaken, especially in this era of AIDS and infectious diseases, and care must be taken to ensure that necessary gloves and equipment as specified are available on each unit.

Employment-at-Will and Wrongful Discharge

Historically, the employment relationship has been considered as a "free will" relationship. Employees were free to take or not take a job at will, and employers were free to hire, retain, or discharge employees for any reason. Many laws, some federal but predominantly state, have been slowly eroding this at-will employment relationship. Evolving case law provides at least three exceptions to the broad doctrine of employment-at-will.

The first exception is a public policy exception. This exception involves cases where an employee is discharged in direct conflict with established public policy (Twomey, 1986). Some examples would be discharging an employee for serving on a jury, for reporting an employers' illegal actions (better known as "whistle blowing"), and for filing a workers' compensation claim.

The second exception involves situations in which there is an implied contract. The courts have generally treated employee handbooks, company policies, and oral statements made at the time of employment as "framing the employment relationship" (Watkins v. Unemployment Compensation Board of Review, 1997).

The third exception is a "good faith and fair dealing" exception. The purpose of this exception is to prevent unfair or malicious terminations, and the exception is used sparingly by the courts. An older case

illustrates its use by the court. In Fortune v. National Cash Register Company (1977), an employee was discharged just before a final contract was signed between his employer and another company for which the employee would have received a large commission. The court held that he was discharged in bad faith, specifically solely to prevent payment of his commission by National Cash Register.

Nurse managers are urged to know their respective state law concerning this growing area of the law. Managers should review institution documents, especially employee handbooks and recruiting brochures, for unwanted statements implying job security or other unintentional promises. Managers are also cautioned not to say anything during the pre-employment negotiations and interviews that might be construed as implying job security or other unintentional promises to the potential employee.

Collective Bargaining

Collective bargaining, also called labor relations, is the joining together of employees for the purpose of increasing their ability to influence the employer and improve working conditions. Usually the employer is referred to as management and the employees, even professionals, are labor. Those persons involved in the hiring, firing, scheduling, disciplining, or evaluating of employers are considered management and may not be included in a collective bargaining unit. Those in management could form their own group, but are not protected under these laws. Nurse managers may or may not be part of management; if they have hiring and firing authority, they are part of management.

Collective bargaining is defined and protected by the National Labor Relations Act and its amendments; the National Labor Relations Board (NLRB) oversees the act and those who come under its auspices. The NLRB ensures that employees are able to choose freely whether they want to be represented by a particular bargaining unit, and it serves to prevent or remedy any violation of the labor laws. See Chapter 10 for a full analysis of this concept.

▋ PROFESSIONAL NURSING PRACTICE: ETHICS

Ethical Theories

Ethics is the science relating to moral actions and one's value system. Many nurses envision ethics as dealing with principles of morality and thus what is right or wrong. A broader conceptual definition of ethics is that ethics is concerned with motives and attitudes and the relationship of these attitudes to the good of the individual. "Ethics has to do with actions we wish people would take, not actions they must take" (Hall, 1990, p. 37). Thus **values** are interwoven with ethics; values are personal beliefs about the truth and worth of thoughts, objects, and behavior.

Ethics may be distinguished from the law as ethics is internal to oneself, looks to the good of an individual rather than society as a whole, and concerns the "why" of one's actions. The law, comprising rules and regulations pertinent to society as a whole, is external to oneself and concerns one's actions and conduct. What did the person do or fail to do as opposed to why did the person act as he or she did? Ethics concerns the good of an individual within society while law concerns society as a whole as opposed to the individual in society. Law can be enforced through the courts and statutes while ethics are enforced via ethics committees and professional codes. Table 3-4 shows the distinctions between law and ethics.

Today, ethics and legal issues often become entwined and it is difficult to separate ethics from legal concerns. Legal principles and doctrines assist the nurse manager in decision making, and ethical theories and principles are often involved in those decisions. Thus the nurse manager must be cognizant of both areas in everyday management concerns.

Many different ethical theories have evolved to justify existing moral principles; these theories are considered normative because they are universally applicable theories of right and wrong. Most normative approaches to ethics fall under the following three broad categories.

Deontological (from the Greek *deon*, or "duty") **theories** derive norms and rules from the duties human beings owe to one another by virtue of commitments made and roles assumed. Generally, deontologists hold that a sense of duty consists of rational respect for the fulfilling of one's obligations to other human beings. The greatest strength of this theory is its emphasis on the dignity of human beings. Deontological theory looks not to the end or consequences of an action, but to the intention of the action. It is one's good intentions, the intentions to do a moral duty, that ultimately determine the praiseworthiness of the action. Deontological ethics have sometimes been subdivided into situation ethics, wherein the decision making takes into account the unique characteristics of each individual, the caring relationship between the person and the caregiver, and the most humanistic course of action given the circumstances.

Teleological (from the Greek *telos*, for "end") **theories** derive norms or rules for conduct from the consequences of actions. Right consists of actions that have good consequences and wrong consists of actions that have bad consequences. Teleologists disagree, though, about how to determine the goodness or badness of the consequences of actions. This theory is frequently referred to as utilitarianism; what makes an action right or wrong is its utility, and useful actions bring the greatest amount of good into existence. An alternate way of viewing this theory is that the usefulness of an action is determined by the amount of happiness it brings. Utilitarian ethics can then be subdivided into rule and act utilitarianism. Rule utilitarianism seeks the greatest happiness for all; it appeals to public agreement as a basis for objective judgment about the nature of happiness. Act utilitarianism tries to determine in a particular situation which course of action will bring about the greatest happiness, or the least harm and suffering, to a single person. As

Table 3-4	DISTINCTIONS BETWEEN LAW AND ETHICS	
	Law	**Ethics**
Source	External to oneself; rules and regulations for society	Internal to oneself; values, beliefs, and individual interpretations
Concerns	Conduct and actions—what did the person do?	Motive and attitudes—why did the person act as he or she did?
Interests	Society as a whole	Individuals within a society
Enforcement	Courts and statutes Boards of nursing	Ethics committees; professional organizations

Adapted from Guido Boards of nursing (1988).

such, act utilitarianism makes happiness subjective (Guido, 1997).

A third ethical theory has slowly been evolving and, while not yet given the full status of a theory, it does assist nurses and healthcare providers struggling with difficult ethical issues. Called **principlism,** this emerging theory incorporates existing ethical principles and attempts to resolve conflicts by applying one or more of the ethical principles. Ethical principles actually control ethical decision making much more than do ethical theories, since principles encompass the basic premises from which rules are developed. Principles are moral norms that nurses demand and strive to implement daily in clinical settings. Each of the principles can be used individually, although it is much more common to see two or more ethical principles used in concert.

Ethical theories are important because they form the essential base of knowledge from which to proceed rather than giving easy, straightforward answers. Without ethical theories, decisions revolve on personal emotions and values. Because most nurses do not ascribe to either deontology or teleology exclusively, principlism is growing in popularity today.

Ethical Principles

Ethical principles that the nurse manager should consider when making decisions include the eight items listed in Box 3-2. Each of these principles can be used by itself, though it is much more common to see more than one ethical principle in practice.

The **autonomy** principle addresses personal freedom and the right to choose what will happen to one's own person. The legal doctrine of informed consent is a direct reflection of this principle. This principle underlies the concept of progressive discipline as the employee has the option to meet delineated expectations or take full accountability for his or her

actions. This principle also underlies the professional nurse's clinical practice as autonomy is reflected in individual decision making about patient care issues as well as in group decision making about unit operations decisions.

The **beneficence** principle states that the actions one takes should promote good. In caring for patients, good can be defined in many ways, including allowing a person to die without advanced life support. Good can also prompt the nurse to encourage the patient to undergo extensive, painful treatment procedures if these procedures will increase both the quality and quantity of life. This principle is used when nurse managers accentuate the employee's positive attributes and qualities rather than focusing on the negative and the employee's failures and shortcomings. Nurse managers also employ this principle when they encourage staff members to excel to their fullest potential.

The corollary of beneficence, the principle of **nonmaleficence,** states that one should do no harm. Many nurses find it difficult to follow this principle when performing treatments and procedures that bring discomfort and pain to patients. Thus the principle of beneficence may be chosen because even pain and suffering can bring about good for the patient. For a nurse manager following this principle, performance evaluation should emphasize the employee's good qualities and give positive direction for growth. Destroying the employee's self-esteem and self-worth would be considered doing harm under this principle.

Veracity concerns truth telling and incorporates the concept that individuals should always tell the truth. The principle also compels that the truth be told completely. Nurse managers use this principle when they give all the facts of a situation truthfully and then assist employees to make decisions. For example, with low patient censuses, employees must be told all the options and then be allowed to make their own decisions about floating to other units, taking vacation time, or taking a day without pay if the institution has such a policy.

Justice concerns the issue that persons should be treated equally and fairly. This principle usually arises in times of short supplies or when there is competition for resources or benefits. This principle is considered with holiday and vacation time and paid attendance at national or local conferences; overall performance should be considered, rather than who is next on the list to attend a conference or to be allowed time off.

Box 3-2

Ethical Principles

- Autonomy
- Beneficence
- Nonmaleficence
- Veracity
- Justice
- Paternalism
- Fidelity
- Respect for others

This principle, **paternalism**, allows one to make decisions for another and often is seen as a negative or undesirable principle. Paternalism assists persons to make decisions when they do not have sufficient data or expertise. Staff members frequently use some degree of paternalism when they assist patients and their family members to decide if surgical procedures should be undertaken or if medical management is a better option. Paternalism becomes undesirable when the entire decision is taken from the patient or employee. Nurse managers use this principle in a positive manner by assisting employees in deciding major career moves and plans.

Fidelity is keeping one's promises or commitments. Staff members know not to promise to patients commitments that they may not be able to keep, such as assuring the patient that no code will be performed before consulting with the patient's physician for such an order. Nurse managers abide by this principle when they follow through on any promises they have previously made to employees, such as a promised leave, a certain shift to be worked, or a promotion to preceptor within the unit.

Many think the principle of **respect for others** is the highest principle and incorporates all other principles. Respect for others acknowledges the right of individuals to make decisions and to live by these decisions. Respect for others also transcends cultural differences, gender issues, and racial concerns. Nurse managers positively reinforce this principle daily in their actions with employees, patients, and peers because they serve as role models for staff members and others in the institution. Nurses also reinforce these principles as they incorporate Watson's Theory of Caring when interfacing with patients and peers. See the theory box below on Watson's Theory of Caring.

Exercise 3-6

The community has been suffering from a severe nursing shortage made worse by a particularly virulent flu that has affected many of the staff members. Upper management is aware of the severity of the shortage and has decreased bed census by 20%; only emergency surgery is being performed until the crisis abates. You are considering reassigning a portion of your critical care staff, including dialysis and emergency care nurses, to the general medical-surgical floors because the crisis is most severe on the general units. None of the staff has been cross-trained specifically to the general units. From an ethical standpoint, how would you begin to achieve this task? How would you select which nurses to reassign and which nurses to retain in the unit? Would you involve the nurses themselves in the decision-making process? Why or why not?

Ethical Decision-Making Framework

Ethical decision making involves reflection on the following: who should make the choice; possible options or courses of action; available options; consequences, both good and bad, of all possible options; rules, obligations, and values that should direct choices; and desired goals or outcomes. When making decisions, nurses need to combine all of these elements using an orderly, systematic, and objective method; ethical decision-making models assist in accomplishing this goal.

There are various models for ethical decision making. All of the models have five to eight ordered steps that start with fully comprehending the dilemma and conclude with evaluation of the implemented option. An example of a traditional model for ethical decision making might include the following steps:

1. Identify the problem
2. Gather data to analyze the causes and consequences of the problem

Watson's Theory of Caring		
THEORY/CONTRIBUTOR	**KEY IDEA**	**APPLICATION TO PRACTICE**
Theory of Caring (Jean Watson)	Caring is a moral ideal rather than a task-oriented behavior whose goal is the preservation of human dignity and humanity in the healthcare system. Caring transcends time and space and has spiritual dimensions.	Nurses have the responsibility to facilitate clients' and peers' development. This can be accomplished by teaching, providing situational support, and recognizing coping skills and adaptation to the environment.
From Watson (1988).		

3. Explore optional solutions to the problem
4. Evaluate these optional solutions
5. Select the appropriate solution from all the options
6. Implement the selected solution
7. Evaluate the results

Perhaps the easiest ethical decision-making model to remember and to implement in practice is the **MORAL model** (see Box 3-3) developed by Thiroux in 1977 and further developed for nursing by Halloran in 1982. Many nurses prefer this method because the letters of the acronym remind nurses of the subsequent steps to take.

Ethical decision making is always a process. To facilitate the process, the nurse manager must use all available resources, including the institutional ethics committee, and communicate with and support all those involved in the process. Some decisions are easier to reach and support. It is important to allow sufficient time for the process so that a supportable option can be reached. The "Research Perspective" on p. 54 shows how nurse administrators make ethical decisions in clinical situations.

Ethics Committees

With the increasing numbers of ethical dilemmas in patient situations and administrative decisions, healthcare providers are using hospital **ethics committees** for guidance. Such committees can provide both long-term and short-term assistance. Ethics committees can provide structure and guidelines for potential problems; serve as open forums for discussion; and function as true patient advocates by placing the patient at the core of the committee discussions.

To form such a committee, the proposed involved individuals should begin as a bioethical study group so that ethical principles and theories can be explored by all potential members. The composition of the committee should include nurses, physicians, clergy, clinical social workers, nutritional experts, pharmacists, administrative personnel, and legal experts. Once the committee has become active, individual patients or patients' families as well as additional representatives of members of the healthcare delivery team may be invited to committee deliberations.

Ethics committees traditionally follow one of three distinct structures, although some institutional committees blend the three structures. The autonomy model facilitates decision making for competent patients. The patient benefit model uses substituted judgment (what the patient would want for himself or herself if capable of making these issues known) and facilitates decision making for the incompetent patient. The social justice model considers broad social issues and is accountable to the overall institution.

In most settings, the ethics committee already exists because there are complex issues dividing healthcare workers. In many centers, ethical rounds, conducted weekly or monthly, allow staff members who may later become involved in ethical decision making to begin reviewing all the issues and to become more comfortable with ethical issues and their resolution.

Box 3-3
MORAL Model for Ethical Decision Making

M Massage the dilemma. Identify and define the issues in the dilemma. Consider the opinions of all the major players in the dilemma as well as their value systems. This includes patients, family members, nurses, physicians, clergy, and any other interdisciplinary healthcare members.

O Outline the options. Examine all the options, including those less realistic and conflicting. This stage is designed only for considering options and not for making a final decision.

R Resolve the dilemma. Review the issues and options, applying the basic principles of ethics to each option. Decide the best option based on the views of all those concerned in the dilemma.

A Act by applying the chosen option. This step is usually the most difficult because it requires actual implementation while the previous steps allow only for dialogue and discussion.

L Look back and evaluate the entire process, including the implementation. No process is complete without a thorough evaluation. Ensure that those involved are able to follow through on the final option. If not, a second decision may be required and the process must start again at the initial step.

Adapted from Thiroux (1977) and Halloran (1982).

Research Perspective

Borawski, D. (1994). Resources used by nurse administrators in ethical decision-making. The Journal of Nursing Administration, 24 (3), 17-22.

Nursing administrative practice involves ethical decision making, often on a daily basis, yet little research has been done concerning resources that these administrators use in ethical decision making. In earlier studies, personal values and previous experience with moral decision making were seen as the highest resources used, followed by the *Patient Bill of Rights*, discussions with colleagues, and institutional ethics committees as resources. Other studies list family, religion, and friends as necessary resources. The majority of these earlier studies were not limited to nurse executives, but incorporated nurses at all levels within institutional settings. The current study was limited to nurse executives within hospital settings.

The Patient Care Administration Ethics Survey (PCAES) was sent to all nursing administrations in North Carolina. The survey tool had two major headings: demographic data and ethical resource data. Both open-ended and closed-ended questions were used, and information sought concerned resources used and whether those resources met the respondent's needs. Of the 159 surveys sent, 102 usable surveys were analyzed.

Respondents were primarily female (91%), with the majority (57%) having been in patient care administration for more than 10 years. Most of the respondents held B.S.N. degrees (28%), master's degrees in nursing (28%), or master's degrees outside of nursing (27%). Most of the master's degrees outside nursing were in business administration or health-related fields.

The number of resources used in ethical decision making ranged from 1 to 12, with the average being 5.9. Findings showed that nurse colleagues were the number one resource used (86%), followed closely by administrative colleagues (83%), personal values (81%), and the *Patient Bill of Rights* (75%). When degrees and responses were evaluated together, nurses with degrees in nursing (A.D.N., B.S.N., and M.S.N.) ranked personal values and nursing colleagues as the most frequently used resources. However, nurses with master's degrees in other fields (M.B.A. or health-related master's degrees) ranked administrative colleagues as their most used resource.

Findings also showed that the majority of respondents (76%) believed that their resources were adequate to meet their needs in ethical decision making. Those who felt that their resources were inadequate expressed the need for institutional ethics committees (or more functional committees), a need for networking with other colleagues, or inadequacy of financial and/or human resources.

This study contrasts with earlier studies regarding resources and ethical decision making. Nursing colleagues were used more frequently than personal values and administrative colleagues. Family and friends, reported in earlier studies, were rarely used as resources by these respondents. Interestingly, the *Patient Bill of Rights* (75%) was used much more often than the American Nurses' Association *Code For Nurses* (57%) by these respondents. The author explained this last finding by reminding readers that the *Patient Bill of Rights* gives more direction about individual autonomy and self-determination—important issues in today's ethical arena.

The recommendations from the study encouraged nurse administrators to pursue continuing professional development in the area of nursing and health care ethics as well as in professional trends. Nurse administrators should also support the development of nursing ethics committees and provide a consultative forum for examining ethical issues.

Nursing administration has emerged as a distinct area of nursing practice. As such, the body of knowledge for nursing administrators must include examination of those elements of administrative practice that are ethical in nature. "As the science of nursing advances, nursing administration can play a major role in structuring the framework for patient care to make the wisest use of scarce resources" (p. 22).

Implications for Practice

Nurse managers need to continue pursuing the following: professional development in the area of nursing and health care ethics; professional trends; and professional standards of ethics. Pursuing these areas will assist nurse managers to implement such practices in their individual institutions.

Future Ethical Concerns for Nurses

Issues of concern in the near future include the whole issue of healthcare reform. With the sweeping ways in which patients are enrolled into managed care and the uncertain future of healthcare delivery in a managed care system, there is great concern that ethical and needed healthcare will prevail (Mohr, 1996).

Other issues of concern involve autonomy and independent practice among nurses, quality of care in home and community settings, and development of nurses as leaders in the healthcare delivery field. Issues that continue to permeate ethical concerns for nurses include the patient's refusal of healthcare, issues surrounding death and dying, nurses' ability to be patient advocates in today's healthcare structure, and the ability to perform competent, quality nursing care in a system that rewards only cost-saving measures and that staffs with fewer and fewer professional nurses. Nursing must begin to address potential issues in a timely manner, lest the profession is unable to address them when needed (Edwards & Roemer, 1996).

Nurses need to begin now to look at the issues, professional values, and expectations, and decide the issues for which they will fight and those that are acceptable. Once identified, strategies for promoting quality nursing care can be delineated.

▋ CHAPTER CHECKLIST

This chapter addresses the issues of legal and ethical interactions with regard to nurse managers. Legislative and legal controls have been established to clarify the boundaries of professional practice and to protect consumers. Thus there are some definite answers and guidelines to assist practitioners from the legal and legislative areas. These controls are constantly evolving, and the nurse manager must continually be aware of these changes as they affect the scope of the practice. Ethics has no such answers. Nor are there rules and guidelines that cover all aspects of human life. Thus nurse managers must explore value systems and become expert in using ethical models, incorporating both ethical theories and principles. The use of a systematic, humanistic approach reduces bias, facilitates decision making, and allows the best working conditions possible from an ethical standpoint.

- Understanding and using legal and ethical principles are key strategies to be integrated into the role of an effective nurse manager.

A Manager's Solution

❓ Staff and managers worked together to devise a plan that would ensure quality patient care, but also require a decreased number of staff per shift. We spent hours consulting with other small rural hospital staff members to see how they had approached such an issue, reviewing legal issues to ensure that quality care would be maintained, and looking at the issue from a principlism approach to ensure that both the patients' and the nurses' ethical values were maintained. We also used the literature to see if there were more effective ways of delivering care, such as requiring all vaginal delivery mothers to use couplet care (rooming-in). After acquiring all this information, we brainstormed possible solutions, throwing out ideas no matter how improbable they appeared at first glance. We then applied a MORAL model approach to the dilemma, creating extensive lists outlining the pros and cons of each possible solution.

The implemented solution was to combine the obstetrical and general medical-surgical unit into a single "nursing" unit. Mothers would be required to keep their newborns in the room, thus employing couplet care; patients would be located on the two units (now one unit) so that nurses could readily care for both sets of patients; and all nurses would receive ongoing education to ensure quality care. This had the advantage of reducing the number of licensed nurses required per shift, enhancing the usage of limited resources, and ensuring that all patients continued to receive quality care. The implemented solution will be evaluated periodically, with a comprehensive evaluation plan enacted at both a 6-month and a 12-month interval. Small changes will continue to be made as problems arise. It was, for us, the best solution, both from a legal-ethical viewpoint and from a realistic viewpoint.

❓ *Would this be a suitable approach for you? Why?*

- Nurse practice acts define the scope of acceptable practice for licensed registered nurses as well as licensed practical (vocational) nurses.
- Legal principles, if effectively integrated into all aspects of nursing management, minimize one's potential legal liability.
  - Malpractice is the failure of a person with professional education and skills to act in a reasonable and prudent manner.
  - Causes of malpractice for nurse managers include:
    - issues of delegation and supervision
    - duty to orient, educate, and evaluate
    - failure to warn
    - staffing issues
  - Liability may be classified as personal, vicarious, corporate, or strict product.
  - Protective and reporting laws ensure the safety or rights of specific groups of people.
  - Informed consent is the authorization by the patient or the patient's legal representative to do something to the patient.
  - Privacy and confidentiality rights protect the patient from unreasonable and unwanted interference and secure the privacy of the patient's medical record.
  - Federal and state governments have enacted a number of employment laws that nurses must understand and follow when dealing with managerial issues. These include:
    - Equal Pay Act of 1963
    - Civil Rights Act
    - Age Discrimination Act of 1967
    - Americans with Disabilities Act of 1990
    - Affirmative Action
    - Equal Employment Opportunity Laws
    - Occupational Safety and Health Act
    - Employment-at-Will and Wrongful Discharge
    - Collective Bargaining
- Ethical theories and principles relate to moral actions and value systems and apply both to patient situations and to management situations.
  - Ethical theories justify existing moral principles and are considered universally applicable.
  - Ethical theories include:
    - deontology
    - teleology
    - principlism
  - Ethical principles exert direct control over professional nursing practice and encompass basic premises from which rules are developed.
  - Ethical principles are:
    - autonomy

- beneficence
- nonmaleficence
- veracity
- justice
- paternalism
- fidelity
- respect for others
  - The "MORAL" model is an easy acronym to remember in ethical decision making.
  - Ethics committees aid in assisting nurses to implement solutions in everyday clinical practice.

TIPS ON LEGAL AND ETHICAL ISSUES

Before applying the information presented in the chapter, the following five tips are offered:

- Read the state nurse practice act carefully to fully comprehend the allowable scope of practice within the given state.
- Consult with risk management, the institutional attorney, or the legal department for a fuller understanding of how federal employment laws pertain to the individual nurse manager.
- Cultivate a group of professional consultants, either within the institution or outside the institution, who can assist with legal-ethical questions. Such a group or even one or two professional consultants may have great insight into issues as they arise and assist in preventing problems in the future.
- Discover who serves on the institutional ethics committee and develop friendships among selected members. Attend the meetings to see how ethical issues are addressed in the institution. Become an active part of the ethical rounds, if such exist in the institution.
- Think before you act. Remember it is always easier to hesitate, even briefly, so that the better approach can be implemented than to try to retract or amend something already done or already verbalized.

TERMS TO KNOW

apparent agency	emancipated minor
autonomy	ethics
beneficence	ethics committees
collective bargaining	expert witness
common law	failure to warn
confidentiality	fidelity
deontological theory	foreseeability

indemnification
independent contractor
informed consent
justice
labor union
law
liability
liable
malpractice
MORAL model
nonmaleficence
nurse practice act

paternalism
personal liability
principlism
privacy
respect for others
respondeat superior
standard of care
statute
teleological theory
values
veracity
vicarious liability

REFERENCES

American Nurses' Association. (1988). *Standards for Nurse Administrators*. Kansas City: The Association.

Beltran v. Downey Community Hospital. (1992). *Medical Malpractice Verdicts, Settlements, and Experts*, 8 (5), 30.

Bishop v. United States, 334 F. Spp.. 415 (D.C. Tex., 1971).

Borawski, D.B. (1994). Resources used by nurse administrators in ethical decision-making. *The Journal of Nursing Administration*, 24 (3), 17-22.

Civil Rights Act, 43 *Federal Register*, 1978, Sec. 703 et. Seq, (1964).

David W. Francis v. Memorial General Hospital, 726 P. 2nd. 852 (New Mexico, 1986).

Edwards, P.A., & Roemer, L. (1996). Are nurse managers ready for the current challenges of health care? *The Journal of Nursing Administration*, 26 (9), 11-17.

Fiesta, J. (1994). Legal update for nurses. Part II: Assigning, delegating, and staffing. *Nursing Management*, 24 (2), 14-16.

Fortune v. National Cash Register Company, 272 Mass. 96, 264 N.E. 2nd. 1251 (1977).

42 USC 12101 et. seq., 12211 (a) and (b) (1) (1990).

Guido, G.W. (1997). *Legal Issues in Nursing*. 2nd ed. Stamford, CT: Appleton & Lange.

Hall, J.K. (1990). Understanding the fine line between law and ethics. *Nursing 90*, 20 (10), 37.

Halloran, M.C. (1982). Rational ethical judgments utilizing a decision-making tool. *Heart and Lung*, 11, 566-570.

Hansen v. Caring Professionals, Inc., 676 N.E. 2nd. 1349 (Ill. App., 1997).

Herrero v. St. Louis University Hospital, 109 F. 3rd. 481 (8th Cir., 1997).

Horton v. Carolina Medicorp, Inc. 472 S. E. 778 (N.C., 1996).

Howard v. North Mississippi Medical Center, 939 F. Spp.. 505 (N.D. Miss., 1996).

Marquis, B.L., & Huston, C.J. (1992). *Leadership Roles and Management Functions for Nurses*. Philadelphia: Lippincott.

Mauro v. Borgess Medical Center, #4:94-CV-05, (Michigan, 1995).

McIntosh v. Brookdale Hospital Medical Center, 942 F. Spp.. 813 (E.D. N.Y., 1996).

Mele v. St. Mary's Hospital of Rochester, Minnesota and Mayo Foundations, (1991). CV-3-87-818. *Medical Malpractice Verdicts, Settlements, and Experts*, 7 (10), 32.

Mohr, W.K. (1996). Ethics, nursing and health care in the age of "re-form." *Nursing and Health Care*, 17(1), 16-21.

Sabol v. Richmond Heights General Hospital, 676 N. E. 2nd. 958 (Ohio App., 1996).

Schank, M.J., Weis, D., & Ancona, J. (1996). Reflecting professional values in the philosophy of nursing. *The Journal of Nursing Administration*, 26 (7/8), 55-60.

Thiroux, J. (1977). *Ethics: Theory and Practice*. Philadelphia: Macmillan.

Trudeau, S. (1992). *Hospital Law Newsletter*, 6 (3), 1.

Twomey, D.P. (1986). A *Concise Guide to Employment Laws*: EEO and OSHA. Cincinnati, OH: South-Western Publishing.

Watkins v. Unemployment Compensation Board of Review, 689 A. 2nd. 1019 (Pa. Commonwealth, 1997).

Watson, J. (1988). *Nursing: Human Science and Human Care—A Theory of Nursing*. New York: National League for Nursing.

Zamudio v. Patia, 956 F. Spp.. 803 (N.D. Ill., 1997).

SUGGESTED READINGS

Cameron, M.E. (1997). Legal and ethical issues: Ethical distress in nursing. *Journal of Professional Nursing*, 13 (5), 280.

Fiesta, J. (1990). The nursing shortage: Whose liability problem? Part II *Nursing Management*, 21 (2), 22-23.

Finkelstein, P. (1996). Best defense is a good offense. *Minnesota Nursing Accent*, 68 (6), 8.

Iversen, J.K. (1997). Combined incident and quality management report. *Home Health Care Management and Practice*, 9 (6), 57-78.

Muller, L. (1997). Management accountability and legal trends. *Nursing Spectrum*, 9 (4), NJ5,7.

Power, K.J. (1997). The legal and ethical implications of consent to nursing procedures. *British Journal of Nursing*, 6 (15), 885-888.

Rhodes, A.M. (1997). Legal issues: Liability for unlicensed assistive personnel, Part 1. *American Journal of Maternal/Child Nursing*, 22 (5), 269.

von Kanel, R.L. (1997). Ethics: Confidentiality: An analysis of the issue. *Plastic Surgery Nursing*, 17 (3), 146-7, 154-5.

CHAPTER

4

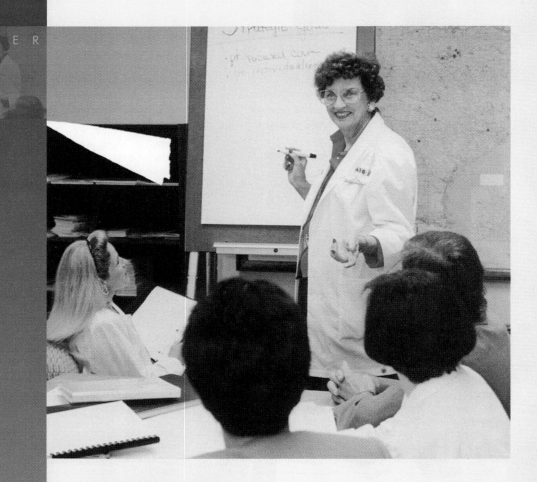

Strategic Planning, Goal Setting, and Marketing

Darlene Steven
RN, MHSA, PhD

This chapter discusses the application of several organizational elements of planning for the future, such as the strategic planning process, goal setting, management by objectives, and marketing. Where appropriate, examples of planning and marketing strategies used in the healthcare field are presented.

Objectives

- Describe the importance of environmental assessment.
- Explain the planning process.
- Outline the purpose of mission statement, philosophy, goals, and objectives.
- Describe goal setting and strategic planning.
- Describe the process of strategic planning in establishing an entrepreneurial business in the healthcare field.
- Explain the importance of marketing plans in the healthcare field.

Questions to Consider

- How is the strategic plan used to implement change in an organization? Provide an example.
- Explain how the mission statement, philosophy, goals, and objectives merge with the strategic plan of the facility.
- How can you influence the direction of your organization by effective planning?
- If you had a "vision" of where your facility should be directed in the future, how would you go about "making your vision a reality"?

A Manager's Challenge
From Judith Shamian, RN, PhD, CHE, Vice-President, Nursing
Mount Sinai Hospital, Toronto, Ontario

In 1991 Mount Sinai Hospital in Toronto, Canada, reviewed the required skill mix (registered nurse/registered practical nurse, nurse's aide) for its patient population. The nursing committee considered the needs of our patients, scope of practice as determined by the regulatory body (College of Nurses of Ontario), knowledge required to care for patients and the existing research with respect to skill mix and care delivery models. The committee then attempted to determine which model would be most effective and efficient in a cost-constrained environment.

What do you think you would do if you were this manager?

INTRODUCTION

The present healthcare system is in a "state of change." The pressure to contain costs in healthcare has resulted in major reforms. In the next decade, "we are going to see a lot more health care delivered in the home through expert systems, through access to the Internet between individuals in their own environments" (Jordan Cohen as cited in *Look at it this way*, 1996, p. 76). Restructuring of our healthcare system includes patient empowerment; comprehensive and coordinated service delivery; efficient and effective use of resources, manpower, and technology; and emphasis on health promotion and prevention. The demographics of our society are also in a state of change and include a dramatic increase in the elderly population.

Nurses have the opportunity to make a difference in planning new strategies for the future and for influencing the direction of healthcare. It is estimated that one in 40 voters is a nurse—we can and will influence the delivery of health services if we are prepared to stand united and speak to government in a unified voice by our lobbying efforts. To achieve this we must be proactive in our stance and efforts. Proactive simply means "aggressive planning," which provides direction for one's efforts and toward which others must then react. Thus greater control is possible so that one's preferred future becomes a probability, not just a possibility.

The importance of thoughtful, deliberate planning in the face of uncertainties cannot be overstated. Wilkinson (1988) offers this insight:

An employee in an organization—manager, supervisor or an [employee] who has no clearly defined, benefit oriented, attainable, measurable objectives is like a ship without a compass or a chart. Such people do not know where they are going, where they should be going, at what rate, at what cost, in what control. They are not managing their working lives or helping others to manage theirs (p. 6).

In this chapter the strategic planning process is described. Planning is followed by an introduction to goal setting and management by objectives. The key concepts of marketing as it relates to the healthcare industry are discussed. Where appropriate and feasible, examples of planning and marketing strategies used in the healthcare field are presented as case studies.

STRATEGIC PLANNING

Definition

Strategic planning is a process that is "designed to achieve goals in dynamic, competitive environments through the allocation of resources" (Andrews, 1990, p. 103).

The strategic planning process shown in Figure 4-1 consists of a series of steps as follows:

- Search of the environment to determine those forces or changes that may affect the work of the organization or that may be crucial to its survival

- Appraisal of the organization's strengths and weaknesses—its potential for dealing with change
- Appraisal of the major opportunities and threats
- Identification and evaluation of the various strategies available to the organization to meet these opportunities and threats
- Selection of the best option that balances the organization's potential with the challenges of changing conditions, taking into account the values of its management and its social responsibilities
- Preparation of the strategy
- Implementation and evaluation of the strategy

Reasons for Planning

To survive in this era of change and restructuring of the healthcare system, thoughtful and deliberate

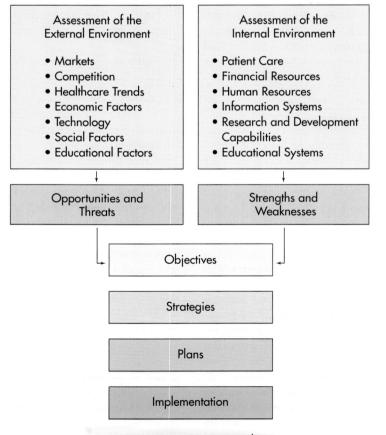

Fig. 4-1 Key steps in strategic planning.

planning becomes a necessity. This process leads to success in the achievement of goals and objectives, gives meaning to work life, and provides direction for operational activities of the organization. Furthermore, planning may result in efficient and effective use of resources and may assist in the formulation of visionary activities and the future direction of the agency. There are numerous reasons why nursing administrators do not plan in a systematic manner: lack of knowledge regarding philosophy, goals, and external and internal operations of the organization; lack of understanding of the planning process; and the fact that time is spent on day-to-day operations rather than on short- and long-range plans.

Phases of the Strategic Planning Process

Strategic planning is an "open systems approach to steering an enterprise over time through uncertain environmental circumstances" (Andrews, 1990, p. 103). The strategic planning process is proactive, vision directed, action oriented, creative, innovative, and oriented toward change.

Strategic planning is based on the assumptions that

". planning is an inherently desirable activity in which administrators should engage; strategic planning has yielded desirable results in education, business and other disciplines; and strategic planning concepts borrowed from other disciplines apply to nursing" (Andrews, 1990, p. 103).

The term *strategic planning process* usually entails the development of a plan of action for 3 to 5 years. The initial phase is the most difficult.

Phase 1: Assessment of the External and Internal Environment

External environmental assessment. Assessment of the external environment is the initial phase in the strategic planning process. The economic, demographic, technological, social, educational, and political factors are assessed in terms of their impact on opportunities and threats within the environment. Healthcare managers can assess the impact of competitors on their environment and thus plan and monitor their own operations and develop other creative and visionary programs. For example, if the government were to introduce a nonlicensed community support worker whose role would be to provide com-

plete home care for the individual in a home setting (i.e., total patient care, dressing change, medication administration, cleaning of house including windows, banking, and even specialized care including dialysis), this would have tremendous impact on the present roles and responsibilities of registered nurses and their assistants.

Exercise 4-1

What is your opinion about the economic situation in the city in which you live? What are the demographics of the area? What are the educational resources?

Internal environmental assessment. The internal assessment of the environment includes a review of the effectiveness of the structure, size, programs, financial resources, human resources, information systems, and research and development capabilities of the organization. The management team involves all levels of staff in this process and focuses on the purpose of the organization, the mission, the capabilities, skills and relationships of various professional and related staff, and the weaknesses and strength of staff in such areas as leadership, planning, coordination, research, and staff development.

Phase 2: Review of Mission Statement, Philosophy, Goals, and Objectives

Mission statement. A mission statement reflects the purpose and direction of the healthcare agency or a department within it. A statement of philosophy provides direction for the agency and/or department within it. The content usually specifies beliefs regarding rights of individuals, beliefs regarding health and nursing, expectations of practitioners, and commitment of the organization to professionalism, education, evaluation, and research. The importance of the mission statement cannot be overstated, yet it is questionable how many individuals in an organization when questioned directly could enunciate the key points in the mission statement or the philosophy of a healthcare setting.

Covey (1990) relates that the mission statement is vital to the success of an organization. He believes that everyone should participate in the development of the mission statement . . . "the involvement process is as important as the written product and is the key to its use" (p. 139). Covey relates the belief system of IBM: individual, excellence, and service—everyone in this organization is committed to these values. This illustration of a mission statement is worthy of further consideration by healthcare agencies. "An organizational mission statement—one that truly reflects the deep shared vision and values of everyone within that organization—creates a unity and tremendous commitment" (p. 143).

Exercise 4-2

Select a clinical organization with which you have been affiliated. How effective is the structure? (Does the organization operate effectively and efficiently?) What overall human resources are present (e.g., various titles and numbers of people)? What information systems are used? Now apply those same questions to the nursing component only.

Covey cites the example of a hotel where all staff participated in the development of the mission statement outlining "uncompromising personalized service" from housekeepers, waitresses, desk clerks, and kitchen staff. Each one carried out the mission statement with no supervision—offering at any time to assist patrons with any difficulties. This can be contrasted to a simple request clients might make regarding dietary practices that may not be met in an institutional setting.

Goal-setting. Goal-setting is the process of developing, negotiating, and formalizing the targets or objectives that an employee is responsible for accomplishing (Curtis, 1994).

Locke, a leading authority on goal setting, and his colleagues (1981) expand on this concept:

The concept is similar in meaning to the concepts of purpose and intent. . . . Other frequently used concepts that are also similar in meaning to that of goal include performance standard (a measuring rod for evaluating performance), quota (a minimum amount of work or production), work norm (a standard of acceptable behaviour defined by a work group), task (a piece of work to be accomplished), objective (the ultimate aim of an action or series of actions), deadline (a time limit), and budget. (Locke, et al, 1981, cited in Kreitner & Kinicki, 1992, p. 219)

Goals assist nurse administrators and other members of the healthcare team to focus attention on what is relevant and important and to develop strategies and actions to achieve the goals. Research conducted in several countries (Australia, Canada, England, West Germany, Japan, and the Caribbean) found that goal setting tends to work differently in various cultures (Locke, et al, 1981).

Exercise 4-3

Review a healthcare organization's mission statement. Tell a colleague in your own words what that statement means in general; then give specific examples of how it translates to nursing.

Practical insights from these studies that are important to nurse administrators are that specific goals are more likely to lead to higher performance than vague or very general goals such as "do your best." Feedback, or knowledge of results, is likely to motivate individuals toward higher performance levels and commitment to the achievement of goals.

Three key steps in implementing a goal setting program include the following:

1. Set goals that are specific and adhere to a deadline.
2. Promote goal commitment by providing instructions and support to employees and managers.
3. Support the achievement of goals with appropriate feedback as soon as possible.

Objectives. The ability to write clear and concise objectives is an important aspect of nursing administration. Characteristics of well-written objectives include the following:

1. The objective statement is properly constructed.
   - It begins with the word "to" followed by an action verb.
   - It specifies a single result to be achieved.
   - It specifies a target date for its attainment.
2. The objective is measurable.
3. The objective can be easily understood by those required to achieve its attainment.
4. The objective conforms to the following criteria: achievable, attainable, measurable, outcome oriented, and specific.

Phase 3: Identification of strategies

The third phase of the strategic planning process involves identifying major issues, establishing goals, and developing strategies to meet the goals. Strategy "determines how the organization will go about attaining their vision. Put another way, how should it exploit the external opportunities and internal strengths and counter external threats and internal weaknesses?" (Curtis, 1994, p. 85). All departmental managers are involved in this process and are responsible for preparing a detailed plan of action, which may include the following: development of short- and long-term objectives, formulation of an-nual department objectives, resource allocation, and preparation of the budget.

Phase 4: Implementation

In the fourth phase of the strategic plan, the specific plans for action are implemented in order of priority. This entails open communication with staff in regard to the priorities for the next year and subsequent periods, formulation of revised policies and procedures in regard to the changes, and formulation of area and individual objectives related to the plan. The specific plans to be focused on included market, program, operating plans and budget, and human resource plans.

Phase 5: Evaluation

At set periods the strategic plan is reviewed at all levels to determine if the goals, objectives, and activities are on target. As stated previously, it is important to consider that objectives may change as a result of legislation, budget cutbacks, and change in structure or other environmental factors. Therefore optional activities may need to be adapted to the situation. For example, one agency was informed that there had to be a decrease in the budget of $500,000 in the next 6 months. Although the savings was realized, the staff were involved in the development of creative methods for ensuring the changes necessary occurred. Savings were realized with organizational restructuring, the elimination of nursing supervisors, and changes in medication administration to a unit dose system (Migliore & Gunn, 1995; Kaplan & Norton, 1996; Galpin, 1997; Liedtka, 1997).

Exercise 4-4

You are a staff nurse at a public health department in a small rural town. The director of nursing has assigned you to work on a planning committee. The purpose of the committee is to devise long- and short-term departmental goals.

The population of the town is 25,000, and the chief industry is agriculture. It is estimated that 8000 more people will move there in the next 5 years; a majority will be immigrants from Asia and Mexico.

The health department currently has four full-time baccalaureate nurses, and the state has not approved additional funding for this year.

Considering the concepts of strategic planning you have just read, what would be a specific strategic plan for your department? How will you determine between long-term and short-term plans? What additional information will your committee need to realistically plan for the next 5 months and the next 5 years?

An example of a strategic plan of action for the development of a women's health center is in the appendix at the end of this chapter.

■ MARKETING

Marketing may be defined as the "analysis, planning, implementation, and control of carefully formulated programs designed to bring about voluntary exchanges of values with target markets for the purpose of achieving organizational objectives" (Harvey, 1990, pp. 186-187). Social marketing emphasizes "nontangible products such as ideas, attitudes, and lifestyle changes, as opposed to the more tangible products and services that are the focus of business marketing" (Blair, 1995, p. 528). Social marketing is used in a number of health promotion activities undertaken by nurses. Kotler and Clarke (1987), authorities in marketing for nonprofit agencies, cite a number of benefits for marketing by healthcare providers, including "increased consumer satisfaction, improved resource attraction, and improved organizational efficiency. The underlying assumption is that marketing helps manage the exchange of goods and services in a more efficient manner" (Hoffman, 1997, p. 67). Marketing principles have been used successfully in antismoking campaigns and participation in exercise programs to decrease the risk of cardiovascular disease. "Nurses have been an active force in disseminating information about cancer detection, immunization, safe sexual practice, and occupational safety" (p. 67).

A number of authors have addressed marketing concepts in the literature (Kotler & Clarke, 1987; Kotler & Andreasen, 1991; Arnold & Fisher, 1996; Blattberg & Deighton, 1996; Gallagher, 1996; Pitt, Berthon, & Watson, 1996; van Dam & Apeldoorn, 1996; Achrol, 1997; Ho et al, 1997; Hoffman, 1997; Kotler et al, 1997; Menon & Menon, 1997; Teas & Palan, 1997; Vitell & Ho, 1997; Woodruff, 1997).

An example of a needs assessment as a marketing strategy for a community health nursing organization is presented in the research box.

In this section, the marketing process will be reviewed.

Strategic Marketing Planning Process

The strategic marketing planning process is similar in nature to the strategic planning process and the nursing process. A comparative chart outlining the steps in the process is in Figure 4-2, p. 65.

Research Perspective

Colangelo, R., & Goldrick, B. (1991). Needs assessment as a marketing strategy: An experience for baccalaureate nursing students. Journal of Nursing Education, 30(4), 168-170.

Sample, Setting
The objective of the project was to conduct a needs assessment using the concepts of marketing and to identify health needs of a community.

Sample Size
N = 200 over the age of 20 years.

Methodology
A community needs assessment questionnaire was developed using focus groups to brainstorm ideas. A demographic data sheet was used to assess age, marital status, educational level, number of dependent children, and town of residence.

Findings
One hundred forty-nine questionnaires were completed. A total of 41% of the respondents were not familiar with the agency and the services provided. Of those who responded to the survey, the services used were health screening and counseling, transportation to medical appointments, health education, Meals-on-Wheels, ill child day care for working parents, and adult day care.

Implications for Practice
A marketing orientation holds that the main tasks of community health nurses are to determine the needs of the community and to provide services with regard to the design of programs, pricing, and provision of competitively viable products and services. Practitioners and students must develop a knowledge base in planning and marketing and must strive to access opportunities for community involvement at various levels.

Kotler and Andreasen (1991) outline the steps in the strategic marketing planning process:

- Analyze the organization-wide mission, objectives, goals, and culture to which the marketing strategy must contribute.
- Assess organizational strengths and weaknesses to respond to threats and challenges presented by the external environment.
- Analyze the future environment the marketer is likely to face with respect to public served, competition, and the social, political, technological, and economic environment.
- Determine the marketing mission, objectives, and specific goals for the relevant planning period.
- Formulate the core marketing strategy to achieve the specified goals.
- Put in place the necessary organizational structure and the systems within the marketing function to ensure proper implementation of the designed strategy.
- Establish detailed programs and tactics to carry out the core strategy for the planning period, including a timetable of activities and the assignment of specific responsibilities.
- Establish benchmarks to measure interim and final achievements of the program.
- Implement the planned program.
- Measure performance and adjust the core strategy, tactical details, or both as needed (pp. 69-70).

Assessment

Determining organization-level missions, objectives, and goals
A marketing plan is developed by the top-level managers and advisory board to:

1. Determine the organization-level long-term culture, mission, objectives, and goals.
2. Assess the organization's likely future external environment.
3. Assess the organization's present and potential strengths and weaknesses (p. 70).

Analyzing organizational strengths and weakness
In the marketing process an environmental assessment is conducted to identify and research assessment of the target market. An example of this is con-

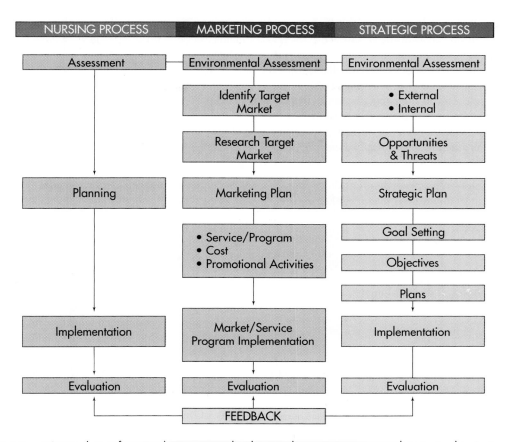

NURSING PROCESS	MARKETING PROCESS	STRATEGIC PROCESS
Assessment	Environmental Assessment	Environmental Assessment
	Identify Target Market	• External • Internal
	Research Target Market	Opportunities & Threats
Planning	Marketing Plan	Strategic Plan
	• Service/Program • Cost • Promotional Activities	Goal Setting
		Objectives
		Plans
Implementation	Market/Service Program Implementation	Implementation
Evaluation	Evaluation	Evaluation
	FEEDBACK	

Fig. 4-2 *Marketing framework as compared with using the nursing process and strategic planning.*

ducting a needs assessment of the services presently provided by an agency to develop new services or promotional activities to meet the needs of the population being served.

Kotler and Andreasen (1991) state that the:

. . . marketing audit is a comprehensive, systematic, independent and periodic examination of an organization's marketing environment, objectives, strategies, and activities with a view of determining problem areas and opportunities and recommending a plan of action to improve the organization's strategic marketing performance (p. 80).

An audit may consist of interviews with key staff, review of documents, observation of staff, visits to other competitors, and overview of advertisements, brochures, and other documents as deemed appropriate.

Analyzing External Threats and Opportunities

A marketer operates in an "external environment that is constantly changing" (Kotler & Andreasen,

1991, p. 88). The three components of the external environment are (1) the public environment, which consists of groups and organizations that have an impact on the organization (i.e., public, media, regulatory agencies); (2) the competitive environment, which consists of other organizations that vie for the attention and loyalty of clientele; and (3) the macroenvironment, consisting of demographic, economic, technological, political, and social forces to which the organization must adapt.

Setting marketing mission, objectives, and goals

Kotler & Andreasen (1991) compare the essence of the development of mission, objectives, and goals to financial management. If one is managing an investment portfolio, then one must decide whether to sell stocks or change from stocks to real estate. The same holds true for the marketing manager who "is constantly evaluating the portfolio against changing market conditions and changing performances of individual units" (p. 109).

Planning

The environmental assessment is followed by the development of a marketing plan. This plan outlines the service/program to be provided, a detailed budget-cost analysis, and the promotional activities designed to promote the program. Predicting the "future" is difficult in turbulent times. Forecasting allows the manager to plan for future and anticipated problems (Urban, Weinberg, & Hauser, 1996). The process incorporates:

- Assessment of the present situation
- Identification of strengths and weaknesses
- Outline of the driving forces in the environment
- Development of optional scenarios
- Identification of the preferred action
- Development of a plan of action
- Implementation of the plan of action
- Evaluation

Morrison & Metcalfe (1996), in their article titled, "Is Forecasting a Waste of Time?", state:

Concern over the usefulness of . . . forecasts can usually be traced back to a concern over being called to task over their accuracy. While a more co-operative style of management might be hoped for, this `target shooting' image of forecasting is still common. . . .

Forecasts should be estimates of how accurately a situation can be forecast, provide alternative futures, be considered more for their impact in convincing managers of the need for change, be a learning experience, be cost effective, and be used for their ritualistic purpose. Rather than using the `shooting at a target' metaphor, it may be more appropriate to consider forecasters as being like art teachers, helping line [and clinical managers] to paint updated pictures of their future (p. 33).

Implementation

The implementation phase includes establishment of the program and promotional activities designed to communicate benefits of the service/program to patients. Forms of promotion may include media releases, brochures, pamphlets, newsletters, and "word-of-mouth" advertising.

Evaluation

The evaluation may incorporate satisfaction surveys, interviews with clients, and further research studies designed to assess reasons why clients are using or not using the service/program or product. Feedback is an essential component of the marketing process.

The following example presents steps in the strategic marketing planning process in relation to the delivery of breast cancer screening services to women in a widespread rural area of Ontario, Canada.

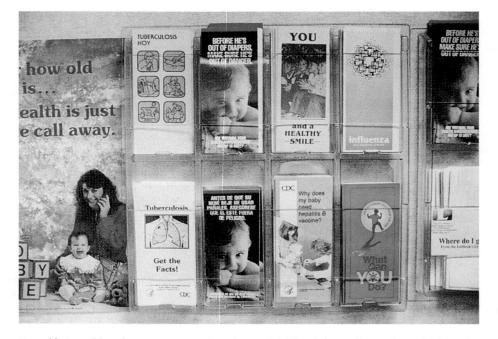

Pamphlets and brochures are promotional materials that inform clients about the benefits of a healthcare agency's programs and services.

A Manager's Solution

[?] The committee recommended implementation of an "all RN skill mix." Strategies were developed to present this recommendation to senior management, the Board of Directors, unions, and other stakeholders. Furthermore, the change to all RN staff needed to be cost- and quality-effective. The necessary approvals and support were granted by the Board and senior management. Over 50 registered practical nurses were laid off. The notion of an all-RN staff being cost and quality-effective is being challenged from time to time. To reevaluate the relevance of this policy, the following is examined: (1) type of patient we care for; (2) current scientific literature; (3) regulatory issues; (4) organizational and economic benefits; and (5) cost and clinical effectiveness of various nursing skill mix models. The most recent review in 1997 concluded that more than ever an "all-RN staff" is the preferred skill mix for our patients in providing high-quality care in a cost-effective and efficient manner.

Judith Shamian

[?] *Would this be a suitable approach for you? Why?*

CHAPTER CHECKLIST

Strategic planning is critical to the effectiveness of any organization. Nurse leader managers must be aware of the critical elements to facilitate the process. Setting goals and defining marketing strategies for product lines are part of the role professional nurses must perform to achieve effective organizational results in creating a niche in healthcare services.

■ The planning process leads to success in the achievement of goals and objectives, gives meaning to work life, and provides direction for the organizational activities of the organization.
■ Strategic planning is similar in nature to the nursing process and involves:
  • assessment of the environment (internal and external)
  • appraisal of the organization's strengths and weaknesses
  • identification of the major opportunities and threats

  • development of strategies to meet these opportunities
  • implementation and evaluation of the strategy
■ Marketing strategies will play a vital role in healthcare settings in the year 2000 as competition increases to provide services and programs to the public. Steps in the strategic marketing planning process are:
  • assessment
  • planning
  • implementation
  • evaluation
■ Nurses can play a pivotal role in the development of visionary programs and services that meet the needs of the population.

TERMS TO KNOW

marketing   strategic planning

TIPS FOR PLANNING, SETTING GOALS, AND MARKETING

■ Be clear about the organization's mission and vision.
■ Read and listen to wide sources of data to determine what is happening and what trends could affect you and your organization.
■ Be clear about your role in the organization and its success.
■ Think about what messages others need to hear about you and your services.

REFERENCES

Achrol, R. (1997). Changes in the theory of interorganizational relations in marketing: Toward a network paradigm. *Journal of the Academy of Marketing Science*, 25(1), 56-71.

Andrews, M. (1990). Strategic planning: Preparing for the 21st century. *Journal of Professional Nursing*, 6(2), 103-112.

Arnold, M., & Fisher, J. (1996). Counterculture, criticisms, and crisis: Assessing the effects of the sixties on marketing thought. *Journal of Macromarketing*, 16(1), 118-133.

Blair, J. (1995). Social marketing: Consumer focused health promotion. *AAOHN Journal*, 43(10), 527-531.

Blattberg, R., & Deighton, J. (1996, July). Manage marketing by the customer equity test. *Harvard Business Review*, 74, 136-144.

Colangelo, R., & Godrick, B. (1991). Needs assessment as a marketing strategy: An experience for baccalaureate nursing students. *Journal of Nursing Education*, 30(4), 168-170.

Covey, S. (1990). *The seven habits of highly effective people.* Toronto: Simon & Schuster.

Curtis, K. (1994). *From management goal setting to organizational results: Transforming strategies into action*. Westport, CT: Quorum Books.

Gallagher, S. (1996). Promoting the nurse practitioner by using a marketing approach. *Nurse Practitioner*, 21(3), 30, 36, 37, 40.

Galpin, T. (1997). Making strategy work. *Journal of Business Strategy*, 18(1), 12, 13, 15.

Harvey, J. (1990). Integrating marketing into health care organizations. In J. Dieneman: *Nursing administration: Strategic perspectives and application*. Norwalk, CT: Appleton & Lange.

Ho, F., Vitell, S., Barnes, J., & Desborne, R. (1997). Ethical correlates of role conflict and ambiguity in marketing: The mediating role of cognitive moral development. *Journal of the Academy of Marketing Science*, 25(2), 117-126.

Hoffman, S. (1997). Marketing professional services. *Journal of Professional Nursing*, 13(2), 67.

Kaplan, R., & Norton, D. (1996, January). Using the balanced scorecard as a strategic management system. *Harvard Business Review*, 74, 75-85.

Kotler, P., & Andreasen, A. (1991). *Strategic marketing for nonprofit organizations*. Englewood Cliffs, NJ: Prentice Hall.

Kotler, P., Armstrong, G., Cunningham, P., & Warren, R. (1997). *Principles of marketing*. Scarborough, ON: Prentice Hall.

Kotler, P., & Clarke, R. (1987). *Marketing for health care organizations*. Englewood Cliffs, NJ: Prentice Hall.

Kreitner, R., & Kinicki, A. (1992). *Organizational behaviour*. Boston: Irwin.

Liedtka, J. (1997). Everything I need to know about strategy I learned at the national zoo. *Journal of Business Strategy*, 18(1), 8-11.

Locke, E., Shaw, K., Saari, L., & Lantham, G. (1981). Goal setting and task performance: 1969-1980. *Psychological Bulletin*, 90(1), 125-152.

Look at it this way. (1996). *Hospitals and Health Networks*, 70(14), 66-70, 72, 74, 76.

Menon, A., & Menon, A. (1997). Enviropreneurial marketing strategy: The emergence of coporate environmentalism as market strategy. *Journal of Marketing*, 61, 51-67.

Migliore, R., & Gunn, B. (1995). Strategic planning/management by objectives. *Hospital Topics*, 73(3), 26-32.

Morrison, M., & Metcalfe, M. (1996). Is forecasting a waste of time? *Journal of General Management*, 22(1), 28-34.

Pitt, L., Berthon, P., & Watson, R. (1996). From surfer to buyer on the WWW: What marketing managers might want to know. *Journal of General Management*, 22(1), 1-13.

Teas, R, & Palan, K. (1997). The realms of scientific meaning: Framework for constructing theoretically meaningful nominal definitions of marketing concepts. *Journal of Marketing*, 61, 52-67.

Urban, G., Weinberg, B., & Hauser, J. (1996). Premarket forecasting or really-new products. *Journal of Marketing*, 60, 47-60.

van Dam, Y., & Apeldoorn, P. (1996). Sustainable marketing. *Journal of Macromarketing*, 16(2), 45-56.

Vitell, S., & Ho, F. (1997). Ethical decision making in marketing: A synthesis and evaluation of scales measuring the various components of decision-making in ethical situations. *Journal of Business Ethics*, 16, 699-717.

Wilkinson, R. (1988). Whether your face fits or not . . . it's the results that matter. *Supervision*, 49(12), 6-8.

Woodruff, R. (1997). Customer value: The next source for competitive advantage. *Journal of the Academy of Marketing Science*, 25(2), 139-153.

SUGGESTED READINGS

Bhide, A. (1996). The questions every entrepreneur must answer. *Harvard Business Review*, 74, 120-130.

Brown, C. (1996). The do's and don'ts of writing a winning business proposal. *Black Enterprises*, 6, 114-116, 120, 122.

Bryson, J. (1995). *Strategic planning for public and nonprofit organizations*. San Francisco: Jossey-Bass Publishers.

Burke, R. (1996, March). Virtual shopping: Breakthrough in marketing research. *Harvard Business Review*, 74, 120-131.

Crow, G. (1996). The business of planning your practice: Success is no accident. *Advanced Practice Nursing Quarterly*, 2(1), 55-61.

Finnigan, S. (1996). Getting started in business: From fantasy to reality. *Advanced Practice Nursing Quarterly*, 2(1), 1-8.

Haag, A. (1997). Writing a successful business plan. *AAOH Journal*. 45(1), 25-32.

Hammer, M. (1996). *Beyond reengineering: How the process centered organization is changing our work and our lives*. New York: Harper Collins.

Hendry, C., Arthur, M., & Jones, A. (1995). *Strategy through people*. New York: Routledge.

Hunt, S. (1996). Marketing midwifery education: Findings from a survey. *Midwifery*, 12, 31-36.

Ingstrup, O. (1995). *The strategic revolution in executive development: What does it mean for your organization?* Ottawa: Canadaian Centre for Management Development.

McDermott, W. (1996). Foresight is an illusion. *Long Range Planning*, 29(2), 190-194.

Porter, M. (1996, November). What is strategy? *Harvard Business Review*. 74, 61-78.

Shrivastava, P., Huff, A., & Dutton, J. (1995). *Advances in strategic management*: Part A. Greenwich, CT: Jai Press Inc.

Shrivastava, P., Huff, A., & Dutton, J. (1995). *Advances in strategic management*: Part B. Greenwich, CT: Jai Press Inc.

Treacy, M., & Wiersema, F. (1997). *The discipline of market leaders*. Menlo Park, CA: Addison-Wesley.

Turnini, N. (1995). Business plans: An effective tool for making decisions. *Nursing Leadership Forum*, 1(4), 116-121.

Wichman, W. (1995). Mapping out effective annual business plans. *Bank Marketing*, 27, 48-52.

Appendix

CASE STUDIES: THE STRATEGIC PLAN OF ACTION AND THE STRATEGIC MARKETING PLANNING PROCESS

Case Study 1: Establishing a Women's Health Center

Five nurse practitioners have conducted an assessment of their community and identified that there is a need for a specific health center for women with

Strategic Plan of Action for the Development, Implementation, and Evaluation of a Women's Health Center

OBJECTIVE	ACTIVITIES	RESPONSIBLE COUNCIL	TIME FRAME
1. To develop a women's health center in a remote rural community	1.1 To conduct a needs assessment	Nurse practitioners	January 1999
	1.2 To conduct a literature review related to each of these topics • Women's health • Entrepreneurship • Programs related to women's health	Nurse practitioners and students	January 1999
	1.3 To form an advisory committee comprising community representatives to oversee the development and implementation of the center	Nurse practitioners	February 1999
	1.4 To develop the organizational structure, mission statement, philosophy, and objectives and revise accordingly	Nurse practitioners and advisory committee	February-April 1999
	1.5 To develop policy and procedure manuals for staff	Nurse practitioners	Ongoing
	1.6 To determine the business structure of the organization (i.e., legalities regarding partnerships, corporations, and proprietorship)	Nurse practitioners	Ongoing
	1.7 To develop a budget		January 1999-ongoing
	1.8 To develop a business site for the organization • All renovations • Office equipment • Supplies • Special healthcare equipment • Filing and billing systems	Consultants and nurse practitioners	February 1999
	1.9 To develop a marketing program (newspapers, telephone, radio messages, signs, and direct mailings)	Nurse practitioners	February 1999-ongoing
2. To implement and evaluate the effectiveness and efficiency of these programs	2.1 To develop patient questionnaires related to satisfaction regarding care provided	Nurse practitioners	March 1999-ongoing
	2.2 To develop cost-effective analysis studies to evaluate each of the programs being provided	Nurse practitioners	Ongoing
	2.3 To collect and collate data related to utilization of services by clientele	Nurse practitioners	Ongoing

a target of elderly, immigrant, and minority women; adolescents; aboriginal, disabled, isolated, and rural women; economically disadvantaged women; and women in mid-life. The particular issues to be addressed are mental health (stress and substance abuse), violence against women (including rape, incest, and wife abuse), reproductive health issues, occupational and environmental issues, nutrition and fitness, and chronic medical conditions.

Goal
The overall goal of this project is to enhance the health of women via health promotion and counseling in a remote rural community.

Objectives
- To provide comprehensive, holistic programs for women that address their specific needs
- To enable women an opportunity to make informed decisions about their healthcare
- To allow women to increase control over factors that affect their health and level of "wellness"

Action Plan
The first phase of the project would entail the development of an advisory committee comprising members of various community agencies directed toward assisting women, i.e., Multicultural Association, Aboriginal Services, Social Planning Council, Medical Association, Health Unit, Health Council, Council for Positive Aging, and consumers.

Focus groups in the community would be offered the opportunity to meet with the nurse practitioners for the purpose of providing information on program needs. The development of specific services to be offered would be finalized in this phase. A preliminary draft of services to be provided includes family planning, sexually transmitted diseases/AIDS, birthing/maternity care that is culturally sensitive, premenstrual syndrome, menopause, obesity/eating disorder programs, stress management programs, and counseling services. It is anticipated that the clinic would also serve as a resource center and provide a wide range of health promotional materials (books, journals, pamphlets, and videos) on the above-mentioned topics. Phase II would consist of renovations to a building site that was donated. Equipment and resources would be purchased at this time.

Hiring and development of staff would begin in Phase 3.

Case Study 2: Strategic Marketing Planning Process for Delivery of a Breast Screening Program

Breast cancer is the leading cause of morbidity and premature death. More than 4000 women develop breast cancer in the province of Ontario and 1700 die annually (it is estimated that one in eight women are affected). The incidence of breast cancer is increasing with the subsequent increase in the age and size of the population. If prevention of this disease is not realized, the number of deaths will continue to rise.

In 1989 the Ministry announced that $15 million would be dedicated to the Ontario Breast Screening Program.

It is important to note that Northwestern Ontario encompasses a vast area of land, the land is rugged, and during the winter months some areas may only be reached by icy roads. The multicultural community with a large native population has approximately 21,000 women aged 50 to 69 years.

The overall purpose of the program was to deliver high-quality comprehensive and coordinated services to the women aged 50 to 69 years in Northwestern Ontario. The mission statement, overall goal, and objectives for the program are in Box 4-1.

Application of Strategic Marketing Planning Process for Delivery of a Breast Cancer Screening Program

Step 1: Situational Assessment
One of the first activities was to establish an advisory committee comprising representatives from the medical community, oncologists, nurses, radiologists, and community agencies (Council on Positive Aging, Canadian Cancer Society, District Health Council, Multi-Cultural Centre, District Health Units, Native Community, and other agencies) to oversee the assessment, development, implementation, and evaluation of the program.

As this was a new program, the external resources in the community were evaluated. Thunder Bay, a regional center, has four mammogram machines, and two mammogram machines were located in other cities; however, travel time to access these facilities was as long as 10 to 12 hours. A proposal was written for funding purposes outlining the overall goal of the program, objectives, background information related to the area and other programs available, and a potential description of the proposed breast cancer screening program.

The most appropriate mode of delivery for this program would be via a mobile van that contained a reception area, an examination room, and the mammography machine. In requesting the mobile van, it was important to the committee that the van be designed so as to withstand extreme cold weather and that the mammogram machine be portable enough to be transported by plane if necessary so as to reach remote northern communities.

The difficulty in obtaining funding for this type of operation was incredible. Lobbying efforts on behalf of the committee ensued. The minister of this region was invited to a meeting of the advisory committee, and the need was apparent, since the van (costing approximately $350,000) and the mammogram machine (costing $150,000) were funded.

Step 2: Marketing Plan

The overall goal of the program was to integrate health promotion strategies and medical practice in order to reduce mortality from breast cancer by 40% using breast cancer screening of women aged 50 to 69 years. The advisory committee developed a strategic plan of action for development, implementation, and evaluation of the project, including specific timelines for hiring a medical coordinator, administrative coordinator, health promotion officer, and staff (registered nurses to conduct breast examination, technicians, and support staff). Costs for each activity were clearly delineated. In addition, a detailed promotional campaign was designed.

Step 3: Implementation

A health promotion coordinator was hired to relate the activities of the program, initiate media coverage, develop pamphlets (a number of the pamphlets have been translated to Ojibwa, Oji-Cree, and other languages), and promote groups in the area to use the service.

The health promotion coordinator organized a promotional campaign in each community, prior to

---

Box 4-1

Mission Statement, Goals, and Objectives of the Northwestern Ontario Breast Cancer Screening Program

Mission Statement

To reduce the leading cause of cancer deaths in women by delivering a comprehensive, organized, and evaluated breast cancer screening program for women between ages 50 and 69 years. In accordance with Ontario's health goals, the Cancer Care Ontario is committed to deliver a program that is sensitive to women's needs, building on health-promoting behaviors, and fostering partnerships with interest groups in the community.

Overall Goal

To integrate health promotion strategies and medical practice so as to reduce mortality from breast cancer by 40% using breast screening of women aged 50 to 69 years.

Objectives

- To detect breast cancer earlier than would occur if organized screening was not available
- To develop and implement a community mobilization plan for the program
- To develop and implement a social marketing plan, including a health education component for the program

- To establish protocols and standards for healthcare professionals associated with the program
- To establish protocols for the interaction of the target population with the program
- To develop and implement training and technical assistance for those associated with the delivery of the program
- To develop a partnership with healthcare professionals that will facilitate program delivery
- To establish a regional breast screening service so that all women in the target population have equal access to breast screening
- To ensure that a minimum of 70% of women in the target population participate in screening every 2 years
- To document the follow-up of all women in whom an abnormality has been detected
- To provide screening that is sensitive and acceptable to the target population
- To evaluate the program on a continual basis, including needs assessment and measurement of process, economic, and outcome variables

the van visiting a certain area. Flyers, brochures, and newsletters about the service were delivered to each household by volunteers. Posters were on exhibit in each of the community agencies. Staff visited each of the communities to promote the service and answer any questions posed by health professionals and members of the community.

A grand opening of the program was held in the community auditorium in Thunder Bay, and there was extensive media coverage throughout Northwestern Ontario. The benefits of the program were outlined to the women in the area.

The response to the program was overwhelming. To date, the program has been so successful that the region has been targeted as a diagnostic center.

Step 4: Evaluation

Each year the medical director, the administrative co-ordinator, and the health promotion coordinator prepare a business plan, which is presented to the advisory committee for review. The plan is reviewed every 3 months. Research will be conducted in the near future to assess why recruitment in certain areas is under 70%. A research project has been completed to assess the "Knowledge, Attitudes, Beliefs & Practices Regarding Breast Screening and Cervical Cancer Screening in Selected Ethno-Cultural Groups in Northwestern Ontario." Cultural, socioeconomic, and physician gender differences were evident in breast self-examination, mammograms, and cervical screening practices. For example, a number of the aboriginal women interviewed stated that "they would not see a male physician and hesitated having a Pap smear or their breast examined because these were their 'private' parts."

Exercise 4-5

Select a clinical agency where you have affiliated. Recall what their "special" services/products are. Recall who their target populations are. Make a summary statement of your recollections. Now go to that organization and peruse the literature in the lobby. Does the literature reaffirm your statements? What is different? After you have read the literature, determine what the mission is, how the organization has positioned itself in the community, and how the mission and targets have impact on nursing.

In summary, the success of this program depended on the "vision," commitment to high-quality service, consumer orientation, marketing, and dedication of advisory committee members, the community, the public, and the staff of the breast cancer screening program.

▌ REFERENCES

Abelsohn, J. (1996). Nursing is their business. *Registered Nurse Journal*, 9-11.

Blouin, A., & Brent, N. (1995). The nurse entrepreneur: Legal aspects of owning a business. *Journal of Nursing Administration*, 25(6), 13-14.

Brokaw, L. (1996). The business plan: Dream vs. reality. *Executive Female*, 19, 60-71.

Croft, A. (1994). Entrepreneurship: The realities of today. *Journal of Nurse Midwifery*, 39(1), 39-42.

Elkins, L. (1996). Tips for preparing a business plan. *Nation's Business*, 84,60R-61R.

Fulscher, R. (1996). A no-fail recipe: Winning business proposals. *Journal of Property Management*, 61, 62-66.

Hau, M. (1997). Ten common mistakes to avoid as an independent consultant. *AAOHN Journal*, 45(1), 17-24.

Jabez, A. (1996). Partners in care. *Nursing Standard*, 10(4), 25-27.

Kets de Vries, M. (1996). The anatomy of an entrepreneur: Clinical observations. *Human Relations*, 49(7), 853-883.

Lambert, V., & Lambert, C. (1996). Advanced practice nurses: Starting an independent practice. *Nursing Forum*, 31(1), 11-21.

Marselle, R. (1997). *The nurse entrepreneur: A literature review.* Unpublished paper, Nursing Leadership, N4350, Lakehead University, Thunder Bay, ON.

Paine, L. (1994). Managing for organizational integrity. *Harvard Business Review*, 72, 106-117.

Patterson, S. (1994). Becoming an entrepreneur. *Canadian Nurse*, 90(2), 53-54.

Shea, C. (1996). Entrepreneur for our times: An interview with Karen Zander. *Journal of American Psychiatric Nurses Association*, 2(1), 23-30.

Stevens, M. (1995). Seven steps to a well prepared business plan. *Executive Female*, 18, 30-31.

The self employed nurse, (1994). (On-line; available: http://www.mabc.ca.122.htm.)

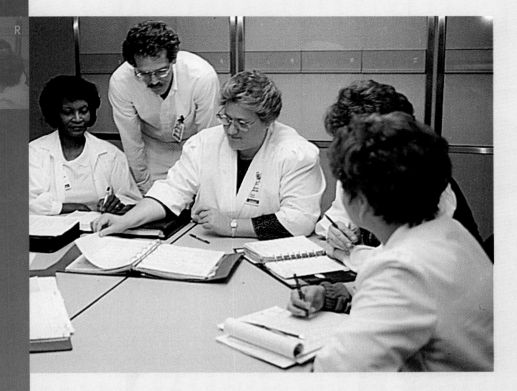

Leading Change

Kristi D. Menix
RN, EdD, CNAA

This chapter describes the general nature of change and innovation and the processes, responses, principles, and strategies typically involved in creating and leading change in healthcare organizations. The manager's role of **change leader** and **innovator** entails anticipating and creating change that involves managing its dynamics. The need for the change leader to create and facilitate change, not just react to imposed change, and to ensure staff empowerment in order to achieve change outcomes is emphasized throughout. The terms *leader* and *manager* are used interchangeably to mean the nurse responsible and accountable for achieving a defined set of work outcomes through the efforts of an employee group for a 24-hour period. The terms **change** and **innovation** are also used synonymously to refer to an alteration in the work environment that is new or different from what existed previously.

Objectives

- Analyze the general characteristics of change in open systems organizations.
- Relate the models of planned change to the process of low-level change.
- Relate chaos, cybernetics, and learning organization theories to high-level change.
- Evaluate select strategies to common responses to change.
- Relate the desirable qualities of effective change leaders.

Questions to Consider

- What is your view of change? What is your usual response to unexpected change? What is your usual response to deliberate, planned change? What is your response to ambiguity?
- Do you actively seek involvement to achieve improved practice and management outcomes?
- What kinds of activities and behaviors do you possess that could be applied to promote change through staff participation?
- What strategies do you use to support continuous learning by staff?

A Manager's Challenge

From a City Health Department Manager in the Southwest

Change in the mission of the City Health Department resulted from pressures exerted by the City Council and City Management in response to changes in the healthcare environment and public policies. The department had to reduce its multiple clinical services, case management, dental care, and services for women and children to two clinics that provided immunization and sexually transmitted disease services. Generally, passive surveillance had to become very active. Administration needed to focus heavily on the core functions of public health—assessment, policy development, and quality assurance. Thus this change became an internal issue that affected every person and every system. How to help everyone see things through the eyes of the city council in a nonthreatening way challenged my many years of management experience. The large staff had been managed by multiple supervisory layers. Many staff feared losing their positions or doing jobs not anticipated. Some left before personnel decisions were made. Other who stayed became uncooperative, saying, "It's not my job." Gossip fueled the already uncertain future of the department. How could I produce the required results?

What do you think you would do if you were this manager?

▌ INTRODUCTION

Change is a natural social process of individuals, groups, organizations, and society. The forces of change originate inside and outside healthcare organizations. Change today is constant, inevitable, pervasive, and unpredictable, and varies in rate and intensity, which unavoidably influences individuals, technology, and systems at all levels of the organization.

Because most healthcare organizations operate as open systems, they are receptive to external environmental influences originating from a rapidly changing healthcare delivery system. Organization-wide change depends on the organization's stage of development, degree of flexibility, and history of response to change, as well as the maturity of its systems. The role of leaders/managers is to lead change efforts using thinking that is systems- and theory-based, tolerant of ambiguity, and mindful of the whole picture. Thus the management of change in organizations is moving from less emphasis on long-range planning approaches to a greater focus on managing the forces, such as information and relationships, in the change situation to achieve outcomes. **Change management** refers to the overall processes and strategies used to moderate and manage the preparation for, impact of, responses to, and outcomes for conditions new and different than what existed previously.

CONTEXT OF THE CHANGE ENVIRONMENT

The transformation of healthcare delivery is occurring rapidly, creating contextual alteration in **change situations,** such as the factors of time, information, decision making, and planning (Begun & White, 1995; Porter-O'Grady, 1997). The use of **planned change** approaches for high-level, or highly complex, accelerated, unpredictable change situations may not be as effective as they are for low-level, low-complexity change in more stable environments (Nutt, 1992). Nursing entities, as open systems, need to begin viewing their work in less bureaucratic, inflexible ways and open themselves up to responding with flexibility and creativity to today's dynamic environment (Begun & White, 1995).

Nursing is a key component of healthcare delivery, a partner with multiple care providers, and a pivotal player in open systems organizations. "In order for the nursing profession to strategically adapt in a rapidly changing environment, it is important to consider its current 'dominant logic' as a source of structural inertia. A system's dominant logic is a screen that filters information deemed relevant by historical antecedents and by those analyzing the data" (Begun & White, 1995, p. 5). Using chaos theory components, Begun and White (1995) suggest that nursing in various areas is too stable, thus too unresponsive and unable to adapt to the influences of rapid change. They believe that nursing must change its entrenched, inflexible thinking and acting typical of bureaucratic

structures. Box 5-1 shows guidelines for altering the dominant logic. For example, because of environmental uncertainty and the need to be responsive, the nursing leader should envision several outcome scenarios to move toward (rather than have limited, rigid goals) within the context of the possibilities of changing circumstances (J.W. Begun, personal communication, July 8, 1997).

Planned change models, or linear approaches, can provide the elements for directional, more incremental, low-level, low-complexity change, such as reorganizing the storage of unit supplies or getting a task force to recommend inservice offerings for unit clerks. High-level change, on the other hand, is characteristically more fluid and complex because of the number of and interaction among multiple players and influences. Change leaders must manage the forces of the change situation while considering several desired outcomes, which can lead to more creative results (Wheatley, 1992; Begun & White, 1995). Nonlinear approaches are found in complexity/chaos, cybernetic, and learning organization theories. They offer helpful approaches for understanding dynamic, open-system healthcare organizations and for guiding change leaders in managing these accelerated, less certain change environments (Menix, 1997).

PLANNED CHANGE USING LINEAR APPROACHES

Most planned change models advocate that change can occur in a sequential and directional fashion when guided by effective change leaders. Planned

---

Box 5-1
Guidelines for Altering the Dominant Logic

DECREASE	INCREASE
Long-term forecasting	Short-term forecasting
Pre-planned strategies	Emergent strategies
Emphasis on past successes	Search for new opportunities
One future vision	Multiple scenarios
Rigid, permanent structures	Self-organizing, temporary structures
Structural isolation in the work place	Structural interdependence in the work place
Stability of leadership	Leadership turnover
Standardization	Innovation, experimentation, diversity
Insulation from other professions and marketplace	Cooperation and competition
Marketplace "passivity"	Marketplace "aggression"
Expectation of job security	Self-learning

From Begun & White (1995). P. 10.

change models, such as those of Lewin (1947), Lippit, Watson, & Westley (1958), and Havelock (1973), explain the nature of change processes as well as offer systematic problem-solving methods designed to achieve change. Rogers' (1995) innovation-decision model highlights individual change. Planned change can be useful for low-level change in more stable, less changing environments; however, flexibility in implementing the plan and moderating the factors, as is advocated by nonlinear approaches, can improve the overall outcomes.

Lewin (1947) suggested that an analysis of change situations (force field analysis) includes identifying **barriers** (elements that hinder) and **facilitators** (elements that support). These elements may be people, technology, structure, or values. For change to be effective, facilitators must exceed barriers.

He (1947) describes change as having three stages: *unfreezing, experiencing the change,* and *refreezing.* "Unfreezing" refers to the awareness of an opportunity, need, or problem for which some action is necessary. This phase may occur naturally as a progressive development or it may result from a deliberate activity as a first step in planning a change. When the current way of giving report is ineffective and errors occur in delivering care, the staff's awareness brings to light the need for a change. As in the case of the manager interviewed in the "Manager's Challenge," external pressure for a new mission resulted in initial awareness of "unfreezing" by the health department personnel.

Exercise 5-1

Identify facilitators and barriers and rate their potential effect on the attainment of the change in the following situation: Administration wants the pediatric neurology unit to merge with the pediatric cardiac unit for improved cost-effectiveness. Staff nurses and managers from both units reluctantly compose the merger planning committee, along with the appointed chair, the organization's powerful personnel director. Administration says that a new facility will be provided to house the merged units.

"Experiencing" the change or solution leads to incorporation of what is new or different into work and interpersonal processes (Lewin, 1947). Again, deciding to begin to use the change or being thrust into the change can result in potential acceptance of the new way.

"Refreezing" occurs when the participants in the change situation accept and use the new attitude or behavior like a new habit (Lewin, 1947). Acceptance is assumed once most staff integrate the change into work processes. Surveys or other data collection measures conducted at various points after the implementation of a designated change can assess the level of acceptance by the participants of change.

Though Havelock's (1973) six-stage model for planning change had particular application to educational entities (see theory box), it shows similarities in the elements of the directional phases recommended by other planned change models. Two adjuncts to Havelock's model advocate development of the effective **change agent** and use of his model as a rational problem-solving process. The rational problem-solving process is *"how* change agents can organize their work so that successful innovation *will* take place" (p. 3). A change agent is an individual who leads a change process.

Lippitt, Watson, and Westley's (1958) model suggests seven sequential phases to use to plan change (see theory box). Inherent in this model is the change agent's appraisal of the "change and resistance forces which are present in the client system at the beginning of the change process as well as others which may be revealed as the process advances. Being continuously sensitive to the constellation of change forces and resistance forces is one of the most creative parts of the change agent's job" (p. 92).

The innovation-decision process (Rogers, 1995) describes an individual's choosing over time to accept or reject a new idea for use in practice (see theory box for Rogers' model of innovation-decision process). According to Rogers' work, the individual's decision-making actions pass through five sequential stages. The decision to not accept the new idea may occur at any stage. The change agent can, however, facilitate movement by others through these stages by encouraging the use of the idea and providing information about its benefits and disadvantages.

▌ NONLINEAR CHANGE

Chaos Theory

Organizations can no longer rely on rules, policies, and hierarchies to get work accomplished in inflexible ways. Healthcare organizations "cannot control long-term outcomes . . ." (McDaniel, 1996, p. 8) according to chaos theory perspectives because of the rapidly changing nature of human and world factors. Organizations are open systems operating in complex, fast-changing environments. The assertions of **chaos theory** are that "organizations are potentially

Theories for Planned Change

KEY CONTRIBUTORS	KEY IDEA	APPLICATION TO PRACTICE
Six Phases of Planned Change Havelock (1973) is credited with this planned change model.	Change can be planned, implemented, and evaluated in six sequential stages. The model is advocated for development of effective change agents and use as a rational problem-solving process. The six stages* are: 1. Building a relationship 2. Diagnosing the problem 3. Acquiring relevant resources 4. Choosing the solution 5. Gaining acceptance 6. Stabilizing the innovation and generating self-renewal	Useful for low-level, low-complexity change.
Seven Phases of Planned Change Lippitt, Watson & Westley (1958) are credited with this planned change model.	Change can be planned, implemented, and evaluated in seven sequential phases. Ongoing sensitivity to forces in the change process is essential. The seven phases[†] are: 1. The client system becomes aware of the need for change. 2. The relationship is developed between the client system and change agent. 3. The change problem is defined. 4. The change goals are set and options for achievement are explored. 5. The plan for change is implemented. 6. The change is accepted and stabilized. 7. The change entities redefine their relationships.	Useful for low-level, low-complexity change.
Innovation-Decision Process Rogers (1995) is credited with formulating this process.	Change for an individual occurs over five phases when choosing to accept or reject an innovation/idea. Decisions to not accept the new idea may occur at any of the five stages. The change agent can promote acceptance by giving information about benefits and disadvantages and encouragement. The five stages[‡] are: 1. Knowledge 2. Persuasion 3. Decision 4. Implementation 5. Confirmation	Useful for individual change.

*From Havelock (1973).
[†]From Lippitt et al (1958).
[‡]From Rogers (1995).

chaotic" (Thietart & Forgues, 1995, p. 19). Nonhuman induced responses are characterized by random-appearing yet self-organizing patterns. In other words, "order emerges through fluctuation and chaos" (Limerick, Passfield, & Cunningham, 1995, online). Typically, organizations will experience periods of stability interrupted with periods of intense transformation. Though not predictable in the long run, small changes in the internal or external environment can result in significant consequences to organizational work processes and outcomes. Chaos theory further explains that the conditions present in a particular organizational change will not occur again in the same form (Preismeyer, 1992; Limerick, Passfield, & Cunningham, 1995; Thietart & Forgues, 1995).

Wheatley (1992) and CRM Films (1997a, 1997b) proposes that organizations have always been self-organizing systems with the potential for self-renewal, but that humans, employees, and leaders/managers have exercised bureaucratic premises such as control, prediction, and emphasis on structure and elements of the whole, rather than on the relationship of the parts in forming a whole. She commanded leaders to act, think, and lead in terms of nonlinear perspectives, particularly in three major interrelated, interacting domains: information as "currency" or vital "air"; relationships as pathways to building teams and generating new information; and vision as a "field of vision" within which all members of the organization share values and beliefs in the development of organizational direction. Continuous learning by personnel as a matter of organizational philosophy further promotes adaptation to accelerated change.

Learning Organization Theory

Learning organizations are organizations that place emphasis on flexibility and responsiveness (Senge, 1990). Specifically, complex organizations (open systems) that are trying to survive in an unpredictable healthcare environment can best respond and adapt to external and internal forces when members of the organization enact their work with others using a learning approach. Enactment of Senge's "five disciplines" is essential to achieving learning organization status. Disciplines mean the critical and interrelated elements that compose a grouping that can only function effectively when all elements are present, linked, and interacting. For example, without the tires, a car with a working engine and other essential operational features could not be driven as designed. And without the knowledge of the interrelatedness of the car's

operational features, one might not be able to take the right action to use this transportation.

Senge's (1990) five disciplines of learning organizations include systems thinking, personal mastery, mental models, building shared vision, and team learning. He includes *dialogue* as the methodology to promote the individual, group, and organizational learning process. *Systems thinking* refers to the need for the organization to view the world as a set of multiple visible and invisible parts that interact constantly. When the organization values and facilitates development of the deeper aspirations of its members in addition to professional proficiency, it successfully matches organizational learning and personal growth or *personal mastery*. Each individual and each organization bases its activities on a set of assumptions, beliefs, and "pictures" about the way the world should work. When these invisible *mental models* are uncovered and consciously evaluated, it is possible to begin to determine in a "learningful" (p. 9) way their influence on work accomplishment. *Building shared vision* occurs when leaders involve all members in moving personal visions of the future into a consolidated yet ongoing vision common to members and leaders. *Team learning* refers to the need for cohesive groups to learn together in order to benefit from the abilities of each member to enhance the overall outcomes of the team's efforts. Summarily, Senge (1990) views dialogue or ongoing, two-way communication as essential to development of the five disciplines.

Resilience

Resilience and hardiness are qualities also needed by organizations and leader/managers to respond quickly and continuously to a dynamic organization and environment (Deevy, 1995). The characteristics of resilience are "manifested by certain beliefs, behaviors, skills, and areas of knowledge" (Connor, 1993, p. 238). A hardy, resilient person is someone who is flexible, focused, positive, organized, and proactive.

An example of the application of chaos and learning organization theories is a community hospital that has been sensitive to and adapted to environmental influences such as incremental changes in reimbursement policies and accreditation policies. Adaptation involved times of fluctuation, then stability. The advent of managed care induced by major insurance players may not have been predictable, but it has had significant consequences for the financial survival of the community hospital. New reimbursement strategies have forced the community hospital and competitive hospitals in the same community to seek consolidation in order for all to survive. Accelerated change of such magnitude has created change that appears chaotic without order. However, all hospitals are becoming transformed, and some order is present in the middle of perceived general chaos. It is likely that these exact conditions will not occur again for these same hospitals. Hospital administrators and other personnel have assumed a "learning" philosophy to enact multiple changes for adaptation, notably financial survival. Resilience assists in promoting adaptation.

MAJOR CHANGE MANAGEMENT FUNCTIONS

Planning, organizing, implementing, and evaluating are functions by which change can be created to reach a specific **change outcome.** Feedback functions in conjunction with the four management functions as a way to learn the status of the change process.

Planning is simply looking ahead to decide how to achieve some result, goal, or outcome. Envisioning several possible outcome scenarios provides flexibility. Planning is a critical function ideally completed before implementation. Putting plans for change in writing can establish a visual method to communicate ideas, decisions, and responsibilities to a group or an individual staff member, or those who will be affected by the process or by the outcome of the process. A written plan is a tool, if used as such, to communicate the change process.

Assessing the current and desired situation is part of the initial and ongoing planning activity and also provides the data that clarify the conditions and direction of the advancing plan. It is important to carefully assess factors in the change situation that predictably will support or interfere with the progress of a change. This chapter's "Research Perspective" illustrates the use of research methods to identify what nurses believe will facilitate or interfere with their integration into a new hospital setting. Using this force field analysis technique (Lewin, 1947), the change leader, in collaboration with the change participants, tries to reduce the barriers and promote the facilitators throughout the change process.

Organizing entails making decisions about reaching outcomes in terms of time, personnel, materials, communication, or other activities and resources. For reasons of efficiency, it is important to weigh the costs and benefits of options to reach several possible change outcomes. Organizing builds clarity into the plan by formalizing the desired sequence and means of accomplishing the change.

Exercise 5-2

Identify the appropriate step(s) in the management process for each number below. From the perspective of a manager applying these same functions to a change process, consider the manager's responsibility to orient a new staffing coordinator. Ideally, the manager, the new staffing coordinator, and the assistant nurse manager will map out in writing (1) the goals of the orientation, the activities (2) for meeting the

---

Research Perspective

George, V.M., Burke, L.J., & Rodgers, B.L. (1997). *Research-based planning for change.* The Journal of Nursing Administration, *27*(5), 53-61.

The purpose of this descriptive study was assessment of the attitudes and perceptions of licensed nurses transitioning from an acquired hospital by the nursing administration of the acquiring hospital. Identifying existing barriers could then facilitate appropriate change management while merging two nursing staffs from different professional governance models and organizational cultures. Job security emerged as the major advantage of the move. Fears included lack of honesty and respect, unequal treatment, and loss of autonomy. Suggestions made to ensure a successful transition included the desire for the acquiring hospital to involve the staff, be respectful and honest, and conduct the transition gradually.

Implications for Practice

Various research methods, including attitudinal surveys guided by attributional theory, can identify the causes individuals believe to explain why experiences happen to them or others. When individuals perceive themselves to be "cognitively appropriate, their ability to transfer and maintain their behavior in subsequent situations is strengthened" (p. 55). Learning these attributes by exploring attitudes and perceptions helps designers of change to proceed with appropriate change management approaches.

*Compare this same article from a different perspective. Turn to p. 142.

Exercise 5-2—cont'd

goals, and a schedule (3) for accomplishing them. The assistant nurse manager and staffing coordinator agree to meet (4) as needed as well as to meet weekly to review progress (5) and address informational or confidence need (6). Part of this plan includes the option to alter the plan based on unexpected changes (7). The staffing coordinator will begin the position in 2 weeks (8) and put the pre-arranged outline of activities (9) into action (10). The assistant nurse manager's responsibility will be to guide and support (11) the education of the new staffing coordinator. Unexpected occurrences, such as the staff coordinator being absent for a few days, will create the need to modify (12) the goal, activities, or time frame of the orientation plan (dynamic quality of process). New information (feedback) guides the overall process.

Implementing ideally occurs *after* a plan is established. However, unexpected change may sometimes require immediate action. Plans made quickly after the change can facilitate handling the effects of the change. Successful implementation, or putting the plan into action, depends on the appropriateness of the change and the involvement of the change participants. It is important to remember that a change in one part of a system can affect the function in other related systems.

Evaluating entails judging the degree to which the change outcomes are met. Monitoring is the ongoing observation of the aspects of the change process by which problems can be recognized and corrected early. Deciding whether or not an outcome has been fully or partially met occurs in the final stage of the change process.

Effective change leaders gather accurate, comprehensive, timely information continuously about the progress of the **change process.** Access to this feedback is accomplished by establishing communication networks that act as self-regulating monitors of specific types of information, known as cybernetics theory. Analysis of this negative feedback can determine where the course of the accelerated change situation has veered away from its progress toward desired outcomes or if some action is needed to facilitate continued progress (Ashby, 1957; Cadwallader, 1959). Subsequently, this feedback provides change participants with guidance for future actions. Some general feedback mechanisms include computerized data findings, staff meeting discussions, and informal/formal observations. Negative feedback sources reside in the reports of exceptions, such as incident reports, variances in budget expenditures, or new reimbursement policies. Multiple sources of positive feedback produce information to build a picture of success for the change process.

RESPONSES TO CHANGE

Change, whether proactively initiated at the level of change or imposed from external sources, has impact on people, technology, and systems. Effective change leaders anticipate possible responses and apply strategies to deal with them for the best possible change outcomes. Answering the self-assessment questions in Box 5-2 can show how receptive one is to change and innovation.

Human Side of Change

Responses by individuals and groups may vary from full acceptance and willing participation to open rejection of all or part of the change process. Of course, some individuals never accept change. The initial reception to change may be, but is not always, reluctance and resistance. Resistance and reluctance are common when the change threatens personal security. For example, changes in the structure of an agency can result in position changes for personnel. Changing positions from critical care nurse to home health nurse can result in the nurse feeling temporarily incompetent and isolated. Specifically, responses to such changes may be behavioral (Rogers, 1983; Bushy & Kamphuis, 1993), emotional (Perlman & Takacs, 1990), or covert (hidden) or overt (visible) (New & Couillard, 1981).

Rogers' (1983) ideal and common patterns of individuals' behavioral responses to change outline how recognition of these responses can facilitate an effective change process. For example, *innovators* thrive on change, which may be disruptive to the unit stability; *early adopters* are respected by their peers and thus are sought out for advice and information about innovations. Individuals fitting the characteristics of the *early majority* category prefer doing what has been done in the past but eventually will accept new ideas; *late majority* persons are openly negative and will agree to the change only after most others have accepted the change. *Laggards* prefer keeping traditions and openly express their resistance to new ideas; *rejectors*, through their active opposition to change, even sabotage, can interfere with the overall success of a change process. The manager's challenge is to deal with these behavioral patterns of individuals so as to influence and channel their responses into behaviors that will support the change process. Individuals moving through change may also experience an emotional grieving of 10 possible stages resulting from the loss of their former employment situation (Perlman and Takacs, 1990). These 10 phases are equilibrium, denial, anger,

Box 5-2			
Self-Assessment: How Receptive to Change and Innovation Are You?			

Read the following items. Circle the answer that most closely matches your attitude toward creating and accepting new or different ways.

	Yes	Depends	No
1. I enjoy learning about new ideas and approaches.	**Yes**	**Depends**	**No**
2. Once I learn about a new idea or approach, I begin to try it right away.	**Yes**	**Depends**	**No**
3. I like to discuss different ways of accomplishing a goal or end result.	**Yes**	**Depends**	**No**
4. I continually seek better ways to improve what I do.	**Yes**	**Depends**	**No**
5. I frequently recognize improved ways of doing things.	**Yes**	**Depends**	**No**
6. I talk over my ideas for change with my peers.	**Yes**	**Depends**	**No**
7. I communicate my ideas for change with my manager.	**Yes**	**Depends**	**No**
8. I discuss my ideas for change with my family.	**Yes**	**Depends**	**No**
9. I volunteer to be at meetings when changes are being discussed.	**Yes**	**Depends**	**No**
10. I encourage others to try new ideas and approaches.	**Yes**	**Depends**	**No**

If you answered "yes" to 8 to 10 of the items, you are probably receptive to creating and experiencing new and different ways of doing things. If you answered "depends" to 5 to 10 of the items, you are probably receptive to change conditionally based on the fit of the change with your preferred ways of doing things. If you answered "no" to 4 to 10 of the items, you are probably not receptive, at least initially, to new ways of doing things. If you answered "yes," "no," and "depends" an approximately equal number of times, you are probably mixed in your receptivity to change based on individual situations.

bargaining, chaos, depression, resignation, openness, readiness, and re-emergence. Each phase is characterized by varying energy levels, attitudes, and willingness to engage in new change activities. Making the transition from the former work situation to a new situation brought about by change can progress due to the passage of time, empathetic listening by others, and understanding the reasons for the change (Muller-Smith, 1993). The nurse manager's challenge is to be sensitive to an employee's stage of loss and transition by responding with appropriate interventions, such as active listening, informing, and problem solving.

Responses may be hidden (covert) or visible (overt) to the observer (Bushy & Kamphuis, 1993). Some nurses may verbalize their dissatisfactions; others may quietly accommodate the change.

Systems and Technology Side of Change

Organizational systems and technology can both influence and be influenced by change. System responses to change may emerge in work processes as evidenced by signs of more or less efficiency or effectiveness. Changes in the type of personnel or tech-

nology used to deliver care and different from what was done before may lead to an initial response of confusion, then to a period of adaptation by the personnel and other systems. The quality of care may change as well as the morale of personnel. Productivity and safety outcomes may be different. Correction of the breakdowns in the affected work processes can restore efficient and effective functioning.

Summarily, the human side of managing change refers to personnel responses to change that either facilitate or interfere with change processes. The systems and technological side of managing change refers to reactions that influence the efficiency and effectiveness of work processes and outcomes. The change leader's challenge is to monitor, recognize, and apply appropriate strategies to minimize responses that are destructive and maximize those that support the dynamics of an ongoing change.

STRATEGIES

The change leader uses various strategies to facilitate both planned and nonlinear change processes. **Strategies** are approaches designed to achieve a particular purpose based on consideration of the character of these responses. Strategies such as education and communication, participation and involvement, facilitation and support, negotiation and agreement, and manipulation, co-optation, and coercion can be used individually or in combination with each other (Kotter & Schlesinger, 1979). As supported by learning organization theory, the change leader uses vision development, relationship building, and information management strategies as needed. The intent of the change leader and those supporting the change is to promote the continued movement toward acceptable change and outcomes, and decrease and eliminate, if possible, any harmful resistance to the change. The key to using the various strategies effectively is to learn to match the appropriate strategies with the demonstrated behavior as it relates to the circumstances of the change situation.

Communication and education refer to interchanges among the change leader, the change participants, and others for the purpose of integrating the elements of the change process. They involve interacting in various ways. Staff meetings and informal discussions are ways to keep people informed and clarify change activities. Active and empathetic listening is essential. Early explanation and education, especially of informal leaders, can facilitate change.

It is critical to involve the individuals who will be most affected by the change. Empowerment through participation and involvement promotes ownership of both the process and the decisions made during the process. In the "Manager's Solution" (p. 86), the nurse manager cited this strategy to be the most effective way to garner support and acceptance for a change.

Facilitation and support strategies are typically used to reassure and assist those in the change situation who do not accept a change because of anxiety and fear. When personal security is threatened or when loss and grief are experienced, people tend to want to keep on doing what they have always done. A staff member with financial problems may believe that a new benefit plan will leave less take-home pay. The change leader can reassure that person by providing the actual calculation to show the fear is unfounded.

Individuals or groups in the change situation may have the power or resources to adversely affect the success of a particular change. Negotiation and agreement strategies can revise these terms of the change to accommodate the involved parties.

Co-optation usually entails manipulated involvement through an appointed or assigned role. An example of this strategy is appointing a highly resistant individual to a change task force that necessitates more active involvement in the change process. Manipulation appeals to the motivational needs of others and influences them to participate in change when they might not do so on their own initiative. Expecting staff to be cooperative by participating in a pilot project of the proposed change on a 3-month basis can reduce barriers of resistance.

Coercion involves the use of power to force others to make a change, particularly when time is critical to implementation. An example would be offering to retain a staff member's position during staff reductions if that individual accepts certain conditions could be viewed as coercion.

Creating a vision (different from an imposed organization mission) shared by all the change participants or change teams (Senge, 1990) involves dialogue to continually redefine the future, whether it be for the organization or for a project. Development of a set of possible outcomes rather than rigid pursuit of one outcome opens the possibilities to respond to unpredictable environmental influences (Begun & White, 1995). Change leaders build work environments that support the time needed as well as accept varied beliefs and their given meanings (Senge, 1990; Wheatley, 1992).

Information management by the change leader focuses on delivery of the right information to the right place at the right time. Sound assessment of environmental influences and decision making depend on accurate and current information (Wheatley, 1992).

Understanding how individual capabilities and potential can facilitate creative solutions to projected organizational outcomes is essential to change management. Formal position titles become irrelevant. Matching specific individuals with the demands of an appropriate project, for example, can lead to more creative sharing, thinking, and creating. Peers can become coaches and teachers for each other.

The responses of employees influence change processes in both positive and negative ways. Wheeler (1995) discussed the need for organizations to facilitate employees' timely transition from what is familiar to what is unknown. She recommended three managerial strategies to promote healthy responses to change: (1) encourage development of the future in specific terms; (2) engage in more face-to-face interaction and other methods that connect personnel, managers, and all facets of the organization; and (3) insist on participation in change at all levels from the beginning.

Finally, McDaniel (1996) advocates that change leaders in healthcare organizations meet the challenges of managing change by applying 12 recommendations: (1) dispense with controlling and planning; (2) operate on the margin between order and disorder; (3) develop new organizations with the help of everyone; (4) allow individual autonomy; (5) encourage information sharing among staff; (6) promote staff's knowledge of others' work; (7) stimulate open learning through discussions generating "creative tension" (p. 22); (8) consider the organization's structure as dynamic; (9) help staff discover their goals; (10) encourage cooperation, not competition; (11) approach work from a smarter view, not harder; and (12) uncover values continuously to form organization-wide visions (McDaniel, 1996).

The strategies discussed are useful when used appropriately. It is important to recognize cognitive responses or concerns, for example, that can be met with education, information, or other forms of communication. When the issue is motivational, the more effective strategies to use may be manipulation or coercion. Participation, facilitation, and support can be choices to address the emotional components of accepting change, such as fear, anxiety, or grief. Effective change leaders develop work environments that support continuous individual and group learning. Rather than rigidly applying strategies to ensure the implementation of planned change elements, change leaders stay focused on the dynamics of change. Greater success in attaining what may be changing outcomes can be achieved by managing information, relationships, and visions.

Typically, combinations of strategies are applied simultaneously, rather than using only one strategy. Table 5-1 captures a view of selecting appropriate strategies to fit the ongoing needs and responses associated with leading followers in change.

ROLES AND FUNCTIONS OF CHANGE LEADERS

Managing the dynamics of change is one of the key roles of change leaders. Understanding the appropriate application of related functions, principles, and strategies can assist in meeting the challenges of any kind of change on the change continuum from **low-complexity change** to **high-complexity change.** Box 5-3 highlights some of the characteristics of effective change agents (Langford, 1990) or change leaders. Flexibility, timing, credibility (Menix, 1997), and knowledge needed in the change situation are other desirable qualities.

Change leaders and innovators, usually members (insiders) within healthcare organizations, use their personal, professional, and managerial knowledge and skills to lead change. Other effective change leaders, such as respected members of the community (outsiders), can also facilitate change. Informal members of the organization can also play important change leader functions.

Being an effective change leader requires the use of excellent communication (Langford, 1990) and interpersonal skills. Knowing how to establish relationships, interact with others, empower change participants and manage conflict is critical to the achievement of change outcomes (Menix, 1997). Change participants who are empowered and who share the creation of change that affects them directly usually integrate change more fully. Assertive communication projects self-confidence. Giving and receiving information that includes clear explanations encourages receptivity to the change process. Persistence and persuasion can communicate the change leader's commitment to the change outcome.

Because the human, systems, and technological responses to change are unpredictable, flexibility, timing, and conflict management by the change leader can keep the change on course. It is important to deal with potential or real conflict in effective ways. Understanding the interrelatedness of change and group dynamics assists the change leader in selecting appropriate strategies. Change participants are members of unique work cultures, so the change leader's selection of strategies to manage responses considers the culture's dominant values and beliefs. Managing a change to fit the preferences of a group's culture can facilitate acceptance of a particular change.

Change participants tend to be more receptive to new ideas when they originate from someone the participants trust (Langford, 1990). This credibility allows change leaders to sometimes make independent decisions without negative responses. However, actively participating in the change situation creates role modeling opportunities that can encourage involvement and acceptance of change. Change participants translate the behavior of the change leader into what is expected of them. The ultimate goal is a coordinated movement of manager, staff, and other participants toward the adoption of something new or different. For example, a manager who experiences the use of the new computerized medication dispenser may be more likely to earn the respect of the change participants.

Table 5-1	MATCHING STRATEGIES TO SITUATIONS												
Situation	Education	Support	Facilitation	Communication	Participation	Negotiation	Manipulation	Co-optation	Coercion	Learning	Visioning	Relationships	Information
Staff not sure of next best step in change process	✓	✓	✓	✓						✓	✓	✓	✓
Two staff members reluctantly try change	✓	✓	✓	✓	✓	✓				✓		✓	✓
Staff has heard rumors about new program	✓			✓						✓	✓		✓
Several staff members propose a different method		✓	✓		✓					✓	✓	✓	✓
One nurse consistently lags behind in accepting a change	✓		✓		✓					✓	✓	✓	✓
A group of staff expresses loss of previous roles		✓	✓	✓						✓		✓	✓
Three staff members challenge the need for a change	✓		✓	✓	✓	✓				✓	✓		✓
Staff member avoids change task force membership				✓		✓			✓	✓		✓	✓
Four staff members have become change agents with manager	✓	✓	✓	✓	✓					✓	✓	✓	✓
A group of staff verbalizes satisfaction with status quo	✓		✓	✓	✓	✓	✓	✓		✓	✓	✓	✓
One nurse disrupts the change process with other ideas	✓			✓	✓	✓	✓	✓		✓	✓	✓	✓
Two nurses try to get others to oppose change	✓		✓			✓	✓	✓	✓				

Exercise 5-3

Recall a work or personal situation where a particular individual tried to get you or a group to do something but did not succeed. Why did you or they decide not to cooperate? Think about the following factors: Was the idea silly, inappropriate, or unsafe? Was the person making the suggestion not known, not understood, or not trusted? Was the person making the suggestion unaware of the real situation, not part of carrying out the idea, or had he or she not received permission to influence activities? Can you see that change agents and innovators need specific qualities and abilities to be effective?

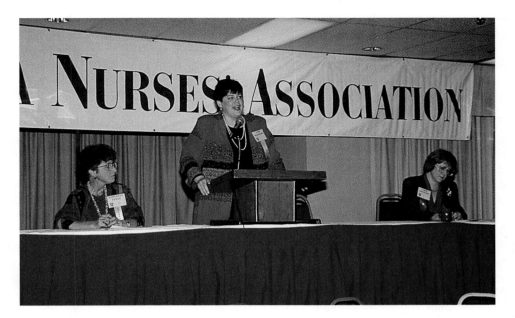

Change leaders within health care organizations use personal, professional, and managerial knowledge and skills to lead change.

Box 5-3
General Characteristics of Effective Change Agents

- Is a respected member of organization (insider) or community (outsider)
- Possesses excellent communication skills
- Understands change process
- Knows how groups function
- Is trusted by others
- Participates actively in change processes
- Possesses expert and legitimate power

Adapted with permission from Langford (1990).

Expert power coupled with the legitimate power of authority and responsibility formally bestowed by the organization or informally granted by the change participants enhances the designated change leader's opportunity for leading a change process effectively (Langford, 1990). How the change leader uses these power bases, expertise and legitimacy, will influence how committed the change participants are to achieving change outcomes.

▌ PRINCIPLES

Principles are assumptions and general rules that guide behavior and processes. Principles are useful

for creating and leading change successfully. Principles that characterize effective change implementation are provided in Box 5-4.

Box 5-4
Principles Characterizing Effective Change Implementation

- The recipients of change feel they own the change.
- Administrators and other key personnel support the proposed change.
- The recipients of change anticipate benefit from the change.
- The recipients of change participate in identifying the problem warranting a change.
- The change holds interest for the change recipients and other participants.
- Agreement exists within the work group about the benefit of the change.
- The change agent(s) and recipients of change perceive a compatibility of values.
- Trust and empathy exist among the participants of the change process.
- Revision of the change goal and process is negotiable.
- The change process is designed to provide regular feedback to its participants.

Adapted from Harper (1993).

A Manager's Solution

❓ Change was guided by a planned change approach for the best outcomes. I chose Lewin's model of change. I also reviewed literature and talked to senior city managers. Early and ongoing activities involved negotiations to educate and persuade the City Council about outcomes the department wanted. Throughout the transition I held meetings, conducted strategic planning sessions, wrote proposals, and "wandered around" to promote communication. My initial responsibilities, however, centered on communicating the nature of the external pressures imposing change and then overcoming the emotional resistance from staff. Proactive efforts, part of the planned change, helped empower staff and encourage their participation in making the transition. Initially, when resistance was intense, staff meetings served to promote awareness of the need to change. At one meeting, small teams of staff envisioned what the health department could and should look like with the new mission. The most effective "unfreezing" occurred, however, when staff took part in an exercise to identify how departmental services did indeed duplicate services provided by other entities in the community. It was only then that staff members became active change agents in the change process to recreate the City Health Department. Over a period of 18 months, the department moved to delivering more traditional public health services with less focus on clinical services. The staff became 14 positions fewer and was managed by only two supervisory layers. I attribute much of my success in moving the department to this new level to embracing the change myself, then using Lewin's model, staff empowerment approaches, joint problem solving with top administration and staff, active listening, frequent explanations, and patience and empathy for the feelings experienced during the state of flux. The existing staff has reached new levels of growth and commitment. Now I can characterize the department as consolidated and stable.

❓ *Would this be a suitable approach for you? Why?*

Exercise 5-4

Prepare an actual or hypothetical change that is meaningful to you in your personal, work, or school life. Select a change that allows you an opportunity to apply the linear (planned) and nonlinear principles of change. Draft a hypothetical or actual plan for change, drawing on the chapter content and paying particular attention to the array of change principles discussed. Share your plan and the rationale used with peers or a small group of other healthcare providers. Ask for their comments and suggestions. (If you need a hypothetical change to work with, consider this one: You are the assistant manager for a home health agency. The agency administrator just informed you by memorandum that in 1 month, because of new reimbursement rules, the agency will begin caring for patients receiving chemotherapy. How will you prepare for this change?)

▌ CHAPTER CHECKLIST

Change is an unavoidable constant in the rapidly changing healthcare delivery system. As a result, uncertainty is an element in most healthcare institutions. Creating and leading change and innovation rather than merely reacting can promote overall organizational effectiveness.

The nature of accelerated change demands flexibility and responsiveness to environmental pressures, rather than thinking and acting in more rigid ways. Planned change as a linear approach to managing change can be useful for dealing with low-complexity change. Nonlinear approaches offered by chaos, learning organization, and cybernetic theories focus more on managing the dynamic elements of higher complexity change situations.

- Planned change occurs in sequential stages, according to planned change theorists:

Lewin:
- Awareness of need for change
- Experience of change
- Integration of change

Lippitt, Watson, and Westley:
- The client system becomes aware of the need for change.
- The relationship is developed between the client system and change agent.
- The change problem is defined.
- The change goals are set and options for achievement are explored.
- The plan for change is implemented.
- The change is accepted and stabilized.
- The change entities redefine their relationship.

Havelock:
- Building a relationship
- Diagnosing the problem
- Acquiring relevant resources
- Choosing the solution
- Gaining acceptance
- Stabilizing the innovation and generating self-renewal

Rogers:
- Knowledge
- Persuasion
- Decision
- Implementation
- Confirmation

■ Nonlinear change occurs in a different manner according to nonlinear change theorists.

Chaos theory
- Organizations as open systems
- Non-human-induced self-organizing patterns
- Periods of stability interrupted with intense transformation
- Small changes resulting in significant consequences
- Conditions in one situation not occurring in same form

Learning organization theory
- Emphasis on flexibility, responsiveness, and learning
- Five disciplines interrelated by dialogue
  - Systems thinking
  - Personal mastery
  - Mental models
  - Building shared vision
  - Team learning
- Resilience
  - Manifested by beliefs, skills, behaviors, and knowledge
  - Personal qualities:
    - Flexible
    - Focused
    - Positive
    - Organized
    - Proactive

Major change management functions
- Planning
- Organizing
- Implementing
- Evaluating
- Feedback/cybernetics

■ The human responses to change manifest in various behavioral patterns that may help or hinder movement toward achievement of the change outcome.

- Innovators
- Early adopters
- Early majority
- Late majority
- Laggards
- Rejectors

■ Multiples strategies are used selectively to promote involvement by the participants of change and to facilitate the overall change process:
- Education and communication
- Participation and involvement
- Facilitation and support
- Negotiation and agreement
- Manipulation and co-optation
- Coercion
- Information management
- Relationship facilitation
- Vision development
- Learning continuously

■ Effective change leaders, both formal and informal, display these characteristics in the change situation:
- Displays leadership
- Is a respected, credible member of organization or community
- Possesses excellent communication skills
- Understands change process
- Knows how groups work
- Is trusted by others
- Participates actively in change
- Possesses expert and legitimate power
- Empowers others
- Is flexible
- Establishes positive relationships
- Manages conflict
- Displays appropriate timing

■ Principles guide change:
- Change ownership
- Anticipated benefits as change consequence
- Negotiability between change leader and participants
- Benefits of feedback to change process

▍TIPS IN LEADING CHANGE

■ Whether involved in planned (low-complexity) or nonlinear (high-complexity) change, create a group of outcome scenarios with prospective actions to achieve.

■ Expect that people will respond differently to change, which may either keep movement toward the outcome on course or slow it down.

- People who assume the role of continuous learner will cope better with accelerated change.
- People involved in change may assume roles of followers or leaders and may emerge from informal formal, or internal/external sources (the formal leader may not be the change agent all of the time).
- The need to rigidly moderate all aspects of a change process can result in lesser outcomes in contrast to the allowance of ambiguity with management of dynamic qualities that can promote creative movement toward change outcomes.

TERMS TO KNOW

barrier	chaos theory
change	facilitator
change agent	high-complexity change
change leader	innovation
change management	innovator
change models	learning organization
change outcome	low-complexity change
change process	planned change
change situation	strategy

REFERENCES

Ashby, W.R. (1957). *An Introduction to Cybernetics*. New York: John Wiley & Sons.

Begun, J.W., & White, K.R. (1995). Altering nursing's dominant logic: Guidelines from complex adaptive systems theory. *Complexity and Chaos in Nursing*, 2 (1), 5-15.

Bushy, A. and Kamphuis J. (1993). Managing change; strategies for continuing education. *The Journal of Continuing Education in Nursing* 23, 197-200.

Cadwallader, M.L. (1959). The cybernetic analysis of change in complex social organizations. *The American Journal of Sociology*, 65, 154-157.

Connor, D.R. (1993). *Managing at the speed of change*. NY: Villard Books.

CRM Films. (1997a). *Leadership and the New Science* [review of the video program]. Best Sellers Series. (available: 2215 Faraday Avenue, Carlsbad, CA, 92008, 1-800-421-0833).

CRM Films. (1997b). *Lessons from the New Workplace*. [review of the video program]. Best Sellers Series. (available: 2215 Faraday Avenue, Carlsbad, CA, 92008, 1-800-421-0833.

Deevy, E. (1995). *Creating the resilient organization*. Englewood Cliffs, NJ: Prentice Hall.

George, V.M., Buske, L.J., and Rodgers, B.L. (1997) Research based planning for change. *The Journal of Nursing Administration*, 27, (5) 53-61.

Harper, C.L. (1993). *Exploring Social Change*. 2nd ed. Englewood Cliffs, NJ: Prentice-Hall.

Havelock, R.G. (1973). *The Change Agent's Guide to Innovation in Education*. Englewood Cliffs, NJ: Educational Technology Publications.

Kotter, J., & Schlesinger, L. (1979, March-April). Choosing strategies for change. *Harvard Business Review*, 57, 106-114.

Langford, T.L. (1990). *Managing and being managed: Preparation for reintegrated professional nursing practice*. 2nd ed. Lubbock, TX: Landover.

Lewin, K. (1947, June). Frontiers in group dynamics: Concept, method, and reality in social science, social equilibria and social change. *Human Relations*, 1(1), 5-41.

Limerick, D., Passfield, R., & Cunnington, B. (1995). Towards an action learning organization. [on-line; available: http://www.mcb.co.uk/services/articles/liblink/tlo/limerick.htm.]

Lippitt, R., Watson, J., & Westley, B. (1958). *The Dynamics of Planned Change*. New York: Harcourt, Brace.

McDaniel, R.R. (1996). Strategic leadership: A view from quantum and chaos theories. In Duncan, W.J., Ginter, P., & Swayne, L. (eds.). *Handbook of Health Care Management*. Oxford, England: Basil Blackwell Publishing.

Menix, K.D. (1997). Validation of change management concepts by nurse managers and educators: Baccalaureate curricular implications. Unpublished doctoral dissertation, Texas Tech University, Lubbock.

Muller-Smith, P.A. (1993). Managing the neutral zone. *Journal of Post Anesthesia Nursing*, 8(4), 290-292.

New, J.R., & Couillard, N.A. (1981, March). Guidelines for introducing change. *The Journal of Nursing Administration*, 17-21.

Nutt, P.C. (1992). *Managing Planned Change*. New York: Macmillan.

Perlman, D., & Takacs, G.J. (1990). The 10 stages of change. *Nursing Management* 21(4), 33-38.

Porter-O'Grady, T. (1997). Quantum mechanics and the future of healthcare leadership. *The Journal of Nursing Administration*, 27(1), 15-20.

Priesmeyer, H.R. (1992). *Organizations and Chaos: Defining the Methods of Nonlinear Management*. Westport, CT: Quorum Books

Rogers, E.M. (1983). *Diffusion of Innovations*. 3rd ed. New York: The Free Press.

Rogers, E.M. (1995). *Diffusion of Innovations*. 4th ed. New York: The Free Press.

Senge, P.M. (1990). *The Fifth Discipline*. New York: Doubleday.

Thietart, R.A., & Forgues, B. (1995). Chaos theory and organization. *Organization Science*, 6(1), 19-31.

Wheatley, M.J. (1992). *Leadership and the New Science*. San Francisco: Berrett-Koehler.

Wheeler, M. M. (1995, Jan.-Feb.). The human side of change. *Canadian Journal of Nursing Administration*, 26-32.

SUGGESTED READINGS

Bennis, W.G., Benne, K.D., & Chin, R. (1984). The planning of change. 4th ed. Fort Worth: Holt, Rinehart & Winston.

Bettis, R.A., & Prahalad, C.K. (1995). The dominant logic: Retrospective and extension. *Strategic Management Journal*, 16, 5-14.

Bhola, H.S. (1994). The CLER Model: Thinking through change. *Nursing Management*, 5, 59-63.

Boynton, D., & Rothman, L. (1996). Charge nurses: Critical change agents for successful restructuring. *Recruitment, Retention, & Restructuring Report*, 9(2), 2-5.

Coeling, H.V., & Simms, L.M. (1993). Facilitating innovation at the nursing unit level through cultural assessment, part I: How to keep management ideas from falling on deaf ears. *The Journal of Nursing Administration*, 23(4), 46-53.

Coeling, H.V., & Simms, L.M. (1993). Facilitating innovation at the unit level through cultural assessment, part 2. Adapting managerial ideas to the work group. *The Journal of Nursing Administration*, 23(5), 13-20.

Dianis, N.L., Allen, M., Baker, K., Cartledge, T., Gwyer, D., Harris, S., McNemar, A., Swayze, R., Wilson, M., & Walker, P.H. (1997). Merger motorway: Giving staff the tools to reengineer. *Nursing Management*, 28(3), 42-47.

Fishman, C. (1997, April/May). Change. *Fast Company*, 64-74.

Hagerman, Z.J. (1994). Evaluation of two planned change theories. *Nursing Management*, 25(4), 57-62.

Havelock, R.G., & Zlotolow, S. (1995). *The change agent's guide*. 2nd ed. Englewood Cliffs, NJ: Educational Technology Publications.

Kowalski, K. (1996). Shifting the organizational culture. *Capsules and Comments in Perinatal and Women's Health Nursing*, 2(1), 23-28.

Lutjens, L.R.J., & Tiffany, C.R. (1994). Evaluating planned changed theories. *Nursing Management*, 25(3), 54-57.

Manion, J. (1994). The nurse intrapreneur: How to innovate from within. *American Journal of Nursing*, 94, 38-42.

Marquardt, M.J. (1996). *Building the Learning Organization*. New York: McGraw-Hill.

McNemar, A., Swayze, R., Wilson, M., & Walker, P.H. (1997). Merger motorway: Giving staff the tools to reengineer. *Nursing Management*, 28(3), 42-47.

Porter-O'Grady, T., & Wilson, C.K. (1995). *The Leadership Revolution in Health Care*. Gaithersburg, MD: Aspen.

Pryjmachuk, S. (1996). Pragmatism and change: Some implications for nurses, nurse managers and nursing. *Journal of Nursing Management*, 4, 201-205.

Schein, E.H. (1995). Building the learning consortium. [on-line; available: http://learning.mit.edu/res/wp/.]

Schein, E.H. (1996a). Organizational learning as cognitive redefinition: Coercive persuasion revisited. [on-line; available: http://learning.mit.edu/res/wp/10010.html.]

Schein, E.H. (1996b). Three cultures of management: The key to organizational learning in the 21st century. [on-line; available: http://learning.mit.edu/res/wp/10011.html.]

Schwartz, K., & Tiffany, C.R. (1994). Evaluating Bhola's Configurations Theory of Planned Change. *Nursing Management*, 25(6), 56-61.

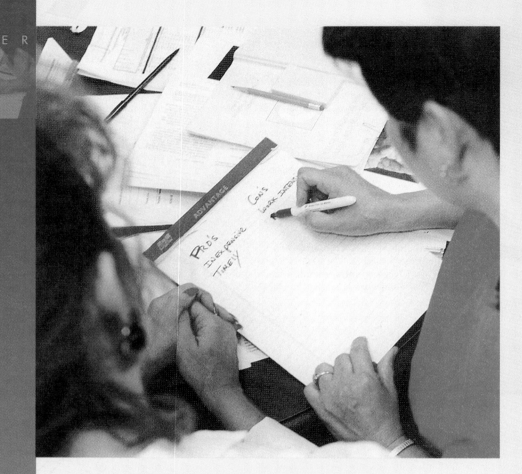

Problem Solving and Decision Making

**Rose Aguilar
Welch**
RN, MSN, EdD

This chapter describes the key concepts related to problem solving and decision making. The relationship between these essential skills and critical thinking is also explored. This chapter explains the primary steps of the problem-solving and decision-making processes and offers analytical tools that are helpful in planning and visualizing decision-making activities. It also presents strategies for individual or group problem solving and decision making. These strategies may be applied to both personal and professional situations.

Objectives

- Utilize a decision-making format to list options to solve a problem, identify the pros and cons of each option, rank the options, and select the best option.
- Evaluate the effect of faulty information gathering on a decision-making experience.
- Investigate the decision-making style of a nurse leader/manager.
- Design a flowchart for a personal or professional project.
- Increase skills in problem solving and decision making.

Questions to Consider

- Why are problem-solving and decision-making skills important for professional nursing practice?
- How can you enhance your skills in problem solving and decision making?
- What is the relationship between critical thinking ability and skill in problem solving and decision making?

A Manager's Challenge
From the Director of Nursing at a Regional Medical Center in the Western United States

Working in the Medical Center in today's competitive managed care marketplace presents many challenges associated with increasing patient satisfaction, while decreasing costs. Many patients have their first contact with a hospital through the Department of Emergency Medical Services (DEMS), and this first impression can have an impact on whether they return to the hospital for continued treatment. Unfortunately, for my hospital, satisfaction with DEMS was decreasing. Specifically, we were receiving complaints from patients, families, and staff regarding perceived safety and security in the Emergency Room (ER) areas. The DEMS treated many victims of gang violence, and known gang members were frequently seen roaming the halls of the hospital and were suspected of defacing elevators and bathrooms with graffiti. Tension in the waiting room would increase as friends and members of the victims' families would arrive and see members of the "other" gang who were also in the waiting room (many times the victims received in the ER were from both gangs in the fight). This could occasionally result in verbal or physical fights breaking out in the waiting room and necessitated involving the police. This environment did not feel "safe" to anyone and resulted in decreased patient and staff satisfaction. Our challenge was to effectively and efficiently improve this situation.

What do you think you would do if you were this manager?

▌ INTRODUCTION

Problem solving and **decision making** are vital abilities for nursing practice. Not only are these processes involved in managing and delivering care, but also they are essential for engaging in planned change. Myriad technological, social, political, and economic changes have had a dramatic effect on healthcare and nursing. Increased patient acuity, shorter hospital stays, and the rise of ambulatory and home healthcare are some of the changes that require nurses to make rational and valid decisions that achieve results. In addition to the focus on achieving results, more emphasis is now placed on making decisions that are people oriented and cost-effective.

Nurses at all levels must possess the basic knowledge and skills required for effective problem solving and decision making. These competencies are especially important for nurses with leadership and management responsibilities.

Problem solving and decision making are not synonymous terms. However, the processes for engaging in both behaviors are similar. Both skills require **critical thinking**, which is a higher cognitive process, and both can be improved upon with practice.

Decision making is a purposeful and goal-directed effort using a systematic process to choose among options. Not all decision making begins with a problem situation. Instead, the hallmark of decision making is the identification and selection of options. For example, the nurse manager of a home health agency is strategizing ways to empower his/her staff nurses. The options she is considering include allowing the staff to make out the schedule, perform self-evaluations, or have more input in the formulation of agency policy.

Problem solving, which includes a decision-making step, is focused on trying to solve an immediate problem. A problem can be viewed as a gap between "what is" and "what should be." In addition, there is the dissatisfaction that the problem creates for individuals and/ or groups. For example, a nurse educator complains to a unit manager that the staff nurses rarely attend the inservice classes or continuing education programs that are offered. In attempting to address this issue, the parties will gather and examine information in an effort to define the problem and identify possible solutions.

As previously mentioned, effective problem solving and decision making are predicated on an individual's ability to think critically. Although critical thinking has been defined in numerous ways, the National Council for Excellence in Critical Thinking Instruction defines it as the "intellectually disciplined process of actively and skillfully conceptualizing, applying, analyzing, synthesizing, or evaluating information gathered from, or generated by, observation, experience, reflection, reasoning or communication, as a guide to belief and action" (Paul, 1995, p. 110). Critical thinking is not an isolated process. It is manifested whenever a nurse asks "why," "what," or "how." A nurse who questions why a patient is restless is thinking critically. Compare the analytical abilities between a nurse who assumes a patient is restless because of anxiety related to an upcoming procedure and a nurse who asks if there could be another explanation and proceeds to investigate possible causes. According to Bette Case (1994), "we apply critical thinking when we make professional and personal decisions as individuals, and when we participate in collaborative decision-making processes with others" (p. 101).

For more information on the critical thinking movement, visit the following sites on the World Wide Web (WWW):

- Center for Critical Thinking and Foundation for Critical Thinking at Sonoma State University (http://www.sonoma.edu/cthink)
- California Academic Press (http://www.calpress.com)

Deguzon and Lunney (1995) suggest using clinical journals as a tool to monitor one's thinking processes. The goal of the exercise is to improve problem-solving and decision-making abilities by reflecting on the thinking that led to specific actions and outcomes. The authors recommend including both content and thinking processes when writing on a clinical issue or situation. Moreover, they propose questions that should be asked to facilitate thinking about thinking. These include the following:

- What data led me to my conclusions?
- What assumptions did I have about this situation?
- What would I do differently next time and why?

For example, instead of a nurse recording "I held Mrs. Smith's digoxin at 9 a.m.," the journal entry might say something like "I held Mrs. Smith's digoxin at 9 a.m. because her apical pulse was only 65 beats per minute (*data*). In addition, the patient complained of two episodes of diarrhea within the past 24 hours (*data*). These are possible signs of digoxin toxicity (*assumption*). I held the dose until I could notify the physician. The physician supported my decision to hold the dig., and ordered labs to check the dig. level and lytes. Since Mrs. Smith is elderly and lives alone, I should have questioned her and her family in more detail about how she takes her meds. at home because she might not be taking her medications properly (*what I would do differently next time and why*).

Not only can individuals use clinical journals for self-improvement, but also nurse managers can use them for staff development. Nurse managers or educators might employ this approach to obtain data on the problem-solving and decision-making skills of staff nurses. However, Deguzon and Lunney (1995) caution that confidentiality of the journal information should be respected and feedback to the journal writer should be supportive, not evaluative.

It is important for managers to assess their staff members' ability to think critically and enhance their knowledge and skills through staff development programs, coaching, and role modeling. Attitudes, or the disposition to think critically, can be enhanced by establishing a positive and motivating work environment.

Creativity is essential for the generation of options or solutions. Creative individuals are able to conceptualize new and innovative approaches to a problem or issue by being more flexible and independent in their thinking.

The model depicted in Figure 6-1 demonstrates the relationship among decision making, problem solving, creativity, and critical thinking. Critical thinking is the concept that interweaves and links the others. An individual, through the application of critical thinking skills, engages in problem solving and decision making in an environment that can promote or inhibit these skills. It is the manager's task to model these skills and promote them in others. The Research box suggests a specific strategy to help others develop these skills.

PROBLEM SOLVING

Before attempting to solve a problem, a manager must ask certain key questions:

1. Is it important?
2. Do I want to do something about it?
3. Am I qualified to handle it?
4. Do I have the authority to do anything?
5. Do I have the knowledge, interest, time, and resources to deal with it?
6. Can I delegate it to someone else?
7. What benefits will be derived from solving it?

If the answer to questions one through five is "no," why waste time, resources, and personal energy? At this juncture a conscious decision is made to ignore the problem, refer or delegate it to others, or consult or collaborate with others to solve it. On the other hand, if the answers are "yes," the decision maker chooses to accept the problem and thus assume responsibility for it.

Methods of Problem Solving

The main principles for diagnosing a problem are know the facts, separate the facts from interpretation, be objective and descriptive, and determine the scope of the problem. Managers also need to determine how to establish priorities for solving problems. For example, does a manager tend to work on problems that are encountered first, that appear to be the easiest, or that take the shortest amount of time to solve, or that may have the greatest urgency?

Common methods for problem solving include trial and error, experimentation, and purposeful inaction ("do nothing") approaches. Often, inexperienced managers use trial and error by trying one intervention after another until one method seems to address the problem. For example, patients' visitors have been complaining about the restrictive visiting hours in nurs-

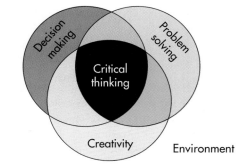

Figure 6-1 Problem-solving and decision-making model. (Adapted from Sullivan & Decker [1992].)

ing units. Without an in-depth analysis of the problem, an inexperienced manager institutes different visiting policies until one seems to generate the least amount of complaints. Trial and error is the simplest technique, but it is often time-consuming and may not be effective, especially if the problem is complex.

Scientific experimentation involves studying the situation under controlled conditions often using trial periods or pilot projects. It is useful when additional information is needed to understand the problem further. Although the likelihood of achieving positive outcomes is greater, sufficient time is required for the experimental approach to be effective.

To utilize an experimentation approach in the above example, after gathering data on the specific nature of the visitors' complaints, the manager might institute one visiting policy in one unit and a different visiting policy in another unit. After a designated period of time, visitor satisfaction might be assessed through a survey, questionnaire, or interviews, and the results compared.

After identifying the problem, the decision maker must decide whether it is significant enough to require intervention and whether it is even within his or her control to do anything about it. Sometimes new managers feel they need to "solve" every problem brought to their attention. There are situations such as some interpersonal conflicts that are best resolved by the individuals who "own" the problem. Known as purposeful inaction, a "do nothing" approach might be indicated when problems should be resolved by other persons or if the problem is beyond the manager's control. Consider the following *scenario*:

Research Perspective

Lamond, D., Crow, R., Chase, J., Doggen, K., & Swinkels, M. (1996). Information sources used in decision making: Considerations for simulation development. International Journal of Nursing Studies, 33, 47-57.

This research study illustrates the global importance of problem solving and decision making for professional nursing practice. The researchers questioned the validity of traditional simulation techniques used to assess decision making, as such approaches usually focus on identifying the outcome or product of the decision making, not the thinking that led to the decision. They propose that by adding a "think aloud" component to simulations such as case studies, one can more accurately assess the thinking processes used for problem solving and decision making. This involves asking the subject to verbalize everything that he or she is thinking while engaged in the problem-solving and decision-making task.

To verify the validity of their assumption, the researchers sought to identify the primary sources of information used by nurses when making conclusions about assessment data. Their sample consisted of a convenience sample of 114 medical and surgical nurses from four hospitals in southwest England. Using semi-structured interviews that were taped and transcribed, the researchers elicited the primary sources of information the nurses used to make assessment judgments. Content analysis of the 104 taped interviews that were suitable for analysis revealed four major themes for nurses' information sources. They are verbal information, observation, prior knowledge, and written information. Of these themes, the most often used information source was verbal information at 41%, followed by observation (21%), prior knowledge (20%), and written information (17%). The researchers also noted that while medical nurses and surgical nurses used verbal and written information in a similar manner, surgical nurses tended to use observation and prior knowledge slightly more often than medical nurses.

Implications for Practice

Based on the findings, the researchers concluded that to ensure a valid process for examining decision-making processes, it is important to determine how the simulation is constructed. Perhaps a written case study as the sole information source is not sufficient because it is not "close enough to reality" for the nurse who may rely on verbal information sources (p. 55). The authors caution against using simulations that present information in a format that the nurse does not generally use. Clearly, one must take care not to generalize the researchers' findings, and further research is warranted. Nevertheless, presenting real-life examples in simulations that nurses can relate to is more likely to accurately assess their problem-solving and decision-making skills.

Mary complains to the nurse manager that Sam, a fellow nurse, was rude and abrupt with her during a hallway interchange. How should the nurse manager handle Mary's complaint? Should the manager discuss the problem with Sam? Should Mary be present during the discussion? What are the possible risks or benefits of such an approach? Alternatively, should the manager assist Mary in developing her communication skills so that Mary can solve the problem herself?

Some decisions are "givens" because they are based on firmly established criteria in the institution, which may be based on the traditions, values, doctrines, culture, or policy of the organization. Every manager has to live with mandates from persons higher in the organizational structure. Although a manager may not have the authority to control certain situations, he or she still may be able to influence the outcome. For example, due to losses in revenue, administration has decided to eliminate the clinical educator positions for the nursing units and place the responsibility for clinical education with the senior staff nurses. It is beyond the manager's control to reverse this decision. Nevertheless, the manager can explore the staff nurses' fear and concerns regarding this change and facilitate the transition by preparing them for the new role.

In these examples, it is a misnomer to refer to the approach as "do nothing," since there is deliberate action on the part of the manager. This approach should not be confused with the laissez-faire (hands off) approach taken by a manager who chooses to do nothing when intervention is indicated.

Exercise 6-1

Using the decision-making format presented in the box on page 97 list other options for this scenario and the advantages and disadvantages of each approach. Rank the options in order of most desirable to least desirable and select the best option. Determine how you would implement and evaluate the chosen option.

Problem-Solving Process

The traditional process for problem solving is illustrated in Figure 6-2. This figure gives the appearance of a sequential and linear process. But, like the nursing process, the problem-solving process is a dynamic one. These steps are described in more detail in the following section.

Define the problem, issue, or situation

The most common cause for failure to resolve problems is the improper identification of the problem; therefore problem recognition and identification is considered the most vital step. The quality of the outcome is dependent on the accurate identification of the problem. Problem identification is influenced by the information available; by the values, attitudes, and experiences of the decision makers; and by time. Sufficient time should be allowed for the collection and organization of data. All too often an inadequate amount of time is allocated for this essential step, resulting in unsatisfactory outcomes.

In work settings, problems often fall under certain categories that have been described as the four Ms: manpower, methods, machines, and materials. For example, does the problem relate to work load issues, lack of resources, or lack of training? Other categories for work-related problems can include, but are not limited to, the following:

- Power struggles or "turf wars"
- Poor communication
- Legal or ethical issues
- Work conditions
- Unsatisfactory performance
- Staff interactions and relationships

After the general nature of the problem is identified, individuals can then focus on gathering and analyzing data to resolve the issue.

Exercise 6-2

Consider a situation in which an unsatisfactory outcome or decision was made based on inaccurate or incomplete information. How could this have been avoided, and what would you recommend to prevent this from occurring in the future?

Gather data

Assessment, through the collection of data and information, is done continuously throughout this dynamic process. The data gathered consist of objective (facts) and subjective (feelings) information. Information gathered should be valid, accurate, relevant to the issue, and timely. Moreover, individuals involved in the process must have access to information and adequate resources in order to make cogent decisions.

Analyze data

Data are analyzed to further refine the problem statement and identify possible solutions or options. It is important to differentiate a problem from the symptoms of a problem. For example, a nurse manager is dismayed by the latest continuous quality improvement (CQI) report indicating nurses are not documenting patient teaching. Is this evidence that patient teaching is not being done? Is lack of documentation the actual problem? Perhaps it is the symptom of the actual problem. On further analysis the manager may discover that the lack of a specific form for documentation of patient teaching is the problem. By distinguishing the problem from the symptoms of the problem, a more appropriate solution can be identified and implemented.

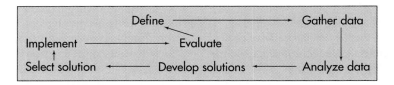

Figure 6-2 The problem-solving process.

Develop solutions

The goal of generating options is to identify as many choices as possible. Occasionally the quality of outcomes is hampered by rigid "black and white" thinking. A nurse, unhappy with her work situation, but who can think of only two options—stay or quit—is displaying this type of thinking.

Being flexible, open-minded, and creative is critical to being able to consider a range of possible options. Everyone has preconceived notions and ideas when confronted with certain situations. Putting these notions on hold and considering other ideas is beneficial, although it is difficult to do. However, asking questions such as the following can allow a person to consider other viewpoints:

- Am I jumping to conclusions?
- If I were (insert name of role model), how would I approach it?
- How are my beliefs and values affecting my decision?

Select solution

The decision maker should then objectively weigh each option according to its possible risks and consequences, as well as positive outcomes that may be derived. Criteria for evaluation might include variables such as cost, effectiveness, time, and legal or ethical considerations. The options should be ranked in the order in which they are likely to result in the desired goals or objectives. The solution selected should be the one that is most feasible and satisfactory and has the least undesirable consequences. Nurses must consider whether they are picking the solution because it is the best solution or because it is the most expedient. Being able to make cogent decisions based on thorough assessment of a situation is an important yardstick of a nurse's effectiveness.

Implement

The implementation phase should include a contingency plan to deal with negative consequences, should they appear. In essence, the decision maker should be prepared to institute "plan B" should the need arise.

Evaluate

Considerable time and energy are usually spent on identifying the problem or issue, generating possible solutions, selecting the best solution, and implementing the solution. However, not enough time is typically allocated for evaluation and follow-up. It is important to establish early in the process how evaluation and monitoring will take place, who will be responsible for it, and when it will take place.

Take the previous example of the manager who instituted new visiting policies in response to visitor complaints. To ensure that this action was effective in solving the problem, an evaluation and monitoring plan should be developed in advance. In collaboration with the nursing staff, the manager would determine when follow-up surveys should be distributed; who will be responsible for their distribution, collection, and analysis; and how the findings will be communicated to appropriate personnel.

DECISION MAKING

The primary steps of the decision-making process are similar to those of the problem-solving process. The phases include defining objectives, generating options, identifying advantages and disadvantages of each option, ranking the options, selecting the option most likely to achieve the predefined objectives, implementing, and evaluating. Box 6-1 contains a form that can be used to complete these steps.

A poor-quality decision is likely if the objectives are not clearly identified or if they are inconsistent with the values of the individual or organization. The essential step of defining the goal, purpose, or objectives is illustrated in the following excerpt from Alice's Adventures in Wonderland by Lewis Carroll.

One day Alice came to a fork in the road and saw a Cheshire cat in a tree. "Which road do I take?," she asked. His response was a question: "Where do you want to go?" "I don't know," Alice answered. "Then," said the cat, "it doesn't matter."

Decision Models

The decision model that a nurse uses depends on the circumstances. Is the situation routine and predictable or complex and uncertain? Is the goal of the decision to conservatively make a decision that is just "good enough" or one that is optimal? Examples of decision models or theories are presented in the theory box on p. 98.

To illustrate decision theories, consider the following scenario. Staff nurses on a medical-surgical unit have complained that excessive time is spent documenting on numerous flowcharts and forms, often charting the same information in several places. Their frustration over charting is exacerbated by the inaccessibility of the medical records on the unit. A **satisficing decision** might involve the expedient option of separating the nursing forms from the medical record and placing them on a clipboard for easy

---

Box 6-1

Decision-Making Format

Issue/problem: _____

Objective: _____

Options:

_____

_____

_____

_____

Analysis of options:

Option	Advantages	Disadvantages

Rank priority of options (1 being most preferred)

_____

_____

Select the best option (Implementation Plan)

_____

_____

Evaluation plan

_____

_____

---

access. However, an optimizing decision might involve creating a multidisciplinary task force to investigate the feasibility of streamlining or eliminating forms, hence reducing redundant charting.

Decision-Making Styles

The decision-making style of a nurse manager is similar to the leadership style that the manager is likely to use. A manager who leans toward an autocratic style may choose to make decisions independent of the input or participation of others. This has been referred to as the "decide and announce" approach. On the other hand, a manager who uses a democratic or participative approach to management involves the appropriate personnel in the decision-making process. Participative management has been shown to increase work performance and productivity, decrease employee turnover, and enhance employee satisfaction.

Recker, Bess, and Wellens (1996) describe a shared governance model used in 16-bed critical care and 10-bed intermediate care units that exemplifies a participative management style. They propose a shared governance model that asks managers and "followers" to consider who is responsible for making decisions, who is involved or affected by the problem, who should be consulted regarding the problem, who needs to be informed in order to support the decision, and who needs to approve the decision (p. 48-D).

Any decision style can be used appropriately or inappropriately. Like the tenets of situational leadership theory, the situation and circumstances should dictate which decision-making style is most appropriate.

In their classic book, *Leadership and Decision Making*, Vroom and Yetton (1973) provide a useful model for defining the most appropriate leadership style based on the characteristics of the problem.

Although it is beyond the scope of this chapter to describe the model in detail, the salient points are presented. The five primary leadership methods identified by Vroom and Yetton (1973, pp. 21-30) are presented in Table 6-1. Eight variables or "decision rules" assist the decision maker in selecting which of the five leadership styles is most appropriate, as follows:

Decision Model Theories

THEORY/CONTRIBUTOR	KEY IDEA	APPLICATION TO PRACTICE
Normative or prescriptive	Used when information is objective, and routine decisions are involved or the problem is structured. Options are known and predictable.	Situations that fall under this category can be handled using agency policy, standard procedures, or analytical tools.
Descriptive or behavioral	Used when information is subjective, nonroutine, and unstructured. Uncertainty exists because options or outcomes are either unknown or unpredictable.	Situations that fall under this category are best handled by gathering more data, using past experience, employing creative approaches, or following a group process.
Satisficing	Decision maker selects the solution that minimally meets the objective or standard for a decision. It is the more conservative method compared to an optimized approach.	This process is the most expedient and may be the most appropriate when time is an issue.
Optimizing	Decision maker selects the solution that maximally meets the objective or standard for a decision. Usually this process involves accessing the pros and cons of each known option as well as listing benefits and costs associated with each option. The goal is to select the most ideal solution.	This process is more likely to result in a better decision, but takes longer.

Table 6-1	VROOM AND YETTON'S LEADERSHIP METHODS

Method	Characteristics
Autocratic I (AI)	Manager independently solves problems and makes decisions based on information at hand
Autocratic II (AII)	Manager obtains information from others before solving problems and making decisions; only information is sought from others, not opinions
Consultive I (CI)	Manager discusses the problem with others *individually* to obtain information and recommendations; the decision made may or may not reflect their suggestions
Consultive II (CII)	Manager discusses the problem with others as a *group* before making decisions that may or may not reflect their suggestions
Group II (GII)	Manager functioning as a discussion leader discusses the problem with the group; the group decides the action to be taken

Adapted from Vroom and Yetton (1973).

1. The importance of the decision quality to institutional success
2. The degree to which the manager possesses the information and skills to make the decision
3. The degree to which the followers have the necessary information to generate a quality decision
4. The degree to which the problem is structured
5. The importance of follower commitment
6. The likelihood that an autocratic decision would be accepted
7. The strength of follower commitment to institutional goals
8. The likelihood of follower conflict over the final decision

The autocratic method results in more rapid decision making and is appropriate in crisis situations or when groups are likely to accept this type of decision style. However, followers are generally more supportive of consultive and group approaches. Although these approaches take more time, they are more appropriate when conflict is likely to occur, when the problem is unstructured, or when the manager does not have the knowledge or skills to solve the problem.

Exercise 6-3

Interview a colleague about his or her decision-making style. What decision-making process does he or she use? What barriers or obstacles to effective decision making has he or she encountered? What strategies does he or she use to increase the effectiveness of the decisions made?

Factors Affecting Decision Making

Numerous factors affect individuals and groups in the decision-making process. The perception of the problem can be influenced by internal and external factors. Internal factors include variables such as the decision maker's physical and emotional state; personal characteristics; values; past experiences; interests, knowledge, and attitudes. External factors include environmental conditions and time. Decision-making options are externally limited when time is short or when the environment is characterized by a "we've always done it this way" attitude.

One's values affect all aspects of decision making from the statement of the problem to how evaluation will be carried out. Values are determined by one's cultural, social, and philosophical background.

Certain personality factors such as self-esteem and self-confidence affect whether one is willing to take risks in solving problems or making decisions. Ask yourself, "Do you prefer to let others make the decisions? Are you more comfortable in the role of 'follower' than leader? If so, why?" Characteristics of an effective decision maker reported in the literature include courage, a willingness to take risks, self-awareness, energy, creativity, sensitivity, and flexibility.

Exercise 6-4

Reflect on your own strengths and limitations as a problem solver and decision maker. List them in two columns, and identify strategies for working on the limitations and capitalizing on the strengths.

GROUP PROBLEM SOLVING AND DECISION MAKING

There are two primary criteria for effective decision making. First, the decision must be of a high quality; that is, it achieves the predefined goals or objectives. Second, the decision must be accepted by those who are responsible for its implementation.

Variables that influence the quality of decisions include the following:

- Was the information used factual, complete, and relevant to the situation?
- What were the behavioral characteristics of the decision makers?
- Were they able to process the data?
- Is the decision defensible in that the solution generated can be justified?
- Did the benefits of the decision outweigh the risks that were involved?
- How well did the decision solve the problem or meet the identified need?

Higher-quality decisions are more likely to result if groups are involved in the problem-solving and decision-making process. When individuals are allowed input into the process, they tend to function more productively and the quality of the decision is generally superior.

Research findings suggest the characteristics of effective groups include the following: followers are involved, the group is moderately cohesive, there is equal participation and communication among members, active verbal participation from members is encouraged, minimal self-oriented behavior is observed, and members are trained in group process (Pankowski, 1984).

In deciding to use the group process for decision making, it is important to consider group size and composition. If the group is too small, there will be a limited number of options generated and fewer points of view will be expressed. Conversely, if the group is too large, it may lack structure and consensus becomes more difficult. Homogeneous groups may be more compatible; however, heterogeneous groups may be more successful in problem solving. Research has demonstrated that the most productive groups are those that are moderately cohesive. If groups are too cohesive, excessive time may be spent on socialization and camaraderie. If they are not cohesive enough, goals may not be achieved (Pankowski, 1984).

For groups to be able to work effectively, the group facilitator or leader should carefully select members on the basis of their knowledge and skills in problem solving. Individuals who are aggressive, are authoritarian, or manifest self-oriented behaviors tend to decrease the effectiveness of groups. Furthermore, the leader should provide a nonthreatening and positive environment in which group members are encouraged to actively participate. Using tact and diplomacy, the facilitator can control aggressive individuals who tend to monopolize the discussion and can encourage more passive individuals to contribute by asking direct, open-ended questions. Providing positive feedback such as "You raised a good point," protecting members and their suggestions from attack, and keeping the group focused on the task are strategies that create an environment conducive to problem solving.

The advantages of group decision making are numerous. The adage "two heads are better than one" illustrates that when individuals with different knowledge, skills, and resources collaborate to solve a problem or make a decision, the likelihood of a quality outcome is increased. More ideas can be generated by groups than by individuals functioning alone. Additionally, when followers are directly involved in this process they are more apt to accept the decision because they have an increased sense of ownership or commitment to the decision. Implementing solutions becomes easier when individuals have been actively involved in the decision-making process. Involvement can be enhanced by making information readily available to the appropriate personnel, requesting input, establishing committees

and task forces with broad representation, and using group decision-making techniques.

The group leader must establish with the participants what decision rule will be followed. Will the group strive to achieve consensus (100% agreement) or will the majority rule? In determining which decision rule to use, the group leader should consider the necessity for quality and acceptance of the decision. Although achieving both a high-quality and an acceptable decision is possible, to do so requires more involvement and approval from individuals affected by the decision.

Groups will be more committed to an idea if it is derived by consensus rather than as an outcome of individual decision making or majority rule. Consensus requires that all participants agree to go along with the solution. Although achieving consensus requires considerable time, it results in both high-quality and high-acceptance decisions.

Majority rule can be used to compromise when 100% agreement cannot be achieved. This method saves time, but the solution may only partially achieve the goals of quality and acceptance. In addition, majority rule carries certain risks. First, if the informal group leaders happen to fall in the minority opinion, they may not support the decision of the majority. Certain members may go so far as to build coalitions to gain support for their position and block the majority choice. After all, the majority may represent only 51% of the group. In addition, group members may support the position of the leader even though they don't agree with the decision because they fear reprisal or they wish to obtain the leader's approval. *In general, as the importance of the decision increases, so does the percentage of group members required to approve it.* Decisions made by individuals acting alone take the least amount of time but also result in decisions low in both quality and acceptance (McFarland, Leonard, & Morris, 1984).

To secure the support of the group, the leader should maintain open communication with those affected by the decision and be honest about the advantages and disadvantages of the decision. The leader should also demonstrate how the advantages outweigh the disadvantages, suggest ways the unwanted outcomes can be minimized, and be available to assist when necessary.

Although group problem solving and decision making have distinct advantages, involving groups also carries certain disadvantages and may not be appropriate in all situations. As previously stated, group decision making requires more time. In some situ-

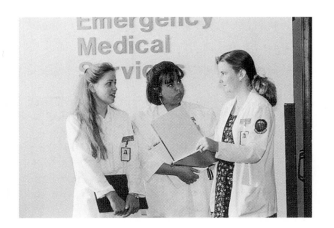

To be part of the solution, followers must be part of the problem-solving process.

Exercise 6-5

Consider the last time you were involved with a group in a problem-solving or decision-making session. Did you suggest something only to hear people say, "It will never work," "Administration won't go for it," "What a dumb idea," "It's not in the budget," "If it ain't broke, don't fix it," or "We tried that before"? Think of other "killer phrases" that stifled creativity and caused resentment. For example, if you are involved in groups that tend to stifle creativity and input through verbal and nonverbal behaviors, try this approach. Agree that when "killer phrases" are used, an individual assigned as a "killer phrase" monitor will ring a bell. This will raise individuals' levels of awareness and put a halt to behaviors that can stifle creativity and cause bruised egos.

ations this may not be appropriate, especially in a crisis situation requiring prompt decisions.

Another disadvantage of group decision making relates to unequal power among group members. Dominant personality types may influence the more passive or powerless group members to conform to their points of view. Furthermore, individuals may expend considerable time and energy defending their positions so that the primary objective of the group effort is lost.

Groups may be more concerned with maintaining group harmony than engaging in active discussion on the issue and generating creative ideas to address it. Group members who manifest a "groupthink" mentality are so concerned with avoiding conflict and supporting their leader and other members that important issues or concerns are not raised. Failure to bring up options, explore conflict, or challenge the status quo results in ineffective group functioning and decision outcomes.

Strategies

Strategies exist to minimize the problems encountered with group problem solving and decision making. These strategies include brainstorming, nominal group techniques, and the Delphi technique.

Brainstorming can be an effective method for generating a large volume of creative options. Often, creativity and idea generation are stifled by the premature critiquing of ideas. When members use inflammatory statements, euphemistically referred to as "killer phrases," the usual response is for members to stop contributing.

The hallmark of brainstorming, a right-brain activity, is to list all ideas as stated without critique or discussion. The group leader or facilitator should encourage people to tag onto or spin off ideas from those already suggested. One idea may be piggybacked off others. Ideas should not be judged nor should the relative merits or disadvantages of the ideas be discussed at this time. The goal is to generate ideas, no matter how seemingly unrealistic or absurd. It is important for the group leader or facilitator to cut off criticism and be alert for nonverbal behaviors signaling disapproval.

Since the emphasis is on the volume of ideas generated, not necessarily the quality, solutions may be superficial and fail to solve the problem. Group brainstorming also takes longer, and the logistics of getting people together may pose a problem.

The nominal group technique, a method designed by Delbecq Van de Ven and Gustafson in 1971, allows every group member the opportunity for input into the decision-making process (Sullivan & Decker, 1992). Although the group is physically present, participants are asked not to talk to each other as they write down their ideas to solve a predefined problem or issue. After a period of silent generation of ideas, generally no more than 10 minutes, each member is asked to share an idea that is displayed on a chalkboard or flip chart. Comments and elaboration are not allowed during this phase. Each member takes a turn sharing an idea until all ideas are presented, after which discussion is allowed. Members may "pass" if they have exhausted their list of ideas. During the next step, ideas are clarified and the merits of each idea are discussed. In the third and final step, each member privately assigns a priority rank to each op-tion. The solution chosen is the option that receives the highest ranking by the majority of participants. The advantage of this technique is that it allows equal participation among members and minimizes the influence of dominant personalities. The disadvantages of this method are that it is time-consuming and it requires advance preparation. In addition, it requires that the group physically come together.

A method that avoids the problem of getting people together, yet retains the advantages of group decision making, is the Delphi technique. This technique was developed by the Rand Corporation in 1950 to forecast technological developments (Whitman, 1990). It involves systematically collecting and summarizing opinions and judgments from respondents on a particular issue by use of interviews, surveys, or questionnaires. Opinions of the respondents are repeatedly fed back to them with a request to provide more refined opinions and rationales on the issue or matter under consideration. Between rounds, the results are tabulated and analyzed in order to report the findings to the participants. This allows the participants to reconsider their responses. The goal is to achieve a consensus. An example of the Delphi technique appears in Box 6-2.

With this process occurring before the strategic planning retreat, the participants came together already in agreement about the goals for the nursing department. This provided a sense of accomplishment before the retreat began and saved time.

There are different variations on the Delphi technique. Nevertheless, the procedure generally calls for anonymous feedback, multiple rounds, and statistical analyses.

One advantage of this technique is the ability to involve a large number of respondents because the participants don't need to assemble together. Indeed, participants may be located throughout the country or world. Also, the questionnaire or survey requires little time commitment on the part of the participant. This technique may actually save time because it eliminates the "off-the-subject" digressions typically encountered in committee meetings. In addition, the Delphi technique avoids the negative or unproductive verbal and nonverbal interactions that can occur when groups work together. Although the Delphi technique has its advantages, using the Delphi technique may result in a lower sense of accomplishment and involvement as the participants are detached from the overall process and do not communicate with each other.

Box 6-2
The Delphi Technique

Before a strategic planning retreat for middle managers, a nurse administrator sought to obtain consensus on the future goals for the nursing department. The administrator distributed in advance the agency philosophy, mission statement, goals and objectives, long-range plans, trends, and future forecasts. The middle managers were asked to review the documents and develop up to three goals congruent with the agency's philosophy.

In the next step, the administrator compiled the list of goals proffered by the managers. For the second round, the administrator asked the managers to rate the goals in order of preference, number one being the most preferred. Furthermore, they were asked to provide a brief rationale for their selection. The results of the second round were fed back to the managers with the narrative comments.

In a third round, the managers were asked to take the feedback into consideration and rank the goals in order of priority. This process was repeated until consensus or the predefined level of agreement was achieved.

DECISION-MAKING TOOLS

Several decision-making tools, sometimes referred to as models, exist to aid a nurse manager in planning a decision-making process or selecting the best decision among the available options. The most common quantitative tools include decision grids and payoff tables. These tools are most appropriately used when information is available and options are known.

Decision grids facilitate the visualization of the options under consideration and allow comparison of options using common criteria. Criteria, which are determined by the decision makers, may include time required, ethical or legal considerations, equipment needs, and cost (see Figure 6-3). The relative advantages and disadvantages of the different options should be listed for each option.

Payoff tables require the manager to establish the cost-versus-benefit relationships and the probabilities of certain outcomes using current information and historical data. To illustrate, the manager of a hospital education department is evaluating whether it is better to retain the services of an outside consultant to coordinate an advanced cardiac life support course in the hospital or pay the per-person fees to send the staff elsewhere. The type of information this manager might compile includes a breakdown of the costs for both options, equipment needs, benefits of each option, the number of nurses needing the course, future training needs, and the feasibility of training hospital staff to conduct the course.

All nurses, whether they are managers or followers, need adequate problem-solving and decision-making skills to be effective in their roles. In addition to relying on your own knowledge and experience, tips are listed at the end of the chapter for increasing your effectiveness as a problem solver and decision maker.

Exercise 6-6

Design a decision grid for a current situation you are experiencing. Identify the components you need to consider in the decision-making process, such as cost, time, resources, advantages, or disadvantages, for the various options you are considering.

Options Under Consideration	Time	Cost	Legal/ethical Considerations	Equipment Needed

Figure 6-3   Decision grid.

A Manager's Solution

Effective problem solving requires a thorough and complete analysis of the problem. The more information discovered affecting the problem increases the likelihood of a successful resolution. We chose to approach this problem through the DEMS process improvement team (PIT). The PIT is a multidisciplinary team of staff who are involved with or affected by the processes of emergency care. The team included physicians, nurses, registration clerks, chaplains, radiology technicians, security, retired employees, and management. The DEMS PIT had formed as part of the hospital's plan to drive process improvement by involving those staff who actually do the work. This team had a process "owner" (the director of nursing) and a trained facilitator to facilitate the weekly team meetings. Group memory (minutes and action plans) was the joint responsibility of the owner and facilitator. The team was chartered by the Process Improvement Council (PIC) with the mission to improve all processes associated with the provision of emergency services.

The first step we took was to validate the problem. We thought we knew the perceptions of our employees, as well as the patients and family members, but we had no actual data. We surveyed our staff with a written tool designed to measure staff perceptions of safety and tabulated the results. We also worked with the Patient Complaint PIT (another multidisciplinary team chartered by PIC to improve the processes of resolving complaints from patients) to provide us with patient comment cards that were given to patients and displayed in the waiting room for visitors to use. These cards were collected daily and analyzed for content specific to our concerns. Additionally, we used volunteers to sit in the waiting area and record events and interactions of the

Continued.

A Manager's Solution—cont'd

people waiting for service or for family members. In this manner, we collected both qualitative and quantitative data with which to support or refute our perceived problem, The problem was supported by the data. These data now become our baseline data to which we can compare data after changes are implemented. It is important to be able to measure the effectiveness of change so that we can justify the resources used.

The PIT then moved into identifying root causes of the problem. We began by flowcharting the process of obtaining a security officer on demand. Flowcharting processes helps us to identify how many steps are involved in the process. Generally speaking, the fewer the steps, the more effective and efficient the process. A security officer was posted in the ER at specific times of the day, but not at other times. Therefore the process for obtaining a security officer differed according to the time of day, the day of the week, and incidences or needs elsewhere.

Another problem-solving tool that we used was a fishbone. A fishbone (also known as a cause and effect) diagram graphically displays, in increasing detail, all of the possible causes related to a problem to discover its root causes. This tool encourages the team to focus on the content of the problem and not be sidetracked by personal interests of team members. It also collects a snapshot of the collective knowledge of the team and helps build consensus around the problem. The "effect" is generally the problem statement, such as lack of perceived security in DEMS, and is placed at the right end of the figure (the "head" of the fish). The major categories of causes are the main bones and are supported by smaller bones representing issues that contribute to the main causes (see Figure 6-4).

After analyzing causes of the problem, the DEMS PIT was ready to start developing solutions. We surveyed other hospitals to find out how they dealt with security in the DEMS, and we referred to the literature as well. We analyzed our physical area to determine if reconfiguration was possible. The best solution, we soon realized, was reducing the number of steps the staff needed to alert security of a possible problem and to obtain security response. Therefore we relocated the security office to the

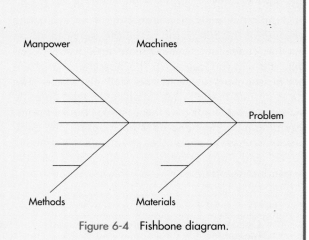

Figure 6-4   Fishbone diagram.

waiting room of the DEMS. The office has bulletproof glass encasing it, but the security officers are visible, as is the bank of video surveillance cameras. The presence of security officers in the DEMS has decreased the number of incidents in the area, and we are hoping that the vandalism of the waiting area bathroom will decrease.

It is important in any problem-solving process to recheck your answers. Patient and visitor complaints are still being collected and analyzed. Staff members have been resurveyed to measure their perceptions of security in the DEMS. The data support increased staff perceptions of security, but reveal further security issues. These new data are being analyzed by the PIT, and action plans continue to be developed. The success of this project depended on the accuracy and completeness of the information obtained. Staff closely involved with the process are the best source of this information, and it is essential that staff be included in the problem solving. Staff learn the effectiveness of problem-solving tools, and management learns much more about the actual processes involved in patient care. Both staff and managers gain knowledge, but more importantly, both realize that they are part of one team and that the success of this team depends on their combined knowledge.

Would this be a suitable approach for you? Why?

CHAPTER CHECKLIST

The ability to make good decisions and encourage effective decision making in others is a hallmark of nursing leadership and management. A nurse manager is in a good position to facilitate effective decision-making by individuals and groups. This requires good communication skills, knowledge of the vagaries of group dynamics, and the ability to foster an environment conducive to effective problem solving, decision making, and creative thinking.

- The main steps of the traditional problem-solving process include:
  - define the problem, issue, or situation
  - gather data
  - analyze data
  - develop solutions and options
  - select solution
  - implement
  - evaluate
- A decision-making format involves:
  - listing options
  - identifying the pros and cons of each option
  - ranking the options in order of preference
  - selecting the best option
- If you want to make sound decisions or solve problems effectively, information gathered must be:
  - accurate
  - relevant
  - valid
  - timely
- The situation and circumstances should dictate the leadership style used by managers to solve problems and make decisions. Analytical tools that are helpful in planning and illustrating decision-making activities include:
  - decision grids
  - gap analysis exercises
  - problem definition exercises
  - fishbone analysis

TIPS FOR PROBLEM SOLVING AND DECISION MAKING

- Seek additional information from other sources even if it doesn't support the preferred action.
- Learn how other people approach problem situations.
- Talk to colleagues and superiors who you believe are effective problem solvers and decision makers. Observe these positive role models in action.
- Read journal articles and relevant sections of textbooks to increase your knowledge base.
- Risk using new approaches to problem resolution through experimentation.

TERMS TO KNOW

creativity

critical thinking

decision making

problem solving

satisficing decision

REFERENCES

Case, B. (1994). Walking around the elephant: A critical thinking strategy for decision making. *The Journal of Continuing Education in Nursing*, 25, 101-109.

Deguzon, C.E., & Lunney, M. (1995). Clinical journal: A tool to foster critical thinking for advanced levels of competence. *Clinical Nurse Specialist*, 9, 270-274.

Lamond, D., Crow, R., Chase, J., Doggen, K., & Swinkels, M. (1996). Information sources used in decision making: Considerations for simulation development. *International Journal of Nursing Studies*, 33, 47-57.

McFarland, G.K., Leonard, H.S., & Morris, M.M. (1984). *Nursing Leadership and Management*. New York: John Wiley.

Pankowski, M.L. (1984). Creating participatory, task-oriented learning environments. *New Directions for Continuing Education*, 1124.

Paul, R.W. (1995). *Critical Thinking: How to Prepare Students for a Rapidly Changing World*. Santa Rose, CA: Foundations for Critical Thinking.

Recker, D., Bess, C., & Wellens, H. (1996). A decision making process in shared governance. *Nursing Management*, 27, 48A-B, 48D.

Sullivan, E.J., & Decker, P.J. (1992). *Effective Management in Nursing*. Menlo Park, CA: Addison-Wesley.

Vroom, V.H., & Yetton, P.W. (1973). *Leadership and Decision-Making*. Pittsburgh: University of Pittsburgh Press.

Whitman, N.I. (1990). The committee meeting alternative: Using the Delphi technique. *Journal of Nursing Administration*, 20(7/8), 30-36.

SUGGESTED READINGS

Boney, J., & Baker, J.D. (1997). Strategies for teaching clinical decision making. *Nurse Education Today*, 17(1), 16-21.

Deguzon, C.E., & Lunney, M. (1995). Clinical journal: A tool to foster critical thinking for advanced levels of competence. *Clinical Nurse Specialist*, 9, 270-274.

Paterson, B.L. (1995). Developing and maintaining reflection in clinical journals. *Nurse Education Today*, 15(3), 211-220.

Recker, D., Bess, C., & Wellens, H. (1996). A decision making process in shared governance. *Nursing Management*, 27, 48A-B, 48D.

Stark, J. (1995). Critical thinking: Taking the road less traveled. *Nursing*, 25(11), 52-6.

Stuart, C.C. (1997). Education. Reflective journals as a teaching/learning strategy: A literature review. *British Journal of Midwifery*, 5(7), 434-438.

Managing the Organization

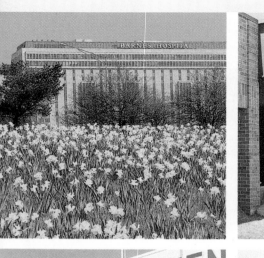

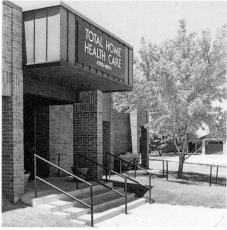

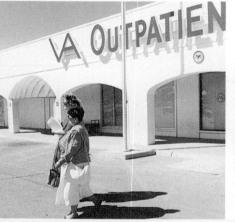

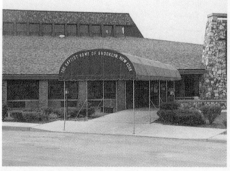

Healthcare Organizations

Carol Alvater Brooks
RN, DNSc, CNAA

This chapter presents an overview of the healthcare organizations that are emerging in a time of rapid change. Characteristics that have differentiated types of organizations are presented, as are issues that are altering these characteristics. Economic, social, and demographic factors that are driving change are discussed. A major emphasis is placed on management and leadership responses that professional nurses must consider in planning the delivery of nursing care in the changing environment. Professional nursing students, as well as followers, leaders, and managers engaged in active practice, must be aware of the changing dynamics if they choose to be appropriately responsive.

Objectives

- Relate characteristics that are used to differentiate healthcare organizations.
- Classify healthcare organizations by major types.
- Analyze economic, social, and demographic forces that are driving the development of healthcare organizations.
- Explain implications for nursing leadership and management role functions of healthcare organization evolution.

Questions to Consider

- What are the changes that have taken place in healthcare organizations in your geographic region in the past 5 years?
- What changes have taken place in specific characteristics of ownership, service orientation, teaching status, and financing of healthcare organizations in your community?
- What economic, social, and demographic factors are forces that are driving the development of healthcare organizations in your community?
- What leadership and management functions are nurses performing in relationship to the evolution of healthcare organizations in your geographic region?

A Manager's Challenge

From the Director of Case Management at a Tertiary Care Facility in the Northeast

As a Director of Case Management in a tertiary care facility, it is a challenge to be innovative in keeping the costs of care within the capitated rates agreed on between the third-party payers and the institution that employs me. A concomitant challenge is to be certain that clients who are discharged have the supports in place in the community to lead a safe and comfortable life. Many clients lack the social and emotional supports to cope with their dependencies. Frequently the agency spends thousands of dollars to bring a client from an acute state to a stable state, only to find that the client is unable to maintain that stable state in the community and is repeatedly readmitted for acute care services.

What do you think you would do if you were this manager?

INTRODUCTION

Healthcare organizations make up the healthcare system, which provides the totality of services offered by all of the health disciplines. Economic, social, and demographic factors affect the purpose and structuring of the system, which in turn affect the mission, philosophy, and structure of healthcare organizations.

In the past, healthcare organizations provided two general types of services: illness care (restorative) and healthcare (preventive). Illness care services help the sick and injured. Healthcare services promote better health and illness and accident prevention. Although most organizations (such as hospitals, clinics, public health departments, community-based organizations, and physicians' offices) have provided both illness and wellness services, the focus has been on illness. Recent economic, social, and demographic changes have placed emphasis on the development of organizations that focus on health (wellness and prevention) so as to meet consumers' needs in more cost-effective ways. Emphasis is being placed on the role of the nurse both as a designer of these restructured organizations and as a healthcare leader and manager within the organizations.

Nurses practice in many different types of healthcare organizations. Nursing roles develop in response to the same social, economic, and demographic factors that shape the organizations in which they work. As the largest group of healthcare professionals providing direct and indirect care services to consumers, nurses have an obligation to present unified direction for the development of healthcare, social, and economic policies that shape healthcare organizations.

CHARACTERISTICS AND TYPES OF ORGANIZATIONS

The healthcare industry is made up of many types of organizations. Since the process of healthcare system development is in a continual state of evolution, issues surround both the characteristics used to differentiate healthcare organizations and the types of organizations.

Institutional Providers

Hospitals and long-term and rehabilitation facilities have traditionally been classified as institutional providers. Major characteristics that differentiate institutional and other types of healthcare organizations are (1) services offered, (2) ownership, (3) financial provisions, (4) teaching status, (5) length of direct service provision, (6) geographic location, and (7) accreditation and licensure status.

Services offered is a key characteristic used to differentiate institutional providers. They range from specialty institutions limited to providing services for a specific disease entity or population segment to those referred to as general, which provide a full range of services for all segments of the population. Examples of specialty hospitals are those limited to psychiatric care, burn care, children's care, women's and infants' care, and oncology care. Another aspect is the duration of services offered. Some services are short term, such as those provided in acute care institutions where patients are discharged as soon as their conditions are stabilized. Others are long term, such as those provided by some geriatric organizations that provide care services from onset of impairments until death. Many institutions, however, are multiunit and have components of both short-term and long-term services; they may provide acute care, home care, hospice care, ambulatory clinic care, day surgery, and an increasing number of other services such as day care for dependent children and adults or focused services such as Meals-on-Wheels. Healthcare networks is a term used to refer to units connected with institutions that either are owned by the institutions or have cooperative agreements with the institutions to provide a full spectrum of wellness and illness services ranging from **primary care** (first access care) to **secondary care** (disease restorative care) through **tertiary care** (rehabilitative or long-term care). Table 7-1 describes the continuum of care and the units of healthcare organizations that provide services in the three phases of the continuum.

Ownership designated as either **private** or **public** is a second characteristic used to classify healthcare organizations. Private institutions are those directed and supported by private citizens. Multihospital systems, which are defined as two or more institutional providers having common owners, represent a significant development that has taken place in the last two decades. Public institutions are government-owned organizations providing health services to groups of people under the support and direction of the local, state, or federal government. Public institutions' ser-

Table 7-1	CONTINUUM OF HEALTHCARE ORGANIZATIONS	
Type of Care	**Purpose**	**Organization or Unit Providing Services**
Primary	Entry into system Health maintenance Long-term care Chronic care Treatment of temporary nonincapacitating malfunction	Ambulatory care centers Physicians' offices Preferred provider organizations Nursing centers Independent provider organizations Health maintenance organizations School health clinics
Secondary	Prevent disease complications	Home health care Ambulatory care Nursing centers
Tertiary	Rehabilitation Long-term care	Home health care Long-term care Rehabilitation centers Skilled nursing facilities Assisted living programs

vices are often provided without cost to specially designated clients such as veterans and prisoners. They may also be offered at a reduced rate to the medically indigent. These organizations are directly answerable to the sponsoring government agency or boards and indirectly responsible to elected officials and taxpayers who support them. Examples of these at the federal level are Veterans, Army and Navy, Indian, Marine, and prisoner healthcare organizations. State-supported organizations may be health service teaching facilities, chronic care facilities, and prisoner facilities. Local supported facilities include county- and city-supported facilities. Table 7-2 shows how several common healthcare organizations are classified.

Exercise 7-1

Using the local telephone directory, determine the types and numbers of primary care, secondary care, and tertiary care services available. Table 7-2 is an example of a format for collecting data.

Financial provisions, referred to as operating either for profit or **not for profit**, are another characteristic that classifies organizations. Operating without profit means that funds are redirected into the organization for maintenance and growth rather than as dividends to stockholders. These organizations are required to serve people regardless of their ability to pay. Not-for-profit organizations located in impoverished urban and rural areas have frequently been economically disadvantaged by the amounts of uncompensated care that they provide. Some states,

such as New York, have created charity pools to which all not-for-profit organizations in the state are required to contribute in order to offset financial problems of the disadvantaged institutions. Tax exempt not-for-profit organizations that meet health needs of the public may also be referred to as voluntary agencies. Although not-for-profit organizations have been tax-exempt, the continuation of this exemption is being debated (Theisen & Pelfrey, 1993). The owners of these organizations include churches, communities, industries, and special interest groups such as labor unions.

Organizations that operate for profit are also referred to as proprietary organizations. These investor-owned hospitals serve only people who can pay for their services either directly or indirectly through organizations such as private or public insurers, known as **third-party payers.** Owners may be individuals, partnerships, corporations, or multisystems. Many for-profit organizations, like the not-for profit ones, receive supplementary funds through private and public sources to provide special services and research. This funding is the means for them to provide financial assistance to clients who can afford ordinary care, but are not in a position to finance catastrophic occurrences such as vital organ failure, birth of premature or sick infants, or bone marrow transplants for metastatic disease.

Investor-owned multihospital systems are becoming increasingly popular. Nursing homes, home care, psychiatric services, and health maintenance

Table 7-2	**CHARACTERISTICS AND TYPES OF HEALTHCARE ORGANIZATIONS**					
			Characteristics			
Healthcare Organization	Type	Services	Own	Fin	Tchg	Multi
Veterans Administration	Instit	General	Fed	NP	Y	Y
Upstate Medical Center	Instit	General	State	NP	Y	Y
Community General	Instit	General	Private	NP	N	Y
Shriners Burn Hospital	Instit	Specialty	Private	NP	N	N
Prepaid Health Plan	Ambu group HMO	General	Private	NP	N	N
Public Health Department	Commun	General	State	NP	N	N
Eastside Women's and Infants' Project	Commun	Specialty	State	NP	N	N
Brookdate Geriatric Corporation	Instit	Long term	Private	NP	N	Y

Key:
Ambu = ambulatory
Commun = community
Fed = federal
Fin = financing

HMO = health maintenance
    organization
Instit = institution
Multi = multiunit
N = No

NP = nonprofit
Own = ownership
Tchg = teaching status
Y = Yes

organizations (HMOs) are frequently units in such systems.

Teaching status is a fourth characteristic that is used to classify healthcare organizations. The term **teaching institution** is applied to academic health centers such as the Massachusetts General Hospital in Boston, Massachusetts, and to affiliated teaching hospitals that provide only the clinical portion of a health education institution's teaching program. Traditionally these programs have received government reimbursement to cover the costs to the institution of the educational program that are not covered by typical fees for patient care. Costs include financial coverage for salaries of physicians who supervise students' care delivery and participate in educational programs such as teaching rounds and seminars. Currently these expenses are reimbursed based on a formula that takes into consideration the cost of caring for low-income and uninsured patients who populate academic teaching programs. Revisions in this reimbursement are occurring as states reduce subsidies for the education of physicians.

Exercise 7-2

Return to the data started in the first exercise and add financial and teaching status information.

Consolidated Systems

Healthcare organizations are being organized into **consolidated systems** both through the formation of multihospital systems that are for profit or not for profit and through the development of networks of independently owned and operated healthcare organizations.

Consolidated systems tend to be organized along five levels. The first includes the large national hospital companies, most of which are investor owned; they include Columbia, Hospital Corporation of America, and Humana. The second level involves large voluntary affiliated systems such as Voluntary Hospitals of America, an organization that represents over 500 hospitals in the country, providing them with access to capital, political power, management expertise, joint venture opportunities, and linkages with health insurance services. The third level involves regional hospital systems such as Southwest Health Care System in New Mexico and Intermountain Health Care System in the Salt Lake area. The fourth level involves metropolitan-based systems such as Henry Ford in Detroit and the New York Health and Hospital Corporation. The fifth level is composed of the special interest groups that own and operate units organized along religious lines, teaching interests, or related special interests that drive their activities. This level often crosses over the regional, metropolitan, and national levels already described. An example of the fifth level is the Sisters of Mercy Health Corporations, which has its headquarters in Farmington Hills, Michigan, and has hospitals in Michigan, Iowa, and Indiana. Among the reasons for creating multiunit systems are increasing the power of the units in competing for clients, influencing public policy, and obtaining funding in an increasingly competitive and complex marketplace (Shortell, Kaluzny & associates, 1988).

ACQUISITIONS AND MERGERS

Economic forces in the shape of capitated payments and managed care are driving responses of healthcare organizations' reorganizing, restructuring, and reengineering to decrease waste and economic inefficiency. Many organizations are forming multiinstitutional alliances that integrate healthcare systems under a common organizational infrastructure. These alliances are accomplished through acquisitions or mergers. Acquisitions involve one organization directly buying another. Mergers involve combining two or more organizations and their assets to form a new entity. Mergers can also happen within organizations as departments or patient care units come together. People, structure, culture, and political issues or organizational change can be very traumatic and lead to dysfunctional outcomes unless managed. Diania et al (1997) have developed a work transformational model to facilitate the merger process based on transformation theory. Elements of structuring to meet the need generated by continuous restructuring are further discussed in Chapter 9.

NETWORKS

Predictions are that by the year 2000, markets with 100,000 or more residents will be served by one to three health **networks**. The networks will likely follow one of three organizational models: public utilities, for-profit businesses, or loose alliances. Public utility models will be set up and governed just like today's public utilities, for example, the county water department. They will be aimed at serving large regional populations such as Benefits Healthcare, Great Falls, Montana. In most markets, two or three competing markets will emerge that will require significant capital, causing many traditional not-for-profit providers to shift to for-profit status. Systems taking this approach are George Washington University, Washington, D.C.; Sharp HealthCare, San Diego; and University Hospital, Oklahoma City. Loose alliances will take the shape of loosely connected "virtual" networks that emulate integrated health systems through contracts and linked computer systems. Current alliances are West Tennessee Healthcare, Jackson, Tennessee, and PennCare, Allentown, Pennsylvania.

AMBULATORY-BASED ORGANIZATION

Many health services are provided on an ambulatory basis. The organizational setting for much of this care has been the group or private physician's office. A growing form of group practice is prepaid group practice plans, referred to as **managed care** systems, which combine care delivery and financing and provide comprehensive services for a fixed prepaid fee. A goal of these services is to reduce the cost of expensive acute hospital care by focusing on out-of-hospital preventive care and illness follow-up care. Group practice plans take various forms. One form has a centralized administration that directs and salaries physician practice, such as HMOs.

The HMO is a configuration of health agencies that provide basic and supplemental health maintenance and treatment services to voluntary enrollees who prepay a fixed periodic fee without regard to the amount of services used. To be federally qualified, an HMO company must offer hospital and outpatient services, treatment and referral for drug and alcohol problems, laboratory and radiological services, preventive dental services for children under age 12 years, and preventive health services in addition to physician services.

Independent practice associations (IPAs) are a form of group practice in which physicians in private offices are paid on a **fee-for-service** basis by a prepaid plan to deliver care to enrolled members. Preferred provider organizations (PPOs) operate similarly to IPAs in that contracts are developed with private practice physicians, but here fees are discounted from their usual and customary charges. In return, physicians are guaranteed prompt payment.

Nurse practitioners' leadership in managing patients in these group practices has contributed greatly to their success. Examples of this can be found by reviewing literature related to nurses' activities at the Kaiser Permanente HMO in California and the Harvard Community Health Plan in Boston, Massachusetts.

A growing number of freestanding ambulatory centers are developing. These organizations include surgi-centers, urgent care centers, primary care centers, and imaging centers.

Exercise 7-3

Again return to the data started in the first exercise and add information about the status of multiunit systems being in place.

Community Services

Community services, including public health departments, are focused on treatment of the community rather than the individual. The historical focus of these organizations has been on control of infectious agents and provision of preventive services under the auspices of public health departments. Funds are allocated to local health departments by local, state, and federal governments for personal health services that include maternal and child care, communicable diseases such as AIDS and tuberculosis, children with birth defects, and mental healthcare. Monies are also allocated for environmental services such as ensuring that food services meet established standards and for health resources such as control of reproduction, promotion of safer sex, and breast cancer screening programs. Local health departments have been provided some autonomy in designating the usage of funds that are not assigned to categorical programs.

School health programs whose funds are also allocated to them by local, state, and federal governments have traditionally been organized to control infectious disease outbreaks, to detect and refer problems that interfere with learning, to treat on-site injuries and illnesses, and to provide basic health education programs. Increasingly, schools are being seen as primary care sites for children.

Visiting nurse associations, which are voluntary organizations, have provided a large amount of the follow-up care for patients after hospitalization and for newborns and their mothers. Some are organized by city, and others serve regions.

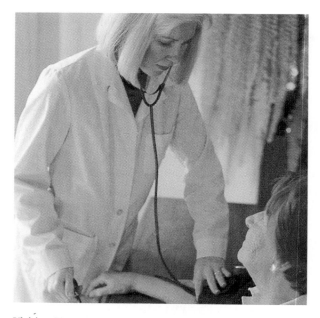

Visiting Nurse Associations provide follow-up care at home for many.

Other Services

Although hospitals, nursing homes, health departments, visiting nurse services, and private physician offices have made up the traditional primary service delivery organizations, it is important to recognize the increasing role being played by other organizations that may be freestanding or units of hospitals or other community organizations. These include subacute facilities and a proliferating number of home health agencies and hospices. This rapid growth was spurred by the implementation of the prospective pricing system, which resulted in early discharge of many patients from acute care facilities. These patients require highly technical continuing nursing care to maintain a stable status. The focus of these organizations is on the care of individuals and their family and significant others in contrast to a focus on the community as a whole. Many of these organizations are functioning as PPOs, and this is expected to be a continuing pattern in the future.

Nursing Centers

Nursing centers, which are nurse owned and operated and where care is provided by nurses, are another rapidly developing community-based organization (Murphy, 1995). Many nursing centers are administered by schools of nursing and serve as a base for faculty practice and research and clinical experience for students. Others are owned and operated by groups of nurses. These centers have a wide variety of missions. Some focus on care for specific populations such as the homeless or on care for people with AIDS, such as the organization connected with the University of Colorado Health Sciences Center School of Nursing. Others, such as the one at Pace University in New York, have taken responsibility for university health services. Some have assumed responsibility for school health programs in the community; and others operate employee wellness programs, hospices, and home care services. Some are freestanding, and others, like St. Mary's Carondolet in Tucson, which is operated as an HMO, are units of hospitals. Church-affiliated organizations, sometimes operating as parish (shul) nursing, are another part of the growing movement of nursing-run organizations (Nakamura, 1997).

Other organizations are the self-help/self-care organizations. These organizations also come in various forms. They are frequently composed of and directed by peers who are consumers of health services. Their purpose is most often to enable patients to provide support to each other and raise community consciousness about the nature of a specific physical or emotional disease. AIDS support groups and Alcoholics Anonymous are two examples.

Home Health Organizations

Home health organizations may be hospital based, nursing home based, or freestanding and may be for profit or not for profit (Stulginsky, 1993). In addition, professional nurses with expert skills in assessing patients' self-care competencies and building structures to overcome patients' and families' social and emotional deficits in providing sick and palliative care are needed to meet home care needs. Home care agencies staffed appropriately with adequate numbers of professional nurses have the potential to keep the elderly, disabled, and chronically ill comfortably and safely at home. An increasing number of restrictions on home care by managed care companies are threatening the adequate performance of this function.

Subacute Facility

Now that hospitals are discharging patients so quickly, a new kind of facility—the subacute facility—is emerging. Many of these new facilities are just old-style nursing homes refurbished with the high-tech equipment necessary to deal with patients who have just come out of surgery or who are still acutely ill and have complex medical needs. Others are newly built centers or new businesses that have taken over hospitals which were shut down in the merger mania of the last several years. Largely run by for-profit companies, this industry is now worth $1 billion, and it is projected that it will be worth $10 billion by the year 2000 (Gordon, 1997).

Hospice

Hospices can be located on inpatient nursing units like the kind commonly found in Canada, the United Kingdom, and Australia or in the community or residential centers. The concept of hospice or palliative care was launched at St. Christopher Hospice in London. It is not a special place where terminally ill patients go to die. Hospices confirm rather than deny the reality of death. Hospice and palliative care programs express the belief that patients should be helped to die in comfort and dignity (Siebold, 1992).

Supportive and Ancillary Organizations

Organizations involved in the direct provision of healthcare are supported by a number of other organizations whose operations have a significant effect on provider organizations as well as on the overall performance of the health system. These organizations include regulatory and planning organizations, third-party financing organizations, pharmaceutical and medical equipment supply corporations, and various educational and training organizations.

Exercise 7-4

Identify supportive and ancillary organizations operating in your community. Can you determine if nurses are playing roles in those organizations and what functions are incorporated into existing nursing roles? How?

Regulatory and Planning Organizations

A subset of supportive and ancillary organizations is the regulatory and planning organizations. These organizations set standards for healthcare organizations' operation, ensure compliance with federal and state regulations developed by governmental administrative agencies, and investigate and make judgments regarding complaints brought by consumers of the services and the public. They are responsible for licensing organizations based on their ability to comply with all standards contained in health codes and for ensuring that the organizations and their personnel continue to meet those standards. Compli-

ance with established standards is necessary for authorization to receive Medicare and Medicaid funding from both state and federal governments. Public agencies sometimes approve private organizations as surveyors for compliance based on their ability to meet certain criteria. Nursing leaders have played active roles in establishing standards and ensuring that organizations comply with standards both in their roles as members of healthcare organizations providing direct and indirect services to clients and as members of, or advisors to, regulatory agencies.

In addition to roles of approving organizations to function as providers of care and to receive public funds for their services, regulatory and planning agencies influence decisions regarding capital construction, cost and charges for service, personnel standards, quality of services, and working conditions (among other things).

Three private organizations that play significant roles in both establishing standards and ensuring care delivery compliance with standards are the Joint Commission on Accreditation of Healthcare Organizations (JCAHO), The National Committee for Quality Assurance (NCQA), and the Community Health Assessment Program (CHAP) established by the National League for Nursing. All three organizations have met federal requirements for deemed status, which means that federal agencies will accept their inspection approvals as authorization for continuing payment of federal funds for services. Individual states, because of states rights provisions, make their own decisions as to whether to accept their approvals. More information on these bodies can be obtained through websites (http://jcaho.org., and http:// www.ncqa.org., and http://www.chapinc.org).

A third group of regulatory organizations is composed of peer review organizations (PROs) that are mandated by federal regulation to be organized in each state for the purpose of monitoring hospital service utilization and quality of care of Medicare patients. These organizations, like all others, are in a continuous state of evolutionary transformation brought about by the changing needs related to healthcare delivery. Nurses have played key roles in developing, implementing, and evaluating the review processes of these regulatory agencies.

Third-Party Financing Organizations

Organizations that provide for financing healthcare make up a second subset of supportive and ancillary organizations. The government, by financing mechanisms such as Medicare and Medicaid, represents the largest third-party organization involved in health-care provision.

Private health insurance carriers, who account for most of the remaining financing, are composed of non-profit and profit-making components. Blue Cross and Blue Shield represent the nonprofit components. The Blues have led the move of insurers from fee-for-service insurance to managed care. This has been both a cost reduction mechanism and a marketing response to the managed care concept introduced by HMOs and arrangements discussed previously in relation to physician practice agreements. Commercial insurance companies such as Metropolitan, Prudential, and Aetna represent the private sector.

Roles of third-party financing organizations have major effects both on the actual delivery of healthcare and in shaping that delivery through political influence. Proposals of a single national payer system and of group insurance purchase by consumer-constituted health alliances are changes under consideration for these organizations. These proposals are generated by the constantly escalating percentage of the gross national product (GNP) that is devoted to healthcare costs and the increasing percentage of the population that is uninsured. Reconfiguration of the third-party payer system and its organizations will in turn bring about restructuring of healthcare organizations responsible for service delivery. Understanding the interrelated changes in healthcare organizations can be gained by examining the results of the 1982 enactment of the Tax Equity and Reimbursement Act (TEFRA) by Congress, introducing the prospective payment system for Medicare reimbursement. One of the results was the rapid development of home care organizations in response to the early discharges engendered by the system's financial incentives and the institution of financial penalties if clients had to be readmitted within certain time periods.

Pharmaceutical and Medical Equipment Supply Systems

A third subset of the supportive and ancillary organizations are the pharmaceutical and medical equipment supply organizations. About one-tenth of all healthcare expenditures are allocated to drugs and medical equipment. When other healthcare supply organizations, such as healthcare information system corporations, are considered, the estimated percentage may rapidly escalate toward the one-quarter mark. Nurses, as primary users of these products, play a significant role in healthcare organizations in setting standards for safe and efficient products that

meet both consumers' and organizations' needs in a cost-effective manner. Supply organizations frequently seek out nurses as customers and as participants in market surveys for the design of new products, services, and marketing techniques. Nurses are employed by these organizations as designers of new products, marketing representatives, and members of the sales force. Examples of the roles played by nurses can be seen by studying the Hewlett Packard Company, which employs nurses to design new products and market them through production and distribution of a newsletter and ongoing continuing education presentations.

Professional Organizations

Another subset of the supportive and ancillary organizations is the professional organizations whose primary purposes are to protect and enhance the interests of the service delivery organizations and their professional and nonprofessional workers. These organizations, because of their tremendous influence on the healthcare delivery system, must be considered in any discussion of healthcare organizations. Professional organizations operate at the local, state, and national level and perform a number of functions, including protection and support through political lobbying; education; and development and maintenance of standards for caregivers, resources, environment, and care. Examples of these are the American Nurses Association, the American Medical Association, and the American Hospital Association. In addition to the professional organizations, labor organizations representing healthcare organization employees are playing a significant and increasing role in healthcare organization development.

FORCES THAT INFLUENCE HEALTHCARE ORGANIZATION DEVELOPMENT

The radical restructuring of the healthcare system that is required to reduce the continuing escalation of economic resources into the system and to make healthcare accessible to all citizens will necessitate ongoing changes in healthcare organizations. Healthcare organizations, functioning as corporate actors, are a major repository of power within the healthcare system. As previously discussed, healthcare expenditures represent a significant percentage of the gross national product (GNP), and as federal and state governments continue to be major purchasers of care, the influence of healthcare corporate actors will increase. Healthcare organizations and their leaders can actively influence their environment and therefore can create and manage the future of the organizations. Demonstration of the professional nursing organizations' ability to influence their environment has been shown by the many points in Nursing's Agenda for Health Care Reform (ANA, 1991) included in the President's Health Security Plan (1993). Economic, social, and demographic factors provide the input for future development and act as the major forces driving the evolution of healthcare organizations.

Economic factors

The complexity of controlling costs is and will remain a major issue driving development of the healthcare system. Perhaps the most immediate change will be in the increasing direct involvement of industrial corporations as healthcare costs rise and as the financing of mandated employee benefit programs remains a major concern. This involvement is presently taking the form of initiating audits of employee healthcare utilization and designing of benefits packages to control utilization. A form of a benefit package, previously referred to in the discussion of third-party insurers, is managed care, which uses specific standards for approving diagnostic testing, medical treatment, and technological interventions, and periods of time for use of inpatient and community service. Another form of control of healthcare organization services is the development of local coalitions composed of community health providers, consumers, and corporations, acting to unify business initiatives in healthcare cost containment and to provide consumers with input into health planning and policy development. Wellness programs designed to modify consumers' use of and demand for services such as health promotion campaigns, ergonomic programs to reduce work-related injuries such as carpal tunnel syndrome, and fitness and exercise programs are other industrial corporate initiatives being introduced to reduce costs. Nurses are playing key roles in managed care and in organizing and directing wellness programs.

There are many implications for the economy of nurses in healthcare organizations. Development of strategies that allow clients to become empowered controllers of their own health status is primary among these. Responsive structural changes in service delivery will be needed to maintain congruence with new missions and philosophies developed in response to changes. Continuous evaluation will be needed to access cost and quality outcomes related to change. Issues of quality care and access to care will require a continual focus so that bottom line costs do not overshadow quality care provisions. Nurses have a major role to play in demonstrating that access to care and quality management are essential components of cost control. With the increasing involvement of industry, business management techniques will assume greater emphasis in healthcare organizations. Nurse leaders and managers will need to go beyond obtaining education in business techniques to gaining skill in adapting the knowledge to meet the specific needs of delivery of cost-effective quality care. One example of an integrated community health system is described in this chapter's "Literature Perspective."

Social factors

Increasing consumer attention to disease prevention and promotion of healthy lifestyles is redefining relationships of healthcare organizations and their clients. Clients are becoming increasingly active in their care planning, implementation, and evaluations, and are seeking increased participation with their providers. Nursing's history of work with the development of interactive strategies with clients places nurses in a position to assume leadership roles in this area of organizational development.

Demands will be made of healthcare organizations for more personal, responsive, and coordinated care. Leadership will need to be taken by nurses to redesign roles and restructure nursing departments. Evidence of the leadership needed in changing roles to meet these needs through the development of support and assistant services is illustrated by reports from the University of Minnesota Hospital and Clinic in Minnesota (Jeska & Rounds, 1996). Strategies introduced were a staff counseling specialist role to support staff through personal and professional stress and a healthy work environment initiative to address the importance of a work environment where employees feel valued, respected, and heard.

Demographic factors

Resources of geographic regions, such as regional employment status, incomes of the populations, and age of the country's population, are chief among the demographic factors influencing the design of healthcare organizations.

Economic and demographic characteristics of many rural communities result in a larger number of

Literature Perspective

Cummings, K. & Abell R. (1993). Losing sight of the shore: How a future integrated health care organization might look. Health Care Management Review, 18(2), 39-51.

This article presents a vision of the integration of a community healthcare system on a continuum of care that begins with birth and ends after death. Integration and accountability are presented as key elements of the future healthcare system. Elements to be integrated are administration, management, education programs, clinical services, and public health services. Accountability resides with both the care providers and the community. An array of services, connection of the services with events, and understanding of community motivation are essential elements of the system.

Implications for Practice

An integrated system, such as the one this article describes, would be patient focused and sensitive to the patient's concerns and understanding. Central components of the system would include wellness through education, early diagnosis and treatment, and patient responsibilities. Nurses' work could be restructured from an inpatient care setting to a community-based system. Nursing can also take advantage of opportunities to demonstrate its value in integrated healthcare organizations. New paradigms will also be necessary as frameworks for developing nursing roles in new healthcare organizations in order to ensure that nursing value is recognized and rewarded.

---

uninsured and underinsured citizens in rural areas (President's Health Security Plan, 1993). Geographic isolation frequently limits access to necessary health services and impedes recruitment of health personnel. Community-based rural health networks that provide primary care linkages to urban health centers for teaching, consultation, personnel sharing, and high technological services provision are one solution to meeting needs in rural areas. Federal and state funding, which includes incentives for healthcare personnel to work in rural areas, is another approach. Strategic planning by nursing has provided the means of economically responding to needs of rural communities in some institutions (Smith, Sat, & Piland, 1993).

The largest influence exerted on healthcare organizations comes from the aging of the population. By the year 2025, it is predicted that over 18% of the population will be over 65 years of age. Increasing numbers of the population are in the group classified as "the old old," those over 80. Recent information shows that this segment of the population does not have the dependency needs society anticipated. Despite these findings, the aging of the population is creating a need for more long-term beds, supportive housing, and community programs. To meet these emerging needs of the elderly, new healthcare organizations will continue to evolve, be evaluated, and be restructured based on findings. New roles for nurs-

es as leaders and managers of elderly care are evolving, such as the roles being played by advanced nurse practitioners in directing the care of clients who have become members of geriatric corporations.

Another major impact on the system will come from the increasing number of poor people who are able to afford care to meet only their most basic needs, if that. The need to create means to cover a broader array of basic healthcare expenses assumes increasing importance because of the increase in expenses caused by not treating a minor problem, such as high blood pressure, until it results in a high-cost illness such as a cerebral vascular accident. This lack of healthcare provision is compounded by the number of people excluded from coverage due to preexisting health conditions and job loss. Means of financing care will change as partial solutions to these problems; those changes will affect existing healthcare organizations.

A SYSTEMS THEORETICAL PERSPECTIVE

Systems theory produces a model that explains the process of healthcare organization evolution (see Figure 7-1). Systems theory presents an explanation of organizational evolution that is similar to biological evolution. This theory sees organizations as sets of

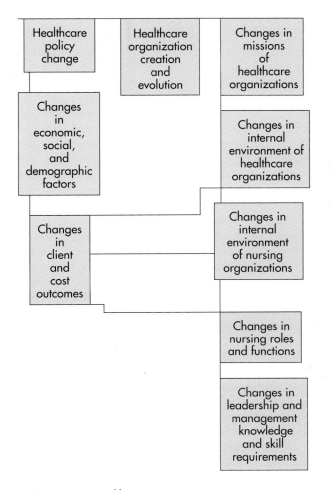

Figure 7-1   Healthcare organizations as open systems.

which put a cap on reimbursing expenses incurred by hospitalized patients. These internal organizational developments placed pressure on the external environment to create mechanisms to respond to increasing percentages of the population with self-care deficits who were returning to the community.

This open systems approach to organizational development and effectiveness emphasizes a continual process of adaptation of healthcare organizations to external driving forces and a response to the adaptations by the external environment, which generates continuing inputs for further healthcare organization development. This open system is in contrast to a closed system approach that views a system as being sufficient unto itself. The effects of external forces on internal structures of healthcare organizations are discussed in Chapter 9.

Exercise 7-5

Think about the changes you can quickly identify in your community. How will they influence healthcare organizations?

NURSING ROLE AND FUNCTION CHANGES

The implications for the increasing leadership and management skills and knowledge that nurses will need are clear in the evolving development of healthcare organizations. They are linked vertically in providing a continuum of individualized care based on client need and horizontally in making efforts to increase their economic viability and their influence in designing and implementing healthcare policy.

Leadership and management roles for nursing are proliferating in the changing healthcare organizations that are developing in response to environmental driving forces. Nurses are finding the proportion of jobs in the community increasing. Nurses need new knowledge and skills to coordinate the care of clients with the many disciplines and organizational units that are providing the continuum of care to clients. Nurses are needed who can engage in the political process of policy development, coordinate care across disciplines and settings, use conflict management techniques to create win-win situations for clients and providers in resolving the healthcare system's delivery problems, and use business savvy to market and prepare financial plans for the delivery of cost-effective care.

The fact that healthcare organizations function as open systems requires that nurses be continuously alert to assessing both the internal and external

interdependent parts that together form a whole (Thompson, 1967). The survival of the organization, as portrayed throughout this chapter, is dependent on its evolutionary response to changing environmental forces; it is seen as an open system. The response to environmental changes brings about internal changes (see Chapter 9), which in turn produce changes that alter environmental conditions. The changes in the environment in turn act to bring about changes in the internal operating conditions of the organization.

A very simplified example of this can be seen by again studying the implementation of the prospective payment system that was caused by the economic driving force of healthcare cost escalation. Ambulatory surgery, same-day admissions, and hospital- and community-based home care organizations are some of the internal healthcare organization changes caused by this environmentally driven policy change, environment for the forces that act as inputs to changes needed in healthcare organizations and for the effects of changes that are made. Awareness of the changing statuses of healthcare organizations and ability to play a leading role in creating and evaluating adaption in response to changing forces will be a central function of nurse leaders and managers in healthcare organizations. Nurses will need to develop a foundation of leadership and management knowledge that they can build on through a planned program of continuing education.

A Manager's Solution

❓ As a master's student, I had become aware of a local community nursing center that was run by a faculty member of the College of Nursing and that served many of the hospital's patients. Several meetings with the center's director resulted in the initiation of a pilot program to coordinate the care of discharged patients with the community nursing center. The center set up wellness plans with all clients discharged with chronic conditions. The plans had a framework of four goals that clients accepted as their own and contracted with the center to achieve. The goals related to (1) promotion of the clients' understanding of their disease, (2) development of self-care skills and knowledge, (3) enhancement of abilities to carry out the activities of daily living appropriate for their age and physical condition, and (4) limitations of need to use the services of the acute care facility for acute episodes of their illnesses. Patients who participated in the referral program and accomplished the goals had no further episodes requiring acute care. As a result of the success of the program in reducing the use of the acute care facility and thus helping the hospital to stay within the capitated rates negotiated with managed care companies, the hospital is in the process of contracting with the nursing center for the continuing nursing care services to their clients.

Cheryl Noetscher

❓ *Would this be a suitable approach for you? Why?*

▍CHAPTER CHECKLIST

Knowledge of types of healthcare organizations and characteristics used to differentiate healthcare organizations provides a foundation for examining the operation of the healthcare system. Understanding the economic, social, and demographic forces driving changes in healthcare organizations identifies needs that organizations must be designed to fit. A recognition that alterations in the environment and in healthcare organizations are mutually interactive is necessary to determine the effects of change and the next steps that need to be taken in response to the constant changes. Changes in focus of nursing roles and settings in which nurses provide service are changing the leadership and management knowledge and skills that nurses need. These changes are part of a continual evolution that demands a foundation in leadership and management knowledge that serves as a basis for future development.

- ■ Key characteristics that differentiate types of healthcare organizations are:
  - profit or nonprofit status
  - public or private ownership
  - teaching status
  - geographic location
  - clinical services provided
  - number and types of units operated
  - relationship with a healthcare network
- ■ Major types of healthcare organizations are:
  - institutions
  - ambulatory based
  - community based
  - third-party payers
  - regulatory and planning agencies
  - pharmaceutical and medical equipment suppliers
  - professional organizations
- ■ Economic forces driving development of healthcare organizations are:
  - high and continuing, escalating percentages of the gross national product composed of healthcare costs
- ■ Social forces driving development of healthcare organizations are:
  - a focus of society that is changing from illness to health (wellness)
  - an increasing demand by individuals that they participate in designing their own customized care plans

- Demographic forces driving development of healthcare organizations are:
  - increasing percentage of society that is composed of the elderly
  - increasing percentage of poor people who do not have the financial resources to have access to care
  - inability of isolated rural areas to provide ready and economical access to needed health services
- Implication of healthcare organization evolution for leadership and management role functions of professional nurses:
  - increased ability to attune to the altered environmental driving forces that predict and direct changes necessitated in healthcare organizations
  - increased ability to attune to the healthcare organization's internal environment in order to predict and direct changes required in both the internal and external environment
  - knowledge and skill in both influencing the development of and in developing healthcare policy at the federal, state, local, and organizational levels
  - knowledge and skill in coordinating and collaborating with peers and other disciplines providing services within a point of service and in networks created by the interconnection of many points of service
  - skill in utilizing business knowledge in planning and evaluating delivery of healthcare in healthcare organizations that must market cost and outcome effectiveness in order to survive
  - knowledge and skill in planning and directing group work, which promotes optimal health statuses with minimal utilization of personnel and material resources

TIPS ON HEALTHCARE ORGANIZATIONS

- Knowledge of economic, social, and demographic changes is essential to redesigning healthcare organizations to meet society's needs.
- Consolidation of healthcare services into large networks that will provide all levels of care necessitates the development of communication systems that provide information on clients receiving services at the various points of care in the network.
- Diversified positions will be available for professional nurses in the various organizations that are developing to enhance the provision of care.
- New configurations of healthcare delivery will demand that professional nurses continually develop new knowledge in leadership and management.

TERMS TO KNOW

consolidated systems
fee for service
managed care
network
not for profit
point of service
primary care

private
public
secondary care
teaching institutions
tertiary care
third-party payers

REFERENCES

American Nurses' Association. (1991) *Nursing's Agenda for Health Care Reform.* Washington, D.C.: The Association.

Cummings, K., & Abell, R. (1993) Losing sight of the shore: How a future integrated health care organization might look. *Health Care Management Review,* 18(2), 39-51.

Diania, N., Allen, M., Baker, K., Cartledge, T., Gwyer, D., Harris, S., McNemar, A., Swayze, R., Wilson, M., & Hinton, P. (1997). "Merger motorway: Giving staff the tools to reengineer. *Nursing Management,* 28(3), 42-47.

Gordon, S. (1997). *Life Support: Three Nurses on the Front Line.* Boston: Little, Brown.

Jeska, S., & Rounds, R. (1996). Addressing the human side of change: Career development and renewal. *Nursing Economics,* 14(6), 339-345.

Murphy, B., ed. (1995). *Nursing Centers: The Time Is Now.* New York: National League For Nursing Press. Pub. No. 41-2629.

Nakamura, P. (1997). Parish nursing on the rise: A growing movement responds to the need of people for wellness. *The Living Church,* 3/16/97, 14-16.

Network News. (1997). *Hospitals and Health Networks,* 3/20/97, 28-29.

President's Health Security Plan. (1993). New York: Random House.

Shindul-Rothchild, J., & Duffy, M. (1996). The impact of restructuring and work design on nursing practice and patient care. *Best Practices and Benchmarking in Healthcare,* 1(6), 271-282.

Shortell, S.M., Kaluzny, A.D. & associates (1988). *Health Care Management: A Text In Organization Theory and Behavior.* 2nd ed. New York: John Wiley.

Siebold, C. (1992). *The Hospice Movement: Easing Death's Pain.* New York: Twayne Publishers.

Smith, H.I., Sat, A.M., & Piland, N. (1993). Nursing department strategy, planning and performance in rural hospitals. *Journal of Nursing Administration,* 23(4), 23-33.

Stulginsky, M.M. (1993). Nurses' home health experiences. *Nursing and Health Care,* 14(8), 402-407.

Theisen, B.A., & Pelfrey, S. (1993). The advantage and risks of being a tax-exempt, non-profit organization. *Journal of Nursing Administration,* 23(2), 36-41.

Thompson, J.D. (1967). *Organization in Action.* New York: McGraw-Hill.

SUGGESTED READINGS

Etheridge, P. (1997). The Carondelet experience. *Nursing Management,* 28(3), 26-28.

Glick, D., Hale, P., Kulbok, P., & Shettig, J. (1996). Community development theory: Planning a community nursing center. *Journal of Nursing Administration, 20*(7/8), 44-50.

Kast, F.E., & Rosenweiz, J.E. (1991). General systems theory: Applications for organizations and management. In Ward, M.J., & Price, S.A., eds. *Issues in Nursing Administration: Selected Readings.* St Louis: Mosby, pp. 60-73.

Kellar, N., Martinez, J., Finis, N., Bolger, A., & VonGunter, C.F. (1996). Characteristics of an acute inpatient hospice palliative care unit in a U.S. teaching hospital. *Journal of Nursing Administration, 26*(3), 16-20.

Kerikes, J., Jenkins, M.L., & Torrisi, D. (1990). Nurse managed primary care. *Nursing Management, 28*(3), 44-48.

Mark, B.A., Sayler, J., & Smith, C. (1997). A theoretical model for nursing systems outcomes research. *Nursing Administration Quarterly, 20*(4), 12-27.

Porter-O'Grady, T. (1996). The seven basic rules for successful redesign. *Journal of Nursing Administration, 26*(1), 46-55.

Shindul-Rothchild, J. & Duffy, M. (1996). The impact of restructuring and work design on nursing practice and patient care. *Best Practices and Benchmarking in Healthcare 1,* 271-282.

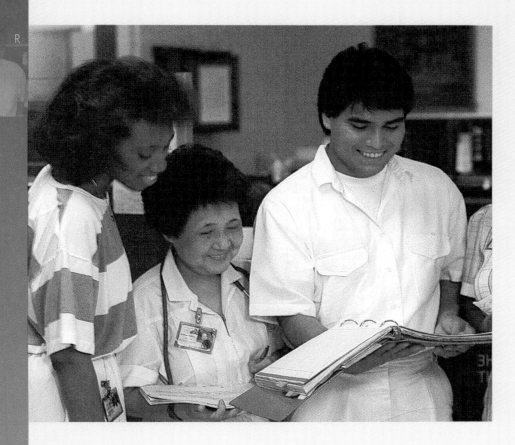

Cultural Diversity
in Healthcare

Dorothy A. Otto
RN, EdD

Ana M. Valadez
RN, EdD,
    CNAA, FAAN

This chapter focuses on the importance of cultural considerations for patients and staff. Although it does not address details about any specific culture, it does provide guidelines for actively incorporating cultural aspects into the roles of leading and managing. It presents concepts and principles of transculturalism, describes techniques for managing a culturally diverse work force, emphasizes the importance of respecting different lifestyles, and discusses the effects of diversity on staff performance. This chapter also contains exercises and scenarios to promote an appreciation of cultural richness.

Objectives

- Use concepts and principles of culture, cultural diversity, and cultural sensitivity in leading and managing situations.
- Analyze differences between cross-cultural, transcultural, multicultural, and intracultural concepts.
- Describe common characteristics of any culture.
- Illustrate the richness of cultures as they relate to personnel and clients through storytelling.
- Evaluate individual and societal factors involved with cultural diversity.
- Compare and contrast values and beliefs about illness that affect management of nursing care interventions involving patients from specific cultures.
- Use tools to address personnel and patient cultural diversity.

Questions to Consider

- Why is it necessary to understand values, beliefs, and rituals held by culturally diverse personnel and patients?
- What implications would "cultural sensitivity" have for you as a nurse manager?
- In what ways do health-related or personal problems vary with the culture of patients and personnel?
- What specific tools could you use to incorporate cultural diversity into your practice setting?

A Manager's Challenge
From a Nurse Manager at a Southwestern Cancer Center

I had a Filipino registered nurse whose name was Alma. She worked here about 8 years and was very good with the patients. She had a 66-year-old man from Saudi Arabia who was hospitalized for sarcoma in the rehabilitation section of our unit. He came from California and spoke English as his second language. He had no family living in the States. He was bedridden and would panic about bedtime for fear of being left alone. He would shake his bedside rails and call out loudly, "Alma," "Alma." She talked with me about him and his "severe insecurity at night." He would become tearful when she would leave his room to take care of other patients.

What do you think you would do if you were this manager?

INTRODUCTION

The American Nurses' Association (ANA, 1993, 1997) has a long and shining history supporting human rights as well as the nursing work force. As early as 1972 the profession supported numerous efforts to eliminate discriminatory practices against specific patients and nurses. In 1993 the ANA took further action that provided a giant step for assuring human rights for everyone. The House of Delegates in an action report agreed that the ANA, along with state constituencies, ethnic minority organizations, and other influential groups such as Nursing Organization Liaison Forum (NOLF), should develop programs to promote an effective, diverse, and multicultural nursing work force. The House of Delegates also requested

the ANA to sponsor a plenary session during the 1994 convention. The session was designed to address multiethnic and multicultural awareness, as well as sensitivity in the nursing work force. At the 1997 House of Delegates meeting a resolution introduced by the Ohio Nurses' Association was accepted by the House. The resolution addresses the problem of racism in the attitudes of nurses toward patients of different ethnic groups as well as toward their fellow professionals. The House of Delegates requested that the ANA take a strong position stating that racism in the work place will not be tolerated.

American healthcare has consistently focused on individuals and their health problems. We have failed some people as a group in recognizing their cultural differences, beliefs, symbolism, and meaning of illness. Frequently, the clients whom healthcare practitioners care for are newcomers to healthcare in the United States. This is true also for new staff. They are neither acculturated nor assimilated into the cultural values of the dominant culture. The knowledge base necessary for providers to recognize and manage cultural differences of clients and staff must be addressed.

Cultural differences that create conflicts and misunderstandings which may result in inferior medical care are addressed by Galanti (1991). For example, consider what communication barriers might occur when an Egyptian physician and a Filipino nurse take care of a Mexican patient.

Gropper (1996) provides critical incidents to delineate a situation that could lead to a cultural misunderstanding. Through these incidents a person's behavior in his or her professional life may be changed as the cultural encounter inculcates cultural sensitivity.

Lipson, Dibble, and Minarik (1996) indicate that culture is influenced by intersections of forces larger than the individual and by shared values of what constitutes ethical professional practice. This is not a "cookbook," but a set of general guidelines to alert nurses in the hospital or community settings to the similarities and differences within and among the groups represented in the guidebook.

The National Advisory Council on Nurse Education and Practice Report (preliminary) to the Secretary of the Department of Health and Human Services (DHHS) clearly addresses the underrepresentation of racial/ethnic minority groups in the overall basic registered nurse work force. The report sets forth a policy goal that federal resources should be used to guarantee that the composition of the basic nurse work force reflects the overall composition of society. This equalization is crucial if we are to deliver meaningful, appropriate nursing services.

MEANING OF DIVERSITY IN THE ORGANIZATION

Leading and managing cultural diversity in an organization means managing personal thinking and helping others to think in new ways. Managing problems that involve culture, whether institutional, ethnic, gender, religious, or any other kind, requires patience, persistence, and much understanding. An organization's culture is significantly affected by the stories that circulate within it. Stories have symbolic power.

Exercise 8-1

Think of a recent event in your work place, such as a project, task force, celebration, or the like. What meaning did people give the event? Was it viewed as being a symbol of some quality of the work place, such as its effectiveness, its values and beliefs, or its innovativeness?

Staff who know what is valuable to the clients and to themselves can act accordingly and feel good about it. Having a clear mission, goals, rewards, and acknowledgment of efforts leads to a greater productivity and work effort from a culturally diverse staff that aspires to unity and uniqueness.

When assessing personnel diversity, the nurse manager can ask these three questions:

- What is the composition of the unit's work force?
- What is the cultural representation of the work force?
- What kind of team-building activities do they need to create a cohesive work force for effective healthcare delivery?

Box 8-1 lists some of the techniques that may be effective when managing a culturally diverse work force.

CONCEPTS AND PRINCIPLES

What is culture? Does it exhibit certain characteristics? What is cultural diversity and what do we think of when we refer to cultural sensitivity? **Culture** is a way of life that is developed and communicated by a group of people and consists of their ideas, habits, attitudes, customs, and traditions (Simons, Vazquez, and Harris, 1993).

The Institute on Black Chemical Abuse (1993) cited four inherent *characteristics of culture*:

1. It develops over time and is responsive to its members and their environment.
2. Its members learn it and share it.
3. It is essential for survival and acceptance.
4. It changes with difficulty.

For the nurse manager these characteristics are important to keep in mind because the underlying thread in all four of them is that staff and patients' cultures have been with them all of their lives. Their individual culture is viewed as normal and the challenge is for the nurse manager to view it also as normal and to assimilate it into her or his existing work force.

Cultural diversity is the term used currently to describe a vast range of cultural differences among people who are different from each other. **Cultural sensitivity**

Box 8-1
Techniques for Managing a Culturally Diverse Work Force

- Have patience. Treat all questions as equally important even though they may be common everyday knowledge to you.
- Be cognizant that foreign or minority staff may not consider themselves deprived or of lesser socioeconomic status than the majority.
- Do not treat gender bias or those with different lifestyles as needing intervening techniques to change behaviors. Assume they are happy with their choice.
- Do not assume emotional outbursts represent anger. This may be a natural communication style for different groups.
- Treat compliments from your staff with respect. Avoid feeling that they are trying to request a special favor from you. In some cultures, compliments are used quite often to demonstrate respect.
- Do not assume that physical features denote a specific race or ethnic identify. Some Hispanics demonstrate Asian features, while some Puerto Ricans or Jamaicans may be mistaken for African Blacks.
- Take the time to know your colleagues. Make time for conversational chats that will facilitate learning about each other.
- Always remember that the less you know about your staff, the more difficult your job will be as an effective manager.
- Be aware that people in your work force may at one time or another have actually felt a part of an oppressed group. Give them a feeling of value and dignity.

describes the affective behaviors in individuals, the capacity to feel, convey, or react to ideas, habits, customs, or traditions unique to a group of people.

Cultural differences are particularly important to Hispanics, whether they originate from Spain, Mexico, or Central or South America. Castillo (1996) wrote of first-generation groups having stronger ties to traditions and customs from their country of origin than second and third generations. Values change as new generations of a culture group adopt the new country's views over time.

In the Black culture, a strong family value system is in evidence. Blacks are more likely to be an integral part of the family structure, receive support from family, and be viewed positively by younger Blacks. In addition, Blacks have a high affiliation and belief in religion, and the church is used as a support system for daily life and during a crisis. Data have shown that some Blacks have lifelong disadvantages of lower economic status, less education, substandard housing, and poorer health status. Consider this question: How will a growing population of Black female elders, who will need assistance with daily living and management of health problems, influence the family support network, the treatment of the aged, and be the family caregiver (Sayles-Cross, 1996)?

A model developed by Campinha-Bacote (1994), entitled "Culturally Competent Model of Care," identifies cultural competence in four constructs: awareness, knowledge, skill, and encounter. Individuals must examine their own biases and prejudices toward other cultures during the awareness process. The skill of conducting a "culturological" assessment is learned while assessing one's values, beliefs, and practices in order to provide culturally competent services. The process of cultural encounter encourages direct engagement in cross-cultural interactions with individuals from other cultures. This process allows the person to validate, negate, or modify his or her existing cultural knowledge. It provides a culturally specific knowledge base from which he or she can develop culturally relevant interventions. Campinha-Bacote believes that individuals must view themselves in the process of "becoming" culturally competent rather than "being" culturally competent.

Nurse managers who ascribe to a positive view of culture and its characteristics acknowledge cultural diversity among clients and staff. Cultural competence includes providing culturally congruent care to clients while simultaneously balancing a culturally diverse staff. For example, cultural diversity might mean being sensitive or being able to embrace the emotions of a large multicultural group comprised of staff and patients. Unless we know the differences, we cannot come together and make decisions in the best interest of the patient.

Exercise 8-2

Think about differences in people's values and how they affect healthcare. What do people who are 20 years old value as compared with those who are 50? What are the values of two people of the same age but who have very different socioeconomic statuses? Visit the public library and look through magazines that are geared toward men and those geared toward women. What values do you see reflected there? How does all this affect healthcare?

Transculturalism sometimes has been considered in a narrow sense as a comparison of health beliefs and practices of people from different countries or geographic regions. However, culture can be construed more broadly to include differences in health beliefs and practices by gender, race, ethnicity, economic status, gender preference, age, and disability or physical challenge. Thus when concepts of transcultural care are discussed, we should consider differences in health beliefs and practices not just between and among countries, but between genders, and among races, ethnic groups, different economic strata, and so on. This requires us to consider multiple factors about any individual, whether patient or employee.

For example, in the medical intensive care unit of the Veterans Affairs Medical Center in Houston, Texas, one of the staff nurses thought of an ingenious idea to help patients who faced temporary physical challenges because they were intubated and on ventilators. This young Filipino nurse developed a "talking board" that allowed patients to point to words that reflected their needs, such as "turn me," "I have pain," or "I am cold." As the patients became stronger and were able to write, they used part of the talking board to write their needs in their own words.

The range of attitudes toward culturally diverse groups can be viewed along a continuum of intensity (Lenburg et al, 1995, p. 4):

hate . . . contempt . . . tolerance . . . respect . . . celebration/affirmation

Two questions that are addressed by Lenburg and others in becoming culturally competent should be considered by practicing nurses (p. 10):

- What has more influence on health and illness behavior—a group's cultural characteristics or the political and economic context in which it exists?
- Is it the cultural characteristics of clients that affect their behavior in the healthcare system or the knowledge and behavior of providers?

Variables that may influence the nurse's response may include how the illness is perceived by the culture and the cultural competency of the healthcare provider.

Leininger (1990) identified several major theoretical premises relating to transcultural nursing theory that nurse managers and staff can follow (see theory box):

Culturally based care values, beliefs, and practices are essential to human growth, living and survival; health values, beliefs, and practices are derived from the culture, and vary between and within cultures; health and care concepts are identifiable by cultural groups and are linked together by cultural values and action patterns; features of social structure are powerful forces influencing health and care in any culture; and, folk and professional care and health values and action patterns are identifiable in a given culture.

Perhaps *communication* is the most important factor that reflects who we are, how we react, and how we approach problems and interpret them. How close we stand to each other is a variable of culture. So are hand gestures, intonation and inflections, slang (see Box 8-2),

Box 8-2
Slang Terms and Their Meanings

TERM	MEANING
"Spent weekend on the Chesterfield"	On the sofa
"You can't act like a wilting violet"	A wimp
"Doing this dopey thing"	Mindless, meaningless
"Clueless"	Doesn't know
"Birds don't marry fishes"	Don't marry outside your race
"It's a disaster"	Chaos
"Peace out"	Goodbye, see ya
"Lip lard"	Lipstick
"Down with my homies"	Out with friends (African American)
"Yo"	What's up?
"Bakwas"	Nonsense talk (India)
"Ciao"	Good-bye (Italy)
"Puti"	White American (Philippines)
"De poca madre"	Cool, neat mother (Mexico)

Cultural Care Theory

THEORY/KEY CONTRIBUTOR	KEY IDEA	APPLICATION TO PRACTICE
Leininger (1991) is credited with developing a theory of culture care.	The theoretical framework embraces the idea that cultural constructs are embedded in each other and their application is broad and holistic. Care is viewed as culturally defined in every culture with predictors defining health or illness.	When patients are given "human caring," the person's cultural characteristics will be addressed and incorporated into the overall plan of care.

patterns of exchange (your turn/my turn variations), use of adjectives (greater in women than in men), and facial expressions. As one nurse manager said, "When we address culture and its embracing parameters, we all bring our own baggage with us. That means that each of us views the world from an individual perspective." All of us have misunderstood or stereotyped people who are different from us, especially in communication styles. What we have done is to expect similar groups to exhibit the same behaviors or norms, thus grouping them into a special cultural "species." Nurse managers need to ensure that ineffective communication by staff with clients and other staff does not lead to misunderstandings and eventual alienation. The staff needs to be able to communicate with clients of various cultures. An understanding, cohesive work force avoids use of foreign language with patients when they do not verbally comprehend that language. For example, in terms of communication between staff and patients, many times it may be the difference in language or the heavy accent of the nurses. Patients may lack understanding or, depending on the way they were raised, they may have feelings about a certain group of individuals. Body language is also different. People living in the United States tend to use slang; people of other origins may think it means one thing when in reality it means something else. Also, their personalities are different. One person may see a warm greeting as shaking someone's hand, when this might be taboo in another person's country.

Exercise 8-3

Consider the patient who is admitted to the postpartum unit after delivery of her third baby. You see that the mother has no right forearm and hand. The patient is aware of your observation, and she comments, "We have our first daughter." What are your reactions to the mother's physical disability? What would you say in response to the patient's comment?

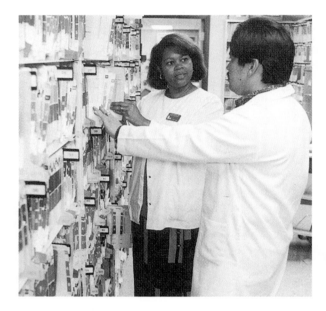

Respecting cultural diversity fosters cooperation and supports sound decision making.

Exercise 8-4

During one of your staff (or student) meetings have the staff members share with each other at least one or two slang words that may have a different meaning for different groups of people. Following the staff meeting have one of your staff post on the employees' bulletin board a list of words discussed in the staff meeting and their meanings (similar to the list shown in Box 8-2, "Slang Terms and Their Meanings"). Allow everyone to continue to add slang words that patients or staff use that may create confusion or misunderstanding.

INDIVIDUAL AND SOCIETAL FACTORS

Nurse managers must work with staff to foster respect of different lifestyles. To do this, nurse managers need to accept three key principles: **multiculturalism,** which refers to maintaining several different cultures; **cross-culturalism,** which means mediating between cultures, and **transculturalism,** which denotes bridging significant differences in cultural practices.

According to Simons, Vazquez, and Harris (1993), some of the most difficult cultural differences to understand arise from gender. This is so because our concept of gender resides deep within our individual psyche and is similarly deeply embedded in our social context. However, a person's sexual orientation—heterosexuality, homosexuality, bisexuality, or celibacy—should not cause him or her to be treated unfairly or discriminated against in the work place.

There is a vast developing body of literature about homosexuality and bisexuality. Simons, Vazquez, and Harris (1993) offer the following suggestions to help guide the manager's practice:

Assume that these persons are already a part of your organization and that you and others are already dealing with them successfully; value the unique perspective that many people have gained by being homosexual, bisexual, or celibate, for example, their increased sensitivity to oppressed groups. Dealing with the misunderstandings and irritants that arise from gender differences is as important as dealing with overt sexual harassment. (p. 185)

Thus the norm for gender recognition should be that males or females be hired, promoted, rewarded, and respected for how successfully they do the job, not because of who they are, where they come from, or whom they know.

Exercise 8-5

Observe the following: How are people who are celibate for religious purposes treated? What about people who are celibate for other reasons? How are homosexual, heterosexual, and bisexual persons treated? Spend a few minutes writing down your thoughts.

In today's work place, female-male collaboration should provide powerful models for the future. Gender does not determine response in any given situation. Yet men reportedly seem to be better at figuring out what needs to be done, whereas women are best in collaborating and getting others to collaborate in accomplishing a task. Men tend to take neutral, logical, and objective stands on problems, while women become involved in how the problems affect people. It is important to recognize that women and men bring separate perspectives to resolving problems, which can help them function more effectively as a team on the nursing unit. Men and women must learn to work

together and value the contributions of the other and the differences they bring to any situation.

Kanter (1993) asserts that managerial uncertainty that was traditionally found is being reduced. She believes that as uncertainty is reduced, so is the need for homogeneity, thus making it possible to accept different kinds of people in managerial positions. The reduction of uncertainty in the nurse manager's job is quite evident because computers make it possible to program many nurse manager tasks, such as client care plans, staffing patterns, and aspects of forecasting.

Accessibility to healthcare in America is linked to specific social strata. This challenges nurse managers and followers who strive for worth, recognition, and individuality for clients and staff regardless of their ascribed economic and social standing. Beginning nurse managers and followers may feel that the knowledge they bring to their job lacks "real life" experiences that provide the springboard to address staff/patient/client needs. In reality, although lack of experience may be a bit hampering, it is by no means an obstacle to addressing individualized attention to staff and patients. The key is that if the nurse manager and staff respect people and their needs, economic and social standing becomes a moot point. Nurse managers must be cognizant of divergent views about healthcare as a right for all people rather than a privilege for a few. Healthcare services are moving from a largely unicultural to a multicultural approach.

LEARNING THROUGH ROLE MODELING

Traditionally, beginning nurse managers have learned many aspects of clinical *role modeling* from faculty and later from expert practitioners. Roberson (1993) writes:

Would it be realistic to hope to learn all the multitude of diverse cultural beliefs in the health arena? No, of course not. What is realistic, however, is for each and every nurse to incorporate principles of transcultural nursing into practice just as you do with other specialized knowledge, such as principles of psychiatric-mental health nursing. Thus, nurses can avoid ethnocentric behaviors. (p. 6)

Ethnocentrism, believing one's own values are the best, most desired, or preferred, is the basis of "cultural imposition," according to Leininger (1990). Ethnocentrism is viewed as a major concern in nursing. Leininger defines cultural imposition as "the tendency of nurses to impose their values, beliefs, and practices on another culture" (p. 55). Such practice occurs from nurses' lack of awareness about the different cultures and nurses' ethnocentric tendencies.

Exercise 8-6

Consider doing a group exercise to enhance cultural sensitivity. Ask each group member to write down four to six cultural beliefs that he or she values. When everyone has finished writing, have the group members exchange their lists and discuss why these beliefs are valued. When everyone has had a chance to share their lists, have a volunteer compile a single all-encompassing list that reflects the values of your work force. (The key to this exercise is that many of the values are similar or perhaps even identical.)

EFFECTS OF DIVERSITY ON STAFF PERFORMANCE

Failure to address cultural diversity leads to negative effects on performance and staff interaction, as described in this chapter's "Research Perspective." Nurse managers can find many ways to address this issue. For example, in relation to performance, a nurse manager can make sure messages about patient care are received. This might be accomplished by sitting down with the staff nurse and analyzing the situation to make sure that understanding has occurred. In addition, the nurse manager might use a communication notebook that allows the nurse to slowly "digest" information by writing down communication areas that may be unclear. For effective staff interaction, the nurse manager can also make a special effort to pair mentors and mentees who are of different ethnic backgrounds. This strategy works because the mentor is able to pick up on mentee clues that allow her or him to draw out information that leads to a therapeutic interaction for both mentor and mentee.

Mancini (1997) speaks to the need for nurse managers and supervisors to be ever-vigilant of attitudes and behaviors that encourage racial-ethnic stereotypes and inhibit communication and trust. She believes a culturally skilled manager who understands and values differences can ultimately build trust and enhance communication, as well as production and motivation in his or her team.

Nurse managers must address communication and motivational issues when working with employees of different backgrounds. Lowenstein and Glanville (1996) challenge nurse managers to use their pivotal positions to confront cultural conflict and render effective conflict resolution. While nurse managers must set the tone, the staff (followers) share in the responsibility for creating a climate that lends itself to open discussions about cultural differences.

RICHNESS OF CULTURES

In many health facilities the staff members, as well as the clients, have a variety of multiculturally diverse backgrounds. Nurse managers must understand and

---

Research Perspective

Chen, Y.-L. (1996). Conformity and nature: A theory of Chinese American elders' health promotion and illness prevention processes. *Advances in Nursing Sciences, 19*(2), 17-26.

Using grounded theory methodology, this study was conducted to generate a theory that best describes beliefs and behaviors of Chinese elders regarding health promotion and illness prevention. Sample size included 21 Chinese elders (11 women) ranging in age from 60 to 90 years. Data collection included two structured interviews in the elders' home, observations during the interviews, personal diary, and the researcher's notes. Analysis of data revealed an emerging theory—conformity with nature. Interrelated subprocesses of the theory included harmonizing with the environment, following bliss, and listening to heaven.

Applications to Practice

- The emergent theory of conformity offers nurses a philosophical insight for understanding the Chinese elders' views and practices relating to health promotion and disease prevention.
- Tenets of the theory can assist nurses in designing health-related programs for populations at risk.
- Nurses should be cognizant of the implications the theory has for nursing practice: use of natural resources, avoidance of disagreement with caregivers, and high emphasis on family input when planning for the care of the Chinese elder.

appreciate the richness of cultures. They should work toward consensus building that offers the staff a practice area that promotes quality care for clients.

Although the literature has addressed multicultural needs of patients, it is sparse in identifying effective methods for nurse managers to use when dealing with multicultural staff. Differences in education and culture can impede patient care, and uncomfortable situations may emerge from such differences. For example, staff members may be reluctant to admit language problems that hamper their written communication. They may also be reluctant to admit their lack of understanding when interpreting directions. Psychosocial skills may be troublesome as well because non-Westernized countries encourage emotional restraint. Staff may have difficulty addressing issues that relate to private family matters. For example, non-Asian nurses may have difficulty accepting the intensified family involvement of Asian cultures. The lack of assertiveness in some cultures and the subservient physician-nurse relationships are other issues that provide challenges for nurse managers.

Exercise 8-7

As part of your "team-building" activities, plan a luncheon with your staff that includes each team member's favorite "homemade" recipe. Ask each person to briefly write or discuss why the recipe is meaningful to him or her, i.e., "we always had it at Christmas," "my grandma said it cured all ailments," or "my dad thought it was gourmet cooking." Share recipes if requested.

Husting (1995) believes that management has a responsibility to address cultural issues because healthcare work forces are rapidly changing. All workers bring to the work place their own values, beliefs, and behaviors. Diversity of these values and beliefs can be in conflict and create a work environment that is not conducive to worker effectiveness and quality client care. The author proposes a model that can help management address a culturally diverse work force and assist in moving them to a culturally congruent work place environment. The model's characteristics include discussing ethnocentricity and moving on to recognizing and respecting diverse views of culture. The outcome of the model is equal worker partnerships, that is, capitalizing on the best aspects of all cultures for an effective harmonious work setting.

The Canadian Nurses Association *Code of Ethics for Registered Nurses* (March 1997) identifies "fairness" as one of its values in which it states, "Nurses provide care in response to need regardless of such factors as race, ethnicity, culture, spiritual beliefs, social or marital status, gender, sexual orientation, age, health status, lifestyle or physical attributes of the client" (p. 17). This comprehensive statement has salient implications of applicability in any country.

Quality of life and human care are difficult to accomplish without knowledge of the group's culture (Leininger, 1994). Her view of cultural care is from a transcultural perspective, that is, examining values, beliefs, and symbols of particular cultures. Accordingly, "quality of life" must be addressed from an emic (inside) cultural viewpoint and compared with an etic (outsider) professional's perspective. By comparing and contrasting these two viewpoints, more meaningful nursing practice interventions will evolve. This comparative analysis will require nurses to include in their cultural studies worldwide, global views taking into account the social and environmental context of different cultures.

Exercise 8-8

Assess several clinical settings. Do these settings have programs related to cultural diversity? Why? What are the programs like? If there are no programs, why do you think they have not been implemented?

DEALING EFFECTIVELY WITH CULTURAL DIVERSITY

Nurse managers hold the key to making the best use of cultural diversity. Managers have positions of power to begin programs that enrich the diversity among staff. For example, it is possible to capitalize on the knowledge that all staff bring to the client for better quality care outcomes. One method that can be used is to allow staff to verbalize their feelings about particular cultures in relationship to personal beliefs.

The National Advisory Council on Nurse Education and Practice Report (preliminary) to the Secretary of DHHS has documented that 9% (206,835) of the 2.2 million registered nurses in 1992 came from racial or ethnic minority backgrounds. The breakdown of minorities included 90,611 Blacks/non-Hispanics; 75,785 Asian/Pacific Islanders; 39,411 Hispanics; and 9,988 American Indians/Alaskan Natives. While the data from the report acknowledge that the racial/ethnic growth of registered nurses has kept pace with the growth in the total number of nurses, the proportion is less than the proportion of minorities in the United States. The only exception is the Asian/Pacific Islander registered nurse population. However, the majority of Asian/Pacific Islander registered nurses are foreign educated rather than graduates from United States nursing programs.

Generalizations can lead to *stereotypes* such as believing that all Hispanics are Roman Catholics, all Jewish people are orthodox in their dietary practices, all whites are WASPs (white, Anglo-Saxon Protestants), or all Asians eat rice. Nurse managers must develop synergism and high morale for a culturally diverse staff. An excellent way to do this is for the nurse manager to use group projects. For example, two or three staff members could be present at a patient care conference. The nurse manager can facilitate the presentation by providing coffee and a relaxed environment. Buttons that convey messages, such as "I'm on a winning team" or "Caring is my job," are high morale boosters for staff.

A program at the Veterans Affairs Medical Center, Houston, Texas, called "Caught Caring" has been a tremendous morale booster for the staff. The unit "caught caring" is awarded a plaque and given a pizza party by top management. In addition, the staff's pictures are proudly displayed near the human resources service. If synergism and high morale are accomplished, they can lead to increased quality of care coupled with positive staff attitudes, thereby lessening cultural stereotyping. Valuing cultural diversity is the key element of an effective manager.

Exercise 8-9

Holiday celebrations have cultural significance. What is the cultural meaning of the specific holiday? How do staff or others celebrate these days?

Araw Ng Mga Patay	All Saints Day, Philippines, November 1
Chinese New Year	China, Chinatowns; January-February (varies with Chinese calendar)
Cinco de Mayo	Independence Day, Mexico, May 5
Ramadan	Muslim/Islamic festival, India, ninth month of Muslim year
Dipavali/Diwali	Hindu festival of lights, India, October-November
Hanukkah/Chanukah	Jewish festival of lights, US, December
Christmas	Compare countries and dates, US, December 25
Kwanzaa	African-American, US, between Christmas and New Year's Day
Boxing Day	Worker's Recognition, Canada, Australia, Great Britain, December 26
Martin Luther King, Jr.	Civil rights, US, January 20

The establishment of *mentoring programs* should be done so that all staff can expand their knowledge about cultural diversity. Programs that address the staff's cultural diversity should not try to make people of different cultures pattern their behavior on the prevailing culture. Nurse managers must select carefully those mentors that ascribe to transcultural, rather than ethnocentric, values and beliefs. A much richer staff exists when nurse managers build on the valuable culture of all staff and when diversity is rewarded. The pacesetter for the cultural norm of the unit is the nurse manager. For example, to demonstrate commitment to cultural diversity, a nurse manager could use whatever programs are sponsored by his or her institution. The nurse manager might make a special effort to ensure that programs such as African-American, Asian-American, and Hispanic days are recognized by the staff. Staff who are active participants in these programs can then be given positive reinforcement by the nurse manager. These activities promote a better understanding and appreciation of individuals' cultural heritage.

Continuing education programs should assist nurses in learning about the care of different ethnic groups. To enhance the development of knowledge related to culturally competent care for diverse and marginalized populations, Meleis et al (1995) identified 10 recommendations. For example, with other appropriate organizations (e.g., Philippine Nurses' Association of Metropolitan Houston) and institutions (e.g., M.D. Anderson Cancer Center), sponsor or encourage the development of a yearly workshop or conference on cross-cultural nursing for faculty and nursing service personnel who have had limited preparation in the area of cultural care (p. 22). Another approach might be to offer a course, such as "Cultural Beliefs in Healing."

A nurse manager may encounter a situation that requires choices or decisions. Kavanaugh's and Kennedy's (1992) Interactive Decision Model presented in Figure 8-1 provides a framework to understand interactive situations in healthcare settings. Every situation involves behavioral choices, although they may or may not be perceived or considered acceptable. Problem-solving communication progresses from the situation through choices that facilitate direct intervention, respectful encounter, and mutual interaction. The Interactive Decision Model illustrates the two-way potential for the flow of communication. Opportunities exist for reassessment of the situation and its accompanying

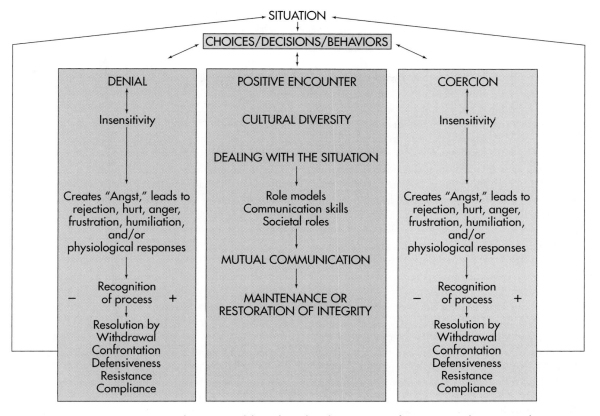

Figure 8-1 Interactive decision model. (Adapted with permission from Kavanagh & Kennedy [1992].)

decisions. However, the bidirectional aspect of the process may also increase the potential for choosing avoidance or coercion as a means for responding to the situation. Some decisions may lead to more productive outcomes than others. All decisions effect outcomes of some type. Mutual communication, as shown in the center of the model, is the most productive approach in situations involving diversity and cultural factors. Untenable or prejudicial beliefs or attitudes about diversity may include ethnocentricism that is based on age, sex, race, national origin, or any other stratifying category.

Exercise 8-10

Identify a situation in which care to a culturally diverse client had positive or negative outcomes of care. If a negative outcome resulted, what could you do to make it a positive one?

Sensitive or controversial issues are often addressed by behaviors that represent avoidance and/or coercion. Whether conscious or unconscious, there is a lack of acknowledgment of the similarities or differences about the issue or person. Avoidance precludes any opportunities for open discussion and potential for change. It is important to realize that avoidance can be a powerful and controlling strategy and that situations do not vanish because they are avoided. Aspects of the situations may eventually resurface. If the situation becomes intolerable, frustration and anger most likely will occur. Various responses are possible, and insistence that the issue is no longer visible in the setting does not imply its resolution.

Coercion is acted out through the use of power or status to persuade people to act in specific ways. Although coercion is not a negative behavior, it can lead to negative consequences through the inequity of power. Coercive tactics limit choices and may result in powerlessness, although the importance of the outcome varies greatly. For example, the use of coercion in a situation may result in anger, which is a normal

Box 8-3
Problem-Solving Communication: Honoring Cultural Attitudes Toward Death and Dying

Scenario #1—Staff and a Patient's Family
What nurses often call interference with the care of a client frequently reflects family attitudes toward death and dying. Often, Hispanic families rush to the hospital as soon as they hear of a relative's illness. Since most Hispanics believe that death is the passing of oneself to a life that offers tranquility and everlasting happiness, being at the bedside offering prayers and encouragement is the norm rather than the unusual. The nurse manager, herself a non-American-educated nurse manager, had worked extensively at helping her staff to understand different cultures. A consensus compromise was worked out between the staff and family. The family, consisting of three generations, was given the authority to decide what family members could stay at the loved one's bedside and for how long. By doing this the family felt they had control of the environment and quickly developed a priority list of family members who could stay no more than 5 minutes at the patient's bedside. As the family member left the bedside, his or her task was to report the condition of their loved one to other family members "camping" in the visitors' lounge. Although their loved one did not survive a massive intracranial hemorrhage, all of the family felt a part of the "passage of life" by their loved one.

Scenario #2—A Nurse Manager and Another Staff Member
Eastern world cultures that profess Catholicism as their faith celebrate the death of a loved one 40 days after the death. The nurse manager needs to recognize that time off for the nurse involved in this celebration is imperative. Such an occurrence had to be addressed by a nurse manager of Asian descent. The nurse manager quickly realized that the nurse, whose mother died in India, did not ask for any time off to make the necessary burial arrangements, but rather waited 40 days to celebrate his mother's death. The celebration included formal invitations to a church service, as well as a dinner after the service. One day during early morning rounds the nurse explained how death is celebrated by Eastern world Catholics. The Bible's description of the Ascension of the Lord into heaven 40 days after his death served as the conceptual framework for the loved one's death. The grieving family believed their loved one's spirit stays on earth for 40 days. During these 40 days the family holds prayer sessions that will assist the "spirit" to prepare for its ascension into heaven. When the 40 days have passed, the celebration previously described marks the ascension of their loved one's spirit into heaven.

Because this particular unit truly espoused a multicultural concept, the nurses had no difficulty in allowing the Indian nurse 2 weeks of unplanned vacation so that his mother's "passage of life" could be accomplished in a respectful, dignified manner.

response to feelings of powerlessness that result from being or feeling controlled. Passivity and aggression often perpetuate the situation, and persons may not recognize the impact of their actions.

It is important to know that choices, decisions, and behaviors reflect learned beliefs, values, ideals, and preferences. The goal of mutual communication is maintenance or restoration of personal integrity and recognition of worth and respect of individuals or groups.

The two scenarios described in Box 8-3 illustrate how problem-solving communication can promote mutual understanding and respect. The first scenario involves a compromise between staff members and a patient's family, and the second involves a nurse manager and a staff member from a different culture.

Exercise 8-11

Identify a situation involving a staff member in which a request was made that requires a culturally sensitive decision. What have you observed about religious or ethnic practices in regard to this decision?

Passages of life that culminate in happy events also can challenge the nurse manager—for example, the *quinceñera* observed by Hispanic families. This event is the celebration for 15-year-old girls to be introduced into society. The nurse whose daughter is celebrating this event must have time to make plans for this festive celebration. Because of the significance of the celebration and the pride that the parents take in their daughter, it is common practice to invite "key" staff personnel to the *quinceñera*. This is one more example of how culture influences nurses and nursing.

A Manager's Solution

[?] As her nurse manager, I discussed the problem with her and she came up with the suggestion of making a contract with him concerning his nursing care. She let him know each day she was working and what she would be doing for him. She reminded him of his call bell (made sure he could use it); and left his room door opened slightly so he could see the nurses' station and know that he was not alone; she was here. She reassured him that between 9:00 and 10:00 PM he would be ready for a good night's sleep. Both the nurse and I monitored the patient to allay his fears as much as possible and to keep his contract with his nurse to achieve a successful outcome.

[?] *Would this be a suitable approach for you? Why?*

CHAPTER CHECKLIST

All potential or current nurse managers must acknowledge and address cultural diversity among staff and patients. Culture lives in each of us. It determines how we think, what we value, how we behave, and how we communicate with each other. In everyday work activities, the nurse manager must be able to:

- Assess personnel diversity and use techniques to manage a culturally diverse work force.
- Lead staff with a clear understanding of principles that embrace culture, cultural diversity, and cultural sensitivity.
- Be able to communicate effectively with staff and clients from diverse cultural backgrounds:
  - Recognize slang terms that have different meanings in different cultures.
  - Understand that nonverbal behaviors also carry different connotations depending on one's culture.
- Describe basic characteristics of any culture.
- Appraise factors, both individual and societal, inherent in cultural diversity:
  - Three key principles relate to respect for different lifestyles:
    - Multiculturalism refers to maintaining several different cultures simultaneously.
    - Cross-culturalism refers to mediating between two cultures (one's own and another).
    - Transculturalism denotes bridging significant differences in cultural practices.
  - Sexual orientation and gender recognition are important factors to consider in dealing fairly with all patients and staff members.
- Use tools that clarify personnel and client cultural diversity effectively:
  - Mentoring programs can help staff expand their knowledge of cultural diversity.
  - Continuing education programs can help nurses learn about caring for different ethnic groups in ways that honor their beliefs.
  - The interactive decision model is an intervention tool that can promote two-way communication, especially when conflict and confrontation are likely.
- Appreciate the cultural richness found among staff and patients/clients.

TIPS FOR DEALING WITH CULTURAL DIVERSITY

Being a nurse manager in a country that views its strength in its population's cultural diversity requires special skills. The nurse manager needs to:

- Ascribe to effective techniques for managing a culturally diverse work force
- Appreciate and encourage programs that address cultural diversity of staff
- Assist staff in problem solving special cultural needs of patients/clients
- Embrace three key principles relating to culture: multiculturalism, cross-culturalism, and transculturalism
- Commit to lifelong learning about culture for self and staff

TERMS TO KNOW

cross-culturalism	ethnocentrism
cultural diversity	multiculturalism
cultural sensitivity	transculturalism
culture	

REFERENCES

American Nurses' Association. (1997). *Summary of Proceedings of 1997 House of Delegates.* Washington, D.C.: The Association.
American Nurses' Association. (1993). *Summary of Proceedings of 1993 House of Delegates.* Washington, D.C.: The Association.

Burner, O., Cunningham, P., & Hatter, H. (1990). Managing a multicultural staff in a multicultural environment. *Journal of Nursing Administration*, 20(6), 30-34.

Campinha-Bacote, J. (March 1994). Cultural competence in psychiatric mental health nursing: A conceptual model. *Nursing Clinics of North America*, 29(1), 1-8.

Castillo, H.M. (1996). Cultural diversity: Implications for nursing. In Torres, S. *Hispanic Voices: Hispanic Health Educators Speak Out*. New York: NLN Press. Pub. No. 14-2693.

Chen, Y.-L. (1996). Conformity and nature: A theory of Chinese American elders' health promotion and illness prevention processes. *Advances in Nursing Science*, 19(2), 17-26.

Code of Ethics for Registered Nurses. (March 1997). Ottawa, ON: Canadian Nurses' Association.

Galanti, G. (1991). *Caring for Patients from Different Cultures: Case Studies from American Hospitals*. Philadelphia: University of Pennsylvania Press.

Gropper, R.C. (1996). *Culture and the Clinical Encounter: An Intercultural Sensitizer for Health Programs*. Yarmouth, ME: Intercultural Press, Inc.

Husting, P.M. (August 1995). Managing a culturally diverse workforce. *Nursing Management*, 26(8), 26, 28-29.

Institute on Black Chemical Abuse. (1993). Eighth Annual Summer Institute, Minneapolis: The Institute.

Kanter, R.M. (1993). *Men and Women of the Corporation*. 2nd ed. New York: Basic Books.

Kavanagh, K.H., & Kennedy, P.H. (1992). *Promoting Cultural Diversity: Strategies for Health Care Professionals*. Newbury Park, CA: Sage Publications.

Leininger, M.M. (Spring 1994). Quality of life from a transcultural nursing perspective. *Nursing Science Quarterly*, 7(1), 22-28.

Leininger, M.M. (1991). *Culture Care Diversity & Universality: A Theory of Nursing*. New York: National League for Nursing. Pub. No. 15-2402.

Leininger, M.M. (1990). Culture: The conspicuous missing link to understanding ethical and moral dimensions of human care. In Leininger, M., ed. *Ethical and Moral Dimensions of Care*. Detroit: Wayne State University.

Lenburg, C.B., Lipson, J.G., Demi, A.S., Blaney, D.R., Stern, P.N., Schultz, P.R., & Gage, L. (1995). *Promoting Cultural Competence in and Through Nursing Education: A Critical Review and Comprehensive Plan for Action*. Washington, D.C.: American Academy of Nursing.

Lipson, J.G., Dibble, S.L., & Minarik, P.A. (1996). *Culture and Nursing Care: A Pocket Guide*. San Francisco: UCSF Nursing Press.

Lowenstein, A.J., & Glanville, C. (1996). Cultural diversity and conflict in the health care workplace. *Nursing Economics*, 13(4), 203-209, 247.

Mancini, M.E. (1997). Managing cultural diversity. In Vestal, K.W. *Nursing Management: Concepts and Issues*. 2nd ed. Philadelphia: Lippincott.

Meleis, A.I., Isenberg, M., Koerner, J.E., Lacey, B., & Stern, P. (1995). *Diversity, Marginalization, and Culturally Competent Health Care Issues in Knowledge Development*. Washington, D.C.: American Academy of Nursing.

National Advisory Council on Nurse Education and Practice Report 1996 (preliminary) to the Secretary of the Department of Health and Human Services on the Basic Registered Nurse Workforce. Washington, D.C.

Roberson, M. (September 1993). Defining cultural and ethnic differences to a changing patient population. *American Nurse*, 25(8), 6.

Sayles-Cross, S. (1996). Aging, caregiving effects and black family caregivers. In Johnson, R.W. *African American Voices: African American Health Educators Speak Out*. New York: NLN Press. Pub. No. 14-2631.

Simons, G., Vazquez, C., & Harris, P.R. (1993). *Transcultural Leadership: Empowering the Diverse Workforce*. Houston: Gulf Publishing.

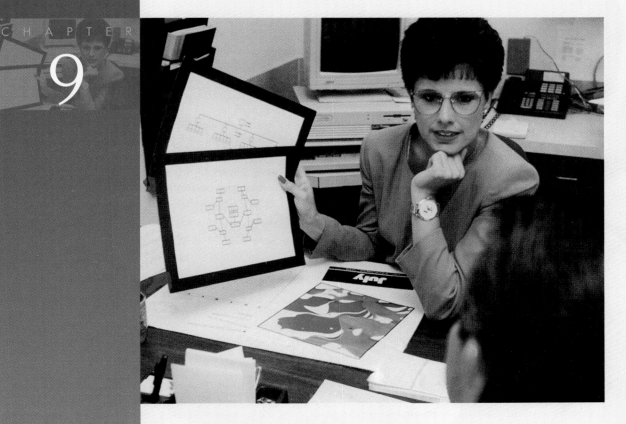

Understanding and Designing Organizational Structures

**Carol Alvater
Brooks**
RN, DNSc, CNAA

This chapter explains key concepts related to organizational structures and provides information on designing effective structures. This information can be used to help new managers function in an organization and to design structures that support work processes. An underlying theme is designing organizational structures that will respond to changes taking place in the current healthcare environment.

Objectives

- Analyze the relationship between vision statements, mission, philosophy, and organizational structure.
- Analyze six factors that influence the design of an organizational structure.
- Relate three types of organizational structures with three distinguishing characteristics of each.
- Evaluate the three forces that are necessitating reengineering of organizational systems.

Questions to Consider

- What is the nursing organization's reason for being?
- What are the beliefs and values regarding patients, patient care, and the workers?
- What characteristics of the nursing organization's structure would best serve patients' and workers' needs and support work processes?
- Who in the nursing organization makes decisions about staffing, work hours, and conditions of employment?
- Where are decisions regarding patient care issues made?

A Manager's Challenge

From a Clinical Nurse Manager of Women's and Newborn Services at a Suburban Hospital in the Western United States

Our 125-bed community-based suburban hospital had always been part of a larger city-based tertiary care facility with Catholic sponsorship. A few years ago, faced with significant competitive forces, our two hospitals, three additional regional hospitals with the same sponsorship, and all affiliated outreach clinics and services formed a new integrated organization with three city-based hospitals under Adventist sponsorship. A new system was born! There were many questions at all levels of the organization concerning structure, decision-making authority, degree of centralization, and the blend-

ing of two distinct religious and cultural traditions. Amidst all of this corporate-wide change, we were acutely aware of new organizational issues for maternity care. Maternal-newborn services had been organized previously within its service line at the two Catholic hospitals. This had also been the case at two of the three Adventist hospitals. The challenge was to decide to what degree, if any, we wanted and needed to work together within our specialty.

What do you think you would do if you were this manager?

INTRODUCTION

Professional nurses work mostly in organizations. Learning to determine how an organization accomplishes its work, how to operate productively within an organization, and how to influence organizational processes is essential to survival.

"Organization" as it is used here refers to the structure that is designed to support organizational processes. The mission or reason for the organiza-

tion's existence influences the design of the structure, for example, to meet healthcare information needs of a designated population, to prepare patients for a peaceful death, or to provide supportive and stabilizing care to an acute care population. Another key factor influencing structure is the philosophy, which expresses the values and beliefs that members of the organization hold about the nature of their work, about the people to whom they provide service, and about themselves and others providing the services.

Exercise 9-1

Consider how you might use the information in the Introduction: (1) to analyze an organization that you are considering joining to determine if it fits your professional development plans, (2) to assess the functioning of an organization that you are already a member of, (3) to make a plan to reengineer the structure or philosophy to better accomplish the mission of the organization.

VISION STATEMENTS

Vision statements are future-oriented, purposeful statements designed to identify the desired future of an organization. They serve to unify all subsequent statements toward the view of the future. Typically, vision statements are brief, consisting of only one or two statements. Within this context, mission and philosophy statements are crafted.

MISSION

The first order of business is the statement of the organization's reason for being. This statement is the foundational assertion from which subsequent statements flow. The **mission** identifies the organization's customers and the types of services offered, such as education, supportive nursing care, rehabilitation, acute care, and home care. It enacts the vision statement.

The mission statement sets the stage by defining the services to be offered, which identify the kinds of **technologies** and human resources to be employed. Hospital's missions are primarily treatment oriented; ambulatory care group practices combine treatment, prevention, and diagnosis-oriented services; long-term care facilities are primarily maintenance and social support oriented; and nursing centers are oriented to promoting optimum health statuses for a defined group of clients. The definition of services to be provided with its implications for technologies and human resources greatly influences the design of the **organizational structure.**

Nursing, as a profession providing a service within a healthcare agency, formulates its own mission statement that describes its contributions to achieve the agency's mission. A purpose of the nursing profession is to provide nursing care to clients. The statement should define nursing based on theories that form the basis for the model of nursing to be used in guiding the process of nursing care delivery. Nursing's

mission statement tells why nursing exists. It is written so that others within the organization can know and understand nursing's role in achieving the agency's mission. The mission should be reviewed for accuracy and updated routinely by professional nurses providing care. It should be known and understood by other healthcare professionals, by clients and their families, and by the community. It indicates the relationships between nursing and patients, agency personnel, the community, and health and illness. This statement provides direction for the evolving statement of philosophy and the organizational structure.

Units that provide specific services such as intensive care, cardiac services, or maternity services also formulate mission statements that detail their specific contributions to the overall mission.

PHILOSOPHY

Philosophy states the values and beliefs held about the nature of the work required to accomplish the mission and the nature and rights of both the people being served and those providing the service. It states the nurse managers' and nurse practitioners' vision of what they believe nursing management and practice are and sets the stage for developing goals to make that vision a reality. It states the beliefs of nurse managers and nurse practitioners as to how the mission or purpose will be achieved. For example, the mission statement may incorporate the provision of individualized care as a purpose and the philosophy would support this purpose through expression of a belief in the responsibility of nursing staff to act as patient advocates and to provide quality care according to the wishes of the patient, family, and significant others. Philosophy both shapes and reflects the organizational culture.

Organizational culture is exemplified by behaviors that illustrate values and beliefs. Examples include rituals and customary forms of practice, such as celebrations of promotions, publications, degree attainment, professional performance, weddings, and retirements. Another example is the characteristics of the people who are recognized as heroes by the organizational members.

Philosophies are evolutionary in that they are shaped both by the social environment and by the stage of development of professionals delivering the service. The nursing staff reflects the values of the times and the values acquired through their education in their statements of philosophy. Technology development such as that of information systems also shapes the philosophy. For example, information systems can provide people with data that allow them greater control over their work; workers are consequently able to make more decisions and take more autonomous action. Philosophies require updating to reflect the extension of rights brought about by such changes.

Mission and Philosophy for a Neurosurgical Unit

Mission Statement

This unit's purpose is to provide quality nursing care for neurosurgical patients, during the acute phase of their illness, which facilitates their progression to the rehabilitation phase to cultivate a multidisciplinary approach to the care of the neurosurgical patient; and to provide multiple educational opportunities for the professional development of neurosurgical nurses.

Philosophy

The philosophy is based on Roy's Adaptation Model and on the American Association of Neurosurgical Nursing Conceptual framework.

Patients

We believe

- It is the right of the patients to make informed choices concerning their treatment.
- Patients have a right to high-quality nursing care and opportunities for improving their quality of life regardless of the potential outcomes of their illness.
- The patient/family/significant other has a right to exercise personal options to participate in care to the extent of individual abilities and needs.

Nursing

We believe

- Neuroscience nursing is a unique area of nursing practice because neurosurgical interventions and/or neurological dysfunction impacts all levels of human existence.
- The goal of the neuroscience nurse is to engage in a therapeutic relationship with his or her patients, to facilitate adaptation to changes in physiological, self-concept, role performance, and interdependent modes.
- The ultimate goal for the neuroscience nurse is to foster internal and external unity of patients in order to achieve optimal health potentials.

Nurse

We believe

- The nurse is the integral element who coordinates nursing care for the neurosurgical patient using valuable input from all members of the patient care team.
- The nurse has an obligation to assume accountability for maintaining excellence in practice.
- The nurse has three basic rights: human rights, legal rights, and professional rights.
- The nurse has a right to autonomy in providing nursing care based on sound nursing judgment.

Nursing Practice

We believe

- Nursing practice must be supported by and support activities in practice, education, research, and management.
- Insofar as possible patients must be assigned one nurse who is responsible and accountable for that individual care throughout their stay on the neurosurgical unit.
- The primary nurse is responsible for consulting and collaborating with other healthcare professionals in planning and delivering patient care.
- The contributions of all members of the nursing team are valuable, and an environment must be created that allows each member to participate fully in the delivery of care in accord with his or her abilities and qualifications.
- The nursing process is the vehicle used by nurses to operationalize nursing practice.
- Data generated in nursing practices must be continually and consistently collected and analyzed for the purpose of managing the quality of nursing practice.

Courtesy of Neurosurgery 7B, State University of New York Health Science Center, Syracuse, New York; Williams Painter, Nurse Manager, and Jocelyne Van Nest-Kinne, Teaching Assistant, Syracuse University College of Nursing.

Obtain a copy of a philosophy of a nursing department and identify behaviors that you observe on a unit of the department that relate or do not relate to the beliefs and values expressed in the document.

Developing a philosophy can be an activity used for **reengineering** a nursing care delivery system. A group process of development provides a method of stating a believed-in ideal and envisioning methods to make that ideal a reality. Box 9-1 shows an example of a philosophy developed for a neurosurgical unit with the leadership of a nurse manager and clinical instructor.

FACTORS INFLUENCING ORGANIZATIONAL DEVELOPMENT

Organizational structure defines how work is organized, where decisions are made, and the authority and responsibility of workers. Structure is a map for communication and decision-making paths. As organizations change through acquisitions, mergers, and downsizing, it is essential that structures change to accomplish revised missions.

Alexander and Bauerschmidt (1987) use contingency theory (see the box on contingency theory) to explain nursing organizational development. They hypothesize that the **fit** between organizational structure and the technologies employed to accomplish the mission determines the efficiency with which the organizational mission is accomplished.

In units such as intensive care and emergency departments, work is characterized by uncertainty and the need for on-the-spot decision making, which necessitates that workers be given authority to make care decisions. Units providing long-term care and rehabilitation are characterized by similarity in care problems such as immobility, urinary and fecal incontinence, and mental confusion; these units may function more effectively with a structure that provides common direction for dealing with these problems.

The issues in healthcare delivery with their concomitant changes, such as reimbursement regulation and development of networks for delivery of healthcare, have profound effects on organizational structure designs. Consumerism, the demand by consumers of care that the care be customized to meet their individual needs, necessitates that decision making be placed where the care is delivered. Change is ongoing as efforts are made to reduce cost and improve outcomes of healthcare. Increasing knowledge of consumers and greater responsibility for selecting healthcare providers and options have resulted in consumers who demand customized care. Competition for clients is another factor influencing structure design. These three factors—change, consumerism and competition—necessitate reengineering healthcare structures. Reengineering, as described by Hammer and Champy (1993); connotes a complete overhaul of an organizational structure, not merely a "tinkering" with one aspect. Flarey (1995) describes the redesign of nursing care delivery systems that must accompany healthcare organization redesign.

Contingency Theory

KEY CONTRIBUTOR	KEY IDEA	APPLICATION TO PRACTICE
Contingency This theory was developed by Alexander and Bauerschmidt (1987).	All the acts necessary to be performed in clients' care must be considered in designing structures for decision making.	When clients' signs and symptoms are generally unstable, nurses must be able to make decisions on the spot. In situations where the clients are relatively stable, decision making may be placed at a level higher than in the units where care is delivered and directed by policies made at that higher level.

Exercise 9-3

Arrange to interview a nurse employed in a healthcare agency or use your own experience to identify examples of changes taking place that necessitate reengineering such as implementation of diagnosis related groups, development of policies to carry out legislative regulations related to the right to die, or development of labor/delivery recovery rooms for marketing. Identify examples of how previous systems of communication and decision-making are inadequate to cope with these changes.

Technological change, particularly in information services, provides a means of customizing care. Its potential of making all information concerning a client immediately accessible to direct caregivers has profound implications for altering decision-making points.

CHARACTERISTICS OF ORGANIZATIONAL STRUCTURES

Knowledge of characteristics of different types of organizational structures and the theories on which designs are based provide a catalog of options to consider in designing structures that fit specific situations. This knowledge also provides useful information to assist managers in understanding structures in current situations in which they function.

An organization is a group of people working together to achieve a purpose. Organizational theory is based largely on the systematic investigation of the effectiveness of specific organizational designs in achieving their purpose. Organizational theory development is a process of creating knowledge to understand the effect of identified factors, such as organizational culture; organizational technology, which is defined as all the work being carried out; and organizational structure or organizational development. A purpose of such work is to determine how organizational effectiveness might be predicted or controlled through the design of the organizational structure. Although many relationships between the variables mentioned above have been hypothesized, there is a need for research studies that test these relationships. (See the following "Research Perspective" for an example of organizational research being carried out in healthcare organizations.)

Organizational designs are frequently classified by their characteristics of complexity, formalization, and centralization. Figure 9-1 illustrates specialization, centralization, authority, and responsibility.

Complexity concerns the division of labor in an organization, the specialization of that labor, the number of hierarchical levels, and the geographic dispersion of organizational units. Division of labor and specialization refer to the separation of processes into tasks that are performed by designated people. The horizontal dimension of an organizational chart relates to the division and specialization of labor functions attended by specialists.

Research Perspective

George, V., Burke, L., & Rodgers, B. (1997). Research-based planning for change: assessing nurses' attitudes toward governance and professional practice autonomy after hospital acquisition. Journal of Nursing Administration, *27(5): 53-61.*

The purpose of this study was to gain information about nurses' attitudes toward governance and practice autonomy in an acquisition to use in planning for the changes necessitated by the acquisition. Structural contingency theory and attribution theory were used to guide leadership staff's assessment of staff attributes to determine their congruence with concepts valued by the acquiring organization. The survey results described nurses' perceptions of the advantages, concerns, and suggestions for a smooth transition after acquisition. By sharing the findings, both staffs were sensitized to the similarities among staff as well as to their differences. Transition strategies were planned to capitalize on this knowledge.

Implications for Practice

Resistance to new policies, procedures, and standards; passive acceptance of new leadership; limited support for management plans; and failure to integrate with new nursing units are common staff reactions after acquisitions. Little has been written about what variables to assess after an acquisition and how to use these data to plan for change. The process may be useful for nurse leaders, managers, and staff to use as they go through similar transitions.

*Compare this same article from a different perspective. Turn to p. 79.

Hierarchy connotes lines of authority and responsibility. *Chain of command* is a term used to refer to the hierarchy and is depicted in vertical dimensions of **organizational charts.** Hierarchy vests authority in positions on an ascending line away from where work is performed and allows for control of work. Frequently workers are placed on a bottom line of the organization, and authority, which provides for control, is placed in higher levels.

Exercise 9-4

Review a copy of a nursing department's organizational chart and identify the divisions of labor, the hierarchy of authority, and the degree of formalization.

Geographic dispersion refers to the physical location of units. Units of work may be in one building, in several buildings in one location, spread throughout a city, or in different counties, states, or countries. An

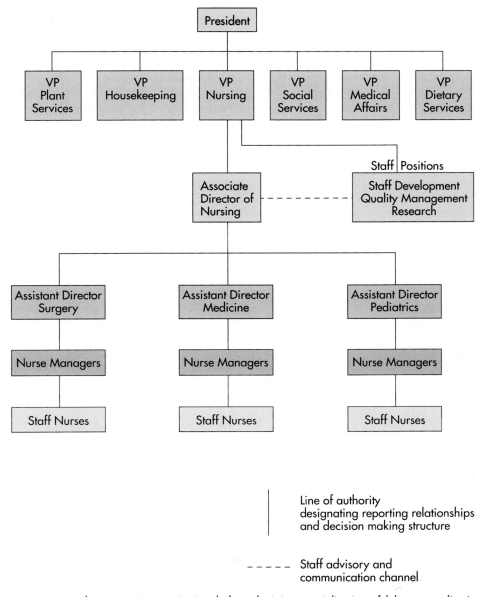

Figure 9-1 A bureaucratic organizational chart depicting specialization of labor, centralization, hierarchical authority, and line and staff responsibilities.

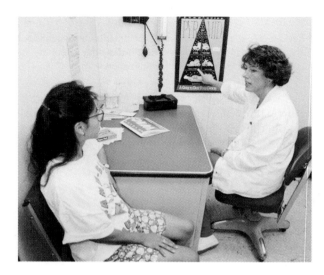

A school health clinic is an example of a geographically dispersed organization.

example of a geographically dispersed organization is Hospital Corporation of America, which owns health-care facilities throughout the world. This aspect of complexity demands creative designs that place decision making related to client care close to the patient and consequently far from corporate head-quarters. A similar type of complexity exists in orga-nizations that deliver care at multiple sites in the community, such as school health programs in which care delivery sites are located in schools that usu-ally are at great distances from the corporate office, which has overall responsibility for the school health program.

Formalization is the degree to which an organiza-tion has rules, stated in policy, that define a mem-ber's function. The amount of formalization varies among institutions.

Exercise 9-5

Review nursing policies in a city health department, a school health office, a home health agency, and a hospital. Are there common policies? Does one of the organizations have more detailed policies than others? Is this formalization con-sistent with the structural complexity?

Centralization refers to the location where a deci-sion is made. In a centralized organization, decisions are made at the top of an organization. In a decen-tralized organization, decisions are made at or close to the patient care level. Highly centralized organiza-tions delegate responsibility without the authority

necessary to carry out the responsibility. An example of this is illustrated by a story related to the writer by a staff nurse who was responsible for a unit that was at full capacity. A request was made to admit an addi-tional patient. The director of nursing was called at home for the necessary permission and had to call the staff nurse for the information necessary for her to make the decision.

TYPES OF ORGANIZATIONAL STRUCTURES

There are three types of organizational structures: **bureaucratic, matrix,** and **flat.** Nursing organizations frequently combine characteristics from the three types, forming a structure that is a **hybrid. Shared governance** is a term frequently used to describe the flat types of structures presently being designed to meet the changing needs of nursing organizations.

Bureaucracy

Bureaucracy evolved from early theories on organiz-ing work. It arose at a time of societal development when services were in short supply, workers' and clients' knowledge bases were limited, and technolo-gies for sharing information were undeveloped. Char-acteristics of bureaucracy arose out of a need to con-trol and were centered around division of processes into discrete tasks. Bureaucratic structures are formal, centralized, and hierarchical and consist of divisions of labor and specialists. Rules, standards, and proto-cols ensure uniform actions and limit individualiza-tion of services and variance in workers' performance. As shown in Figure 9-1, communication and decisions flow from top to bottom, limiting workers' autonomy.

Exercise 9-6

Develop a list of decisions that you as a staff nurse would like to make in order to optimize care for your patients. Determine where those decisions are made in a nursing organization with which you are familiar. Consider such issues as (1) deciding on visiting schedules that meet your own, your clients', and their significant others' needs and (2) determining a personal work schedule that meets your personal needs and your clients' needs, for example, talking to the children of an elderly confused client who work during the day shift, when you are on duty, and visit in the evening.

At the time that they were developed, these char-acteristics promoted efficiency and production. As the general population's and workers' knowledge bases grew and technologies developed, the bureaucratic structure no longer fit the evolving situation. Increasingly, workers and consumers functioning in bureaucratic situations complain of red tape, procedural delays, and general frustration.

Applying the characteristics of bureaucracy to an organization shows the characteristics present in varying degrees. An organization can demonstrate bureaucratic characteristics in some areas and not in others. For example, nursing staff in intensive care units may be granted autonomy in making and carrying out direct client care decisions, but may be granted no voice in determining work schedules or financial reimbursement systems for hours worked. A method of determining the extent to which bureaucratic tendencies exist in organizations is to assess the organizational characteristics of labor specialization (the degree to which client care is divided into highly specialized tasks), centralization (at what level of the organization decisions regarding carrying out work and remuneration for work are made), and formalization (what percentage of actions required to deliver patient care is governed by written policy and procedures).

Bureaucratic structures are commonly called line structures. Line structures usually have a staff component. Line structures have a vertical line, designating reporting and decision-making responsibility, that connects all positions to a centralized authority (see Figure 9-1).

Exercise 9-7

Analyze the decisions identified in Exercise 9-6 from a manager perspective. Is that perspective similar to or different from the original perspective you identified?

Line functions are those that involve direct responsibility for accomplishing the objectives of a nursing department, service, or unit. Staff functions are those that assist the line in accomplishing the primary objectives. Line positions may include staff nurses, licensed practical/vocational nurses, and unlicensed assistive personnel who have the responsibility for carrying out all aspects of direct care. Staff positions may include staff development personnel, researchers, and special clinical consultants who are responsible for supporting line positions through activities of consultation, education, role modeling, and knowledge development, with no authority for decision making. Line personnel have authority for decision making, while staff provide support, advice, and

counsel. Organizational charts usually indicate line positions through the use of solid lines and staff positions through broken lines (see Figure 9-1).

To make line and staff functions effective, the authority for decision making is clearly spelled out in position descriptions. Effectiveness is further ensured by spelling out competencies required for the responsibilities, providing methods of determining whether or not personnel possess the competencies, and providing means of maintaining and developing the competencies.

Matrix Structures

Matrix structures are designed to focus on both product and function. Function is defined as all the tasks required to produce a product that is designated as the end result of the function. In an acute care organization, the desired product may be defined as a satisfactory outcome to the client's problem that necessitated treatment, while the function is defined as all the actions required to produce the product. In a matrix organization, the manager of a unit responsible for a service reports both to a functional manager and to a product manager. For example, a director of pediatric nursing could report both to a chief executive officer (product manager) and to a vice president of nursing (functional manager) (see Figure 9-2).

Matrix structures are very effective in the current healthcare environment. The matrix design enables timely response to the forces in the external environment that demand continual programming and facilitates internal efficiency and effectiveness through the promotion of cooperation among disciplines.

A matrix structure is a hybrid structure that combines both a bureaucratic structure and a flat structure; teams are used to carry out specific programs or projects. A matrix structure superimposes a horizontal program management over the traditional vertical hierarchy. Personnel from various functional departments are assigned to a specific program or project and become responsible to two bosses—their functional department head and a program manager. This creates an interdisciplinary team. Study of a geriatric matrix team program showed that after the program was in place for 1 year, mortality was significantly decreased and the functional ability of patients increased (Newman & Boissoneau, 1987).

A line manager and a project manager function collaboratively. For example, in nursing, there may be a chief nursing executive, nurse managers, and

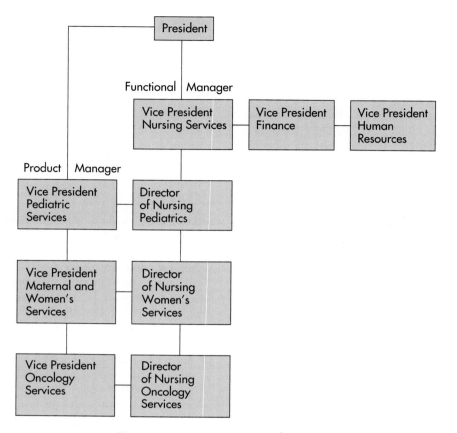

Figure 9-2   Matrix organizational structure.

staff nurses in the line of authority to accomplish nursing care. In the matrix structure, some of the nurse's time is allocated to project or committee work. Nursing care is delivered in a teamwork setting or within a collaborative model. The nurse is responsible to a nurse manager for her nursing care and to a program or project manager when working within the matrix overlay. Well-developed collaboration and coordination skills are essential to effective functioning in a matrix structure. The nature of a matrix with its complex interrelationships requires workers with knowledge and skill in interpersonal relationships and teamwork.

One example of the matrix structure is the patient-focused care delivery model that is being implemented in some facilities. Another example would be the programs focused on specialty services such as geriatric services, women's services, and cardiovascular services. A matrix model could be designed to cover both a patient-focused care delivery model and a specialty service. Other examples are special healthcare facility programs such as discharge planning, total quality management, and cardiopulmonary resuscitation.

Flat Structures

Delegation of decision making to the professionals doing the work, referred to as participatory management, is the primary characteristic of flat organizational structures. The term *flat* signifies the removal of hierarchical layers granting authority to act and placing authority at the action level (see Figure 9-3). Decisions regarding work methods, individual patients' nursing care, and conditions under which workers work are made in the place where the work is being carried out. Decentralization replaces the centralization of decision making at the top of the organization. The solution to the "Manager's Challenge" at the beginning of this chapter is based on the implementation of a flat structure. Providing staff with authority to make decisions at the place of interaction with clients reflects a flat structure.

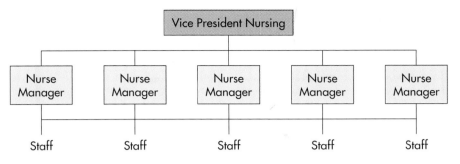

Figure 9-3   Flat organizational structure.

Exercise 9-8

Organizational structures vary in the extent to which they have bureaucratic characteristics. Using observations from your current situations, place a check mark (✓) in the "Present" column beside the bureaucratic characteristics that you believe apply to the agency. What does this analysis indicate about the bureaucratic tendency of the agency? Do the environment and technologies fit the identified bureaucratic tendency? (Consider the state of development of information systems, method of care delivery, clients' characteristics, workers' characteristics, regulatory status, and competition.)

Characteristic	Present
Hierarchy of authority	_____
Division of labor	_____
Written procedures for work	_____
Limited authority for workers	_____
Emphasis on written communication, related to work performance and workers' behaviors	_____
Impersonality of personal contact	_____

Flat organizational structures are less formalized than hierarchical organizations. A decrease in rules and policies allows for individualized decisions that fit specific situations and meet current needs created by consumerism, change, and competition.

The degree of flattening varies from organization to organization. Organizations that are decentralizing frequently retain bureaucratic characteristics. They may at the same time have units that are operating as matrix structures. *Hybrid* is a term applied to organizational structures that operate with characteristics of different types of structures.

Problems with letting go of centralized control, and of top managers changing from boss roles to facilitator roles, are partially responsible for the development of hybrid structures. Managers are unsure of what needs to be controlled, how much control is needed, and which mechanisms can replace control.

Fear of chaos without control predominates. Education that prepares managers to employ leadership techniques that empower nursing staff to take responsibility for their work is one method of eliminating managers' fears. These fears stem from loss of centralized control, as authority with its concomitant responsibilities moves to the place of interaction. The evolutionary development of self-governance structures in nursing departments demonstrates a type of flat structure being used to replace hierarchical control.

Self-Governance

Self-governance goes beyond participatory management through the creation of organizational structures that allow nursing staff to govern themselves. Accountability forms the foundation for designing self-governance models. To be accountable, authority to make decisions concerning all aspects of responsibilities is essential. This need for authority and accountability is particularly important for nurses who treat the wide range of human responses to wellness states and illnesses. The major cause of nurses' dissatisfaction with their work revolves around the absence of this accountability. The magnet hospital study (McClure et al, 1983), which identified characteristics of hospitals successful in recruiting and retaining nurses, found that nursing departments with structures that provided nurses the opportunity to be accountable for their own practice were the major contributing characteristic to success.

Shared governance or self-governance structure designs, sometimes referred to as professional practice models, go beyond decentralizing and diminishing hierarchies. Accountability is determined by needs arising from the services provided to clients. Authority, control, and autonomy are placed in specifically defined areas of accountability. For example, all issues related to nursing practices are dealt with by nursing staff.

All organizations require a foundation for operation. In a shared governance organization, the structure's foundation is the work place rather than the hierarchy. Authority, responsibility, and accountability for all aspects of the work are vested in the nurses delivering care. The management/administrative level serves to coordinate and facilitate the work of the practicing nurses. Areas of accountability, such as quality management, are points of final authority for their designated accountability and are not subject to other sources for approval and mandated performance. Mechanisms are designed outside of the traditional hierarchy to provide for the functional areas needed to support professional practice. These functions include areas such as quality management, competency definition and evaluation, and continuing education. Structures of shared governance organizations vary. Box 9-2 shows three self-governance structures in progressive stages of evolution. As shown, evolution is moving structure beyond committees imposed on hierarchical structures to governance structures at the unit level. Minnen et al (1993) provide an account of one such evolution. The authors describe one hospital's use of a multidisciplinary shared governance system to provide the structure and process support for the change initiated by work redesign.

Shared governance structures require new behaviors of all staff, not just new assignments of accountability. Behaviors required are in the areas of interpersonal relationship development, conflict resolution, and personal acceptance of responsibility for action. Education and experience in group work and conflict management are essential for successful transitions. Porter-O'Grady and George (1996) provide a case study illustrating the dangers of more structure than substance (process) in self-governance models.

Changing nurses' positions from dependent employees to independent, accountable professionals is a prerequisite for (1) the required healthcare organization reengineering, (2) the radical redesign of healthcare organizations that is required to create value for clients and to abandon basic notions regarding the necessity of the diversion of labor, (3) the need for elaborate controls, and (4) the managerial hierarchy on which healthcare organizations have been founded. Structures providing nurses' accountability will meet needs for change, while also meeting consumers' demands and remaining competitive. Fitting nursing process and function with the governance process and determining that organizational structure characteristics fit the technology is an ongoing process.

> **Box 9-2**
>
> ## Self-Governance Structure Evolution
>
> **Phase One**
>
> Representative staff nurses are members of clinical forums, which have authority for designated practice issues and some authority for determining roles, functions, and processes. Managers are members of the management forums, which are responsible for the facilitation of practice through resource management and location. Recommendations for action go to the *executive committee*, which has administrative and staff membership that may or may not be in equal proportion. The nurse executive retains decision-making authority.
>
> **Phase Two**
>
> Representative staff nurses belong to nursing committees that are designated for specific management and/or clinical functions. These committees are chaired by staff nurses or administrators appointed by the vice president of nursing. The nursing committee chairs and nurse administrators make up the nursing cabinet, which makes the final decision on recommendations from the committees.
>
> **Phase Three**
>
> Representative staff nurses belong to councils with authority for specific functions. Council chairs make up the management committee charged with making all final operational organizational decisions.

■ CHAPTER CHECKLIST

Nursing care delivered in healthcare organizations is determined by the mission of the organization in which the care is delivered. Changes occurring in missions affect both the culture of the work place and the philosophies regarding the work required to accomplish the mission. Actualizing new missions and philosophies requires reengineered organizational structures that place decision-making authority and responsibility where care is delivered. Decision-making responsibility requires staff to take responsibility for understanding the organization's mission and to participate in the development of mission and philosophy statements.

- Six factors influencing design of an organization structure are:
  - the types of service performed or the product produced

A Manager's Solution

? Staff representatives, the five nurse managers, and both service line directors began meeting weekly to develop a redesign model. The most significant achievement of that group's work was the respectful, non-competitive process of getting to know one another and the details of each unit's operations. Nurses visited each other's hospitals and shared best practices. Staff developed a unique documentation system incorporating clinical paths. The managers created one charging system to ease contracting with third party payers and to compare financial indicators. We were able to decrease supply costs significantly by agreeing on the same products and negotiating better pricing based on pooled volumes. Statewide, we developed a common "report card" of major quality indicators that are updated monthly. Lactation consultants, parent education coordinators, and NICU nurses collaborated. Now, all departments may use a breastfeeding core curriculum for staff education, one parent handbook is used at all facilities, and all staff have the same foundation of knowledge regarding developmentally supportive care in the NICU.

A new citywide service line director role was created, eliminating two prior positions. As a result, five nurse managers report to three different hospital CEOs. The role has huge challenges but enables one coordinated direction. Neonatal nurse practitioners now meet monthly to network and explore more cost-effective practice models. A citywide physician strategy is in process for maternal-fetal medicine. All staff from the five facilities attend one session of a two day workshop to learn skills and tools related to conflict resolution, communication, and personal accountability. A by-product of these efforts has been that nurses have begun to identify themselves as systemwide nurses, develop friendships across the system, share specialized equipment, and assist each other with staffing crises.

? *Would this be a suitable approach for you? Why?*

  - the characteristics of the workers performing the service or producing the product
  - the beliefs and values concerning the work, the people receiving the services, and the workers that are held by the people responsible for delivering the service
  - the characteristics of people performing the service or producing the product
  - the technologies used to perform the service and produce the product
  - the needs, desires, and characteristics of the consumers using the product or service
- Reengineering, complete overhaul of organizations' structures, is being driven by forces of:
  - change
  - consumerism
  - competition
- Bureaucratic structures are characterized by:
  - a high degree of formalization
  - centralization of decision making at the top of the organization
  - a hierarchy of authority
- Matrix structures are characterized by:
  - dual authority for product and function
  - mechanisms such as committees to coordinate actions of product and function managers
  - success that is dependent on recognition and appreciation of each others' missions and philosophies and commitment to the organization's mission and philosophy
- Flat organizations are characterized by:
  - decision making concerning work performed decentralized to the level where the work is done
  - authority, accountability, and autonomy as well as responsibility for staff
  - low level of formalization in the way of rules with processes tailored to meet individual consumer's needs
- Mission and philosophy determine the characteristics of the organizational structure by:
  - describing the consumers and services as a prescription for the technologies and human resources needed to accomplish the defined purpose (mission)
  - citing values and beliefs that shape and are shaped by the nature of the work, the rights, and responsibilities of workers and consumers (philosophy)
  - designing characteristics that support the service implementation to fulfill the mission and philosophy (structure)

TIPS ON UNDERSTANDING ORGANIZATIONAL STRUCTURES

- The mission of the organization and the mission for the specific unit where a professional nurse is employed or is seeking employment provide knowledge concerning the major focus for the work to be accomplished.
- Understanding the philosophy of the organization and/or unit where work occurs provides knowledge of the behaviors that are valued in the delivery of client care and in interactions with persons employed by the organization.
- Organizational structures describe channels of communication and decision making.
- Matrix organizations usually have two persons responsible for the work so it is important to know to whom you are responsible for what.
- For a self-governance structure to function effectively, it is essential that mechanisms be put in place to promote decision making about client care by persons providing the care.
- Professional nurses in staff or followership positions need to understand mission, philosophy, and organizational structure to maximize their contributions to client care.

TERMS TO KNOW

bureaucratic organization	organizational chart
fit	organizational structure
flat organization	philosophy
hierarchy	reengineering
hybrid organization	shared governance
matrix organization	technology
mission	

REFERENCES

Alexander, J.W., & Bauerschmidt, A. (1987). Implications for nursing administration of the relationship of technology and structure to quality of care. *Nursing Administration Quarterly,* 11(4), 1-10.

Flarey, D.L. (1995). *Redesigning Nursing Care Delivery: Transforming Our Future.* Philadelphia: Lippincott.

George, V., Burke, L., & Rodgers, B. (1997). Research and planning for change: Assessing nurses' attitudes toward governance and professional practice autonomy after hospital acquisition. *Journal of Nursing Administration,* 27(6), 53-61.

Hammer, M., Champy, J. (1993). *Reengineering the Corporation: A Manifesto for Business Revolution.* New York: HarperCollins.

Minnen, T.G., Berger, E., Ames, A., Dubree, M., Baker, W.C., & Spinella, J. (1993). Sustaining work redesign innovation through shared governance. *Journal of Nursing Administration,* 23(7/8), 35-40.

Newman, J.G. & Boissoneau, R. (1987). Team care and matrix organization in geriatrics. *Hospital Topics,* 65(6), 10-15.

McClure, M.L., Poulin, M.A., Sovie, M.D., & Wandelth, M.A. (1983). *Magnet Hospitals, Attrition and Retention of Professional Nurses.* Kansas City: American Nurses' Association.

Porter-O'Grady, T., & George, V. (1996). A nature shared governance system: More structure than substance. *Journal of Nursing Administration,* 26(2), 14-19.

Senge, P. (1990). *The Fifth Discipline: The Art and Practice of the Learning Organization.* New York: Doubleday/Currency.

SUGGESTED READINGS

Deveau, B., & McCabe, D. (1996). Result-oriented committee restructuring. *Journal of Nursing Administration,* 26(10), 35-46.

Graham, P., Constantine, S., Balik, B., Bedore, B., Hoake, M.C.M., Papin, D., Quamme, M., & Rivaid, R. (1987). Operationalizing a nursing philosophy. *Journal of Nursing Administration,* 17(3), 14-18.

Kennedy, S.H. (1996). Effects of shared governance on perceptions of work and work environment. *Nursing Economics,* 14(2), 111-116.

Porter-O'Grady, T. (1996). The seven basic rules for redesign. *Journal of Nursing Administration,* 26(1), 46-53.

Poteet, G., & Hill, A. (1988). Identifying the components of a nursing service philosophy. *Journal of Nursing Administration,* 18(10), 29-35.

Prince, S. (1997). Shared governance: sharing power and opportunity. *Journal of Nursing Administration,* 27(3), 28-35.

Trexler, B. (1987). Nursing department, purpose, philosophy and objectives: their use and effectiveness. *Journal of Nursing Administration,* 17(3), 8-12.

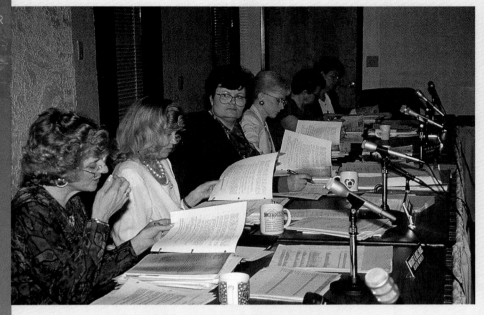

Collective Action

Michael Evans
RN, PhD, CNAA

Fran Hicks
RN, PhD, FAAN

As society has moved toward a more egalitarian environment, employees are expecting and in many situations demanding a greater voice in decisions involving their work life. These decisions involve both the context and the content of their work. Healthcare workers are reminded by policy and preparation to engage the consumer in healthcare decisions. Workers see a direct relationship of these skills to their own situation. They see merit in being part of the decision-making process. Participation in decisions regarding one's practice is an appropriate expectation of a professional nurse. Collective action is one mechanism to achieve that participation. The manager can capitalize on this strategy to accomplish positive outcomes.

Objectives

- Relate the participation of staff nurses in decision making to job satisfaction.
- Analyze the influence that culture has on the selection of a governance model.
- Identify key characteristics of each collective action model: shared governance, work place advocacy, and collective bargaining.
- Distinguish between the rights of individuals included in collective bargaining contracts and the rights of at-will employees.
- Compare the factors that contribute to nurses' decisions to be represented for the purpose of collective bargaining and the decision for no representation.
- Evaluate strategies for their effectiveness in collective bargaining and non–collective bargaining environments.

Questions to Consider

- What is the relationship of nurse participation in decision making and job satisfaction?
- Within the context of labor law, how do the responsibilities of nurses who are supervisors differ from the responsibilities of nurses who are nonsupervisory?
- How can you use collective participation in your nursing practice?
- What would influence you to practice in an organization in which nurses are organized for the purpose of collective bargaining?
- What criteria would you use to select an organization to support you in your practice setting?
- How can you transfer your knowledge of work place advocacy to other forms of advocacy?

 ## A Manager's Challenge

From the Vice President of Patient Services at a Southwestern Metropolitan Hospital

I was a new vice-president for patient services. After several months of assessing the new organization, I determined that I would like to redesign how care is delivered on the patient care unit. Specifically, I wanted to re-evaluate various roles

and possibly redesign certain roles to better meet the need of patients and their families.

What do you think you would do if you were this manager?

■ INTRODUCTION

The excitement of beginning a career in nursing or assuming the position of a manager is balanced by events taking place in healthcare and the impact of these events on nursing and nurses. The knowledge gained about healthcare provides a background for considering issues within healthcare and factors that promote or inhibit the achievement of professional practice.

Nurses are deeply involved in the complex clinical problems of individuals, families, and communities. Nursing practice requires an acquisition, synthesis, and retrieval of knowledge in order to provide competent nursing care. Having the time and resources to engage in this level of preparation for each situation may be viewed as the "high hard ground." The current environment in which nursing practice

occurs may be more akin to "the messy swamps and the pathways between" (Streets, 1990, p. 22).

■ COLLECTIVE ACTION

Collective action is a benign phrase. Inpatient care has historically been delivered through the collective action of shifts of nurses. This pattern requires a level of independence during the shift, and interdependence between shifts and other healthcare professionals. Nurses learn quickly to depend on their colleagues. "In a climate of job insecurity, it is easy to lose sight of our personal power as individuals and our collective power as professionals" (Harris, Ryan, & Belmont, 1997, p. 39). Nurses have been less comfortable with formal collectives. A number of factors may have contributed to this discomfort. As a female-dominated profession, nurses have had less experience in work-ing in groups and, before Title IX, few females partic-ipated in competitive team sports. Women have demonstrated less commitment to the structure of rules. Many women, including nurses, view employ-ment as a job versus a career. For these individuals, the time to work with others to achieve common goals deprives them of personal time. Women have not per-ceived themselves to be powerful. The "good" nurse was considered to be obedient. (The Nightingale Pledge even reinforced obedience: "With loyalty will I endeavor to aid the physician in his work . . .".) This obedience or acquiescence to authority appears to have been transferred to the hospital administration.

Minarick and Catramabone (1993) describe four main purposes of collective participation for nurses: to promote the practice of professional nursing; to establish and maintain standards of care; to allocate resources effectively and efficiently; and to create satisfaction and support in the practice environment. Collective action helps to define and sustain indi-viduals in achieving their purpose. In the absence of collective action the average individual has limited influence in achieving his or her purpose. Perhaps you learned the strength and value of collective ac-tion early in life as you and your siblings banded together to make a request to your parent. The same strategy has probably served you in an organization as you brought together a group of peers to make a point or to plead your case. In nursing practice you may have observed nurses as they identified a prac-tice concern and joined to bring about change. Mason, Talbott, and Leavitt (1993) suggest strategies for building collectives, including developing net-works, developing a collective voice, and cultivating a collective mentality.

Exercise 10-1

Identify three collectives to which you belong. List the purposes of each. How do you feel as a member of these groups?

These strategies require strong leaders and a broad **followership.** Matusak (1997) suggests that the relationship between leaders and followers is symbiotic. The definition for symbiotic derives from science: ". . . two or more very dissimilar organisms form a relationship which depends on the other" (p. 25). Followers and leaders share many character-istics. Successful people move easily between the roles of follower and leader. The knowledge and skills of followers may differ from those of the leader; they are not less. They are knowledgeable of the context and content of their practice. Followers are active, in-volved participants committed to an agreed-upon agenda. They are loyal and supportive to the individ-ual who is setting the pace and the agreed-upon agenda. The absence of followers is personally painful. As one CEO commented: "I didn't necessarily expect to find friends among my vice presidents, but I surely didn't plan on living in a hostile world where key people see my missteps as a chance to add to their power" (Zaleznik, 1989, p. 19).

The change in an initiative or agenda may result in today's leader being tomorrow's follower. The con-verse is applicable: today's follower may be tomor-row's leader. The change may result from the context of the situation. In the operating room the surgeon is the acknowledged leader and the anesthesiologist follows that lead with respect to the extent of the anesthesia. In the event there is a change in the pa-tient's condition, the anesthesiologist becomes the leader and the surgeon may simply step away from the table, an overt act that demonstrates a change in leadership. As healthcare consumers and partici-pants, we salute the clarity.

Exercise 10-2

Identify two groups in which you have been a leader (scouts, Camp Fire, sports). Was your specific role the result of a group decision? How did your role as a leader differ from when you were a follower?

Followers are not submissive partisans blindly following a cultist personality. They are effective group members, not "groupies." They are skilled in group dynamics and accountable for their actions. They are willing and able to question, debate, com-promise, collaborate, and act. Consider potential dif-ferences between being a subordinate in a hierar-chical organization and being a follower committed to one's practice.

Collective action provides a mechanism for achieving professional practice through greater par-ticipation in decision making. The selected gover-nance structure provides the framework for participa-tion. Participation in decision making regarding one's practice is an appropriate expectation for profession-als, provides for greater autonomy and authority over practice decisions, contributes to empowering the professional nurse, and is a major component of job satisfaction. The privilege and obligation to partici-pate are inherent in the discipline. Consistent with the Code for Nurses (ANA, 1985) members of the discipline participate based on their competence. Increasingly, nurses today are expected to be in-formed participants.

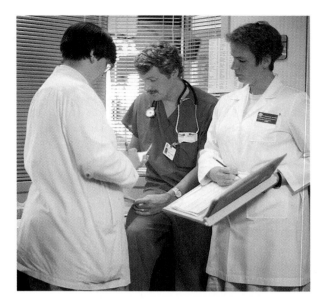

Decision making is at the core of nursing practice.

Not all nurses are interested in or have a desire to participate in decisions. For these nurses, going to work and doing their assigned job may fulfill their expectations. They may not perceive themselves as being in a subordinate position or, if they do, it is not a concern for them. Their orientation is to serve the care recipient. For these individuals, asserting the right and responsibility to participate in decisions may be considered disrespectful to the organization's policies and to the physician. However, participation in practice-related decisions is critical to quality patient care and is essential to autonomy for nursing. Lewis and Batey (1982) define four key concepts: responsibility, authority, autonomy, and accountability.

Responsibility

The history of nursing provides evidence of nurses accepting responsibility or the "charge to act." In the past, this charge took the form of meticulously and unquestioningly following the "physician's orders" and "hospital procedures." The "good nurse" rendered disclosure at the convenience of medicine and management. Progressive healthcare organizations recognize "the rightful power of the nurse to act." The recognition of credentialing, especially certification, has contributed to the exercise of expert power by nurses.

Authority

Authority based on preparation and experience suggests a departure from the tradition of delegating

authority to individual nurses based on the physician's knowledge of the nurse—a knowledge that too frequently was based on personal characteristics and not clinical competence. That statement does not denigrate the collegial relationship between nurse and physician, relationships that are based on mutual respect and trust. There is evidence that patient care improves when these relationships exist.

Autonomy

Autonomy, "the freedom to decide and act," has come about more slowly. In today's cost-containment environment, the effort of all individuals must be maximized. To maximize the efforts of registered nurses, they must have autonomy within their scope of practice. It is unfortunate that autonomy for nurses is based on management's trust of the individual nurse instead of the profession. Multiple studies have indicated that a healthcare organization that provides a climate in which nurses have authority and autonomy retains nurses at a higher rate, is more cost effective, and has evidence of greater client satisfaction than an organization in which such a climate does not exist.

Recruitment and retention are affected by participation, since the "failure on the part of health care delivery organizations, physicians, and policy making bodies to fully recognize the decision making abilities of RNs has contributed to problems in recruiting and retaining nurses, hindered the development of a career orientation in professional nursing, and limited the efficiency and effectiveness of patient care delivery" (USDHHS, 1988, p. vii).

Autonomy encourages innovation and increases productivity. Although automobile manufacturing is a highly mechanized process, management has learned that it is cost effective to give the employee on the shop floor the autonomy to "stop the line" when the potential for error is detected. Stopping the error before it occurs is much more cost effective than recalls and retrofitting. Unlocking minds by providing greater autonomy and diversifying tasks decreases fear, specifically, fear of ridicule, fear of punishment, fear of loss of job, and even fear of favors.

Accountability

Accountability focuses the organization and all its members on the purposes and the outcomes of their collective activities. Accountability requires ownership. "It is not possible to be accountable for what one does not own" (Porter-O'Grady and Wilson, 1995, p. 30). These researchers identify five accountability basics: accountability is about outcomes, not processes; accountability is individually defined; accountability is inherent in the role—it is not delegated; accountability must be clear to all those in related roles; and accountability is the foundation for evaluation.

The value of process is determined by the extent to which individuals observe a particular protocol while accomplishing a goal. Accountability focuses on the achievement of the specified outcome. This shift in thinking has had a tremendous impact on healthcare reimbursement. An example of the shift is evident in patient education. It is no longer acceptable to initial a form indicating that patient teaching has occurred. The criterion now expects that the patient's behavior has changed.

GOVERNANCE MODELS

Nursing **governance** is defined as the methodology or system by which an organized department of nursing within a hospital controls and directs the formulation and the administration of nursing policy. Some type of governance mechanism, a way to provide for nursing services, exists in every nursing department. Governance systems that do not include the involvement of an entity outside of the organization, such as a labor union, can be classified as internal governance mechanisms. Three models of governance will be discussed: shared governance, work place advocacy, and collective bargaining. These models are not mutually exclusive. The governance system is influenced by the overall culture within which the organizational culture is embedded.

The **culture** of the geographic area influences the organizational culture and the selected governance structure. For example, in right-to-work states a model that features collective bargaining may be tolerated more than supported by nurses as well as administration. Box 10-1 summarizes the key factors about these states. The "purity" of geographic cultures has been diluted due to mobility and mass media. However, it is prudent to acknowledge how deeply embedded these cultural influences are within the fabric of American society.

When the respective subcultures are clearly rooted in the mission of the organization (delivery of quality care in a cost-effective environment), the possibility of genuine negotiation or problem solving is enhanced. The presence of congruent subcultures supports healthy relationships. Healthy relationships are an important variable in the development of a strong

> **Box 10-1**
> **Right-to-Work States**
>
> Right-to-work legislation prevents unions from mandating membership by workers in a given organization. In these states, unions are not allowed to mandate membership of employees in a bargaining unit. Therefore unionization is less prevalent. Nurses are less likely to choose unionization as the governance mechanism, since they are less familiar with unions as an option.

internal governance structure capable of supporting a professional practice environment that works well for everyone involved.

Exercise 10-3

> Is your state a right-to-work state? If it is not, what is the nearest state that is a right-to-work state? Are any workers in the right-to-work state organized for the purpose of collective bargaining? How would you describe these workers, e.g., laborer, professional, etc.?

Subcultures form within organizations as "distinct clusters of ideologies, cultural forms, and other practices that identifiable groups of people in an organization exhibit" (Trice & Beyer, 1992, p. 5-1). Nurses and administrators are frequently members of separate subcultures. This phenomenon should not be given a negative connotation. Several factors may increase the distinct ideologies of the two groups, including the presence of a union and the presence of a distant corporate structure. Both factors may be considered external tensions. Traditionally, American organizations have centralized decision making at the top administrative level. The change in organizational culture is toward governance systems with increased opportunity for decision making at the point of service.

When efforts have been made to address nurses' perceptions about job satisfaction, there has been a resulting effect on the relationship between nursing and the top administration of a hospital. Hospitals seeking to increase job satisfaction enhanced the relationship between nurses and the hospital's top administration when nurses were included in identifying the specific areas to be addressed (TNA, 1991). The relationship was damaged when administration addressed the areas without including nurses in the process or when administration did nothing to address

Research Perspective

Moss, R., & Rowles, C. (1997). Staff nurse job satisfaction and management style, Nursing Management. *January, 32-33.*

Job satisfaction for staff nurses is related directly to the perceived management style of managers. In a study of 623 staff nurses from three midwestern hospitals, researchers found that the greater the perceived level of participatory style, the greater the level of job satisfaction of staff nurses. Researchers identified four management styles (exploitative/authoritarian; benevolent/authoritative; consultative; participative). Job satisfaction was higher when the manager's style incorporated characteristics of the participatory style, including loyalty, trust, group problem-solving, and high levels of consideration.

Implications for Practice
The staff nurse's perception of the style is key. As managers begin a process of changing practice and perception, it is necessary to keep the staff informed of proposed changes and to implement changes slowly. Although the known style does not contribute to job satisfaction, there is a sense of security with the known style. Staff who have expected certain behaviors experience unnecessary job stress with a rapid change in style.

job satisfaction. The Research Perspective identifies the important role of managers (see box above).

Exercise 10-4

Identify four factors in your practice (experience) that contribute to job satisfaction. Compare your responses to those of three practicing nurses who are not supervisors and three practicing nurses who are supervisors. Are these commonalities? Are you surprised by the responses?

In the past, nurses have experienced practice environments and working conditions controlled by the medical profession and hospital administration. Increasingly nurses expect a motivating, satisfying work environment that includes a role in decision making. They are no longer willing to participate in organizations in which decisions, clinical and nonclinical, are made by others. Evolving or creating a system that incorporates others in the decision-making process is difficult for many in upper management. Nurses have a long history of zero tolerance for error. Yielding control is frequently associated with the loss of power to manage the error rate (Manthey, 1993). Sharing responsibility and risk requires optimism and trust.

Contractual models provide for nurses to form an organization and contract with the healthcare organization to provide nursing services. Nurses become contract providers instead of employees. Stahl (1997) considers direct contracting to be the "wave of the future" for subacute healthcare organizations. A contractual model can be characterized as a self-

governance model as opposed to a shared governance model.

Shared Governance

Shared governance builds a structure that supports the point of care and sustains ownership and accountability there (Porter-O'Grady, Hawkins, & Parker, 1997). According to these authors, basic principles of shared governance include partnerships, equity, accountability, and ownership. It is more accurate to say that shared governance demands participation in decision making rather than provides for participation. Shared governance creates a framework for ensuring that the processes of empowerment operate effectively throughout a system at every point where work and relationship intersect (Porter-O'Grady & Wilson, 1995).

Staff nurses prefer shared governance models (AHA, 1990). Staff nurses were asked to rate five different consensus-building activities in terms of how they relate to their job satisfaction. In addition to shared governance, the activities included interdisciplinary conferences, interdisciplinary team-building activities, physician-nurse collaborative practice committees, and joint practice. Although shared governance received the highest mean evaluation score, it was planned for implementation by only about 18% of the hospitals that did not have it in place. The following Research Perspective illustrates the value of shared governance.

Some organizations have mislabeled their governance structures. Although they may be labeled

---

Research Perspective

Allen, D., Calkin, J., & Peterson, M. (1988). Making shared governance work: A conceptual model. Journal of Nursing Administration, 17(1), 37-43.

A significant increase in decisional participation can be expected to produce a number of positive outcomes for the employees and the overall organization. They can be expected to become more involved in their practice, their practice becomes more important to them, and they will be more internally motivated and more committed to the organization. These relationships will be stronger for those with strong desires for achievement, responsibility, and autonomy; for those who perceive themselves as decisionally deprived; and for those whose work is difficult and varied. One can anticipate that people may come to value autonomy and responsibility more highly and to find their jobs more challenging. The employee must understand the relationships between performance and reward as well as how their role contributes to the organization and its services. It is essential that staff participate in those decisions which they perceive as being most important to them.

Implications for Practice

Staff nurses and administration can use participative decision making to create a true "win-win" situation while enhancing professional practice. A participative program can increase that challenge if it affects an employees' autonomy. If the intervention promotes variety, taps more of the nurses' abilities, and helps them develop new skills, it can also make their work more challenging and hence more satisfying. Staff nurses who perceive support for their input will be more likely to risk input. By increasing the input of staff nurses into decisions and the issues around which decisions need to be made, there is the potential to improve the cost-effectiveness of care.

"shared governance," they possess few of the characteristics outlined by those who are recognized as experts on the topic. They have developed thinly veiled mechanisms designed to preclude nurses from participating in collective bargaining. There is evidence to suggest that organizations design the systems for that purpose. In 1994 a "National Labor Relations Board administrative law judge ruled that a labor-management cooperative effort at a hospital was illegal. The hospital had established a core group of six employees and supervisors to look into staffing issues. The committee was formed with the purpose of establishing new and innovative ideas including the drafting for a newly created position" (ANA, 1995, p. 11). The mechanism would have diminished the role of the union by "setting up a pattern and practice of dealing with the union on a variety of mandatory subjects." (ANA, p. 11) In today's competitive environment, it is important to be informed and not rush to premature judgment.

Professional practice climates recognize individual performance. Finding organizations that provide a professional practice climate frequently influences a nurse's decision on where to practice (Jones, 1994). The nurse should include in any position search an interview with nurses in the organization to which he or she plans to apply for a position.

Work Place Advocacy

Work place advocacy reflects an array of activities undertaken to address the challenges nurses face in their practice settings. The focus of these activities is on career development, employment opportunities, terms and conditions of employment, employment rights and protections, control of practice, labor-management relations, occupational health and safety, and employee assistance. The objective of work place advocacy is to equip nurses to practice in a rapidly changing environment. Advocacy occurs within a framework of mutuality, facilitation, protection, and coordination. The term "work place advocacy" is an umbrella encompassing activities within the practice setting. The choice of "advocacy" to reflect the framework in which nurses control the practice of nursing is consistent with the goals of the profession. The manifestations of advocacy include (1) assuring relevant information; (2) enabling the selection of information; (3) disclosing a personal view; (4) providing support for making and implementing decisions; and (5) helping determine personal values (Gadow, 1990).

Exercise 10-5

Contact nurses who are not represented by contract. Discuss the strategies they use to influence practice decisions (staffing, skill mix, responsibilities, etc.) and economic decisions (wages, benefits, time off, retirement).

Ensuring Relevant Information

Within the practice setting, nurses must have relevant information to support their practice. Access to information is the basis for initiative, full participation, and sharing information. Clinical nursing practice demands that nurses begin with client information. Today, client information is the beginning of data gathering, not the end. It is equally important for nurses to have information related to occupational health and safety issues, equal employment opportunity information, professional liability, and labor law.

Enabling the Selection of Information

Just as healthcare patients must have relevant information to make good decisions, nurses must be able to select information that is relevant to their practice. The use of clinical data is necessary for client well-being. Data regarding the work place inform nurses of the history of the work place. These data are available through the organization's OSHA 200 logs (Shogren, Calkins, & Wilburn, 1996). Additional information related to injuries is available in Rogers (1996).

Disclosing a Personal View

Nurses and management disclose their views on issues related to the work environment. Disclosure of management's perspective is important. Nurses must be aware of the mission of the organization and knowledgeable of the culture. Peters (1992) describes a German plant in which sharing information in a timely fashion is a critical part of the relationship. In Germany there is a legal requirement that all employees must receive a quarterly situation report, including the balance sheet and the profit-loss statements. Both parties disclose challenges and compromises that influence a maturing relationship. Failing to build on trust jeopardizes the achievement of outcomes.

Healthcare organizations constitute one of the most unsafe work environments in the United States. This environment is characterized by "speed-ups," fewer personnel, fewer full-time personnel, and a propensity to underemploy. An increasingly cynical public holds accountable the "face" of the organization. Frequently, it is the face of a nurse. Violence toward healthcare personnel continues to increase.

Box 10-2
Safety in the Work Place

The Occupational Safety and Health Act of 1970 requires employers to provide a safe and healthy environment. Fire protection, construction and maintenance of equipment, worker training, machine guarding, and protective equipment are specified. Employers are required to familiarize themselves with applicable standards.

The **Centers for Disease Control and Prevention** (CDC) has developed guidelines which assume that all patients are infectious for HIV and other bloodborne pathogens. Although the CDC is not an enforcement agency, its guidelines are adopted as professional practice standards.

There is also an increase in the identified toxins in the work place. It is important for nurses to be involved in addressing work place safety. The organization has a responsibility to ensure a safe environment for staff and patients. Box 10-2 describes two key sources of environmental support.

Providing Support for Making and Implementing Decisions

The support needed to make and implement decisions is achieved through role models, **mentors**, and empowerment. **Role models** may include the nurse who has exquisite clinical skills in assessment. Many nurses have had the opportunity to observe a nurse who seems to "absorb" data when he or she enters a patient's environment. This is a desirable skill. Similarly watching someone who is adroit at the assertive communication skills that transformed an explosive situation into a positive interaction is impressive. The implementation of a primary mentorship program may contribute to the development of these skills. It is clear that a short-term inservice session with an external expert will not achieve the goal. A mentoring relationship is an ongoing, "hands on" process. The value to the organization is in the outcome: The individual will make good decisions.

Exercise 10-6

List the characteristics that you would want a mentor to possess. If you have identified a person you would want as a mentor, ask if he or she is willing to mentor you. Identify any factors that may be a barrier to your seeking a mentorship relationship with the individual. Consider ways that you can address the factor(s).

Nurses are making many difficult decisions in today's healthcare environment. None is more painful than documenting an unsafe assignment. Accepting an unsafe assignment or refusing an assignment is difficult for both the novice and the expert nurse. The ANA (1997) has developed a form that documents the acceptance of an assignment despite objections. The completed form may be useful to nurse managers as they prepare budgets. Experience shows that many unsafe assignments are documented because of a lack of personnel and a lack of training of the existing personnel. Nurses need to prepare themselves to respond when an assignment is inappropriate. Being informed yourself of the procedures for refusing an assignment in practice settings and for accepting an assignment despite objection is important. Consider the consequences of accepting an assignment that is beyond the individual's scope and skills.

Helping Determine Personal Values

You will have an opportunity to determine your own values as a skillful mentor guides your practice. Those who have been the recipient of a successful mentorship have identified a number of positive, frequently occurring behaviors that characterized their mentor; these have been expressed as follows: showed confidence in me; encouraged independent decision making; and their knowledge and energy inspired me (Holloran, 1993).

Empowered individuals are an asset to the organization because they have the power to make decisions within their scope of practice. It is that simple and that complex. **Empowerment** requires redefining the managerial role and a change in behavior by nurses and administrators. The behavior changes to one in which trust replaces distrust and respect replaces disrespect. How will nurses and others determine their own values within various types of decisions if there are inadequate opportunities to practice decision making?

Traditional models have segmented the responsibility for the provision of care and management of resources for that care. Involvement in decision making is critical and can vary from none whatsoever to a high degree of input by nurses in virtually every decision affecting the conditions of employment and their practice. Even those hospitals that operate under some semblance of the traditional model are experiencing a transition toward more involvement of the staff nurse with the emergence of nurse administra-

tors who are prepared by education and experience (Kelly, 1991).

Exercise 10-7

Identify four factors that you consider most empowering in a governance model. Would the presence of one or more of these factors influence you to practice in this environment? Identify four factors that you would consider least empowering in a governance model. Would the presence of one or more of these factors influence you to avoid practicing in this environment?

■ COLLECTIVE BARGAINING

Collective bargaining is defined as "the performance of the mutual obligation of the employer and the representatives of the employees to meet at reasonable times and confer in good faith with respect to wages, hours, and other terms and conditions of employment or the negotiation of any agreement or any question arising thereunder . . ." (Labor Management Reporting Act, 1947, section 8). Like nonhealthcare collective bargaining (Box 10-3), the purpose of collective bargaining by nurses is to secure reasonable and satisfactory conditions of employment, including the right to participate in decisions regarding their practice. These conditions are directly correlated with the quality of care (Flanagan, 1995).

Peters (1992) calls for a decrease in unionism. Naisbitt and Aburdene (1985) pronounce that "The union movement is dead . . . only about 17% of the US work force is organized. In the private sector, only 15% of workers are unionized. In the economically dynamic south and west, only 5% of the work force belongs to a union" (p. 82). Drucker (1986) maintains that the union is accorded legitimacy not accorded to other non-governmental institutions. Accepting and protecting the union's right to strike gives to one group in society a "right to civil disobedience." Toffler (1990) recommends that unions refocus their efforts and consider the autonomous employee who receives little support from individual workers or organized union leadership.

Preventing unionization is considered a responsibility of management by many corporate boards. The message is that unions are bad for business, bad for profits, and bad for workers. Their implicit conclusion is that companies that get unions deserve them. In some organizations, supervisors are urged to identify and report concerted activity such as two or more individuals in action together. There are managers who insist that unions hinder a company's goals of achieving maximum productivity, maintaining profits,

Collective Bargaining in Non-healthcare Industries

Unionization is accepted as a reality in many non-health-related industries. Improved communication and good will cannot eliminate the gap between labor and management. Cooperation between management and labor will remain an illusion unless or until there is sharing of responsibility, power, and profits (Levitan & Johnson, 1983). In 1977 McIsaac recommended that the United States adopt the European model of cooperation between management and labor. Where cooperation and trust exist between the union and the company, the union will be understanding when the company is experiencing financial difficulties. Mills (1983) cites examples of companies in which employees voluntarily accepted wage reductions in order to help the company decrease expenses. In 1996 the Malden Mills continued to assist employees from company funds when the company was unable to produce popular Polartec items due to a fire.

There are those (Reisman & Compa, 1985) who see no benefit to employees for management and the union to have a positive relationship. Heckscher (1988) suggests that the union model is outdated because of trends that have made the public policy framework of unionization less useful. One such trend is the shift to replace blue-collar workers with "knowledge workers." When knowledge workers unionize, they develop organizations that function more like associations than traditional industrial unions. They become involved in activities such as lobbying and coalition-building.

and rewarding individual initiative. Furthermore, there are those who allege that flexibility is a major "union-free" benefit that allows a company and its employees to reach their goals.

Union activity in the healthcare sector has become more aggressive in the recent past due to changes in labor law. The federal role in labor relations is a dynamic, evolving one. The 1935 Wagner Act (National Labor Relations Act) established election procedures for employees to be able to freely choose their collective bargaining representatives. Two years later, the ANA included provisions for improving nurses' work and professional lives. In 1947 the Taft-Hartley Act placed curbs on some union

activity and excluded from coverage employees of not-for-profit hospitals. The Labor Management Reporting and Disclosure Act of 1959, known as the Landrum-Griffin Act, provides for greater internal democracy within unions. The 1974 amendments to the Taft-Hartley Act removed the exemption of not-for-profit hospitals, and employees of these types of organizations have the same rights as industrial workers to join together and form labor unions. The National Labor Relations Act is administered by the National Labor Relations Board (NLRB). In addition to the National Labor Relations Act on the national level, states have laws that further define labor law.

The removal of the exemption for not-for-profit hospitals created a frenzy of activity as traditional industrial unions targeted healthcare facilities. Organizing nurses and other healthcare workers for the purpose of collective bargaining is very attractive because of the numbers of people involved and the decrease in organizing in other sectors. In the United States the number of nurses represented by traditional industrial unions is increasing, and the number of nonnurse labor representatives seems to be increasing. These industrial unions are seeking to represent nurses for the purpose of collective bargaining and to speak for nursing with boards of nursing, regulatory agencies, and the legislature.

Why is there an increase in organizing nurses and other healthcare professionals? Healthcare is a "hot" topic at the state and federal level. The morning newspaper, nightly news, and a continuous parade of "news magazines" have featured countless articles related to health and illness. A television station in Portland, Oregon, proclaims itself as the only local station that has a registered nurse who does the "medical news." Nurses have historically looked to other groups for direction. This direction has been in the form of the physician, the church, the military, the hospital administrator, and perhaps now a trade union. One may paraphrase Willie Sutton when he was asked why he robbed banks: "that is where the money is." Why organize nurses and other healthcare workers? That is where potential members are. As technology replaces unskilled workers, a smaller pool of workers is available for trade union organizing. Declining union membership has been the catalyst for unions to explore other membership bases. NLRB data confirm that organizing campaigns are more successful in healthcare than in other industries. In 1993, the win rate for all industries was 48%, while the win rate in healthcare was 58.3% (*Modern Healthcare*, 1994).

With all this interest in creating units, nurses who seek collective bargaining should carefully consider the representing agent. (See Box 10-4 for suggested screening criteria.)

Historically nurses may have resisted being identified with unions; however, "some RNs now may view unionization as the most promising avenue available to them through which to address professional practice issues and improve their economic and career status" (Wilson, Hamilton, & Murphy, 1990, p. 35). The relationship between management and unions has been adversarial, but exceptions do occur.

Although state nurses' associations (SNAs) have the right to bargain for nurses, the American Hospital Association spent millions of dollars challenging the appropriateness of all RN bargaining units or a unit separate from other organized employees. In a 1991 unanimous opinion, the U.S. Supreme Court upheld the NLRB's ruling that provides for RN-only units. This decision was critical for nursing. At stake was the ability of nurses to control nursing practice and the quality of patient care. Nurses, as others, must be accorded work place rights and the protection that allows them to practice. Nurses must have the freedom to do what the profession and their license require them to do.

The role of the SNA as a collective bargaining representative has been challenged by some health-care organizations based on the presence of statutory supervisors on the SNA board of directors. SNAs have withstood multiple legal challenges (Ketter, 1996). Costly, time-consuming challenges have the effect of denying timely representation to nurses.

The most recent challenge is to label all nurses as supervisors. In the United States the number of nurses represented by traditional industrial unions is increasing and the number of nonnurse labor representatives seems to be increasing. The Supreme Court decision declaring that nurses who assign and direct others are supervisors has the potential to decrease the number of nurses eligible for collective bargaining (McMullen & Campbell-Philipsen, 1995). However, the NLRB ruled in February, 1996 that registered nurses, including charge nurses at an Anchorage hospital, were not statutory supervisors and are protected by federal labor law; in August, 1997 the U.S. Court of Appeals for the Ninth Circuit upheld that decision (Nguyen, 1997). RNs monitor and assess clients as a part of their professional practice, not as a statutory supervisor within the definition of the National Labor Relations Act (ANA, 1997).

Box 10-4

Suggested Criteria for Selecting a Bargaining Agent

- A strong commitment to nursing practice, legislation, regulation, and education
- A well-prepared practice, policy, and labor staff: a minimum of a bachelor's degree in nursing
- Representative of those they represent in both gender and ethnic makeup
- A bargaining agent that is national in scope and local in implementation

---

Nurses as Knowledge Workers

The change from producing a product to providing a service has had many implications for management and labor. In the past, employees in manufacturing were treated like interchangeable cogs: when a cog was broken, it was replaced. A large pool of unskilled workers was available to step forward in the steel mill, the coal mine, and the shop floor. The increased number of technical workers in healthcare seems to be replacing the technical workers in other industries displaced as a result of technology. The move from an industrial model requires knowledge workers. Today's nurses are knowledge workers. The tools of knowledge workers differ. As the knowledge content of the work increases, practice becomes more individualized. The unskilled worker of yesterday did not have a high school diploma. Today, knowledge workers may have multiple college degrees and certifications. As we move into an information society, we might expect fewer organizing activities than would be present in an industrial society.

Yesterday's union leaders could negotiate a contract for thousands of workers and just inform them of the outcome. For example, the executive committee, a governing entity of the organized workers and union staff, could order workers to strike if the executive committee approved. Nurses in Canada demonstrate that solidarity between the union and its leadership does not exist as it did in the past. The union leaders approved an agreement only to have the membership repudiate it. Although an agreement was reached, the anger toward the union leaders endures (Kerr & MacPhail, 1991).

For many nurses the question may be, "Why be represented for collective bargaining?" A collective bargaining contract requires management to bargain. That requirement is not present in noncontract organizations.

Multiple factors have influenced the organizing of nurses, including the belief that a professional collective can contribute to an improvement in professional status; a growing discontent with working conditions; the increased use of unions by other professionals, particularly physicians and teachers; the successes of the activist feminist movement; and the negotiation of contract provisions addressing professional concerns (Flanagan, 1983). More recently, nurses and the general public have become angry as they have witnessed the corporatization of healthcare. Nurses are seeking assistance from an external source in order to balance the assistance they perceive to be available to administration.

Dividends to stockholders have escalated, while nurses have observed a decline in the quality of care, which is attributable to decreased professional nurse staffing. For example, Columbia/HCA developed a plan that would have given its top three officials a bonus of $15.5 million (AJNNEWSLINE, 1996). The increase in the number of conglomerates has increased the "bottom line" focus. This change has resulted in less concern with humanistic factors (Shindul-Rothschild, Berry, & Long-Middleton, 1996). The victims are the public and the providers. As healthcare has become a commodity traded on the stock market, allegiance has shifted from the patient to the stockholder. Healthcare is a labor-intensive industry that manifests many of the ills of other labor-intensive industries: impersonal management, discrimination, favoritism, and arbitrary termination.

Drucker (1986) advocates for a countervailing power between management and labor. A collective bargaining contract can be that countervailing power. Individuals will seek ways to defend themselves from what is perceived to be arbitrary actions. Many nurses fear arbitrary discipline and dismissal. Although there is "whistle blower" legislation (see Box 10-5), the current environment in healthcare places the at-will employee who voices concern about the quality of care in a vulnerable position.

Concerns about discipline, due process, and burden of proof have been used to support collective bargaining. Managers of at-will employees have greater latitude in selecting disciplinary measures for specific infractions. The discipline structure provided by contract treats all employees in the same manner and may decrease the manager's flexibility in designing or selecting discipline. An at-will employee may be terminated at any time for any reason except discrimination (Fiesta, 1997).

Contract language requires management to follow "due process" for represented employees. That

---

> **Box 10-5**
> ### Whistle-blower Protection
>
> "Whistleblowers are employees who disclose information about an agency's violation of a law, rule, or regulation; or a substantial and specific danger to public health or safety. Legal protections vary, depending on the activity reported and where the whistleblower is employed" (Flanagan, 1995). The 1989 Whistle Blower Protection Act protects federal workers. The law does not cover the private sector. Some states have specific laws.

---

is, management must provide a written statement outlining disciplinary charges, the penalty, and the reasons for the penalty. Management is required to keep a record of attempts to counsel the employee. Employees have the right to defend themselves against charges and the opportunity to settle disagreements in a formal grievance hearing. They have the right to have their representative with them during the process. Management must prove that the employee is wrong or in error. In a nonunion environment, the burden of proof is on the employee.

Many nurses have been intimidated by the charge that "unions were unprofessional." These charges have been made by nurse colleagues, hospital management, and physicians. However, today physicians have collective bargaining contracts. Why? They want to have greater control of their practice, improve working conditions, and influence their remuneration. Contracts are a usual part of our present-day environment. They are neither "professional" nor "nonprofessional." There are many adages in our vocabulary that characterize the relationship between parties; they include "a man's word is his bond"; "let's shake on it"; and "I am as good as my word." These expressions convey a trust between the two parties. In today's marketplace, one rarely "shakes on it." The purchase of a house, a car, or consultation results in a contract that details the responsibilities of the parties involved.

Moore (1970), a sociologist, identified the responsibilities of the professional: respect the duty to perform; respect the duty to learn; respect the public interest; and preserve and enhance the image. A labor contract, a collective bargaining agreement, is unrelated to being professional. It is ironic that there are such divided views on the existence of a contract between employer and employee.

Leaders in nursing have consistently maintained that the ANA is the only organization that can speak authoritatively for nursing and nurses. As a professional society, all registered nurses and only registered nurses may hold membership in the SNA. The SNA and ANA represent the interests of the profession, nurses, and healthcare at the state, federal, and international levels. The collective bargaining program of the SNA is designed to implement strategies that maintain or attain improvement in nursing practice in addition to addressing the economic issues.

Lucille Joel, former President of the ANA, provided eloquent support for ANA's involvement. "As long as professionals (nurses) look to collective action to assure public access to quality service, this professional association must offer workplace representation to its members. . . . Where collective bargaining is the model of choice for work place representation, our appeal must lie in something above and beyond what competing unions offer. . . . Where there is a plea for work place representation but collective bargaining is rejected, it becomes critical to give substance and meaning to labor/management coalitions, practice councils, nursing staff organizations, and a variety of other strategies and models that can bring authority, purpose and professional parity" (Joel, 1990, p. 7).

Collective Bargaining	**Non-Collective Bargaining**

Goal

← Safe quality health care →

Context

← State Nurse Practice Act →

← Public policy: including applicable labor law →

Strategies

← Identify shared values →

← Consult State Nurses Association →

← Education of nurses and management →

← Collaboration →

← Identify issues →

← Support groups →

← Public relations →

← Consult SNA →

← Organize for collective bargaining

← Negotiate and administer a legal contract

Employment Status

Employment at will →

← Collective bargaining contract

← Requirement to bargain in good faith

Obtain individual contract →

Desired Outcomes

Input into conditions of work including:

← Input into the way care is delivered →

← Input into practice →

← Input into allocation of resources →

Fig. 10-1 Appropriateness of selected factors to two-employment environments.

If you work in a setting with a collective bargaining agreement, secure a copy. Identify the articles of this contract. Are they practical issues or economic issues? What is the relationship between the two?

Not all nurses are eligible to participate in collective bargaining. The nurse who is a statutory supervisor is excluded. These nurses may hold membership in the same SNA as the nurses in the bargaining unit. They have the same concerns about working conditions, practice standards, and the care delivery environment. Many supervisory nurses may feel that they are unnecessarily placed in an adversarial relationship with nonmanagement nurses in the hospital who are represented by the union. It is unfortunate that the terms of employment within a particular organization may prevent supervisory nurses from maintaining membership in the SNA that represents nurses employed by the hospital. The prohibition is unnecessary and may reflect negatively on the employer.

Canadian nurses have two separate organizations based on a Supreme Court decision. There is a professional association and a union. In the province of British Columbia, the Registered Nurses Association of British Columbia is the professional association and the British Columbia Nurses Union is the union. The professional association focuses on maintaining appropriate standards of nursing care and serving the public interest. The union focuses on the socioeconomic needs of members and is not legally bound to protect the public interest. Strategies that allow the separate organizations to cooperate differ from province to province (Kerr & MacPhail, 1991). "Where collective bargaining is controlled by nurses and where professional values predominate, the greater the likelihood of cooperation between the professional body and the negotiating body" (Conroy & Hibberd, 1983).

Replacing the adversarial system should be the goal of efforts to redesign the work place. The new social order in the work place must be based on a spirit of real cooperation between management and the workers.

Selecting Strategies

Figure 10-1 outlines strategies that are appropriate in two employment environments. Collective bargaining environments use a full range of strategies. The presence of a contract requires the employer to negotiate within a legally binding framework. Noncollective bargaining environments do not provide that assurance.

Professional practice models may exist in both environments. Nurses may feel valued in both environments. The future may hold new relationships, and public policy may continue to include provisions that in the past were negotiated through contracts. Until that occurs, nurses will practice in highly competitive environments. Nurses, and those they serve, will benefit from collective action that uses a wide range of strategies.

CHAPTER CHECKLIST

Collectively nurses possess the knowledge, skills, ability, and numbers to influence decisions. Collective action may take many forms. Geographic and organizational contexts influence the formal and informal structures in which nurses participate. An organization's governance structure establishes the parameters for participation in decision making. The decision

A Manager's Solution

In any redesign effort, involving the staff is critical. I would begin by meeting with the staff and telling them why I would like to begin a redesign process and what I hoped to accomplish from such efforts. I would then set up redesign teams that have a great deal of staff involvement.

Involving the staff is critical for several reasons. First, the most creative solutions for redesign are, most of the time, thought of by the individuals who are actually taking care of patients. Also, staff are more likely to embrace redesign activities if they feel that they have been actively involved in the process. Finally, staff can often anticipate issues or problems with these efforts and help develop solutions before the implementation of redesign.

If I worked in a unionized environment, my approach would not differ except I would meet with the union representatives before initiating the redesign efforts. Again, I would explain what I hoped to accomplish through these efforts, answer any questions or concerns, and ask for their support of the project.

Would this be a suitable approach for you? Why?

to organize for the purpose of collective bargaining represents an important decision for nurses and for the organization in which they practice. A level of tension exists when an external group becomes a part of an organization's decision making processes. External groups may enter as a new management consultant, as a part of a merger, as a new owner, or as a union representing registered nurses. The acceptance and appreciation of the external group are influenced by understanding the rationale for the group's entry and by the respect between the constituencies.

- The purposes of collective participation by nurses are to:
  - promote the practice of professional nursing
  - establish and maintain standards of care
  - allocate resources effectively and efficiently
  - create satisfaction and support in the practice environment (Minarick and Catramabone, 1993)
- Increased autonomy and diversification decrease:
  - fear of ridicule
  - fear of punishment
  - fear of loss of job
  - fear of favors
- Governance models dictate levels of participation. The level of participation in decision making influences job satisfaction.
- Shared governance is characterized by partnerships, equity, accountability, and ownership. The framework for advocacy includes mutuality, facilitation, protection, and coordination. The manifestations of advocacy are:
  - assuring relevant information
  - enabling the selection of information
  - disclosing a personal view
  - providing support for making and implementing decisions
  - helping determine personal values
- The goal of work place advocacy is to equip nurses to practice in a rapidly changing environment
- Collective bargaining is an effective mechanism used by nurses to obtain the right to participate in decisions regarding their practice.
- Represented nurses must be proven wrong or in error. Unrepresented nurses bear the burden of proving themselves.
- Representation for the purpose of collective bargaining, belonging to a union, is neither professional nor unprofessional.
- Nurses who are statutory supervisors are excluded from representation.

TIPS FOR COLLECTIVE ACTION

- Managers and staff alike should understand the 'culture' and the organization's approach to any collective action strategy.
- Some states have laws that are more supportive of "whistle-blowing" than others.
- Use some type of criteria to select a collective bargaining agent, if this is the appropriate strategy.

TERMS TO KNOW

Centers for Disease Control and Prevention	followership
	governance
collective action	labor acts
collective bargaining	mentor
culture	role model
empowerment	shared governance

REFERENCES

American Hospital Association. (1990). *Survey of the Hospital Nursing Strategies Pretest.* Chicago: AHA.

AJNNEWSLINE. (1996). Speaking of Columbia/HCA, nurses ask 'What direction we're going in.' *American Journal of Nursing,* 96, December, p. 69.

Allen, D., Calkin, J., & Peterson, M. (1988). Making shared governance work: A conceptual model. *Journal of Nursing Administration,* 17(1), 37-43.

American Nurses Association. (1985). *A code for nurses with interpretive statements.* Kansas City: ANA.

American Nurses Association. (1995). *Legal developments: ANA's labor & employment newsletter.* March 10, 11.

American Nurses Association. (1997). *What you need to know about today's workplace: An independent study continuing education module.* Washington, D.C.: ANA.

Conroy, M., & Hibberd, J. (1983). Areas for cooperation and conflict between nursing associations and negotiating bodies. In Quinn, S. ed. *Cooperation and Conflict: Caring for the Carers.* Geneva: International Council of Nurses.

Drucker, P. (1986), *The frontiers of management: Where tomorrow's decisions are being shaped today,* New York: Dutton.

Fiesta, J. (1997). Labor law update. *Nursing Management,* 28, January, 27-28.

Flanagan, L. (1983). *Collective Bargaining and the Nursing Profession.* Kansas City: ANA.

Flanagan, L. (1995). *What You Need to Know About Today's Workplace: A Survival Guide for Nurses.* Washington, D.C.: American Nurses Publishing.

Gadow, S. (1990). Existential advocacy: Philosophic foundations of nursing. In Pence, T., Cantrell, J. eds. *Ethics in Nursing: An Anthology.* New York: NLN.

Harris, A., Ryan, M., & Belmont, M. (1997). More than a friend: The special bond between nurses, *American Journal of Nursing,* 97, May, 37-39.

Heckscher, D. (1989). *The New Unionism: Employee Involvement in the Changing Corporation*, New York: Basic Books, Inc.

Holloran, S. (1993). Mentoring: The experience of nursing service executives. *Journal of Nursing Administration*, 22, February, 49-54.

Joel, L. (1990). Workplace representation: Continuing commitment, new choices. *The American Nurse*, March, 7.

Jones, P. (1994). Developing a collaborative professional role for the staff nurse in a shared governance model. *Holistic Nurse Practitioner*, 8, 32-37.

Kelly, L. (1991). Past imperfect: Future perfect? *Nursing Outlook*, 39(2), 53.

Kerr, J., & MacPhail, J. (1991). *Canadian Nursing: Issues and Perspectives*, St. Louis: Mosby.

Ketter, J. (1996). Collective bargaining comes of age. AJN, 96, 62.

Levitan, S., & Johnson, C. (1983). Labor and management: The illusion of cooperation. *Harvard Business Review*, 61, September-October, 8-16.

Lewis, F., & Batey, M. (1982). Clarifying autonomy and accountability in nursing service: Part 2. *Journal of Nursing Administration*, 12, October.

Manthey, M. (1993). "Empowering staff to create a professional practice environment." In *Nursing Leadership: Preparing for the 21st Century*, American Organization of Nurse Executives, Chicago: AHA.

Mason, D., Talbot, D., & Leavitt, J. (1993). *Policy and Politics for Nurses: Action and Change in the Workplace, Government, Organizations and Community*, 2nd ed. Philadelphia: Saunders.

Matusak, L. (1997). *Finding Your Voice: Learning to Lead . . . Anywhere You Want to Make a Difference*. San Francisco: Jossey-Bass.

McIsaac, G. (1977). Thinking ahead: What's coming in labor relations. *Harvard Business Review*, 56, September-October, 22-36.

McMullen, P., & Campbell-Philipsen, N. (1995). The end of collective bargaining for nurses? *Nursing Policy Forum*, 1(1), 34-39.

Mills, D. (1983). When employees make concessions. *Harvard Business Review*, 61, May-June, 103-113.

Minarik, P., & Catramabone, C. (1993). Collective participation in workforce decision making. In Mason, D, Talbott, S, Leavitt, J: *Policy and Politics for Nurses*, 2nd ed. Philadelphia: Saunders.

Modern Healthcare. (1994). Keep employees involved in decision-making process. 24(26):86.

Moore, W. (1970). *The Professions: Roles and Rules*, New York: Russell Sage Foundation.

Moss, R., & Rowles, C. (1997). Staff nurse job satisfaction and management style. *Nursing Management*, 29, January, 32-34.

Naisbitt, J., & Aburdene, P. (1985). *Re-inventing the Corporation: Transforming Your Job and Your Company for the New Information Society*, New York: Warner Books.

National Labor Relations Act (NLRA) *Sec.* 8(5), 29 USCA *Sec.* 158 (5).

Nguyen, B. (1997). Long-awaited Providence ruling upholds right of charge nurses to bargain. *The American Nurse*, 29, September-October, 1, 14.

Peters, T. (1992). *Liberation Management: Necessary Disorganization for the Nanosecond Nineties*. New York: Knopf.

Porter-O'Grady, T., & Wilson, C. (1995). *The Leadership Revolution in Health Care: Altering Systems, Changing Behaviors*. Gaithersburg, MD: Aspen Publishers.

Porter-O'Grady, T., Hawkins, M., & Parker, M. (1997). *Whole Systems Shared Governance: Architecture for Integrations*. Gaithersburg, MD: Aspen Publishers.

Reisman, B., & Compa, L. (1985). The case for adversarial unions. *Harvard Business Review*, 63, May-June, 22-36.

Rogers, B. (1996). Nursing injury, stress, and nursing care. In *Nursing Staff in Hospitals and Nursing Homes: Is it Adequate?* Washington, DC.: IOM.

Shindul-Rothschild, J., Berry, D., & Long-Middleton, E. (1996). Where have all the nurses gone? Final results of our patient care survey. *American Journal of Nursing*, 96, November, 25-39.

Shogren, E., Calkins, A., & Wilburn, S. (1996). Restructuring may be hazardous to your health, AJN, 96, 64-66.

Stahl, D. (1997). Direct contracting: A new wave for subacute care. *Nursing Management*, 28, May, 22-23.

Streets A. (1990). *Nursing Practice—High, Hard, Ground, Messy Swamps and the Pathways in Between*. Geelong, Australia: Deskin University Press.

Texas Nurses Association. (1991). *Increasing Nursing Satisfaction in the Hospital Environment*. Austin: TNA.

Toffler, A. (1990). *Powershift: Knowledge, Wealth, and Violence at the Edge of the 21st Century*. New York: Bantam Books.

Trice, H., & Beyer, J. (1992). *The Cultures of Work Organizations*. Englewood Cliffs, NJ: Prentice-Hall.

U.S. Department of Health and Human Services. (1988). *Secretary's Commission on Nursing: Final Report*. Washington, D.C.: U.S. Government Printing Office.

Wilson, C., Hamilton, C., & Murphy, E. (1990). Union dynamics in nursing. *Journal of Nursing Administration*, 20(2), 35-39.

Zaleznik, A. (1989). *The Managerial Mystique: Restoring Leadership in Business*, New York: Harper & Row, Publishers.

◼ SUGGESTED READINGS

Breda, K.L. (1997). Professional nurses in unions: working together pays off. *Journal of Professional Nursing*, 13, 99-109.

Mohr, W.K. (1997). Outcomes of corporate greed. *Image: Journal of Nursing Scholarship*, 29(1), 39-45.

Powers, J. (1993). Accepting and refusing assignments. *Nursing Management*, 24, September.

Smith, M.H. (1996). NLRB vs. Health Care and Retirement Corporation of America, Inc.: A challenge for the nursing profession. *Nursing Outlook*, 44, 191-196.

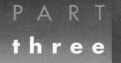

Managing Resources

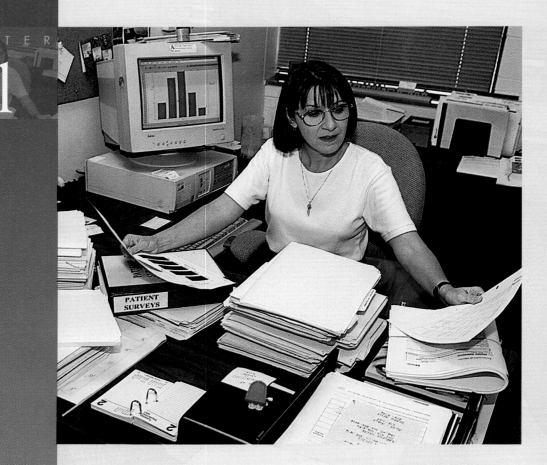

Managing Quality and Risk

Deborah Wendt
RN, MS, CS

Darla Vale
RN, DNSc, CCRN

This chapter's purpose is to explain key concepts and strategies related to quality and risk management. All healthcare professions must be knowledgeable about, and involved in, the continuous improvement of client care.

Objectives

- Apply quality management principles to clinical examples.
- Use the six steps of the quality improvement process.
- Practice using selected quality improvement strategies to:
  - Identify customer expectations
  - Diagram clinical procedures
  - Develop standards and outcomes
  - Evaluate outcomes statistically
- Demonstrate the importance of planning in quality management.
- Differentiate between quality management and risk management.
- Employ the "five why" technique and triangulation method to obtain data about a situation or problem.

Questions to Consider

- How can a staff nurse make effective suggestions to improve nursing practice?
- If a colleague makes a mistake, what can you do to prevent future errors while protecting your colleague's self-esteem?
- How can clients' expectations be used to improve nursing care?

A Manager's Challenge
From the Director of Nursing of a Midwestern Health Department

The Cincinnati Health Department applies the philosophy of total quality management to all its programs and services. Within the community health nursing programs, committees meet regularly to plan, implement, and evaluate quality improvement ideas. These committees are composed of both managers and staff workers, and each focuses on a specific area of nursing service. We have a standards committee, audit committee, documentation committee, and staff development committee. This approach to quality improvement has been very successful in the past and has resulted in the implementation of changes and innovations in nursing care.

However, at a recent staff meeting, nursing supervisors expressed the concern that several quality improvement committees were working on similar projects. This duplication of effort was a waste of the committee members' time and the health department's scarce resources.

What do you think you would do if you were this manager?

▪ INTRODUCTION

Healthcare agencies and health professionals want to provide the highest quality of care with minimal risk to clients. But what is quality care? How can it be measured? As healthcare costs continue to rise, third-party payers and healthcare consumers, as well as health professionals, increasingly ask these questions. The philosophy of quality management and the process of quality improvement strive to answer such questions by redesigning the corporate culture and teaching all employees specific skills for assessment, measurement, and evaluation of client care. Quality management stresses the prevention of client care problems, but, if problems occur, risk management activities focus on reducing the negative impact of such problems.

▪ QUALITY MANAGEMENT IN HEALTHCARE

The path to quality in healthcare has become crowded in the last few years as providers recognize that survival and competitiveness are built on improved client outcomes. Short cuts to quality have been tried, but success depends on a philosophy that permeates the organization and values a continuous process of improvement. The quality management philosophy differs from other evaluation techniques because it focuses on the customer instead of the provider, prevention instead of inspection, and the process instead of the person.

The terms *quality management* and *quality improvement* have evolved from the business philosophy

Table 11-1	PAST, PRESENT, AND EVOLVING QUALITY TERMS		
	Past Quality Terms	**Present Quality Terms**	**Evolving Quality Terms**
	Quality control	Total quality management	Quality management
	Quality assurance	Continuous quality improvement	Quality improvement

known as *total quality management*, which is discussed later in this chapter. Many healthcare organizations prefer to use the term *quality management* or **continuous quality improvement** because *total* quality management can never be achieved. Quality-related terminology or jargon has changed in the last few years. Table 11-1 lists past and present quality abbreviations and terms. These terms are defined in the glossary.

Quality management and **quality improvement** are terms that are sometimes used interchangeably. However, quality management is a philosophy that defines a corporate culture emphasizing customer satisfaction, innovation, and employee involvement. Quality improvement is an ongoing process of innovation, prevention of error, and staff development that is used by corporations and institutions who adopt the quality management philosophy.

BENEFITS OF QUALITY MANAGEMENT

Healthcare systems can benefit in a number of ways from quality management. First, the current financial environment with prospective payments has constrained budgets, which in turn caused a decrease in staff. Greater efficiency and proactive planning while maintaining quality may overcome some of the problems with prospective payments. Second, the abundance of legal malpractice suits emphasizes the need for quality of care. Quality management is based on the philosophy that things should be done right the first time and that improvement is always possible. In the United States this "ideal notion" is sometimes questioned, but in Japan, where quality management flourishes, people are committed to this belief. Third, quality management involves everyone on the improvement team and encourages everyone to make contributions. This style of participative management enhances job satisfaction. Employees feel valued as team members who can really make a difference.

PLANNING FOR QUALITY IMPROVEMENT

Multidisciplinary planning is integral to the quest for quality. Issues are examined from various perspectives using a systematic process. Planning takes time and money; however, quality managers say, "We don't have time *not* to plan." The price of poor planning can be very expensive in both human and dollar terms. Poor planning costs might involve redoing what was originally done poorly, increasing the risk of liability, making costly accidents and errors, risking a negative public image, and increasing employee frustration/turnover. The costs of errors and ineffective nursing actions are considered avoidable costs.

EVOLUTION OF QUALITY MANAGEMENT

Deming lectured about building quality into every product and service during a tour of postwar Japan. Using Deming's 14 points of quality management as a guide, Japan recovered from the devastation of World War II and rapidly gained a reputation for efficient production and excellent products (Anschutz, 1995). A summary of Deming's 14 management points appears in Box 11-1.

During the 1980s the United States faced increased competition for products in a global market. Deming's philosophy was rediscovered by Americans who enthusiastically began applying quality management to business, industrial, educational, and healthcare systems (Anschutz, 1995).

Deming's original management philosophy has been expanded and modified by various management theorists. Crosby stressed conformance to standards and zero defects. According to Crosby, quality improvement is not a program but a permanent process of prevention. Juran developed a structured process for quality improvement and encouraged the use of self-directed quality improvement teams composed of workers. The quality control circle, a team of workers who meet regularly to detect and correct quality prob-

1. Create constancy of purpose for improvement of product and service.
2. Adopt the new philosophy.
3. Cease dependence upon inspection to achieve quality.
4. End the practice of awarding business on the basis of price tag.
5. Improve constantly and forever the systems of production and service.
6. Institute training on the job.
7. Institute leadership.
8. Drive out fear.
9. Break down barriers between departments.
10. Eliminate slogans, exhortations, and targets for the work force.
11. Eliminate numerical quotas for the work force and numerical goals for management.
12. Remove barriers that rob people of pride of workmanship.
13. Institute a vigorous program of education and self-improvement for everyone.
14. Put everyone in the company to work to accomplish the transformation.

From Deming (1986).

lems, was the idea of Kaoru Ishikawa. He valued the use of statistical measurements and believed that all workers should be able to use basic statistics to improve the quality of products (Omachonu & Ross, 1994).

Larrabee (1996) has developed a theoretical model of quality specifically for healthcare. This model suggests that quality, ethics, and economics do not exist in isolation. Rather, they are all directly and indirectly affected by each other. Further information about this model is presented in the theory box on page 172. Figure 11-1 is an illustrated example of Larrabee's theoretical model.

The combination of quality improvement ideas from these theorists is sometimes referred to as **total quality management** or, more simply, quality management. Whichever label is used, the basic tenets of quality management and quality improvement remain the same. These basic principles of quality management are summarized in Box 11-2 and developed further in the next section of this chapter.

QUALITY MANAGEMENT AND QUALITY IMPROVEMENT

Quality management operates most effectively within a flat, democratic organizational structure. Healthcare agencies in the past have often adopted a traditional bureaucratic organizational structure.

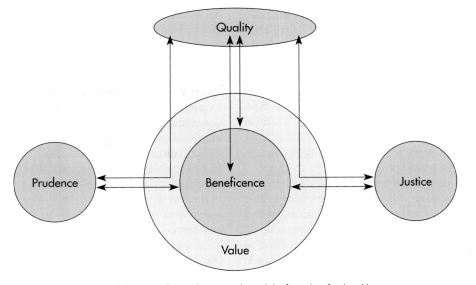

Figure 11-1 Larrabee's theoretical model of quality for healthcare.

Larrabee's Theory		
KEY CONTRIBUTOR	**KEY IDEA**	**APPLICATION TO PRACTICE**
Larrabee (1996) developed a model of quality specifically for healthcare.	Includes both ethical and economic concepts to provide a framework for understanding healthcare quality. The model encompasses the four interrelated concepts of value, beneficence, prudence, and justice (see Figure 11-1). Value is the relative worth or importance, beneficence is promoting well-being without harm, prudence is good judgment and skill in using resources, and justice is fairness.	This theory can help provide balance between efficacy, efficiency, and benefits of healthcare services. More research is needed to test the effectiveness of the model

From Larrabee (1996).

Box 11-2

Principles of Quality Management and Quality Improvement

1. Quality management operates most effectively within a flat democratic organizational structure.
2. Managers and workers must be committed to quality improvement.
3. The goal of quality management is to improve systems and processes, not to assign blame.
4. Customers define quality.
5. Quality improvement focuses on outcomes.
6. Decisions must be based on data.

Within a bureaucratic structure, workers usually specialize in one function or skill and decisions related to that skill are made at the management level above the worker (Heckman, 1996). This type of structure tends to be quite rigid with limited communication across levels of the organization.

Many healthcare organizations have shifted to a different type of corporate structure. This democratic structure, flatter in style with decentralized authority, encourages teamwork and shared leadership among all levels of employees (Heckman, 1996). In a democratic structure, workers can perform more than one function and are involved in decisions related to their areas of expertise (Heckman, 1996). Figure 11-2 on page 173 shows the difference in organizational design between the traditional bureaucratic model and the democratic model.

Involvement

Managers and workers must be committed to quality improvement. Top-level managers retain the ultimate responsibility for quality management, but must involve the entire organization in the quality improvement process. Although some healthcare organizations have achieved significant quality improvement results without system-wide support, total organizational involvement is necessary for a cultural transformation (Boerstler et al, 1996). If all members of the healthcare team are to be actively involved in quality management, a nonthreatening environment must be established. Deming believed that fear was not an effective motivator of employees and even advocated eliminating annual performance reviews because they inhibit creativity (Deming, 1986).

To work effectively in a democratic, quality-focused corporate environment, nurses and other healthcare workers must accept quality improvement as an integral part of their role. When a separate department controls quality activities, healthcare managers and workers often relinquish responsibility and commitment for quality control to these quality specialists. Employees working in an organizational culture that values quality freely make suggestions for improvement and innovation in client care. Exercise 11-1 may help nurses make quality improvement suggestions.

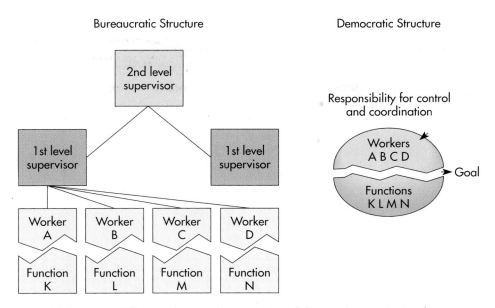

Figure 11-2 Design differences between bureaucratic and democratic organizational structures. (Adapted from Heckman [1996, March].)

Exercise 11-1

Think of a problem or potential problem that exists in the agency where you practice. Describe the problem using as many specific facts as possible. List the advantages to the staff, clients, and agency of correcting this problem. Describe several possible solutions to the problem. Decide who you would contact about this suggestion.

Goal

The goal of quality management is to improve the system, not to assign blame. Managers strive to provide a system in which workers can function effectively. To encourage commitment to quality improvement, nurse managers must clearly articulate the organization's mission and goals. All levels of employees, from nursing assistants to hospital administrators, must be educated about quality improvement strategies.

Communication should flow freely within the organizational structure. To enhance communication, the nurse manager uses a participative or democratic management style. The nurse manager does not micromanage by concentrating on details but leads by demonstrating knowledge, integrity, and commitment to quality care (Omachonu & Ross, 1994).

Quality management improves the system of healthcare delivery. Detection of employees' errors is not stressed. Approximately 85% of all mistakes in the work place are caused by inefficient procedures, policies, or work processes. Only 15% of errors occur because of employee incompetence (Kirk & Hoesing, 1991). When problems occur, intervention should emphasize reeducation of staff rather than imposition of any punitive measures.

Customers

Customers define quality. Successful organizations measure the factors that are most important to their customers and focus their energies on enhancing quality in these areas. As healthcare clients become more sophisticated and view themselves as "consumers" who can take their business elsewhere, they want input into treatment decisions. While a typical patient may not be knowledgeable about a specific treatment, he knows if he was satisfied with the healthcare provider experience.

Every nurse and healthcare agency has internal and external customers. Internal customers are people or units within an organization who receive products or services. A nurse working on a hospital unit could describe clients, nurses on the other shifts, other hospital departments, and nursing managers as internal customers. For a nurse manager, the staff members working under him or her are internal customers. External customers are people or groups outside the organization who receive products or services. For nurses, these external customers may include clients, families, physicians, managed care organizations, and the community at large. Managers and staff nurses can use Exercise 11-2 to identify their internal and external customers.

Exercise 11-2

For 1 week, list every person with whom you interact as a nurse. Which of these people work for your organization? These are the internal customers. Which of these people come from outside the organization? These are the external customers.

Consumer satisfaction with healthcare can be assessed through the use of questionnaires, interviews, focus group discussions, or observation. However, clients cannot always adequately assess the competence of clinical performance. Healthcare providers may use additional tools to assess the safety, effectiveness, and timeliness of patient care (Palmer, 1996).

Focus

Quality improvement focuses on outcomes. Patient outcomes are statements that describe the end results of healthcare (Grohar-Murray & DiCroce, 1997). They are specific and measurable and describe a client's behavior. Outcome statements may be based on client needs, ethical and legal standards of practice, or other standardized data systems. Sources for outcome statements are described further in the next section of this chapter.

Decisions

Decisions must be based on data. The use of statistical tools enables nurse managers to make objective decisions about quality improvement. However, Ishikawa (1985) warned against collecting data merely to support a preconceived idea. In Japan this was one of the most common reasons for poor decision making. Quality information must be gathered and analyzed without bias before improvement suggestions and recommendations are made.

▌ THE QUALITY IMPROVEMENT PROCESS

Quality improvement involves continual analysis and evaluation of products and services to prevent errors and to achieve customer satisfaction. The work of continuous quality improvement never stops because products and services can always be improved. The old adage, "If it ain't broke, don't fix it," conflicts with the main assumption of quality improvement. Improvement is always possible.

Box 11-3

Steps in the Quality Improvement Process

1. Identify needs most important to the consumer of healthcare services.
2. Assemble a multidisciplinary team to review the identified consumer needs and services.
3. Collect data to measure the current status of these services.
4. Establish measurable outcomes and quality indicators.
5. Select and implement a plan to meet the outcomes.
6. Collect data to evaluate the implementation of the plan and the achievement of outcomes.

The quality improvement process is a structured series of steps designed to plan, implement, and evaluate changes in healthcare activities. Many models of the quality improvement process exist, but all contain steps similar to those listed in Box 11-3.

These six steps can easily be applied to clinical situations. In the following example, a community clinic staff uses the quality improvement process to handle client complaints about waiting for appointments.

A community clinic receives a number of complaints from clients about waiting up to 2 hours for scheduled appointments. The clinic secretary and staff nurses suggest to the clinic manager that scheduling clinic appointments be investigated by the quality improvement (QI) committee, which is composed of the clinic secretary, two clinic nurses, one physician, and one nurse practitioner. The clinic manager agrees to the staff's suggestion and assigns the problem to the QI committee. At their next meeting, the QI committee uses a flow chart to describe the scheduling process from the time a client calls to make an appointment until the client sees a physician or nurse practitioner in the examining room. Next, the committee members decide to gather and analyze data about the important parts of the process: the number of calls for appointments, the number of clients seen in a day, the number of canceled or missed appointments, and the average time each client spends in the waiting room. The committee discovers that too many appointments are scheduled because many clients miss appointments. This overbooking frequently results in long waiting times for the clients who do arrive on time. The QI committee also gathers information on clinic waiting times from the literature and through interviews with clients and colleagues. A measurable outcome is written: "Clients will

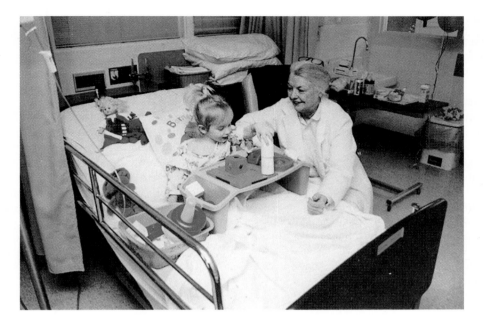

Quality nursing is both caring and compassionate.

wait no longer than 30 minutes for an appointment." After a discussion of options, the team recommends that appointments be scheduled at more reasonable intervals, that clients receive notification of appointments by mail and by phone, and that all clinic clients be educated about the importance of keeping scheduled appointments. The committee communicates its suggestions for improvement to the manager and staff and monitors the results of the implementation of their improvement suggestions. Within 3 months the average waiting room time per client decreased by 30 minutes and the number of missed client appointments decreased by 20%.

Identify Consumers' Needs

The quality improvement process begins with the selection of a clinical activity for review. Theoretically, any and all aspects of clinical care could be improved through the quality improvement process. However, quality improvement efforts should be concentrated on patient care changes that will have the greatest impact. The 80/20 rule applies: 80% of positive improvement in patient care and customer satisfaction will come from changes in 20% of clinical activities (Kirk & Hoesing, 1991).

To determine which 20% of clinical activities are most important, nurse managers or staff nurses may interview or survey patients about their healthcare experiences. What would have helped them at a

particular time? Although many quality improvement activities focus on physical tasks, the caring behavior of nurses may also be studied. The results of the research study (Williams, 1997) highlighted in this chapter's "Research Perspective" on page 176 suggest that patients' perceptions of nurses' caring behavior is related to increased patient satisfaction.

Assemble a Team

Once an activity is selected for possible improvement, a multidisciplinary team implements the quality improvement process. Quality improvement team members should represent a cross section of workers who are involved with the problem. For example, if the activity under review is dinner tray delivery, representatives from the nursing units, nursing assistants, and dietary staff should be on the team. When the activity under review involves medical treatment, physicians should be represented on the team (Anschutz, 1995). Team members may need to be educated about their roles before starting the quality improvement process.

To develop effective quality improvement teams, the work place environment must promote teamwork. Some healthcare facilities are more open to teamwork than others. Nurse managers can use Exercise 11-3 to decide if their clinical facility is ready for quality improvement teams.

Research Perspective

Williams, S.A. (1997). The relationship of patients' perceptions of holistic nurse caring to satisfaction with nursing care. Journal of Nursing Care Quality, 11(5), 15-29.

This correlational study examined the relationship of patients' perceptions of holistic caring and their satisfaction with nursing care in two rural hospitals. Ninety-four hospitalized patients were asked to complete three instruments: the Holistic Caring Inventory, the Pain Thermometer, and the Patient Satisfaction Inventory. Overall, patients reported low satisfaction with nursing care, but patients who perceived the nurses to be caring were more likely to be satisfied with their nursing care.

Implications for Practice

Quality improvement activities often focus on the tasks of nursing care rather than the quality of the nurse-patient relationship. This study suggests that patients' perceptions of nurses as caring individuals are associated with increased client satisfaction. Since patient satisfaction with care is an important quality indicator, nurses and healthcare agencies may need to assess and support the interpersonal aspects of patient care in order to improve patient outcomes.

Exercise 11-3

Ask yourself the following questions pertaining to your system:
1. Is communication between nurses and other disciplines promoted? If so, how?
2. Could the communication process be improved in any way?
3. Does your system encourage nurses to act as a team?
4. Are other disciplines/departments included in team activities?
5. Can the team focus be improved in any way?

Collect Data

After the multidisciplinary team forms, the group collects data to measure the current status of the activity, service, or procedure under review. Various data tools may be used to analyze and present this information. These data tools include flow charts, line graphs, histograms, pareto charts, and fishbone diagrams. The use of empirical tools to organize quality improvement data is an essential part of the quality improvement process. Unfortunately, this step is often omitted (Gilman & Lammers, 1995).

A detailed flow chart is used to describe complex tasks. The flow chart is a data tool that uses boxes and directional arrows to diagram a process or procedure (Longo & Bohr, 1991). Sometimes just diagramming a patient care process in detail reveals opportunities for improvement. The flow chart in Figure 11-3 depicts the process of a home health agency receiving a new patient referral.

Line graphs present data by showing the connection between variables. The dependent variable is usually plotted on the vertical scale, and the independent variable is usually plotted on the horizontal scale. In quality improvement, this technique is frequently used to show the trend of a particular activity over time, and the result may be called a trend chart (Omachonu & Ross, 1994). The line graph in Figure 11-4 illustrates the number of referrals a home health agency receives over the course of a year.

The histogram in Figure 11-5 illustrates the number of home health referrals that come from five different referral sources during 1 year. A histogram is a bar chart that shows the frequency of events.

A bar chart that identifies the major causes or components of a particular quality control problem is called a pareto chart (Omachonu & Ross, 1994). Used frequently in quality improvement, the pareto chart helps the quality improvement team determine priorities. The pareto chart in Figure 11-6 demonstrates that on a medical/surgical unit over a 1-month time period omission of vital signs is the most frequent type of documentation error.

The fishbone diagram, also called the cause-effect diagram, was developed by Ishikawa as a quality control tool. A specific problem or outcome is written on the horizontal line. All possible causes of the problem or strategies to meet the outcome are written in a fishbone pattern. This tool is an effective method of summarizing a brainstorming session. Figure 11-7 uses a fishbone diagram to present possible causes of clients' complaints about extended waits for clinic appointments.

Although quality improvement teams should be able to use these basic statistical tools, more complex

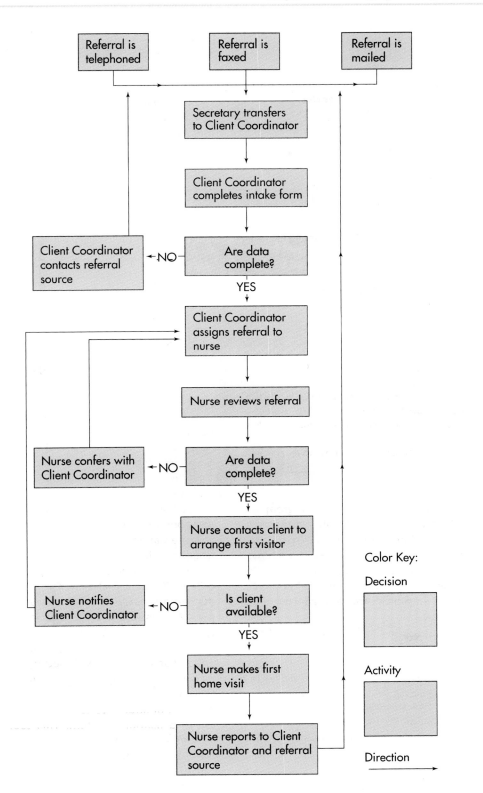

Figure 11-3   Steps in a flow chart diagramming process starting with the time a home health referral is made and ending with the first home visit.

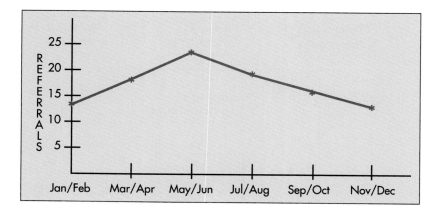

Figure 11-4   Line graph depicting the number of home health referrals received during 1 year.

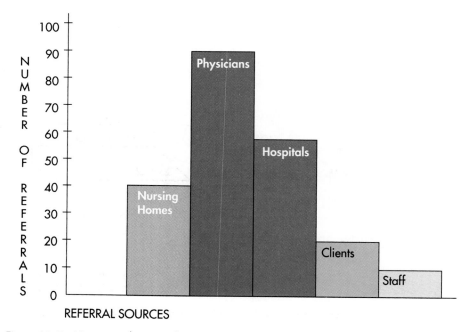

Figure 11-5   Histogram depicting the number of home health referrals received from five sources during 1 year.

analysis is sometimes necessary. In this situation a statistical expert could be included on the quality improvement team or the team may use a statistician as a consultant.

Establish Outcomes

After analyzing the data, the team next sets a goal for improvement. This goal can be established in a number of ways but always involves a standard of practice

and a measurable patient care outcome. The multi-disciplinary team should use accepted standards of care and practice whenever possible. Sources that establish these standards include:

1. State nurse practice act
2. Joint Commission on Accreditation of Healthcare Organizations (JCAHCO) and the Community Health Accreditation Program (CHAP)

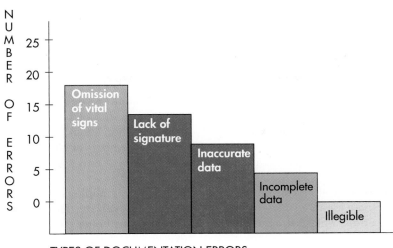

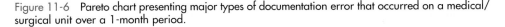

Figure 11-6   Pareto chart presenting major types of documentation error that occurred on a medical/surgical unit over a 1-month period.

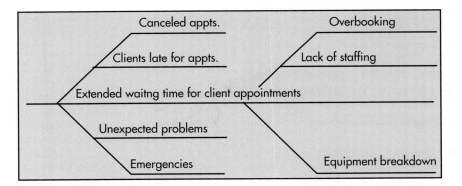

Figure 11-7   Fishbone diagram showing possible causes of extended waiting time for clinic clients.

3. Nationally recognized professional organizations
4. Nursing research
5. Internal policies and procedures
6. Agency for Healthcare Policy and Research (AHCPR)

While individual healthcare organizations may have unique patient needs related to their specific population or environment, many patients and outcomes are similar. One way to evaluate the quality of outcomes is to compare one agency's performance against that of similar organizations. In a process called benchmarking, a widespread search is conducted to identify the best performance against which to measure others. Through this process of comparing the "best practices" against your practice and process, the organization learns more about itself. For example, documentation of discharge teaching can be compared with other institutions and with readmission rates. Unfortunately, the usefulness of the information from other institutions continues to be hampered by differences in terminology. A consistent information system would provide a vast database regarding outcomes of care and resource allocation.

Quality improvement is a data-driven process, so documentation on computers has greatly increased the amount of data available. For example, medication errors within a facility can be analyzed to identify patterns of occurrences as well as consequences. This increased access to data identifies high-risk procedures and systematic errors, which can then be the focus for quality improvement.

Nursing has been a leader in the information system field by developing standardized nursing intervention classification systems. The availability of standardized nursing data enables the study of health problems across populations, settings, and caregivers. Three leading nursing classification systems have been identified: the Nursing Intervention Classification (NIC) System, the Omaha System, and the Home Health Care Classification System (Bowles & Naylor, 1996).

The NIC System is the most universal system designed for use by nurses in all areas of nursing with patients of all ages. This classification consists of interventions that represent both general and specialty nursing practice. Clinical testing for validation and refinement have occurred in various settings, and the standardization of terms continues to develop (Henry et al, 1997).

The two other leading classification systems, the Omaha System and the Home Health Care Classification System, both focus on nursing practice and documentation in home healthcare and nurse-managed care centers (Bowles & Naylor, 1996). Regardless of the classification system used, the consistency of terms is essential in providing a large database across healthcare settings to predict resource requirements and establish outcomes of care.

Discuss Plans

The team discusses various strategies and plans to meet the new outcome. One plan is selected for implementation, and the process of change begins. Since quality management stresses improving the system rather than assigning blame to employees, change strategies emphasize open communication and education of workers affected by the new stan-

dard and outcome. Quality improvement is not possible without continual education of all managers and workers. Even in a cost-conscious environment, staff education is not a luxury but a necessity.

Policies and procedures may need to be written or rewritten during the quality improvement process. Policies should be frequently reviewed and updated so that they do not become barriers to innovation. Communication about the change or improvement to the team members at large is essential.

Evaluate

As the plan is implemented, the team continues to gather and evaluate data to document that the new outcomes are being met. If an outcome is not met, revisions in the implementation plan are needed. Sometimes improvement in one part of a system presents new problems. For example, a school nurse wanted to improve the psychosocial assessment of children with possible family problems. A result of this improvement in care was a greatly increased number of referrals for counseling, which overwhelmed the two school psychologists. The interdisciplinary team may need to reassemble periodically to handle the inevitable snags that develop with the implementation of any new process or procedure. The example that follows illustrates this idea:

A hospital is implementing a pneumatic tube system to dispense medications. A multidisciplinary team was assembled to discuss the process from various viewpoints: pharmacy, nursing, pneumatic tube operation managers, aides who took the medications from the pneumatic tube to the client medication drawers, administrators, and physicians. The tube system is implemented. A nurse on one unit realizes that several patients do not have their morning medications in their med boxes. The nurse borrows meds from another patient's drawer and orders the rest of the meds stat from pharmacy. Other nurses on that unit and other units have the same problem and are doing the same or similar things. Several problems are occurring—some of the medications are being given late, nurses waste precious time by searching other med boxes, the pharmacy charges extra for the stat medications and is overwhelmed with stat requests, and the situation increases the nurses' frustration level. Quality management principles would encourage the nurses to report the problems to the nurse manager or appropriate team member. The pneumatic tube team could compile data such as frequency of missing medications, timing of medication orders, and nursing units involved. The problems are analyzed with a system perspective to effectively solve the late medication problem.

When the change is successfully implemented, the quality improvement team disbands after celebrating their success. One of the crucial tasks of the nurse manager is to publicize and reward the success of each quality improvement team. The nurse manager must also evaluate the work of the team and the ability of individual team members to work together effectively.

Some organizations that have used the quality management philosophy for several years establish permanent quality improvement teams or committees. These quality improvement teams do not disband after implementing one project or idea, but may meet on a regular basis to focus on improvements in one specific area of patient care. In this chapter's "Manager's Challenge" and "Manager's Solution," the director of nursing in a health department describes the use of permanent quality improvement teams and how she prevented duplication of efforts within the quality teams.

QUALITY ASSURANCE

While quality improvement is a comprehensive process to prevent problems, it is naive to suggest the total abandonment of periodic inspection. One such monitoring of healthcare is done with quality assurance programs. **Quality assurance** focuses on clinical aspects of the provider's care, frequently in response to an identified problem. The focus may differ from that of quality improvement, asking questions such as "Did the nurse document the response to the pain medication within the required time period?" instead of "Did the client receive adequate pain relief postoperatively?" The similarities and differences between quality improvement and quality assurance are summarized in Table 11-2.

One of the methods most frequently used in quality assurance is chart review or chart auditing.

Chart audits may be conducted using the records of active and/or discharged patients. Charts are selected randomly and reviewed by qualified health professionals. In an internal audit, staff members from the same hospital or agency that generated the records examine the data. External auditors are qualified professionals from outside the organization who conduct the review. An audit tool containing specific criteria based on standards of care is applied to each chart under review. For example, auditors might compare documentation related to use of restraints with the criterion, "Physician order is obtained for physical restraints within 8 hours of application." Auditors note compliance or lack of compliance with each audit criterion and report a summary of these findings to the appropriate manager or committee for corrective action (Marriner-Tomey, 1996).

Quality assurance staff usually conduct or supervise the chart audits within an agency. Although these nurses are internal auditors, they may not be directly involved with the staff nurses whose charting is under review. Because the focus of the chart audit is on detecting errors and determining the person responsible for them, many staff members tend to view quality assurance as a nuisance or a threat.

RISK MANAGEMENT

Although quality management and risk management are related concepts, quality management emphasizes the prevention of patient care problems, while **risk management** attempts to analyze problems and minimize losses after a patient care error occurs. These losses include financial loss as a result of malpractice or absorbing the cost of an extended length of stay for the patient. They can also include negative public relations and employee dissatisfaction. If quality

Table 11-2	COMPARISON OF QUALITY ASSURANCE AND QUALITY IMPROVEMENT PROCESS	
	Quality Assurance Process	**Quality Improvement Process**
Goal	To improve quality	To improve quality
Focus	Discovery and correction of errors	Prevention of errors
Major tasks	Inspection of nursing activities	Review of nursing activities
	Chart audits	Innovation
		Staff development
Quality team	QA personnel or department personnel	Multidisciplinary team
Outcomes	Set by QA team with input from staff	Set by QI team with input from staff and clients/customers

management was 100% effective, there would be no need for risk management. In the current healthcare environment, however, risk management departments are needed and utilized.

Risk management has blossomed since the malpractice crisis in the 1970s. Before that time, healthcare was assumed to be safe and of high quality except for a very few exceptions. Healthcare professionals were revered, and medical treatment was not questioned. The abundance of liability suits in the 1970s had people doubting the validity of their faith in quality healthcare. The inclusion of risk management standards in the 1990 JCAHO guidelines further emphasized the importance of risk management (Marriner-Tomey, 1996).

The risk management department has several functions. These include the following:

- Define situations that place the system at some financial risk such as medication errors or patient falls.
- Determine the frequency of those situations that occurred.
- Intervene and investigate identified events.
- Identify potential risks or opportunities to improve care.

Each individual nurse is a risk manager. The nurse has the responsibility to identify and report unusual occurrences and potential risks to the proper authority. One method of communicating risks is through incident reporting. Incident reports should be a nonpunitive means of communicating an incident that did cause or could have caused harm to clients, family members, visitors, or employees. These reports should be used to improve quality of care and decrease risk.

Evaluating Risks

In gathering data about unusual occurrences, the risk manager may use the **"five-why" technique.** This technique involves asking "Why" several times to help discover underlying problems that a cursory overview might miss. Risk managers also use a technique called **triangulation.** This technique involves using multiple data sources and data collection techniques. Quantitative methods such as a yes/no questionnaire or chart records are merged with qualitative methods such as an open-ended question interview. This technique is also used in nursing research as a means to gain a broader perspective on nursing questions. Triangulation gives researchers, nurse managers, and risk managers additional information that

might have been missed by using only one method. Triangulation takes more time to conduct and evaluate than just reading an incident report, so it should be used for significant issues.

■ CHAPTER CHECKLIST

Many healthcare organizations are in the process of transforming their system to quality management. Greater efficiency with improved quality is the goal of this approach. Effective quality improvement includes identifying consumer expectations, planning, using a multidisciplinary approach, evaluating outcomes, and changing the system to provide an environment where employees can perform their best. The main principles of quality management and quality improvement are as follows:

- Quality management operates most effectively within a flat, democratic organizational structure.
- Managers and workers must be committed to quality improvement.
- The goal of quality management is to improve systems and processes—not to assign blame.
- Customers define quality.
- Quality improvement focuses on outcomes.
- Decisions must be based on facts.

A Manager's Solution

? After gathering data about the problem of duplication of quality improvement efforts and after consulting with other members of the management team, I decided that there was a lack of communication among the various committee members. To remedy this, we established a "Performance Improvement Council" composed of representatives from each of the original committees. This council meets monthly to exchange information about the progress of each quality improvement committee. The council members strive to avoid duplication of efforts and to encourage collaboration and coordination among the teams. This adjustment in our quality improvement process has allowed us to save time and to maximize the use of our resources.

? *Would this be a suitable approach for you? Why?*

Quality management strives to prevent errors. Quality management requires effective planning. Initially, planning requires both time and money. Quality management saves money in the long run. The quality management philosophy originated with Deming and is being modified by contemporary management theorists.

The major steps in the continuous quality improvement process to evaluate and improve client care are as follows:

- Identify needs most important to the consumer of healthcare services.
- Assemble a multidisciplinary team to review the identified consumer needs and services.
- Collect data to measure the current status of these services.
- Establish measurable outcomes and quality indicators.
- Select and implement a plan to meet the outcomes.
- Collect data to evaluate the implementation of the plan and the achievement of outcomes.

Any process can be improved. Risk management focuses on minimizing loss after a patient care error occurs. Techniques to obtain data include the "five-why" technique and triangulation.

TIPS ON QUALITY MANAGEMENT

- Quality management is based on data—what gets measured and recorded can be improved.
- Concentrate quality improvement energies on factors that are most important to your customers.
- Working together to prevent problems is more effective than fixing problems after they occur.

TERMS TO KNOW

continuous quality improvement
"five why" technique
quality assurance (QA)
quality improvement (QI)
quality management (QM)
risk management
total quality management
triangulation

REFERENCES

Anschutz, E.E. (1995). *TQM America: How America's Most Successful Companies Profit from Total Quality Management.* Bradenton, FL: McGuinn & McGuire.

Boerstler, H., Foster, R.W., O'Connor, E.J., O'Brien, J.L., Shortell, S.M., Carman, J.M., & Hughes, E.F.X. (1996). Implementation of total quality management: Conventual wisdom versus reality. *Hospital and Health Services Administration,* 41(2), 143-159.

Bowles, K.H., & Naylor, M.D. (1996). Nursing intervention classification systems. *Image: Journal of Nursing Scholarship,* 28(4), 303-308.

Deming, W.E. (1986). *Out of the Crisis.* Cambridge: Massachusetts Institute of Technology.

Gilman, S.C., & Lammers, J.C. (1995). Tool use and team success in continuous quality improvement: Are all tools created equal? *Quality Management,* 4(1), 56-61.

Grohar-Murray, M.E., & DiCroce, H.R. (1997). *Leadership and management in nursing.* Stamford, CT: Appleton & Lange.

Heckman, F. (1996). The participative design approach. *Journal of Quality and Participation,* 2(3), 48-51.

Henry, S.B., Holzemore, W., Randell, C., Hsieh, S., & Miller, T. (1997). Comparison of nursing interventions classification and current procedural terminology codes for categorizing nursing activities. *Image: Journal of Nursing Scholarship,* 29(2), 133-138.

Ishikawa, K. (1985). *What Is Total Quality Control? The Japanese Way.* Englewood Cliffs, NJ: Prentice-Hall.

Kirk, R., & Hoesing, H. (1991). *The Nurses' Guide to Common Sense Quality Management.* West Dundee, IL: S-N Publications.

Larrabee, J.H. (1996). Emerging model of quality. *Image: Journal of Nursing Scholarship,* 28(4), 353-358.

Longo, D.R., & Bohr, D., eds. (1991). *Quantitative Methods in Quality Management: A Guide for Practitioners.* Chicago, American Hospital Publishing.

Marriner-Tomey, A. (1996). *Guide to Nursing Management* (4th ed). St Louis: Mosby.

Omachonu, V.K., & Ross, J.E. (1994). *Principles of Total Quality.* Delray Beach, FL: St. Lucie Press.

Palmer, R.H. (1996). Measuring clinical performance to provide information for quality improvement. *Quality Management,* 4(2), 1-6.

Williams, S.A. (1997). The relationship of patients' perceptions of holistic nurse caring to satisfaction with nursing care. *Journal of Nursing Care Quality,* 11(5), 15-29.

SUGGESTED READINGS

Abbott, K.M. (1996). Home care and nursing risk management. *Journal of Nursing Law,* 3(3), 41-52.

Brailer, D.J., Goldfarb, S., Horgan, J., Katz, F., Paulus, R.A., & Zakrewski, K. (1996). Improving performance with clinical decision support. *Joint Commission Journal on Quality Improvement,* 22(7), 443-356.

Case, T. (1996). A quality assessment and improvement system for long-term care. *Quality Management in Health Care,* 4(3), 15-21.

Fannucci, D., Hammill, M., Johannson, P., Leggett, J., & Smith, M. (1993). Quantum leap into continuous quality improvement. *Nursing Management,* 24(6), 28-30.

Feigenbaum, A.V. (1996). Managing for tomorrow's competitiveness today. *Journal of Quality and Participation,* 19(3), 10-17.

Hilliard, L.S. (1997). Manager's corner: Risk management an important component of quality. *Home Care Nurse News,* 4(1), 1,3,5.

Hudock, K.L., Smerker, J., Fisher, C., Taylor, I., Fanning, V., Chapla, J., & Ireland, C. (1997). Benchmarking in home care. *Caring,* 16(2), 77.

Iowa Intervention Project. (1993). The NIC taxonomy structure. *Image: Journal of Nursing Scholarship*, 25(3), 187-192.

Jones, L., & Arana, G. (1996). Forum. Is downsizing affecting incident reports? *Joint Commission Journal on Quality Improvement*, 22(8), 592-594.

King, K. (1996-97, Winter). Using a quality balance sheet to weigh assets and liabilities. *The Journal of Long-term Administration*, 24(4), 15-19.

Koch, M., & Fairly, T. (1992). *Integrated Quality Management: the Key to Improving Nursing Care Quality.* St Louis: Mosby.

Labovitz, G. (1990). *The Quality Advantage.* Burlington, MA: Organizational Dynamics, Inc.

Office of Continuous Quality Improvement, Houston Health Center, University of Texas. (May 2, 1995). Continuous quality improvement (on-line; available at http://www.uth.tmc.edu/ut_general/admin_fin/cqi/index.html).

Patton, S., & Stanley, J. (1993). Bridging quality assurance and continuous quality improvement. *Journal of Nursing Care Quality*, 7(2), 15-23.

Rhinehart, E. (1996). Synergy of quality management and risk management in home care. *Caring*, 15(9), 32-33, 35, 38.

Willoughly, C., Budrearu, G., & Livingston, K. (1997). A framework for integrated quality improvement. *Journal of Nursing Care Quality*, 11(3), 44-53.

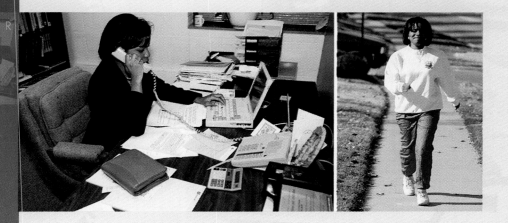

Self-Management: Stress and Time

Fay Carol Reed
RN, PhD

Amy C. Pettigrew
RN, DNS

This chapter examines the concept of self-management—the ability of individuals to gain control of their lives. Four components of self-management are explored: stress management, time management, meeting management, and delegation. Methods for managing stress and organizing one's time are introduced. Practical exercises and suggestions for stress and time management are presented that can be used for personal as well as professional situations in order to reduce stress and enhance efficiency.

Objectives

- Define self-management.
- Explore causes of stress in nursing.
- Analyze selected strategies to decrease stress.
- Assess the manager's role in helping staff to manage stress.
- Evaluate common barriers to effective time management.
- Critique the strengths and weaknesses of selected time management strategies.
- Evaluate selected strategies to manage time more effectively.

Questions to Consider

- Are you currently using self-management strategies?
- What types of activities cause stress for you?
- Can you identify ways to handle stress more effectively?
- What are your highest priority personal and professional goals?
- Does the way you spend your time reflect your priorities?
- Are you drowning in information and paperwork?
- How does a nurse manager successfully use time to attain work goals?

? A Manager's Challenge
From a Nurse Manager at a Midwestern Hospital

As a newly assigned nurse manager, I was expected to manage a medical-surgical unit as well as function as a charge nurse. This responsibility often included acting as team leader and direct care provider. Stress and time management issues evolved out of the dual role expectations. Most of my management duties were deferred to late afternoons after my patient care responsibilities were completed, or to evenings and weekends. I felt stressed and guilty when I had to leave the unit for nurse manager or quality assurance meetings. I was also constantly trying to balance my work life with the demands of my family life.

? *What do you think you would do if you were this manager?*

INTRODUCTION

How many times have you gone to bed at night feeling guilty about not having accomplished anything during the day? How many times have you stopped to wonder what you really want to be when you grow up? **Self-management** is about deciding what you want for yourself, setting goals for your life, developing objectives and short-term outcomes to reach the goals, and finally organizing the time and activities you have to reach them (Weiss, 1986). Self-management is also about finding a balance between quality in career, family, social activities, and self (Griessman, 1994).

To find this balance within ourselves, we must actively engage in taking control of our lives—no one else is going to! The two key strategies introduced in this chapter—stress and time management—constantly interplay with our life goals. We can move in a straight line toward our personal and professional goals if stress or distractions do not interfere. When stress becomes overwhelming, or others rob us of our time, the path suddenly becomes unclear. Time and stress are somewhat of a "chicken and egg" phenomenon—not enough time creates stress, and stress can erode efficiency and thus decrease time on task. The key here lies in our ability to manage both time and stress, not only personally but also professionally.

MANAGEMENT OF STRESS

In the introduction to his book, *Work and Stress*, James D'Amato (1988) wrote, "Stress today has become a focus for behavioral scientists because of the damage it has done and will continue to do" (p. 7). New graduates have often learned about the impact of stress on patients and how to manage its consequences. They are less likely, however, to have considered in any structured manner the stress in their own lives. Yet nearly every sentient being has experienced stress—the exhilaration of a joyous event and the negative feelings and unpleasant physical symptoms that may be associated with a difficult life situation, or even the anticipation of difficulty. Nurses are not immune to stress and its effects, although some attempt to present that appearance and some employing organizations reinforce that stance. Learning what stress is, its dynamics, and some strategies to manage the distress should be part of the personal and professional maturation of nurses. Their human struggle can link nurses with the humanity of their patients, that is, with those who suffer and experience stress.

Definition

In this chapter, *stress* and *distress* will be used interchangeably, although some writers regard stress as neutral and refer to the positive and negative attributes of *eustress* and *distress*, respectively. Stress (or distress) has such meanings as adversity, pressure, and strain (Simpson & Weiner, 1989).

Sources of Stress

Expectations

For many people, perhaps particularly human service providers, work is more than an activity required to earn a salary in order to purchase goods and services. Work is significant not only because it occupies many hours each week but also because most nurses and other healthcare professionals expect to find their work meaningful; if it is not, work may become a source of distress (Zales, 1994).

Often nurses select their profession because they "want to work with people"; however, they are frequently unprepared for the seemingly endless demands of the position. One investigator found, for example, that junior and senior nursing students were able to identify the stressors reported by a group of registered nurses; however, they underestimated the magnitude of the stress. In this study, underestimating the stressors reduced position satisfaction and esteem and increased incidents of depression (Dytell, 1990).

Cherniss (1980) has written that unseasoned nurses imagine a more ideal work place than that which exists. There may be disillusionment when inexperienced nurses learn that they have much to learn and that some periods in the work place have few successes (Cherniss, 1980). Such unrealistic expectations may be a problem for employers, nurse managers, and patients as well as newly hired nurses. In a study of recently employed nurses, McCloskey and McClain (1987) found that 24% of those who had unrealistic expectations left their positions after 18 months of employment. Nurses who resigned their positions

included not only neophytes, but also newly hired, experienced nurses. This finding points to the need for managers to clarify position expectations and the reality of the work setting for new employees. To minimize distress, nurses who interview for positions need to strive to learn whether their expectations can be met by their potential employing agency. Often the best resources are persons in comparable positions rather than human resources personnel.

Change

"Restructuring," "rightsizing," and similar terms encapsulate the dramatic shift in healthcare practices, management, and values. Nurses, as well as other healthcare providers, are reeling from the effects of changes in healthcare financing, all of which are potential stressors. In the work situation, nurses may feel powerless to control their areas of responsibility and to meet ever-increasing new position demands (Zales, 1994).

Although the distress that results from change takes many forms, two underlying patterns appear to be constant. First, nurses feel trapped by conflicting expectations. They expect to furnish care, to meet patients' needs, and to be nurturing. However, organizations require nurses to be managers of patient care and of systems and value their contribution to efficiency and cost-effectiveness. Because nurses cannot comply with both expectations, they experience considerable role conflict, frustration, and distress.

Second, increasing numbers of managers in healthcare agencies have no background in healthcare. According to Czander (1993), as these managers have gained power by controlling financial and other information, professionals have lost the needed authority to control their practice. Loss of autonomy, together with increases in rules and regulations, results in distress for nurses as well as for other clinicians. They feel powerless and devalued.

People

Interpersonal relations can buffer stressors or can become stressors. Outside the work setting, home can be a refuge for harried nurses; however, stresses at home, when severe, can impair work performance and relationships among staff or even result in violence that may invade the work place.

Changes in healthcare delivery systems reduce the number of professional staff to a minimum. Consequently, some nurses lose supportive, collegial relationships that may have been established over many years. Reduction in staff may result in the discharge of some nurses and sever all work relationships, forcing nurses into the loneliness and uncertainty of unemployment. In other situations, nurses are reassigned or "float" to various patient care units requiring that they work with unfamiliar staff. Thus they may feel isolated or become unwillingly involved in dysfunctional politics on the unit. Such situations may also necessitate that nurses work with patients whose requirements for care may be unfamiliar, resulting in further stress related to uncertainty or lack of knowledge.

Persons at the corporate level may also become stressors. Communication may be from the top down with little opportunity for nurses to participate in decisions that affect them directly or that they may need to implement without proper training or support. Distress results from feeling impotent and frustrated.

The position

Most nurses expect, and rightly so, that caring for patients who are chronically or critically ill and for families who have experienced tragedy will be stressful. Nurses expect and are somewhat prepared for such stress. Yet sometimes the care of a suffering human being completely depletes the emotional and physical resources of even wise and experienced nurses.

The current environment in many healthcare agencies, however, is more complex and is often characterized by **overwork** as well as by the stresses inherent in nursing practice. In her book, *Abuse in the Workplace*, Bassman (1992) posited that overwork is the norm in many organizations. It is no longer episodic or related to individual staff members. Commonly, employees experience strong pressures to produce more and more, she wrote, while managers perceive that the employees are not producing enough. In the abusive work place, Bassman continued, the culture of the organization conveys the expectation that work must be the primary commitment. These demands can destroy personal and family life, demoralize employees, and add to the stress inherent in the position. Citing several studies, Bassman concluded that it is doubtful that increased productivity results from overwork. Clearly, this type of organization is stress producing and sounds familiar to many persons who feel overwhelmed by the demands of the work place.

Dynamics of Stress

Stress may be the consequence of unrealistic or conflicting expectations, of the pace and magnitude of change, of human behavior, of the characteristics of the position itself, or of the culture of the organization. Other stressors may be unique to certain environments, situations, and persons or groups. Even

hardy persons are likely to experience the deleterious effect of some stressors.

Although some stress may be motivating and make employees more effective, distress is more often a problem that results in decreased position performance, unpleasant feelings, and sometimes illness (Golembiewski & Munzenrider, 1988). In fact, even anticipation of a stressor can evoke effects that are similar to those that occur when a stressor is actually experienced (Spacapan & Cohen, 1983). The concept of stress and the reactions to it are complex. A substantial review of the literature pertaining to psychosomatic illness by David Oken (1987) illustrates that the understanding of stress and associated concepts such as **coping** or adaptation is evolving. In this review, Oken noted that although there were antecedent studies, Hans Selye's mid-century investigations of the nature of and reactions to stress have been very influential. In his classic theory, Selye (1956) described the concept of stress, identified the **general adaptation syndrome (GAS)** and detailed a predictable pattern of response (see Figure 12-1). Although the stress research methodologies have become more sophisticated and the findings more illuminating, the average employee recognizes the origins of stress and its symptoms. For example, a healthcare agency may make demands on nurses, such as excessive work, which they regard as beyond their capacity to perform. When they are unable to resolve the problem through overwork, with more staff, or by looking at the situation in another way, nurses may feel threatened or depressed. They may also experience headache, fatigue, or other physical symptoms. If the stress persists, such symptoms may increase and they may attempt to cope by becoming apathetic or by quitting their positions. What else can they do? Table 12-1 gives signs of overstress in individuals.

Managing Stress

Individuals respond to stress by eliciting coping strategies that are a means of dealing with stress intentionally to maintain or achieve well-being. These strategies may be ineffective and rely on methods such as withdrawal or substance abuse, or they may be effective in helping to restore a greater sense of well-being and effectiveness. Some of these strategies are discussed here.

Primary prevention

The most effective way to deal with stress is to determine and eliminate its source (Cooper, 1996). Discovering the origin of stress in patient care may be difficult because some environments have changed

Stress Theories		
KEY CONTRIBUTORS	**KEY IDEAS**	**APPLICATION TO PRACTICE**
General Adaptation Syndrome Selye (1956) is credited with developing this theory.	The "stress response" is an adrenocortical reaction to stressors that is accompanied by psychological changes and physiological alterations that follow a pattern of fight or flight. This general adaptation syndrome includes an alarm, resistance, and adaptation or exhaustion.	Change, lack of control, and excessive work load are common stressors that evoke psychologic and physiologic distress among nurses.
Pareto's Law V.F. Pareto in 1892 is credited with this theory (Davis, 1997).	Pareto studied distribution of personal incomes and discovered that 80% of the wealth was controlled by 20% of the population. This ratio carries over into healthcare today—80% of healthcare expenditures are on 20% of the population, or 80% of personnel problems come from 20% of the staff.	In quality improvement, 80% of improvement can by expected by removing 20% of the causes of unacceptable quality or performance. A nurse can also expect that 80% of patient care time will be spent working with 20% of her patient assignment.

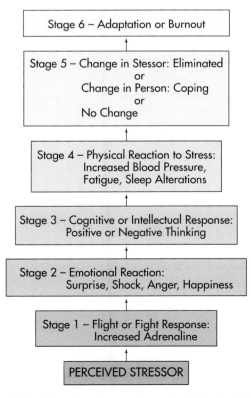

Figure 12-1   The stress diagram. (Based on Selye, H. [1991]).

so rapidly that the nursing staff is overwhelmed trying to balance bureaucratic rules and limited resources with the demands of vulnerable human beings. In their distress, nurses may need to step back and look at the "big picture," to identify the stressor, and then to determine whether it may be eliminated, modified, or perceived differently.

Good managers must have a **systems perspective** that enables them to seek the problem that lies beyond its manifestations. Maslach & Leiter (1997) suggest that employee stress (burnout) may be a sign of organizational dysfunction. The Literature Perspective box emphasizes the importance of recognizing and managing stress. For example, the numbers of staff nurses in an acute care hospital were reduced and unlicensed assistive personnel (UAPs) with minimal training were introduced. The professional staff nurses who managed groups of patients were soon frustrated by the quality and quantity of work accomplished by the UAPs. They used various strategies to cope with the situation, including cajoling and scolding the UAPs, "doing the work themselves," and even resigning their positions in disgust. The UAPs responded by vanishing from the unit as often as possible and even sabotaging the professional nurses.

Table 12-1	SIGNS OF OVERSTRESS IN INDIVIDUALS	
Physical	**Mental**	**Spiritual/Emotional**

Physical signs of ill health:
   a. increased flu, colds, accidents
   b. change in sleeping habits
   c. fatigue
	Dread going to work every day
	
	 Rigid thinking and a desire to go by the rules in all cases; being unable to tolerate any changes
		Sense of being a failure; disappointed in work performance
		
		 Anger and resentment toward clients, colleagues, and managers; overall irritable attitude

Chronic signs of decreased ability to manage stress:
   a. headaches
   b. hypertension
   c. backaches
   d. gastrointestinal problems
	Being forgetful and anxious about work to be done; errors and incidents more frequent
	
	 Returning home exhausted and unable to participate in enjoyable activities
		Lack of positive feelings toward others
		
		 Cynicism toward clients, blaming them for their problems

Use of unhealthy coping activities:
   a. increased use of drugs and alcohol
   b. increased weight
	Confusion about duties and roles	Excessive worry; insecurity; lowered self-esteem
		 Increased family and friend conflict

Literature Perspective

Menninger, W. W. (1996). Practitioner, heal thyself: Coping with stress in clinical practice. Bulletin of the Menninger Clinic, 60(2), 197-205.

Clinicians are subject to special stressors related to caring for vulnerable persons and to sharing their problems. Women may experience added stress related to gender and role and the resultant time pressure associated with career and family responsibilities. Such responsibilities may result in "compassion fatigue." Stressors may be manifest as "body language," including physical or other symptoms such as emotional exhaustion.

Coping with stress involves dealing directly with a situation and overcoming it and/or gaining some distance from it. These approaches provide a sense of control and may furnish a fresh perspective. Reduction of high levels of stress also requires ways to release negative emotion, to engage in outside activities, and to enjoy a social support system. Over time, stress reduction may involve reconsideration of long-term aspirations and priorities.

Implications for Practice
If nurses and other healthcare professionals seek to provide effective care and be available to those persons who are their patients, they must recognize signs of overstress and be responsible for managing it.

One might assume that this problem was one of human relations or of nurses unable to cope with an altered system of delivering nursing care. The problem, however, was a systems problem and violated some good management principles. First, those nurses who were most affected by the decision to use UAPs were not involved in determining what their duties should be. Thus the professional nurses had no "ownership" of the decision and no stake in making it work. Second, the UAPs just "appeared" on the patients' units. The nurses had neither a planned orientation concerning how

Table 12-2	STRESS MANAGEMENT STRATEGIES		
Physical	**Mental**	**Emotional/Spiritual**
Accept physical limitations.	Learn to say no!	Use meditation.
Modify nutrition: high carbohydrate, low caffeine, low sugar.	Use cognitive restructuring and self-talk.	Seek solace in prayer.
Exercise: participate in an enjoyable activity three times a week for 30 minutes.	Use imagery.	Seek professional counseling.
	Develop hobbies or activities.	Participate in support groups.
Make your physical health a priority.	Plan vacations.	Participate in networking.
	Learn about the system and how problems are handled.	Communicate feelings.
Nurture yourself by taking time for breaks and lunch.	Learn communication, conflict resolution, and time management skills.	Identify and acquire a mentor.
Sleep: get enough in quantity and quality.		Ask for feedback and clarification.
Relax: use meditation, massage, yoga, or biofeedback.	Take continuing education courses.	

to assign tasks to the UAPs, nor information about the nature and scope of their training. Third, the professional nurses were told that they were responsible for the care that the UAPs provided, but they had no part in their performance evaluation. The management principle that authority and accountability should be commensurate was violated. In this case the stressors were systems' problems and could have been prevented by the application of accepted management principles.

Secondary prevention

Unpredictable and uncontrollable changes, together with immense responsibility, produce stress for nurses and other healthcare professionals. Consequently, nurses develop symptoms such as anxiety, physical alterations such as headache, and behavioral changes such as immoderate use of alcohol. In situations when stressors cannot be eliminated, it is important to develop strategies to modify the distress (Cooper, 1996). Each nurse must find his or her most effective stress reliever, such as those summarized in Table 12-2. If the stress symptoms are not too taxing, such activities make the situation more manageable and improve the nurses' sense of well-being.

More severe symptoms may require more structured approaches when nurses feel that their well-being is in jeopardy. Planned physical activity appears to reduce stress. Although the specific mechanism by which stress is modified by physical activity has not been fully investigated, Blumenthal and McCubbin (1987) elicited the following explanations from a review of selected literature. First, aerobic exercise appears to modify the cardiovascular responses to stress. Second, exercise is a diversion from stressful thoughts. Third, group exercise may furnish social support, which seems to modify stress. Fourth, physical activity may provide a sense of effectiveness and modify the symptoms of anxiety.

Meditation to elicit the relaxation response may be beneficial. The benefits of practicing relaxation techniques for 20 minutes daily include a feeling of well-being, the ability to learn how tension makes the body feel, and the sense that tension can be controlled. In cases of some stress-related disorders, such as hypertension, biofeedback may be employed to monitor physiological relaxation processes. This technique enables some individuals to better relax and to gain control over selected physiological processes (Beech et al, 1982).

Exercise 12-1 Relaxation Response

This exercise can be used in the middle of a working day, or the last thing at night, or at any time you feel tense or anxious.

1. Find a place away from interruption for 10 minutes.
2. Loosen tight clothes; lie on the floor, a mat, a towel, or a couch, if possible. Close your eyes, and let your body go slack.
3. Starting from the top of your body, work steadily through all your muscles, tightening and then relaxing them.
4. Lift up your head and pull it forward as far as you can, then let it fall back gently.
5. Continuing downward, press your shoulders down hard, then slowly relax them.
6. Open your fingers wide, stretch your arms out to your side, and hold them as tight and hard as you can. Then slowly let them go.
7. With your arms lying at your side, tighten your abdominal muscles as hard as you can, then relax them.
8. Lift your buttocks, tightening them as they go, and then gently let them fall back. Relax the buttocks and spine muscles, thinking consciously of the areas you are working on.
9. Do a mental check to make sure other muscles have not tightened up. Put your heels together and stretch your legs and toes as far as you can, then slowly relax them.
10. Turn on your side and lie that way for 2 to 3 minutes. Sit up slowly and think how you are feeling, and try to keep that feeling as you go back to your activities.

Adapted from Wilson (1990).

Supportive work relationships, as well as nurturing family and friends, may be an important way to buffer the negative effects of a stressful work environment as exemplified in the "Research Perspective" on page 193. Although friendships may be formed with colleagues, the work load and the shifting of staff from one unit to another often makes it difficult to establish and maintain close relationships with peers. However, managers and coworkers who are supportive may improve morale in the work place (Zales, 1994). Nurses who are in a new position or in an unfamiliar geographic area must anticipate that they will benefit from the security of being part of a group that can furnish unconditional acceptance. Without easily accessible family and friends, they need to be intentional about seeking out new, supportive personal relationships. The foregoing efforts may help nurses cope with work place demands that seem to exceed their capacity. Such positive coping strategies may make nurses less likely to adopt such potentially negative coping strategies as withdrawal, lowering their standards of care, and abusing alcohol or other substances. Readers are invited to analyze their stress experiences by completing Exercise 12-2.

Exercise 12-2

Identify what stress you experience and how you usually manage it. Create and complete the following log at the end of every day for 1 week. Review the log and note what situations (people, technology, value conflict, etc.) were the most frequent. Also identify how you most frequently react to stress: physically, mentally, and emotionally/spiritually. *Keeping this diary for a week is helpful to determine what causes you stress and learn about your reactions.*

DATE   _____

SITUATION   _____

YOUR RESPONSE   _____

ACTION   _____

EVALUATION   _____

Tertiary prevention

Sometimes individuals, through their own efforts, are unable to manage stress successfully and require assistance (Cooper, 1996). In such situations, stress-related behavior becomes a persistent problem that seems unresolvable (Beech et al, 1982). Examples of behavior related to stress that feels overwhelming are found in Table 12-1. Coping strategies, such as those described above, furnish temporary relief or none at all. With this level of distress, one can feel overwhelmed, helpless, or at risk for mental or physical illness. This constellation of emotions is frequently called **"burnout."**

Burnout has been defined as " . . . a process in which a previously committed professional disengages from his or her work in response to stress and strain experienced on the job" (Cherniss, 1980, p. 18). The sources of the stressors may exist in the environment, in the individual, or in the unique interaction between the individual and the environment, resulting in perceived stress (Schwartz, Pickering, & Landsbergis, 1996). Some stressors, such as employment termination, appear to be universal, while other stressors, such as meeting deadlines, are more personal. For example, some nurses thrive on goals and timetables while others feel constrained and frustrated and thereby experience distress. Burnout is not an objective phenomenon, as if it were the accumulation of a certain number and type of stressors. How the stressors are perceived and how they are mediated by an individual's ability to adapt are important variables in determining levels of distress.

Nurses who are burned out feel as if their resources are depleted to the point that their well-being is at risk. A self-analysis usually uncovers the characteristics of burnout. First, there is a feeling of *emotional exhaustion*. Leiter (1992) wrote that the etiology of exhaustion is often the unexpected demands of the work place and the nature of professional standards that may be in conflict with the practices and resources of the employing institution. For example, recent graduates may value total, detailed care for individuals and may have little experience in caring for more than two patients simultaneously. When confronted with the responsibility of caring for a group of eight acutely ill patients, they may sustain difficulty adapting to the realities of the work place and emotional exhaustion ensues. Parker and Kulik (1995) found that emotionally exhausted nurses' performance was rated lower by them and by their supervisors and that increased absences for mental health reasons were reported.

A second characteristic of burnout is **depersonalization** (Leiter, 1992), a state that is characterized by an inability to become involved with patients or others. Koeske and Kelly (1995) observed that overinvolvement by helping professionals often results in burnout. The authors recommended an attitude of "detached concern" to avoid ineffectiveness and the decreased morale and position satisfaction that may accompany burnout. A balance of caring without becoming overwhelmed requires a view that although the caregiver cannot be responsible for the outcome of illness, providing care can make a difference (Carmack, 1997). Depersonalization is a form of withdrawal when employees believe they no longer possess the emotional resources to handle interpersonal stressors (Lee & Ashforth, 1996).

Decreased effectiveness is the third hallmark of burnout (Leiter, 1992). This characteristic appears to be related to the desire for control (Lee & Ashforth, 1996). When human service professionals were not free to use their initiative and professional judgment, tension, stress, and burnout occurred (Leiter, 1992). Via complex mechanisms not yet fully understood, prolonged stress and burnout are also related to physiological problems. Some studies have demonstrated a link between the nature of the work place and illness; however, the nature of individual susceptibility to physical changes related to stress has been studied little (Schwartz, Pickering, & Landsbergis, 1996).

Resolving High Levels of Stress

Social support

Peers and followers can be supportive and help to reduce stress via assistance with problem solving and with developing new perspectives. Family and friends

---

Research Perspective

Parker, P. & Kulik, J. (1995). Burnout, self- and supervisor-rated job performance, and absenteeism among nurses. Journal of Behavioral Medicine, *18(6) 581-599.*

This study reported the effect of stress and social support on the development of burnout among nurses. The volunteer subjects were 73 registered nurses who were employed in a Veterans Medical Center. Self-reported data were collected concerning job stress (Nursing Stress Scale), social support for work-related stress (House/Wells Social Support Scale), burnout (Maslach Burnout Inventory), and negative affectivity (Taylor Manifest Anxiety Scale). In addition, job performance was assessed by asking the subjects to rate their own job performance and by asking supervisors to measure the subjects' performance using the same instrument. Data concerning absences and intention to leave their current position were also collected.

Relationships existed among work support, stress, and burnout. Higher levels of burnout were predicted by higher levels of job stress and limited social support. Burnout, specifically emotional exhaustion, was related also to poorer job performance as described by the supervisors and by the nurses themselves. Higher burnout levels were associated also with increased absenteeism, particularly absences for mental health reasons.

Implications for Practice

When their absenteeism for mental health reasons increases, nurses should be alerted to the possibility that it is related to burnout and emotional exhaustion. Behaviors associated with nurse burnout may be related to alterations in interpersonal relationships with patients. Their perceptions of quality of care, while not studied specifically, should be considered.

can provide a safe haven and a vacation from stress. Social isolation increases stress.

Counseling

Persistent unpleasant feelings, problem behavior, and helplessness during prolonged stress suggest the need for assistance from a mental health professional. Examples of problem behaviors include tearfulness or angry outbursts over seemingly minor incidents, major changes in eating and/or sleeping patterns, frequent unwillingness to go to work, and substance abuse. In such cases the above coping strategies afford only temporary relief; nurses with this level of distress feel overwhelmed and believe that their well-being cannot be maintained. In these stressful situations, nurses may feel helpless and must seek professional assistance from a clinical psychologist, psychiatrist, or other mental health worker.

In some organizations, **employee assistance programs** (EAPs) provide counseling and other services for employees either via in-house staff or by contract with a mental health agency. This type of counseling can be effective because the counselors may already be aware of organizational stressors. Although such counseling may be both economical and effective, it is prudent to ask the following questions:

- Will my identity or any information from the sessions be shared in any way?
- What records are kept and how are they stored?
- What type of reports on EAP activity are made to the employer?
- Have there been any claims that confidentiality has been violated?
- What are the limits of confidentiality?

Counseling may begin when satisfactory answers have been obtained and when the counselor and employee have established positive rapport.

Those who seek counseling outside of the work place may be guided in their selection of mental health professionals by a personal physician, by a knowledgeable colleague, or by such publications as the most recent edition of *Directory of Medical Specialists*, which is available in many hospital libraries. When the problem underlying the distress is ethical or moral, a trained pastoral counselor may be helpful. Some clergy are certified in pastoral care or have earned a degree in another discipline such as psychology. Referrals can be obtained from hospital pastoral care departments, or sometimes churches sponsor regional centers where certified counselors are available. When arranging for counseling privately, it is wise to check your health insurance contract for mental health benefits to determine the payment limitations and the type of provider eligible for reimbursement.

Leadership and Management

While social support and counseling can alter how stressors are perceived, time management and good leadership can modify or remove stressors. Perhaps the most important stress modifier is enhancing the control of nursing staff over their environment. First-line managers such as nurses responsible for patient care units have limited formal authority as individuals in most organizations, although managerial groups may be able to influence policy and resource allocation. Individuals can, however, control some environmental stressors on their units. First, leaders can examine their own behavior as a source of subordinates' stress. A review of selected literature (Offermann & Hellmann, 1996) reported that some leaders underestimate the influence of their behavior on subordinates' stress level and that they may attribute observed stress to the environment rather than their own behavior. This review also reported that lower performance and position satisfaction among subordinates was associated with nonparticipative, autocratic leadership styles.

In some cases a controlling style of leadership is appropriate, such as in emergency situations and when working with a large percentage of new and inexperienced employees. For the most part, however, professional nurses need and want the latitude to direct their activities within their sphere of competence. "Letting go" ultimately means that the manager trusts the personal integrity and professional competence of nurse subordinates. It does not mean abdicating responsibility for achieving accepted standards of patient care and agreed-upon outcomes.

Assistance with problem solving is an additional way to reduce environmental stressors. Nurse managers may provide technical advice, direct staff to appropriate resources, or mediate conflicts. Often nurse managers enable staff to meet the demands of their work more independently by providing time for continuing education and professional meetings to enhance competence.

Another way in which managers can reduce stress is to be supportive of staff. Support is *not* equated with being a friend, but with helping staff to accomplish good care, to develop professionally, and to feel valued personally. Encouraging innovation and experimentation, for example, can motivate staff and give them a sense of greater control over their environment. Affirming a good idea or finding resources to study or implement a promising new procedure or proposal by a staff nurse is supportive. In contrast, when staff struggle with overwork and other stressors, support is recognizing the condition and helping the nurses to avoid passive coping strategies, such as feeling helpless or lowering standards of care, in favor of active problem solving. Managers must be sensitive to the distress of the nursing staff and recognize it verbally without becoming counselors, which is in conflict with their role. Support may involve making nursing staff aware of resources that furnish counseling while being careful to avoid diagnostic labels and to maintain strict confidentiality. When distress relates to the personal life of subordinates, managers should focus on the effect of such situations on work place performance, not on the events that have produced the stress.

Finally, managers can enhance the work place by dealing effectively with their own stressors. Maintaining a sense of perspective and even a sense of humor is important. Some stressors, in fact, can be ignored or minimized by posing three questions:

1. "Is this event or situation important?" Stressors are not all equally significant. Don't waste energy on little stressors.
2. "Does this stressor have an impact on me or my unit?" Although some situations that produce distress are institution wide and need group action, others target specific units or activities. Don't borrow stressors.
3. "Can I change this situation?" If not, then find a way to cope with it or, if the situation is intolerable, make plans to change positions or employers. This decision may require gaining added credentials that may produce long-term career benefits.

Keeping stressful situations in perspective can enable patient care managers to conserve their energies to cope with stressful situations that are important, that are within their domain, or that can be changed or modified. Dr. Hans Selye captured the essence of perspective during a speech in New York in the 1970s. His advice, equally relevant today, was: "Remember, you can love puppy dogs, but you cannot love crocodiles."

MANAGEMENT OF TIME

There is a very close relationship between stress management and time management. Time management, per se, is one method of stress prevention or reduction, while stress can decrease productivity and lead to poor use of time, Time management can also be considered a preventive action to help reduce the elements of stress in a nurse's life.

Everyone has two choices when it comes to managing time: organize or "go with the flow." There are only 24 hours in every day, and it is clear that some people make better use of time than others. It is how people use time that makes some people

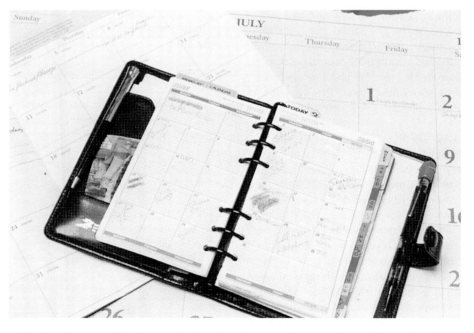

Systems for organizing time include calendars, organizers, and appointment books.

more successful. The current status of healthcare organizations, enmeshed in mergers and work force redesign, has led to more demands (stressors) being placed on care providers and care managers. The effective use of time management skills becomes an even more important tool to achieve personal and professional goals. **Time management** is the use of tools, techniques, strategies, and follow-up systems to control wasted time and to ensure that the time invested in activities leads toward achieving a desired, high-priority goal. More simply put, time management is the ability to use your time on the things that matter (Croft, 1996).

Where Does Your Time Go?

Have you ever wasted time? Time, while a cheap commodity, is our most valuable resource. There are some commonly identified time wasters, and individuals must recognize them in order to guard against them.

Doing too much

Do you try to do too much at once? At work, do you have three or four major projects going simultaneously? Are you a member of more than one organizational committee? Do you have to worry about what will be on the table for dinner while you are hanging an IV and planning a staff meeting? Have you ever completed a nursing intervention and realized that your mind was really somewhere else, and the patient had been ignored? If you think you have too much to do, you probably do! The solution here is to learn to have fewer projects running simultaneously and to concentrate your efforts on one thing at a time. The first step is to limit major commitments and then give each activity your full and undivided attention. Sometimes completing one task before starting another is the most efficient method of getting everything done. **Prioritization** of goals and activities each day is very helpful.

Inability to say "No"

If you are suffering from overload, you probably have gotten there by not being able to say "no." Learning to not say "yes" to every request is difficult, and in the process others may be displeased. If you don't say "no," you may end up spending a great deal of time on projects in which you have no interest, projects that have no relationship to your personal goals and priorities, and projects that are great time wasters. When someone asks you to do something, you need to stop and consider the request. Do you ever want to do the task? If not, then say so. If you wish to do the task but simply do not have the time, consider delegation. However, be honest with the requester—if you simply do not have the time, say so as politely as possible. If you wish to take on the task but at a later date, negotiate. Remember, accepting an assignment you will never be able to complete does not shed a favorable light on you.

Procrastination

Do you put off important tasks because they are not enjoyable? Do you find excuses for not starting or completing tasks? Are you a procrastinator? Engaging in **procrastination**, or doing one thing when you should be doing something else, you give up time to complete your task and therefore limit the quality of the work you produce. There are techniques to help deal with procrastination. First, identify the reason for procrastinating, then make the task your highest priority the next day. Give yourself rewards for attacking the problem (Barkas, 1984). Some people find that they procrastinate when the task ahead is very large. The solution is to break the task down into manageable pieces and plan rewards for accomplishing each of the smaller tasks. Another technique is to select the least attractive element of the task to do first and the rest will seem easy (Bliss, 1976).

Exercise 12-3

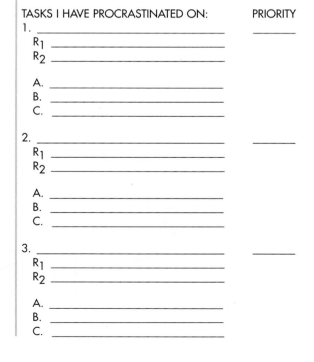

What tasks have you been putting off? Identify three things that you really need to do, that you labeled high priority, yet still have not done.

TASKS I HAVE PROCRASTINATED ON: PRIORITY

1. _____   _____
   R$_1$ _____
   R$_2$ _____

   A. _____
   B. _____
   C. _____

2. _____   _____
   R$_1$ _____
   R$_2$ _____

   A. _____
   B. _____
   C. _____

3. _____   _____
   R$_1$ _____
   R$_2$ _____

   A. _____
   B. _____
   C. _____

Exercise 12-3—cont'd

For each task, write down two reasons why you have been avoiding the work (R_1 and R_2). Prioritize the tasks. Now break each task down into three or more manageable pieces (A, B, and C). Treat yourself to something nice after completing each smaller job!

Complaining

Often the time nurses spend complaining about a task or a particular situation is greater than the time needed to solve the problem. If you find yourself complaining, stop and ask yourself what would be the ideal solution to the problem, and then take the risk to act on it. If the problem is another person, either take the time to talk with the person and get the problem out in the open, or sit down and write a letter to the person discussing your point of view (even if sometimes you do not mail it). If there is a problem within the work place, take the time to think about the problem and generate some possible solutions. Then talk to your manager, but be prepared. By presenting solutions, and not just problems, your manager will see you as interested in contributing to the goals of the organization.

Perfectionism

Perfectionism is the tendency to never finish anything because it is not perfect. This approach tends to consume a great deal of time when your expected outcome is not attainable. Overcoming perfectionism takes considerable effort. However, this does not mean that you should do less than your best. Being aware of perfectionism means that you occasionally need to give yourself permission to do slightly less than a perfect job, such as buying a carryout dinner rather than preparing a four-course dinner after a day at work.

Interruptions

A common distraction from priorities is interruptions. Some interruptions, however, are integral to the positions that you hold, and others can be controlled. A home care nurse with a large case load can expect to be paged at any time. More common, however, are the numerous small interruptions by individuals who want just a "minute of your time" and take 2 minutes getting to the point! Box 12-1 identifies some specific strategies to prevent and control interruptions. The two keys to dealing with interruptions are to resume "doing it now" so that an interruption does not destroy your schedule, and to maintain the attitude that whatever the interruption, it is a part of your responsibility. Every crisis is really an opportunity in disguise. When you make a conscious decision not to worry about the things you cannot control, you have more energy to maintain a positive perspective and to move projects forward.

Disorganization

One of the most serious time wasters of all is disorganization. How many times have you had to spend 5 minutes trying to find something you have

---

Box 12-1

Tips to Avoid Interruptions and Work More Effectively

- Chart somewhere other than in the place you will be most accessible.
- Ask people to put their comments in writing—don't let them catch you "on the run."
- Let the office/unit secretary know the information you need immediately.
- Conduct a conversation in the hall to help keep it short or in a separate room to keep from being interrupted.
- Be comfortable saying "No."
- When involved in a long procedure or home visit, ask someone else to cover your other responsibilities.
- Break projects into small, manageable pieces.
- Get yourself organized.
- Minimize interruptions—e.g., allow voice mail to pick up the phone; shut the door.
- Keep your manager informed of your goals.
- Plan to accomplish high-priority or difficult tasks early in the day.
- Develop a plan for the day, and stick to it. Remember to schedule in some time for interruptions,
- Schedule time to meet regularly throughout the shift with staff for whom you are responsible.
- Recognize that crises and interruptions are part of the position.
- Be cognizant of your personal time-waster habits, and try to avoid them.

misplaced or misfiled? Organization can be a great time saver and is discussed shortly. Remember that the guiding principle is that organization is a process rather than the product. You can spend so much time organizing that you will never get to the task at hand (procrastination). Simple organizing guidelines include eliminating clutter, keeping everything in its place, and doing similar tasks together.

Too much information

The newest time waster to evolve is data proliferation. We are now in the midst of a paradigm shift to the Information Age. The technology within our work place forces us to receive huge amounts of data and to transform these data into useful information. The computer work station, once touted as a time-saving device, has become the driving force behind care delivery. Nurses can view the computer either as a stress-producing slave-driver or as a simple tool to assist them in their daily activities.

Information overload is what happens when you are overwhelmed by too much information, too fast, too often, and you do not have the skills to interpret the data into useful information. Symptoms of information overload can include a sense of inability to keep up with everything; feeling that data keep you from accomplishing your "real position"; inability to proceed from the question or problem to fact finding; complaining of irrelevant information; and taking work home every day (Melanchuk, 1996).

Developing data/information receiving and sending skills can greatly reduce stress and improve efficiency and productivity. Gaining a new appreciation for information is important. Information once again is simply a tool to use to plan action or make decisions.

By learning what information is important, you can learn to use it to your advantage.

Time Management Concepts

Table 12-3 presents a classification scheme for time management techniques. All three levels of prevention techniques have concepts in common. The unifying theme is that each activity undertaken should lead to goal attainment, and that goal should be the number one priority at that time. Useful techniques and strategies for effective time management are discussed later.

Time Management Strategies

Goal setting

The first step in time management is setting goals. If determining long-term goals is difficult for you, consider setting more short-term goals—steps along the way to the long-term goal. Set goals that are reasonable and achievable. Do not expect to reach long-term goals overnight—long term means just that. Give yourself time to meet the goals. Set many short-term goals to reach the long-term goal, thus giving yourself a frequent sense of goal achievement. Annual goals should become monthly goals, monthly goals become weekly goals and weekly goals become daily goals. Give yourself flexibility. If the path you chose last year is no longer appropriate, change it. Write your goals on paper, date the page, and refer to it often to give yourself a progress report (Mayer, 1995).

Setting priorities

Once goals are known, priorities are set, although they may shift throughout a given period in terms of

Table 12-3	CLASSIFICATION OF TIME MANAGEMENT TECHNIQUES	
Level of Technique	**Purpose**	**Actions**
Primary	Designed to promote efficiency and productivity	Organize and systematize things, tasks, and people Basic time management skills
Secondary	Focuses on goal achievement	Assemble a prioritized "to do" list based on goals daily
	Uses the right tool for planning and preparation	Use of tools such as the Franklin Planner
Tertiary	Helps to refocus, to gain control, and to use information appropriately	Develop a personal time management plan

goal attainment. For example, working on a budget may take precedence at certain times of the year, while new staff orientation is high priority at other times. Knowing what the goals and priorities are helps shape the "to do" list. On a nursing unit or as you work in a community setting, you must know your personal goals and current priorities. How you organize work may depend on geographic considerations, patient acuity, or some other schema. Covey, Merrill, and Merrill (1994) identify a particular strategy to assist in prioritization. They state that people generally focus on those things that are important and urgent. By placing the elements of importance and urgency in a grid as shown in Figure 12-2, it is possible to classify all activities as shown.

Typically we tend to focus on those items in cell A because they are both important and urgent and therefore command our attention. Making shift assignments is an A task because it is both important to the work to be accomplished and frequently urgent because there is a time frame during which data about patients and qualifications of staff can be matched. Conversely, if something is neither important nor urgent (cell D), it may be considered a waste of time, at least in terms of personal goals. An example of a D activity might be reading the junk e-mail. Even if something is urgent but not important (cell C), it contributes minimally to productivity and goal achievement. An example of a C activity might be responding to a memo that has a specific time line but is not important to goal attainment. The real key to setting priorities is to attend to the B tasks, those which are important, yet not urgent. Examples of this may be reviewing the organization's strategic plan or participating on organizational committees.

Organization

A number of simple routines for organization can save many minutes over a day and enhance your efficiency. Keeping a work space neat or arranging things in an orderly fashion can be a powerful time management tool. Rather than a system of "pile management," use "file management." The adage "there is a place for everything, and everything in its place" makes for a successful work space. A few hints include (1) plan ahead where things should go (frequently used items should be more accessible); (2) do not use the top of your desk (table, computer station) for storage; (3) create a "to do" folder; (4) create a "to be filed" folder; and (4) regularly schedule time to work your way through the folders (Griessman, 1984). Everyone accumulates a pile of papers that becomes a

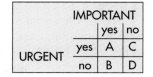

Figure 12-2   Classifications of priorities.

problem over time. Take the time to sort the piles, perhaps tossing a page or two, acting on those things which are urgent, or if all else fails, filing it!

The easiest way to keep a desk neat is to clean off the desk at the end of every day. After cleaning the desk, determine your priority goals for the next day and have the materials ready to work on when you start the next morning.

Time tools

Sometimes the real problem is that the events of the day become the driving force, rather than a planned schedule. Days may become so tightly scheduled that any little interruption can become a crisis. If you do not plan the day, you may find yourself responding to events, rather than prioritized goals. If you think you are a reactor rather than a proactive time user, use a time log to list work-related activities for several days. One reason you may not be able to plan well is that you really do not have a good estimate of how long a particular activity actually takes, or you do not know how many activities can be accomplished in a given time frame.

As the registered nurse's role in care management increases in complexity, the need for organizational tools increases. Tracking the care of groups of clients, either as the member of a care team or in a leadership capacity, can be overwhelming. Each nurse must devise a method for tracking care and organizing time, as well as delegating and monitoring care provided by others. While some nurses depend on a shift flow sheet or Kardex system, others are enjoying the benefit of computerized information tracking systems. The Nurse Tracker currently being beta tested by the Fuld Institute for Technology in Nursing Education (FITNE) is a point-of-service data-based system that will give nurses in community-based roles access to on-line services such as client records from the home, thus saving a great deal of time with phone calls and voice mail.

Dealing with information

The first step in managing information is to assess the source. Once you have identified the sources of your data, you have a better handle on how to deal with the information. Track the who, what, where, and why of the incoming information for a few days. Patterns will begin to emerge, which will start to give clues as to how to deal with it. You can generally predict, using the Pareto Principle, that 80% of your incoming data comes from approximately 20% of your sources.

By developing information-receiving skills, you can quickly interpret the data and convert them to useful information, discarding that which is not needed. Melanchuk (1996) identifies seven skills needed to process data. Initially you should reduce or eliminate that which is useless. Delete the e-mail, toss the memo in the trash, or dispose of it somehow. Next, monitor the information flow and decide what to do with incoming data. Find and focus on the most important pieces, and then quickly focus down on the specific details you need. Identify resources that are most helpful and have them readily available. Be able to sort out the big picture from the masses of data. Finally, know when you have enough information to act (Melanchuk, 1996).

Once you have mastered the receiving end of information, move on to information-sending skills. Remember, your information is another person's data! Try to keep your outflow short and sweet; make it a synthesis of the information. Finally, select the most appropriate mode of communication for your message from the technology available. You may be sending in written form (memo or report), verbal form (face-to-face and presentation), telephone, voice mail, e-mail, or FAX. Remember, the most important skill is to know when you have said enough. Exercise 12-4 will help you consider how you have dealt with information.

Exercise 12-4

Think of the last time you were in the clinical area. How often did you record the same piece of data (for example, a finding in your assessment of the client)? Don't forget to include all steps, from your jotting down notes on a piece of paper to the final report of the day. Unless you were on a totally computerized unit, you may have recorded the same piece of information nearly a dozen times.

■ MEETING MANAGEMENT AND DELEGATION

Two key time management strategies critical to success are managing meetings and delegation, which are discussed in the next two sections of this chapter. Even nurses who may not have extensive management responsibilities usually are in the position of delegating tasks to less skilled workers and can benefit from learning to make the most of meetings, either as the leader or as a group member.

Managing Meetings

Unfocused, poorly managed meetings can waste considerable, valuable time and can frustrate busy staff members. Meetings serve various purposes ranging from creating social networks to setting formal policy. They may be designed to solve problems, disseminate information, seek input, inspire the group, delegate work or authority, or create/maintain a formal power base. Unless the purpose of a meeting is to socialize, the meeting is unlikely to be effective if it is poorly managed. The following tips list several popular techniques and strategies to enhance the productivity and effectiveness of meetings.

Tips for managing meetings effectively

Before scheduling a meeting ask yourself several questions:

- Is this meeting really necessary? What would happen if the meeting never happened?
- Would a phone call or one-on-one meeting better achieve the goal?
- Is this meeting simply informational? If so, would written communication better meet the need? Would a memo or posting an announcement suffice?
- Are the people who really need to attend available to meet?

Schedule meetings right before lunch or at the end of the day. Participants will have an incentive to stick to the schedule. Set a start and stop time, and reward prompt members by starting on schedule. Most of the work of the meeting is accomplished in the first hour. Try to avoid meetings lasting longer than 1.5 to 2 hours.

Select an appropriate setting, where the participants are not readily accessible. If necessary, plan the seating arrangement to prevent inappropriate behaviors such as whispering or other interruptions.

If the group meets over a period of time, have group members set rules for conduct and behavior.

Distribute an agenda. Whenever possible, provide a written agenda to each member in advance of the meeting. Establish and make known the goal of the meeting. Attach all needed preparation reading to the agenda. The more advance reading or preparation required, the earlier members should receive agendas. Different types of agendas can be used for different purposes:

Structured agendas—If a topic is particularly controversial, consider setting a rule that requires any negative comment to be preceded by a positive one.

Timed agendas—Consider setting a specific amount of time to be dedicated to each item on the agenda. If you stick to the schedule, discussion will stay focused and you might possibly make it through the agenda.

Action agendas—Consider submitting an agenda with a description of the needed/desired action, e.g., review proposals, approve minutes, or establish outcomes.

Keep the group on task. Use rules of order to facilitate meetings. *Roberts' Rules of Order* may seem overly structured; however, this structure is particularly helpful when diversity of opinion is likely or important. Specifically, these rules help the person chairing the meeting by setting limits on discussion and using a specific order of priorities to deal with concerns.

Keep minutes and distribute to participants. The minutes provide a record to refer back to if needed and also serve to convey contents to persons unable to attend.

• • •

Planning ahead for the meeting is a group leader's best strategy for a satisfactory experience. Participants must also prepare for meetings. Reviewing the **agenda** (or requesting one in advance if not provided), reviewing preparatory materials, and thinking through agenda items are ways that group members may assist in accomplishing the meeting goals. Meeting participants should be on time for all meetings, or communicate that they will be late or unable to attend. Participants should be prepared to leave on time as well. If a meeting is handled poorly by an immediate supervisor, a committee member could volunteer to be sure that the meeting agendas and minutes are distributed. It is important to recognize that some people deliberately avoid preparing agendas and distributing minutes in an attempt to control the meeting. Exercise 12-5 will help you understand the importance of well-run meetings.

Exercise 12-5

Have you ever sat in a meeting and wondered why you were there? Perhaps you weren't clear about the purpose of the meeting, or where the meeting was heading, or even who was in charge! Analyze what irritated you about the meeting.

Delegating

Delegation is a component of self-management that is a critical strategy for nurse managers and care managers to learn. Appropriate delegation not only increases time efficiency, but also serves as a means of reducing stress. While delegation is discussed in depth in another chapter of this text, it is also appropriate to discuss briefly as a time management strategy. Delegation only works when the delegator trusts the delegatee to accomplish the task and reports findings back to the nurse. It does not save time for the nurse to go back and check or redo everything someone else has done. Delegation requires empowerment of the delegatee to accomplish the task. If the nurse does not delegate appropriately, with clear expectations, the delegatee will constantly be asking for assistance or direction. Delegation can also be a means of reducing stress if used appropriately. If the nurse does not understand delegation and does not use it appropriately, it can be a major source of stress as the nurse assumes accountability and responsibility for care administered by others.

▌ CHAPTER SUMMARY

Self-management is a means to achieve a balance between work and personal life, and it is a way of life developed to achieve personal goals within self-imposed priorities and deadlines (Weiss, 1986). Time management is clock oriented, and stress management is the control of external and internal stressors.

To achieve a balance in life and minimize stressors, nurses must learn to sit back and see their own personal "big picture" and examine their personal and professional goals. Personal priorities also must be established. Stressors and coping strategies need to be identified and employed. By developing these techniques, nurses can gain a sense of control and become far better nurses in the process.

A Manager's Solution

❓ Over a 6-month period I developed a strong trusting relationship with my staff. They knew they could count on my help whenever things got rough. One afternoon the patient care needs slowed down and a staff nurse suggested that I should go to my office and get some administrative work done so I wouldn't have to take it home that night. She assured me that they would

Continued

A Manager's Solution—cont'd

seek me out if the unit got busy again. That's how the pattern of relief got started. Because my staff trusted that I would be immediately available if needed, they were supportive of my going to my office during slack periods. The other half of the equation was that I always made sure to let them know how much I had accomplished and how much I appreciated their concern and consideration. My stress level went down, and more of my administrative duties were actually completed at work.

Things were not always perfect. I still often took work home, but I had more time for myself and my family, and I used my work time more efficiently. The valuing, caring, and trust that were shared between my staff and me far exceeded the stress. The nurses who worked for me saw me as a mentor. They learned how to function in the charge nurse role, as well as how to prioritize and organize patient care. They also learned how to mentor each other, as well as the LPNs/LVNs and corpsmen who worked with them. I would say that what happened to decrease my stress and maximize my time management was a combination of trust and team development. That is what I remember most about that unit—the spirit of teamwork.

Would this be a suitable approach for you? Why?

▌ CHAPTER CHECKLIST

Stress management and time management are two strategies for self-management. Balancing stress means caring for your emotional, physical, and mental needs. Effective delegation, using schedules and calendars and other planners, using time management principles, and managing meetings are key strategies to be integrated into the nurse leader role. By accomplishing self-management, managers, leaders, and followers will find themselves in control of work time and stressors, as well as more confident in achieving both personal and work-related goals.

Stress and overwork are inherent in the nursing profession, and nurses can adapt and cope with stress and time crunches by learning effective ways to care for themselves and to manage time. By assessing and reducing specific stressors and time wasters, nurses will manage to thrive on the healthcare challenges before them. Increasing skills in coping, organization, delegation, and effective time management are vital components of effective leadership. A nurse manager who can role model and support her staff in turbulent times is a true leader.

■ Stress management includes using cognitive and psychosocial activities to decrease the stress or enhance the ability to handle stress.
■ Time management includes using tools and strategies to assure that priority goals are achieved.
■ Signs of excess stress must be heeded to prevent burnout or chronic health problems.
■ Strategies to reduce stress include:
  • Physical
    – Accept physical limitations.
    – Plan physical activity.
    – Maintain adequate physical health, including adequate nutrition.
    – Schedule time for breaks and relaxation.
  • Mental/emotional
    – Use problem identification and solving strategies.
    – Differentiate perceived and "objective" stressors.
    – Evoke the relaxation response via meditation.
    – Recognize stress-induced behavioral changes.
    – Seek social support.
  • Management
    – Maintain awareness of effect of own behavior on others.
    – Develop a participative management style.
    – Practice a systems perspective.
    – Retain a sense of distance from stress.
■ Strategies to improve time management include:
  • Identification of potential time wasters
    – Doing too much
    – Inability to say "no"
    – Procrastination
    – Complaining
    – Perfectionism
    – Interruptions
    – Disorganization
    – Too much information
  • Use of time management strategies
    – Setting priorities
    – Organization
    – Time tools such as time logs, Kardex, and shift flow sheets

- Devising a personal time management system
- Effectively dealing with data and information
- Appropriate delegation
  - Willingness to delegate/be delegated to
  - Giving the delegatee sufficient responsibility and authority
  - Conveying expectations clearly
  - Requiring the delegatee to be accountable
- Strategies to improve meeting management:
  - Distribute meeting agendas and minutes.
  - Schedule meetings appropriately.
  - Use rules of order to facilitate meetings.

TIPS FOR SELF-MANAGEMENT

- Know what your high priority goals are and use them to filter decisions.
- Know your personal response to stress and self-evaluate frequently.
- Make your health a priority and use strategies that keep you in self-control.
- Use organizational systems that meet your needs; the simpler, the better.
- Simplify.
- Refocus on your priorities whenever you begin to feel overwhelmed.

TERMS TO KNOW

agenda
burnout
coping
delegation
depersonalization
employee assistance
  programs
general adaptation
  syndrome (GAS)

information overload
overwork
perfectionism
procrastination
self-management
systems perspective
time management

REFERENCES

Barkas, J.L. (1984). *Creative Time Management: Become More Productive and Still Have Time for Fun.* Englewood Cliffs, N.J.: Prentice-Hall.

Bassman, E. (1992). *Abuse in the Workplace: Management Remedies and Bottom Line Impact.* Westport, CT: Quorum Books.

Beech, H.R., Burns, L.E., & Sheffield, B.F. (1982). A *Behavioral Approach to the Management of Stress: A Practical Guide to Techniques.* New York: John Wiley & Sons.

Bliss, E.C. (1976). *Getting Things Done.* New York: Bantam.

Blumenthal, J.A., & McCubbin, J.R. (1987). Physical exercise as stress management. In Baum, A., & Singer, J., eds. *Handbook of Psychology and Health: Vol. 5. Stress* (pp. 109-135). Hillsdale, NJ: Laurence Erlbaum Associates.

Carmack, B. (1997). Balancing engagement and detachment in care giving. *Image,* 29(2), 139-143.

Chernis, C. (1980). *Staff Burnout: Job Stress in the Human Services.* Beverly Hills: Sage Publications.

Cooper, C. (1996). Stress in the workplace. *British Journal of Hospital Medicine,* 55(9), 560-563.

Covey, S.R., Merrill, A.R., & Merrill, R.R. (1994). *First Things First: To Love, to Learn, to Leave a Legacy.* New York: Simon & Schuster.

Croft, C. (1996). *Time Management.* London: International Thomson Business Press.

Czander, W.M. (1993). *The Psychodynamics of Work and Organizations.* New York: Guilford Press.

D'Amato, J. (1988). *Work and Stress: A Report on How Work Stress Affects the Quality of Life.* New York: Institute for Professional and Personal Development, Publishing Division.

Davis, M. (1997). *The 80/20 Rule.* (On-line; available: http://www.nipltd.com/Main/21a6.htm.)

Dytell, R.S. (1990). The effects of unanticipated work stressors on registered nurses. In Humphrey, J., ed. *Human Stress: Current Selected Research,* Volume 4. New York: AMS Press, 47-55.

Golembiewski, R.T., & Munzenrider, R. (1988). *Phases of Burnout: Developments in Concepts and Application.* New York: Praeger.

Griessman, B.E. (1994). *Time Tactics of Very Successful People.* New York: McGraw-Hill, Inc.

Koeske, G., & Kelly, T. (1995). The impact of over involvement on burnout and job satisfaction. *Journal of Orthopsychiatry,* 65(2), 282-292.

Lee, R., & Ashforth, B. (1996). A meta-analytic examination of the correlates of the three dimensions of job burnout. *Journal of Applied Psychology,* 81(2), 123-133.

Leiter, M. (1992). Burnout as a crisis in professional role structures: Measurement and conceptual issues. *Anxiety, Stress & Coping,* 5(1), 79-93.

Maslach, C. & Leiter, M.P. (1997). *The Truth about Burnout.* San Francisco: Jossey-Bass Publishers.

Mayer, J.J. (1995). *Time Management for Dummies.* Foster City, CA: IDG Books Worldwide, Inc.

McCloskey, J., & McCain, B. (1987). Satisfaction, commitment and professionalism of newly employed nurses. *Image: Journal of Nursing Scholarship,* 19(1), 20-24.

Melanchuk, M. (1996). *Inforelief: Stay Afloat in the Infoflood.* San Francisco: Jossey-Bass.

Menninger, W.W. (1996). Practitioner, heal thyself: Coping with stress in clinical practice, *Bulletin of the Menninger Clinic,* 60(2), 197-205.

Offermann, L.R., & Hellmann, P. (1996). Leadership behavior and subordinate stress: A 360° view. *Journal of Occupational Health Psychology,* 1(4), 382-390.

Oken, D. (1987). Coping and psychosomatic illness. In Baum, A., & Singer, J., eds. *Handbook of Psychology and Health,* Volume 5: Stress (pp. 109-135). Hillsdale, NJ: Lawrence Erlbaum Associates, Publishers.

Parker, P. & Kulik, J. (1995). Burnout, self and supervisor-rated job performance and absenteeism among nurses. *Journal of Behavioral Medicine,* 18, 581-599.

Schwartz, J.E., Pickering, T., & Landsbergis, P. (1996). Work-related stress and blood pressure: Current theoretical models and considerations from a behavioral medicine perspective. *Journal of Occupational Health Psychology,* 1(3), 287-310.

Selye, H. (1956). *The Stress of Life.* New York: McGraw-Hill.

Selye, H. (1991). History and present status of the stress concept. In Monat, A., & Lazarus, R., eds. *Stress and Coping: An Anthology* (pp. 21-36). New York: Columbia University Press.

Simpson, J.A., & Weiner, E.S.C. (1989). *The Oxford English Dictionary,* 2nd ed. Oxford: Claredon Press.

Spacapan, S., & Cohen, S. (1983). Effects and after effects of stressor expectations. *Journal of Personality & Social Psychology,* 45, 1243-1245.

Weiss, D. (1986). *Get Organized: How to Control Your Life Through Self-Management.* New York: AMACOM.

Wilson, J. (1990). *Woman: Your Body, Your Health.* New York: Harcourt, Brace, Jovanovich.

Zales, M. (1994). *Stress in Health and Diseases.* New York: Brunner/Mazel.

SUGGESTED READINGS

Farrington, A. (1997). Clinical management: strategies for reducing stress and burnout in nursing. *British Journal of Nursing,* 6(1), 44-50.

Field, T., Quintino, O., Henteleff, T., Wells-Keife, L., & Delvecchio-Feinberg, G. (1997). Job stress reduction therapies. *Alternative Therapies in Health & Medicine,* 3(4): 54-56.

Maslach, C., & Leiter, M.P. (1997). *The Truth About Burnout.* San Francisco: Josey-Bass Publishers.

Sherry, D. (1996). Clinicians' forum: Time management strategies for the new home care nurse. *Home Healthcare Nurse,* 14, 718-720.

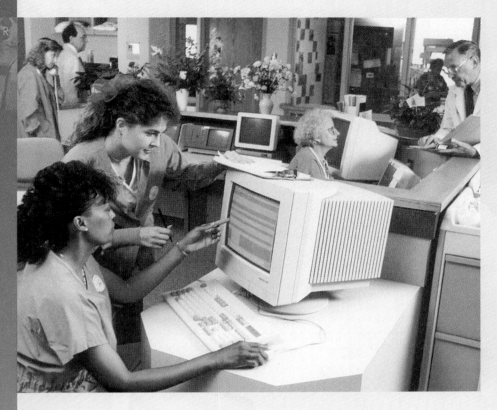

Managing Information and Technology: Caring and Communicating With Computers

Mary N. McAlindon
RN, EdD, CNAA

This chapter identifies and describes current uses of information technology for patient care that allow nurses to use the data gathered at the point of care in the most effective and efficient manner. It discusses types of information technology, the nursing minimum data set, health management, information systems, knowledge technology, and future trends. Such technologies allow nurses to compare and contrast not only current patient data to previous data for the same patient, but also data for other patients with the same diagnosis. The chapter concludes with a look into the future of healthcare technology.

Objectives

- Analyze the three aspects—data, information, and knowledge—used for patient care communication.
- Evaluate three types of computerized information technologies used in nursing.
- Evaluate three uses for biomedical technology.
- Apply the nursing minimum data set to a nursing situation.
- Compare two types of information systems used to provide patient care information.
- Analyze three types of technology for capturing data at the point of care.
- Discuss knowledge systems and their uses for patient care.
- Explore the issues of nurse ethics and patient confidentiality in information technology.
- Predict future trends in information technology useful for healthcare.
- Understand the use of the Internet for healthcare information.

Questions to Consider

- What types of technology do you use in your daily practice?
- How do you use the data gathered in providing healthcare?
- What can be done to improve the communication process while decreasing the amount of time spent in documenting care?
- Are you or your staff members reluctant to try new technologies?
- How do you and your staff approach learning new information technologies?

A Manager's Challenge

From the President and CEO of a Visiting Nurse Association in the Midwest

What do I, as a nurse leader and manager, need to do to take advantage of the advances in technology? I am president of the Visiting Nurse Association that is affiliated with a multiple-entity corporation. This means that our nurses take care of patients in three counties, and some of them drive 150 miles just to get to work. Under the manual documentation system, the nurses must drive to the agency and review the patient charts for new orders, laboratory results, and recent events. They then leave to visit the patients, often driving many miles between calls. At the end of the day they return the charts to the agency so that they can be updated and charges billed. As a result, they see fewer patients in a managed care environment where we are supposed to become more effective and efficient while accomplishing quality outcomes.

What do you think you would do if you were this manager?

■ INTRODUCTION

Technology surrounds us! We find computers being used at the bank, at the grocery checkout, in our cars, on our telephones, and in almost every other aspect of daily living. The purpose of all these technologies is to gather data and provide information. This allows businesses to be more efficient and effective in providing their services. **Information technology** is the use of computers to gather, aggregate, process, and communicate information; it is as useful for the business of healthcare as it is for any other business. The data gathered in the process of patient care provide information about the effectiveness of nursing care for a successful patient outcome. Is the patient better? What did we do to cause this to happen?

■ INFORMATION SCIENCE

Information is the communication or reception of knowledge. Since earliest times nurses have collected, processed, and communicated information about patients. When personal computers were introduced in the 1970s, nurses began to use these electronic tools to assist with communication. Today we combine computer science and information science for managing and processing data, information, and knowledge to support the practice of nursing in the delivery of healthcare.

Information science consists of three aspects of a concept generally called information. These three aspects are data, information, and knowledge. Figure 13-1 illustrates the relationship among these aspects.

Data are discrete entities that describe or measure something without interpreting it. Numbers are data; for example, the number 30, without interpretation, means nothing. Information consists of interpreted, organized, or structured data. The number 30 interpreted as milliliters or as a length of time in minutes or hours has meaning. **Knowledge** refers to information that is combined or synthesized so that interrelationships are identified. For example, the number 30, when included in the statement that "all patients with indwelling catheters longer than 30 days developed infections" becomes knowledge, something that is known.

Data, information, and knowledge constitute the content of professional communication. Nurses deliver and manage patient care through continuous communication with patients, families, other professionals, and staff, and we study the patient's record,

Data $\longrightarrow$ Information $\longrightarrow$ Knowledge

Figure 13-1   Three aspects of information science.

Box 13-1
Using the Information Triad

Several patients in the coronary care unit had fallen at night over the last 3 weeks. This was very unusual, since heart patients do not usually become disoriented at night. The nurse manager became concerned about this and began to look for commonalities among the patients who had fallen. She found that they were all taking the same sleeping medication. She mentioned this at a meeting and found that several other nurse managers had noticed the same situation. Together they contacted the pharmacy who contacted the pharmaceutical representative. He found that the medication dosage had been tested on college students, and that the dose was too high for older, less healthy patients. This is an example of combining data to provide information that when aggregated and processed becomes new knowledge.

---

adding to the observations in it. We monitor instruments that provide current information about the patients. We perform tests and review the results of tests performed by others. All these examples reflect giving and receiving data, information, and knowledge.

The progression from data to information to knowledge occurs quickly in practice as data are interpreted and compared to previous information about the patient to provide knowledge. Much of this value is lost, however, because the data are not stored where others might retrieve and use them to synthesize new knowledge. Box 13-1 provides an example that illustrates combining and interpreting data to provide information, which, when synthesized and re-presented, provides new knowledge.

The *management component of communication* is the ability to collect, aggregate, organize, and represent information in a way that is useful. This is technology—a scientific method for achieving a practical purpose.

Exercise 13-1

Think about the data that you gather every day: the vital signs, intake and output, and the symptoms that you communicate during shift report. What data did you automatically combine or reorganize to help you make a patient care decision? Whom did you report it to?

For example: you are charting vital signs and you notice that the patient's blood pressure is lower than it was yesterday. He is also complaining of nausea and lightheadedness. You check his medications and see that he is receiving apresoline. Based on your processing of the data that you have collected, you make a note to check the blood pressure and other symptoms again and notify the physician if the situation has not changed.

Nurse leaders are the visionaries for the nursing department and for the technology used in healthcare. They must understand the importance and use of the data collected by the staff at the point of care for eventual use in the computerized patient record, which will reach beyond the walls of the institution. Nurse leaders must empower their nurse managers to be knowledgeable users of technology so that the staff is able to use these systems to deliver effective, efficient healthcare. The end product will be improved patient outcomes.

TYPES OF TECHNOLOGIES

As nurses we commonly use and manage three types of technologies: biomedical technology, **information technology**, and **knowledge technology. Biomedical technology** is evidenced in the physiological monitoring that occurs in the critical care units, and the other electronic equipment used in the care of patients. This includes the use of ventilators to assist respirations, and computers used for diagnostic testing, drug administration, and therapeutic treatments. Information technology is processing and using the information gathered in monitoring patient care. The nursing minimum data set provides a framework for gathering data related to patient care through the use of health management information systems. **Knowledge technology** is the use of expert and decision support systems to assist nurses in making decisions about the delivery of patient care. These systems mimic the reasoning of nurse experts in making decisions related to patient care.

Biomedical Technology

Biomedical technology was developed in the mid-1970s to monitor the vital signs of critical care patients. It is now found in all patient care areas of the hospital and has extended to home health and long-term care facilities. This type of technology is used for (1) physiological monitoring, (2) diagnostic testing, (3) drug administration, and (4) therapeutic treatments. Box 13-2 lists the computer capabilities for each of these uses.

Physiological monitoring systems measure heart rate, blood pressure, and other vital signs and include arrhythmia monitors, pressure transducers, and oxygen and carbon dioxide analyzers. Other information captured through these systems includes central venous pressure, temperature, respiratory rate, weight, blood pressure, and pulmonary artery pressure. In addition, these systems often include treatment interventions as they change oxygen or carbon dioxide levels or tidal volume after lung functions that are out of range are diagnosed by the computer.

Continuous arrhythmia monitors and electrocardiograms (ECGs) are used to provide visual representation of electrical activity in the heart. Two types of arrhythmia systems are detection surveillance and diagnostic or interpretive systems. In the detection system the criteria for a normal cardiac rhythm are programmed into the computer, which then continuously surveys the patient's cardiac rhythm for normal and abnormal waveforms. The detection systems also monitor rhythm, rate, and pacemaker artifacts. The computer can audibly and visually alert the nurse when a preset number of abnormal waveforms is reached or when deviations from any other preset limit occurs. These data are stored so that the patient's history can be retrieved.

These systems can also be diagnostic. The computer, after processing the ECG, generates an analysis report. The ECG tracings may be transmitted over telephone lines from the patient's home to the physician's office or clinic. Patients with implantable pacemakers can have their cardiac activity monitored without leaving home.

Many hospitals are using oximetry to continuously monitor arterial oxygenation. This is a simple noninvasive procedure that can detect any trend in the patient's oxygenation status within 6 seconds. The oximeter can measure oxygenation through ear, pulse, or nasal septal oximetry. Ear oximetry measures the arterial oxygen saturation by monitoring the transmission of light waves through the vascular bed of the ear lobe. If low cardiac output causes insufficient arterial perfusion in the ear lobe, a pulse oximeter may be used to measure the wavelengths of light transmitted through a pulsating vascular bed such as a fingertip. As the pulsating bed expands and relaxes, the light path length changes, producing a waveform. Since the waveform is produced from arterial blood, the pulse oximeter calculates the arterial oxygen saturation for every heartbeat without interference from surrounding tissues. If the patient has reduced peripheral vascular pulsations or is taking vasoactive drugs, a nasal probe may be used. This device fits around the septal anterior ethmoidal artery to detect vascular pulsations.

Systems for diagnostic testing include blood gas analyzers, pulmonary function systems, and intracranial pressure monitors. Blood gas analyzers use arterial blood to sense and calculate arterial blood gases, saturation curves, and buffer curves from normal data. These analyzers measure the partial pressures of oxygen and carbon dioxide and the pH of the arterial blood used in the test, enter primary results as soon as they are available, communicate the results quickly, and generate trend analysis for patients throughout their hospitalization.

Box 13-2

Computer Capabilities for Biomedical Technology

1. Process physiological data
2. Store patient documentation
3. Graph data
4. Regulate physiological equipment
5. Process diagnostic equipment
6. Recognize deviations from preset ranges
7. Compare data among patients with similar diagnoses

Adapted from Saba & McCormick (1996).

Pulmonary function systems automate and simplify routine lung mechanics, lung volume, and diffusion capacity measurements. They can store data, calculate results, generate a numeric report, and display volumes graphically.

Intracranial pressure monitoring (ICP) systems monitor the cranial pressure in closed head injury or postoperative craniotomy patients. The ICP, along with the mean arterial blood pressure, can be used to calculate perfusion pressure. This allows for assessment and early therapy as changes occur. When the intracranial pressure exceeds a set pressure, some systems allow ventricular drainage. These systems supplement rather than replace nursing observations of the patient.

Drug administration systems are often used with implantable infusion pumps that administer medications. This equipment can be programmed to deliver medication at a preestablished rate for a defined period. Up to six variations in medication schedules may be stored in the system. These pumps are commonly used for hormone regulation, treatment of hypertension, chronic intractable pain, diabetes, thrombosis, and cancer chemotherapy.

Therapeutic systems may be used to regulate intake and output, regulate breathing, and assist with the care of the newborn. Intake and output systems are linked to infusion pumps that control arterial pressure, drug therapy, fluid resuscitation, and serum glucose levels. These systems calculate and regulate the intravenous drip rate.

Ventilators are used to deliver a prescribed percentage of oxygen and volume of air to the patient's lungs and to provide a set flow rate, inspiratory-to-expiratory time ratio, and various other complex functions. Ventilators also provide sophisticated, sensitive alarm systems for patient safety. Some computer-assisted ventilators are electromechanically controlled by a closed-loop feedback system to analyze and control lung volumes and alveolar gases by a preset inspiratory pressure.

In the newborn nursery, computers monitor the heart and respiratory rates of the babies. In addition, these newborn nursery systems can regulate the temperature of the isolette by sensing the infant's temperature and the air of the isolette. Alarms can be set to notify the nurse when preset physiological parameters are exceeded. Newer systems are used to monitor fetal activity before delivery; these systems monitor the ECGs of the mother and baby, pulse oximetry, blood pressure, and respirations.

The latest developments in biomedical technology include the use of implantable devices such as pacemakers, artificial organ transplants, gene therapy, and even the use of robot servants for people who are disabled. Biomedical technology has an impact on nursing care, since nurses assume responsibility for monitoring the data generated by these devices and assessing their effectiveness.

Nurse leaders must be aware of how these technologies fit into the strategic plan of the institution or corporation for whom they work. They must have a vision for the future and be ready to suggest solutions that will assist nurses across specialties and institutions.

Exercise 13-2

List the types of biomedical technology available for patient care in your organization. List ways that you presently use the information gathered by these systems. Does this information help you care for patients? Can you think of other ways to use the technology? The information? For example, patients with respiratory problems often have frequent arterial blood gases drawn to assess the effectiveness of treatment. Are there instances when the noninvasive pulse oximetry might be used? Nurses spend many hours learning to use the devices and to interpret the information gained from them. Have we come to rely on technology rather than on our own intuition?

Nurse managers must be aware of the latest technologies for monitoring patients' physiological status, for diagnostic testing, for drug administration, and for therapeutic treatments. It is important to identify the data to be collected, the information that might be gained, and the many ways that the data might be represented to provide new knowledge. More importantly, nurses must remember that these systems are tools for our use and do not replace our responsibility for monitoring the patient. Box 13-3 describes the

---

Box 13-3

Characteristics of Nurse-Users of Information Technology

Nurse-users of information are those registered nurses who collect data as part of their patient care activities, interpret it, and make decisions based on their interpretations. As nurses advance from novice to expert practitioner, interpretations of the data become intuitive and automatic, based on previous experience. When the information gained from previously cared-for patients is combined or synthesized so that new interrelationships are identified, nurses gain new knowledge. At this point they begin to think of other uses of data and information for improving patient care.

stages through which nurse-novices pass to become nurse-experts in the use of information technology.

Information Technology

Information technology refers to computers and programs used to process data and information. Computers offer the advantage of organizing, storing, retrieving, and communicating data with accuracy and speed. Patient care data can be entered once and stored in a database called a central data repository, then quickly and accurately retrieved many times and in many combinations by healthcare providers and others. A **database** is a collection of data elements organized and stored together. **Data processing** is the structuring, organizing, and interpreting of data into information. For example, vital signs for one patient can be entered into the computer and communicated on a graph; the vital signs of several patients can be compared to the number of doses of antiarrhythmic medication. The same vital signs can be correlated and used to show a relationship between blood pressures and hypertensive medications for male patients between the ages of 40 and 50 years. Nurses process data continuously, but computers do it faster and more accurately and provide a method of storage so that the data need not be remembered or written in several places on the patient record. Collecting a set of basic data from every healthcare encounter makes sense because comparisons can be made among many patients, institutions, years, or countries, almost in any combination imaginable. The theory box below provides key ideas about information processing.

Information theory

Information theory is a collection of mathematical estimations that are concerned with methods of coding, decoding, sorting, and retrieving information.

The **nursing minimum data set (NMDS)** was defined to establish uniform standards for the collection of comparable essential patient data. It is based on the concept of the uniform minimum health data set (UMHDS), a minimum set of items of information with uniform definitions and categories that meets the needs of multiple data users. UMHDSs have been developed for long-term care, hospital discharge, and ambulatory care, but the hospital set is the only one in widespread use.

The NMDS was developed by Werley et al. (1994) and represents nursing's first attempt to standardize the collection of nursing data. It follows UMHDS criteria in that (1) data items included in the set must be useful to healthcare professionals and administrators and to local, state, and federal planning, regulatory, and legislative bodies; (2) data items must be readily collectible and with reasonable accuracy; (3) data items should not duplicate data available from other sources; and (4) confidentiality must be protected.

Information Theory

KEY CONTRIBUTORS	KEY IDEAS	APPLICATION TO PRACTICE
Tan (1995) describes the elements of information theory as source, transmitter, channel, receiver, and destination.	The information source selects the message or information to be transmitted. An underlying code or set of characters represents the message to be processed by the computer. The transmitter has an encoding function that converts the message to be sent. The communication channel (cable, air waves) provides the medium necessary for the information to be transmitted over distance. The receiver converts the information from its transmitted form, and the destination is the final stage of reception in which the message is decoded so as to be understandable.	The physician enters an order for laboratory tests (*source, message*). The computer program converts the message (*transmitter*). The converted order is sent over the computer network (*communication channel*) to the laboratory (*receiver*), where it is converted and read by the computer system in the laboratory (*destination*).

The purpose of the NMDS is to (1) establish the comparability of patient care data across clinical populations, settings, geographical areas, and time; (2) describe the care of patients and families in various settings; (3) provide a means to mark the trends in the care provided and the allocation of nursing resources based on health problems or nursing diagnosis; (4) stimulate nursing research through links to existing data; and (5) provide data about nursing care to influence and facilitate healthcare policy decision making. Box 13-4 lists the elements of the nursing minimum data set.

The NMDS elements of intervention and outcome are not collected so easily as the demographic and service elements, many of which are captured at patient registration or discharge. Documentation of nursing interventions and outcomes has become crucial for accreditation and for quality management activities.

Research done at the University of Iowa College of Nursing describes a classification of nursing-sensitive patient outcomes that completes the nursing process elements of the NMDS (Maas, Johnson, & Moorhead, 1996; Daly, Maas, & Johnson, 1997). The Nursing-Sensitive Outcomes Classification (NOC) provides standardized patient outcomes for determining the effectiveness of nursing interventions by providing the language for the evaluation step of the nursing process and the content for the outcomes element in the NMDS. This standardizes the language for the outcome element of the NMDS, which can be shared by all healthcare disciplines. Karpiuk, Delaney, and Ryan (1997) report that the nursing resource utilization element of the NMDS was the most difficult to collect because of the variances in each facility.

Nurse managers must be aware of the existence of the NMDS and its usefulness for nursing. Even though some of the elements of information may not be easy to collect on every patient, the data set provides an excellent framework for a patient database.

Exercise 13-3

Examine the elements of the NMDS. Which of them would be collected by patient registration? Which information might you collect? Using a community nursing service, determine through auditing two charts which elements are evident and which are not. For example, in an acute care setting, you have given patient medication several times today. The nursing diagnosis was alteration in comfort due to pain. You probably charted that the patient stated a lessening of the pain within 30 minutes. You have documented an intervention and an outcome, two nursing care elements of the NMDS.

Box 13-4
Elements of the NMDS

Nursing Care Elements
1. Nursing diagnosis
2. Nursing intervention
3. Nursing outcome
4. Intensity of nursing care

Patient Demographic Elements
5. Personal identification*
6. Date of birth*
7. Sex*
8. Race and ethnicity*
9. Residency*

Service Elements
10. Unique facility or service agency number*
11. Unique health record number of the patient
12. Unique number of the principal registered nurse provider
13. Episode, admission, or encounter date*
14. Discharge or termination date*
15. Disposition of patient or client*
16. Expected payer for most of the bill

Elements comparable to those in the UMHDS.
Adapted from Werley, H., Ryan, P., Zorn, C., and Devine, E. (1994). Why the nursing minimum data set (NMDS)? In McCloskey, J., & Grace, H., eds. *Current Issues in Nursing.* St. Louis: Mosby.

Information systems

An information system uses computer hardware and software to process data into information needed to solve problems and answer questions. These systems accept healthcare data, and reorganize and process them to provide information. These data should be gathered at the point of care and the information made available to healthcare providers anywhere that it is needed. This is accomplished by networking computers and information systems to form one large integrated system that consists of all the entities in the enterprise or corporation. These integrated systems might encompass several hospitals, clinics, hospice, home health, and physician practices. Data from all patient encounters with the healthcare system are stored in a central data repository where they are accessible to authorized users located anywhere in the world. These become the computerized patient records, which will contain health data from birth to death.

Nursing leaders must be prepared to make choices that will benefit the staff and patients. These systems must make sense to the people who use them and not increase the work load. Nurse managers should be members of the selection team, so that the systems chosen reflect the work being done. Staff nurses must be aware of the concept of computerized patient records and the importance of the data that they collect as they care for patients.

Integrated information systems

An integrated information system focuses on patient health information. A major function of these systems is to communicate and integrate patient care data and information and provide management support. Health data are entered into the system from computer stations located in the various departments in the organization and stored in a central computer to be accessed by all patient care services.

The nurse manager should be aware of information system configurations: (1) the stand-alone system, (2) the on-line interactive system, (3) the networked system, and (4) the integrated system. **Stand-alone systems** are internal to a department and automate the processes of the department. Because these systems do not communicate with each other, orders may be written as a paper requisition, and a computer in the laboratory processes the test. Results are then returned to the ordering department as a paper report. Statistics important to the department are also reported; the number of tests completed each month, the number done by each technician, and the revenue generated are all important information for the functioning of every department.

On-line interactive systems communicate patient information throughout the organization. Areas in the organization are connected to the **mainframe computer** through handheld devices, cathode ray tubes (CRTs), or terminals (the end point of the mainframe computer). These systems are used to transmit orders to the various departments and integrate patient data in real time. When an order for electrolytes is entered, it is transmitted to a computer in the laboratory that prints the order on a "pick list" for the technician. The blood is drawn and placed in a computer that will process it and send the reports to a central data base where it is available for viewing. Once the order is placed, staff can use a terminal to see if the test is pending, in process, or complete. If it has been completed, results appear on the screen. These systems save phone calls and the time it takes to write the information. They process and generate information needed to provide patient care and to document the patient care process. The entered patient care data are stored and can be retrieved at any time by anyone who has access to the system.

Networked systems consist of several computers that are supported by another computer that acts as a file server. Each of the computers on the network shares a data base stored in the file server. For example, the secretaries in the nursing office are networked to a central computer, the file server. The file server contains the word processing, data base, spreadsheet, and nurse staffing and scheduling programs or applications. Each secretary uses a computer to access these applications, and individual work is stored in the file server. In addition, nurse managers have personal computers in their offices located throughout the hospital, but linked to the file server in the nursing office through the network. They also access these various applications, can make changes to the staffing and scheduling files, and store their work on a file server without leaving their offices. If the system provides electronic mail, anyone with a personal computer or terminal connected to the network can send instant messages to anyone else on the network. This saves time and increases the efficiency of the nurse managers.

Integrated systems are those that link one mainframe containing a central data base with computer devices in all departments in the institution. These systems contain a central data base of patient care information that is written to and accessed by all departments: laboratory, pharmacy, radiology, nursing, physical therapy, occupational therapy, and so on. The programs that link the individual departments must be able to "talk" to one another in order to exchange patient care data. For example, pharmacy needs access to certain laboratory results and the height, weight, and allergy information entered by nursing. This is a straightforward process if the software has been written by one computer vendor; if different systems must be linked, the process is more difficult or may even be impossible.

It is extremely important that nurse leaders, nurse managers, and staff understand the patient care process from a data-information-knowledge perspective. In an information-intensive era, we must be aware of the data we collect, the reasons that we collect them, and the decisions that we make based on them. The new technologies offer an opportunity to examine the way we do things and improve them rather than duplicate them. The storage of the data in a central repository accessible to all patient care providers is essential. Nurses must serve on the committees that choose these information systems for the hospital, for nursing plays the pivotal role in establishing these data bases. Box 13-5 lists elements of the ideal hospital information system for consideration in choosing a system for an institution.

Exercise 13-4

Select a hospital with which you are familiar. Does this hospital have a hospital information system (HIS)? Do you know what nursing information systems are used in this organization? Make a list of the names of these systems and the information that they provide. How do they help you in caring for patients? In making management decisions? If you have either or both systems, think about the communication of data and information between department. Does the nursing system communicate with the HIS? If you do not have computerized systems, think about how data and information are communicated. How might a computer system help you to be more efficient?

As an example, assume that a barium enema has been ordered. Handwritten requisitions are sent to nutritional services, the pharmacy, and the radiology department. With a computerized system, the barium enema is ordered, and the requests for dietary changes, magnesium citrate, and the barium enema itself are automatically sent to the appropriate departments. Radiology will compare its schedule openings with the patient's schedule and automatically place the date and time for the barium enema on the patient's automated Kardex.

Nursing information systems

Nursing information systems (NISs) are systems that use computers to process nursing data. NISs can be stand-alone systems or components of the integrated system. Most are found in nursing administration and practice.

In these systems, direct patient care information is entered, stored, retrieved, processed, displayed, and communicated. The documentation of patient care information and discharge plans may be incorporated for nursing documentation.

Stand-alone nursing documentation systems are becoming obsolete with the development of integrated delivery networks in which all areas of healthcare contribute and share information. Patient information will be entered into the integrated system with the first health encounter, and all data and information from subsequent encounters will be added to the record, which will be accessible to all caregivers.

Nursing administration systems improve the effectiveness of nurse leaders/managers by providing timely and appropriate information. Figure 13-2 lists the essential components of a nursing administration information system. The key to successful administrative

---

Box 13-5
Elements of the Ideal Hospital Information System

1. The hardware is fail-safe.
2. The software requires minimal staff support.
3. The system is integrated wherever possible.
4. Data from the patient care process are gathered at the point of care.
5. The medical record is on-line and almost paperless, and the previous medical record is available on the system.
6. The data base is complete and easy to modify.
7. Physician offices, satellites, and future external sites are interfaced to the system.
8. Data are gathered by instrumentation whenever possible so that only minimal data entry is necessary.

Adapted from McAlindon, Danz, & Theodoroff (1987).

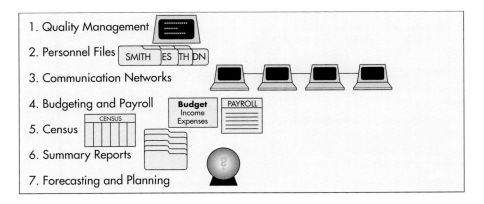

1. Quality Management
2. Personnel Files
3. Communication Networks
4. Budgeting and Payroll
5. Census
6. Summary Reports
7. Forecasting and Planning

Figure 13-2   Essential components of a nursing administration information system. (Adapted from Saba & McCormick [1996].)

applications is the nurse leader's analysis and management of the volumes of information that are available to maintain effectiveness and efficiency.

Quality management and the measurement of efficiency, effectiveness, and patient care outcomes have become necessary for the accreditation and licensing of healthcare organizations. This can be accomplished through documentation of the patient care process. If the computerized care plan (critical path, computerized Kardex) outlines what patient care ought to occur, and nursing documentation confirms that it was done, then the computer is able to monitor and evaluate the patient outcome, an effective and efficient method for documenting quality management activities.

Beginning with the 1994 *Accreditation Manual*, the Joint Commission on Accreditation of Healthcare Organizations (JCAHO) provides a separate chapter that addresses the management of information. Within these standards the goal of information management is to obtain, manage, and use information to enhance and improve individual and organizational performance in patient care. The standards address the identification, design, capture, analysis, communication, and use of information. Under these standards, criteria have been suggested for the selection of information systems. Box 13-6 details what healthcare organizations will need to gather data across departmental

lines, a situation most easily accomplished by an integrated information system.

Other data used by the computer to monitor quality are compiled from staff performance, incident reports, acuity data, and staffing and scheduling statistics. Computerized personnel files generate reminders for license renewal and track position changes to produce reports on budgeting and forecasting trends.

Communication networks are used to transmit information that is entered at one terminal and received by another. These networks are usually part of the integrated system and reduce the clerical functions of nursing. They can provide patient census and locations, results from tests, and lists of medications. Nursing policies and procedures may be entered onto a communication network to be accessible to everyone.

Budgeting and payroll information is usually processed from a combination of data entered by personnel (hourly wages) and the nurse staffing and scheduling system (number of hours worked). These data, when combined with the patient census, provide valuable information for nurse managers. Hours worked should fluctuate with changes in census and acuity data. When the number of staff worked is multiplied by the hourly wage and compared to the census over a period of time, the nurse manager has the information needed to forecast staffing needs.

Summary reports can be written for any of the data entered into the computer. These are especially useful for the JCAHO accreditation process for hospitals and for home healthcare agencies. Incident reports, allergy and drug reaction reports, infection control reports, and utilization review reports are examples of summary reports. Forecasting and planning systems are designed to predict staffing needs, determine trends in patient care, and forecast departmental budgetary compliance.

Nurse leaders/managers must be aware of the differences between nursing information systems and hospital information systems and their limitations. Hospital information systems usually link the information needs of many departments in the organization, while nursing information systems often reflect the manual documentation systems of nursing and do not provide hospital-wide access to patient care information gathered by nursing.

Discussion has focused on information systems for acute care institutions, but many patients are cared for in community settings. Box 13-7 lists types of systems used to support home healthcare. Community

---

Box 13-6

Criteria for Selecting an Information System Based on the JCAHO Standards

An information system must provide:
1. Information confidentiality and security
2. Uniform data definitions such as minimum data sets and standardized classifications
3. Standard format for transmitting data
4. Combining of data and information
5. Sharing of information between systems
6. Linking of clinical and fiscal information
7. Linking to libraries, practice guidelines, and comparative data
8. Patient-specific data
9. Management of verbal orders and authentication of record entries
10. Aggregation of data for use in risk management, quality improvement, decision making, and planning

Adapted from Mills (1995).

health nursing includes health promotion, maintenance, and education as well as coordinated continuity of care. Information systems are also found in community and home health programs where they are used for financial management and billing, statistical reporting, and patient care information systems. These systems can be used within the agency or location or connect the agency to an enterprise integrated data network supporting continuity of care through a computerized patient record. Links would be provided between the patient's home, hospital, and physician office using bedside terminals, voice-activated systems, and laptop computers. Interactive learning would be enhanced, and there would be opportunities for quality outcomes measurement.

Client management includes client demographics, problem lists, and information such as health status. Personnel management describes the types of client care activities performed and provides payroll information. Fiscal information systems include client charges, agency accounts, expenditures, and funding sources. Program management systems allow reporting of information from data entered through all these systems.

Nurses in community health have communicated with their offices and clients through the use of beepers and cellular phones. Day-to-day events are recorded on a Dictaphone or tape recorder and returned to the office for typing into the client record. Nurses caring for patients in the home healthcare industry have many government and insurance requirements for form completion. Computers offer a means of reducing this paperwork burden by allowing direct entry of data in the required format. In recent years the portable palmtop or laptop computer has made recording of patient care information and personnel productivity possible.

These portable computers are used to download files of the patients to be seen during the day from the main data base. During each visit, the computer prompts the nurse for vital signs, assessments, diagnosis, interventions, long- and short-term goals, and medications, based on previous entries in the medical record. The nurses then enter any new data, modifications, or nursing notes directly into the portable computer. At the end of the day, patient care entries are transmitted by telephone to the host computer in the main office, which automatically updates the patient record and prepares any verbal order entry records, home visit reports, federally mandated treatment plans, productivity and quality improvement reports, and other documents for review and signature.

The elimination of the paper trail has been partially accomplished by the placement of computer terminals at the bedside or through the use of hand-held computers. In this way, information can be entered once at the point of care and accessed over and over again. Specific applications most beneficial for documentation at the bedside are vital signs, medication administration, and intravenous fluid administration. Documentation of the patient assessment at the bedside saves time and decreases the likelihood of forgetting to document vital information. Bedside systems that adapt to the nurse's work flow, personalize patient assessments, and simplify care planning are available. Patient care areas with bedside terminals have improved the quality of patient care by decreasing errors of omission, providing greater accuracy and completeness of documentation, reducing medication errors, providing more timely response to patient needs, and improving discharge teaching. These systems shorten or eliminate shift-to-shift communication and eliminate redundant charting of data.

There are advantages and disadvantages in the use of this technology. Bedside terminals must be

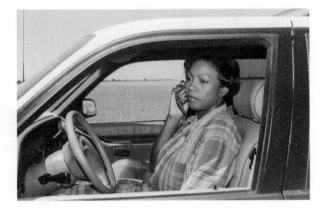

Nurses working in the community often use cellular phones to communicate with their offices.

Box 13-7

Systems to Support Home Healthcare

1. Client management systems
2. Personnel management systems
3. Fiscal management systems
4. Program management systems

Adapted from Saba & McCormick (1996).

suited to patient rooms. They should have quiet fans, must be lighted to be viewed in the dark, and must be either wall mounted or placed on portable stands. Research studies are being conducted to determine the usefulness of bedside technology. This chapter's "Research Perspective" summarizes a study that points to some unanswered questions involving bedside terminals.

Hand-held technology is also used in gathering data at the point of care. These are hand-held computer terminals that have access to the central computers in the institution. Use of these terminals makes it less expensive to equip each caregiver on the shift rather than place a stationary terminal in each patient room. Hand-held terminals are available that offer documentation of care plans, medications, laboratory results, intake and output totals, and patient demographic information at the point of care.

Disadvantages of hand-held technology stem from their portability; they can be put down and forgotten, or dropped and broken, and are a target for theft. There must also be a convenient and adequate place to store them when they are not in use. These terminals are bulky and tiresome to carry, and the display screen is small. Users may enter selections from menus rather than entering text. For example, the appropriate numbers may be entered from a menu

for vital signs, and by pressing a key on the keyboard, a menu for entering intake and output appears for data entry. Many of these terminals must be placed in a host computer so that the data can be downloaded to a central data base, a process that takes approximately 15 minutes per patient.

Wireless messaging (WL) may also change the way we work. Wireless communication is an extension of an existing wired network environment that uses radio-based systems to transmit data signals through the air without any physical connections. These small hand-held computers are connected to a wireless network consisting of internal or external radios, wireless bridges known as access points, a special antenna, and Heliax cabling. These are useful in a reengineered environment where the caregiver goes to the patient rather than the patient going to the caregiver. In these cases, access to on-line patient information must also be mobile. Nurses and physicians can use wireless computing at the bedside to document changes in assessment and place orders. By streamlining the work processes, the need for transfer of information to paper is eliminated.

Wireless systems are also being used by emergency medical personnel to request authorization for the treatments or drugs needed in emergency situations. Laboratories can use WL technology to transmit

Research Perspective

In Saba, V., & McCormick, K. (1996). Essentials of Computers for Nurses (p. 371). New York: McGraw-Hill.

A study reported by the New York University Medical Center Nursing Department on the quality of patient care documentation before and after bedside terminal installation found no significant relationship between the presence of bedside terminals and the quality of documentation. In studying the use of terminals at the nurses' station compared to terminals at the bedside, charting was found to be more timely at the patient's bedside, but the percentage of use was too low for significant benefits to be gained. The conclusion of this study was that nurses, when given a choice of entering information at the bedside or at a central nurses' station, chose not to use the bedside terminal.

Implications for Practice

Reasons for less charting at the bedside in favor of charting at the nurses' station might include:

- Nurses may need time away from the bedside where they can organize thoughts and collaborate with colleagues.
- Nurses may need respite from demands on their time and an opportunity to sit down.
- The charting pathway may need to be redesigned to facilitate capture of data at the bedside.
- Placement of the terminal in the patient's room was determined by available space and may have been inconvenient to use.
- The central nurses' station design as the hub of staff communication and activity as well as terminal availability may not support bedside data entry.

Care facilities that wish to use bedside charting should take these reasons into consideration when designing and implementing the new charting procedure.

laboratory results to physicians; patients awaiting organ transplants are being provided with WL pagers so that they can be notified if a donor is found; and parents of critically ill children carry them when they are away from a phone.

A home monitoring system in use by visiting nurses uses WL technology to enter vital signs and other patient-related information. This information is transmitted to the agency so that treatment plans and bills can be generated.

Voice technology is the ability to control a computer system through voice input by the user. It is the ability of a machine to gather, process, interpret, and execute audible signals by comparing the spoken words with a template already resident in the system. If the patterns match, recognition occurs and a previously stored command is executed by the computer. This allows untrained personnel or those whose hands are busy to work in computer-based environments without touching the computer. These systems recognize about 60,000 words (Bunschoten, 1996), but the speaker must use staccato-like speech, pausing about one-tenth of a second between each clearly spoken word, as these systems must be programmed for each user so that the system recognizes the user's voice patterns.

The management of these technologies is important. Nurse leader/managers must make knowledgeable decisions about the type of technology to use, the education needed, and the proper care and maintenance of the equipment. Important questions to ask include: What data and information do we need to gather? Where do we need to gather it? How difficult is the equipment to use? How soon will it become obsolete?

Exercise 13-5

Think about the data you gather as you go through the day. What data are collected directly from the patient? How do you communicate the data? Based on your answer, which point-of-care technology would you recommend for use in your setting? (For example: "I collect vital signs and intake and output on patients during the day. Sometimes the patients are in the sunroom, sometimes they are sitting in the hallway. I would like to have a portable computer to enter data as they are gathered." Or, "I travel throughout the county assessing the status of newborns. I would like to have a portable computer to enter these data.")

Knowledge Technology

Knowledge technology consists of systems that generate or process knowledge. Computers process symbols; therefore they offer a technology similar to that of the human mind, a knowledge technology. Knowledge technology combines an application of computer science and information science with nursing science to assist in the management and processing of data, information, and knowledge to support the practice of nursing and patient care.

The use of knowledge technology is called **informatics.** Nursing informatics is a specialty for nursing, recognized by the American Nurses' Association. Specialists in nursing informatics recognize that data and information are processed by nurses to make knowledgeable clinical decisions. The processing of information is complex. Information consists of data to which meaning has been attached because they have been organized into a structure that carries meaning that may result in the development of new or different information or knowledge. This new or different knowledge is then used to make decisions.

Knowledge technology relies on **expert systems.** An expert system is a computer program that mimics the inductive or deductive reasoning of a human expert. These programs process knowledge to produce decisions by means of a **knowledge base** and a software application that controls the use of the knowledge (an inference engine). To automate this process, the necessary data elements must be identified and rules for combining the data established. The same data elements are always required, and the same formula or rule is applied in the same way to the same data. The knowledge base contains the knowledge (rules, heuristics) that an expert nurse would apply to the data and information in order to solve a problem. The inference engine controls the use of the knowledge by providing the logic for its use. Box 13-8 illustrates the use of an expert system for giving a maximum dose of pain medication. The knowledge base contains eight items that are to be considered when giving the maximum dose. The inference engine controls the use of the knowledge base by applying logic that an expert nurse would use in making the decision to give the maximum dose.

This decision frame states that IF pain is severe (A), or a painful procedure is planned (B) and there is an order for pain medication (C), and the time since surgery is less than 48 hours (H) and the time since the last dose is greater than 3 hours (G) and there are no contraindications to the medication (D) or history of allergy (E) or contraindication to the maximum dose (F), then the "decision" would be to give the dose of pain medication. The rule or heuristics appearing in this logic are those that expert nurses would apply in making the decision to give

Expert Decision Frame for "Give Maximum Dose of Pain Medication"

The Knowledge Base:
A. Severe pain
B. Painful procedure planned
C. Pain medication order
D. Contraindications to the medication
E. History of allergic reaction to opiate analgesics
F. Contraindication to maximum dose of opiate analgesic
G. Time since last dose
H. Time since surgery

The Inference Engine:
Logic: Give the maximum dose of pain medication
   IF:
(A or B) and (C and H < 48 hours and G > 3 hours) and not (D or E or F)
   OR:
(C and H < 48 hours and G > 4 hours) and not (D or E or F)

pain medication. The inference engine controls the IF logic or knowledge.

One of the benefits of computerized expert systems is that they outperform nonexpert human clinicians, assisting with the decision making for novices, nurses working outside their areas of expertise, and orientees. Because the systems obtain their information directly from patient care documentation, the computer never forgets when a patient needs pain medication or the effectiveness of the last treatment. If the expert system is used in conjunction with an information system, the documentation of observations, care, and patient outcomes can be expected to increase significantly and improve the quality of care.

Nurse managers must be aware of the usefulness of expert systems for nursing. By helping to develop the logic used in the knowledge base through the use of critical thinking skills, changes in current practice can be made for the improvement of patient care.

Exercise 13-6

For example, Mr. Jones' heart rate is 58 beats per minute. Tony is about to give Mr. Jones his Tenormin. When Tony enters Mr. Jones' identification number, and the medication name, the computer warns him that Tenormin should not be given for a heart rate less than 60 beats per minute.

Nurse Attitudes

The attitudes of nurses who use computers are as important as the technology itself. Nurses' attitudes and anxiety toward technology and the use of computers must be explored and areas of acceptance and resistance identified in order for the nursing profession to determine the impact of computer use on the quality of patient care. Negative attitudes toward the use of computers usually lead to resistance to implementation and use of the system. There are several reasons for resistance. The first is economic, since computers are time and labor saving and thus could be associated with layoffs and unemployment. The second reason is psychological, as computers can be ego-threatening. Nurses fear the loss of prestige and status because they do not know how to use computers and a loss of power because the computer contains more information than they have. A third reason is ideological barriers, such as less human contact or the deprivation of personal or professional freedom. A major source of resistance involves confidentiality and perceived interference in the nurse-patient relationship.

Education and training before implementation or during orientation can alleviate the ego threat by equipping staff with the knowledge needed to maintain their status and power. User involvement is necessary during the design, implementation, and evaluation of the systems so that nurses will use the technology to provide quality care. Box 13-9 contains a checklist of objectives for education and training.

▎ PROFESSIONAL ISSUES

Confidentiality

Converting the patient record to a computer-generated document changes the procedures to be followed in maintaining patient confidentiality. With manually generated documents, there is only one copy of the data and caregivers access the chart on the patient care unit. With computerized data, the information may be accessed by any persons with the proper permission.

This makes it mandatory that system users never share the passcodes that allow them access to information in the computerized data base. Each passcode uniquely identifies a user to the system by name and title, gives approval to carry out certain functions, and provides access to data appropriate to the user. When a nurse signs onto a computer, all data and information that are entered can be traced to the passcode. Policies on the use, security, and accuracy of data must be written and enforced.

Ethics

Ethics is a form of thinking about morality, moral problems, and moral judgments. Principles are general action guides for judgment; an ethical principle might be to prevent harm and promote the highest level of health possible. Because of the increasing ability to preserve and maintain human life via the technological interventions, questions dealing with life become complex, both conceptually and ethically. Conceptually, it becomes more difficult to define extraordinary treatment and human life because technology has changed our concepts of living and dying. The ethics problem becomes one of precedence, such as the dilemma of how to relieve pain without hastening death.

A frequent source of ethical dilemmas is the use of invasive technological treatment to prolong life for patients with limited or no decision-making capabilities when there are unlimited choices in determining who shall live and who shall be permitted to die. Healthcare institutions that use technology strive for efficiency and cost-effectiveness with an ethical mandate of the greatest good for the greatest number. The nursing profession holds a holistic orientation and is concerned with individual patient welfare and the impact of technological intervention as it affects the immediate and long-term quality of the patients and their families. Patient advocacy remains an important function of the professional nurse.

Nurse leaders must promote the existence of an ethics committee in their institutions and assign knowledgeable nurses to serve on these committees. Nurse managers must ensure the confidentiality of patient data and information by establishing policies and procedures for the collection and entering of data and the use of security measures such as passcodes. They must also be knowledgeable patient advocates in the use of technology for patient care by referring ethical questions to the organization's ethics committee. Staff nurses must be aware of their responsibilities for the confidentiality and security of the data that they gather and for the security of their passcodes.

FUTURE TRENDS

Because of escalating healthcare costs, insurance companies (third-party payers) and the federal government are supporting new technologies to reduce costs. Managed care, computerized patient records, and the credit-card-like devices that store health history data are technologies of the future. Use of the Community Health Information networks, the Internet and World Wide Web, and telecable will also provide new exciting options for healthcare. Managed care is an effort by the insurance companies, the payers of healthcare, to manage healthcare costs by limiting the care provided for each diagnosis. In the hospital, this means that the number of days a patient is permitted to stay is limited, depending on the diagnosis. If the patient remains longer than the permitted days, the health insurer will not reimburse the costs of the care for the unapproved days. The concept of managed care has caused the redesign of patient care plans to clinical pathways that detail the interventions needed day by day to achieve the outcome of discharge by the final approved day. Data from the clinical pathway form the basis of the computerized patient record.

The **computerized patient record** (CPR) has been mandated by the federal government, and healthcare organizations are expected to adopt this technology by the year 2000. The CPR allows for immediate and complete access to patient information for clinical decision making, outcome evaluation, and coordination of patient care resources and patient flow through the healthcare delivery system. Box 13-10 gives the stages of development for the CPR. The CPR is expected to contain a problem list, health status and functional levels, and clinician rationale for patient care decisions. It will be a "womb to tomb" record of the patient's healthcare. The CPR is necessary because of the need for better access to quality

---

Box 13-10

Stages in Development of the Computerized Patient Record (CPR)

Stage 1. Computerize all areas and functions within the hospital.

Stage 2. Integrate these systems into networks.

Stage 3. Create a data repository of patient clinical information.

Stage 4. Provide clinical access to the repository.

Stage 5. Allow clinicians to enter information/orders into the system.

Stage 6. Develop computer logic for decision support and reminders based on expert system logic.

Adapted from Furfaros, Muchoney, & Anania-Firouzan (1996).

Box 13-11

Smart Card Information

1. Patient classification with a link to insurance plans
2. Emergency care information
3. Recent care encounter data including medications
4. Past care encounter summaries
5. Record locations and electronic address information to the records

Adapted from Elliott (1996).

---

care, patient mobility, and care received from various health professionals.

Furfaros, Muchoney, and Anania-Firouzan (1996) reported a study in which 91% of hospitals surveyed did not have all areas or functions computerized. Their conclusion is that complete CPR systems will not be implemented by the year 2000.

Credit-card-like devices called smart cards store up to eight pages of data on a computer chip. The implementation of computer-based health information systems will lead to computer networks that will store health records across local, state, national, and international boundaries.

The smart card serves as a bridge between the clinician terminal and the central repository, making patient information available to the caregiver quickly and cheaply at the point of service because the patients bring it with them. This will help to coordinate care, improve quality-of-care decisions, and reduce

risk, waste, and duplication of effort. Patients are mobile and consult many practitioners, thereby causing their records to be fragmented. With the electronic smart card, patients and providers and notes can be brought together in any combination at any place. Box 13-11 provides examples of the kinds of data that are recorded on smart cards.

TECHNOLOGIES FOR THE FUTURE

Community Health Information Networks

These technologies for the future will be data links to **community health information networks** (CHINs). A CHIN is an electronic highway providing access to data that are collected and stored in the central data repository. This provides information for healthcare delivery, outcome data, and clinical quality assessment. Figure 13-3 illustrates the concept of the CHIN.

In the CHIN, health data remain in the central data repository of the agency in which it was collected. Authorized staff can view the previous health history for patients admitted to Hospital 1 in Figure 13-3 by retrieving the information in the CPR. The data for the CPR were gathered at the point of care in the physician's office, laboratory, pharmacy, or hospital—wherever a health service was provided. The CHIN will serve as a router to this information. If the staff in Hospital 1 needs previous laboratory results, the CHIN will route the request to the laboratory central data repository and back. This information might also be located on the patient's smart card.

Internet

Another vehicle for health information is the *Internet*. The Internet is a "now" phenomenon that provides health education and other health information. The Internet is a worldwide network of computers that fosters communication, collaboration, resource sharing, and information access. It is a multicultural library that is open all day, every day to ordinary computer users.

The main uses of the Internet are sending and receiving electronic mail (e-mail) and browsing the World Wide Web (www). Mail may be sent to individuals in any part of the world through e-mail if they have an e-mail address, or e-mail of particular interest may be obtained by subscribing to a *listserv*. A listserv is a group of people who have similar interests. Subscribers to a listserv become part of the "conversation." All messages sent to the listserv are for-

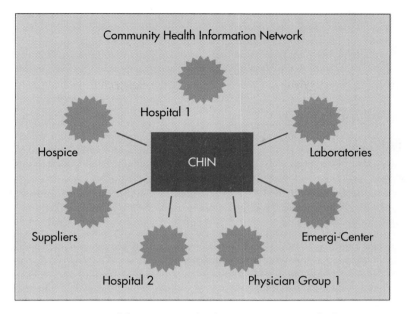

Figure 13-3   Some of the entities involved in CHIN. (From McAlindon [1997].)

warded to all subscribers, who can then read and respond to them.

World Wide Web

The *World Wide Web* is a network of information in the form of text, pictures, video, and sound. Web pages contain text and "links" to other documents filled with information. Links are highlighted or underlined words that are clicked on with the mouse to activate another linked document. Web servers are located all over the world so that you can retrieve information from linked web pages without knowing whether the server is located in Australia, Europe, or California. You will need a software program called a browser to view web pages. Instructions and exercises for finding information on the World Wide Web are located in the workbook section of this text.

Box 13-12 is a list of sites of interest to nurses. This demonstrates a potential path of health information from the user to the Internet. All users will have access to an internal e-mail system (Figure 13-4). All affiliates in the corporation (no matter how distant) will be connected to each other through a wide area network (WAN). Physicians will be able to consult about a patient while accessing the health information in the central data repository through the WAN. Because the WAN is also connected to the Internet, health information could be sent to authorized users anywhere in the world. The firewall protects the information in the central data repository from access by

unauthorized users. It is a network security measure that keeps electronic intruders from accessing an organization's data on its private network. It must also allow members of the organization to reach the Internet.

Exercise 13-7

Assuming you are somewhat familiar with the Internet and the World Wide Web, think about the use of these networks in healthcare. If the data that you collect at the point of care reside in a central data repository, could they be sent to someone over the Internet? Would this be secure? Figure 13-4 might help you with your answer.

Telehealth

Telecommunications and systems technology facilitate clinical oversight of healthcare via the telephone, remote monitoring, information links, and the Internet. An emerging technology called telehealth allows care to occur through two-way interactive video conferencing.

Telehealth is the use of modern telecommunications and information technologies for the provision of healthcare to individuals at a distance and the transmission of information to provide that care. This is accomplished through the use of two-way interactive video-conferencing and high-speed phone lines, fiber optic cable, and satellite transmissions. People sitting in front of the teleconferencing camera can be diagnosed, treated, monitored, and educated by nurses and physicians. ECGs and x-rays can be

---

Box 13-12
Health-Related Web Site Uniform Resource Locators (URLs)

DESCRIPTION	URL
Centers for Disease Control	http://www.cdc.gov
Public mailing lists	http://www.neosoft.com/internet/paml
Information for health professionals	http://www.clark.net/pub/poshank/index.htm
Mayo Clinic site	http://www.mayo.edu
Nursing and health-related resources	http://www.access.digex.net/~nurse/website/htm
Resources for nurses and families	http://pegasus.cc.ucf.edu/%7Ewink
Health on the Net	http://www.hon.ch/
Excellent links to health information	http://www.simmons.edu/~paris/#Mlists
U.S. Department of Health/Human Services	http://www.Healthfinder.gov
Nursing and healthcare resources	http://www.shef.ac.uk/~nhcon

NOTE: URL addresses are case sensitive. Be sure to use capital letters where shown. The sign ~ is called a tilde; it is located next to the number 1 over the tab key on the left side of the keyboard.

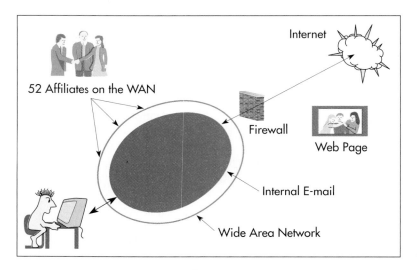

Figure 13-4   Health information path to the Internet.

---

viewed and transmitted. Sophisticated electronic stethoscopes and dermascopes allow nurses and physicians to hear heart, lung, and bowel sounds and to look closely at wounds, eyes, ears, and skin. Ready access to expert advice and patient information is available no matter where the patient or information is located. Patients in rural areas and prisons especially benefit from this technology.

SUMMARY

We have discussed the advances of technology in a managed care environment that will stress wellness and illness prevention, as well as the linking of local and global communities. Care in this new era will focus on empowering patients and their families through information and education. Everyone (families, employers, insurers, providers) will evaluate care based on outcomes. Healthcare in the future will emanate from the home. Clinicians will move beyond the traditional walls of healthcare facilities to become as skilled with wellness maintenance activities and prevention methods as with direct care delivery. Technology has become the bond that links communities together in a rapidly changing world of healthcare, and with technology comes the need for a new set of competencies. Are you prepared for this exciting future?

A Manager's Solution

❓ In an effort to provide the visiting nurses with the information we needed in a timely manner, we purchased an information system suited to community health. Each nurse will have a laptop computer to access a central data repository of patient information. He or she will be able to obtain the information needed to make the scheduled visits while still at home. At the end of the day, the nurse will send the new patient information to the central repository. The computer automatically completes all the required forms and submits charges for the services rendered. Our nurses will no longer have to travel great distances to obtain and submit information, and efficiency, effectiveness, and patient outcomes will be improved.

❓ *Would this be a suitable approach for you? Why?*

▌CHAPTER CHECKLIST

Science and technology give us the means but not the ends, and nurses are the key personnel in the healthcare system to mediate the interaction among science, technology, and the patient because of their unique roles as caregivers who preserve the patients' humanity. The challenge for the profession is to continue to provide human and moral care that gives life, health, and death their meaning in a technological organization that strives for efficiency and cost-effectiveness. Nurse leaders, managers, and staff must provide leadership in managing information and technology to meet the challenge.

■ Information is the communication or reception of knowledge. It consists of three aspects of the concept of communication:
  • data
  • information
  • knowledge
■ Nurses commonly manage three types of information technology:
  • biomedical
  • information
  • knowledge
■ Biomedical technology includes the use of:
  • physiological monitoring
  • diagnostic testing
  • drug administration
  • therapeutic testing to gather patient care data
■ Information technology refers to computers and programs that are used to process data and information.
■ Use of the nursing minimum data set provides a framework for gathering data so that they can be retrieved and compared across time.
■ Healthcare information systems possess patient care data to provide information.
■ Integrated information systems focus on organizational functions and may consist of:
  • stand-alone systems
  • on-line interactive systems
  • networked systems
  • integrated systems
■ Nursing information systems are used within nursing for patient care documentation and often do not communicate with other departmental information systems, although these systems may be interfaced to the hospital information system.
■ Information systems for nursing administration provide information for:
  • quality improvement
  • personnel files
  • communication networks
  • budgeting and payroll
  • patient census
  • summary reports
  • forecasting and planning
■ Computer terminals to capture data at the point of care have improved communication by providing immediate access to information.
■ The use of knowledge technology, which mimics the information processing of the expert nurse, is called informatics.
■ The computerized patient record contains healthcare information for each individual from birth to death, allowing immediate and complete access to health information.
■ Smart cards are credit-card-like devices that store up to eight pages of data. These cards and the information they provide help to coordinate care across local, state, national, and international boundaries— wherever patients may need access to healthcare.
■ Confidentiality issues have become important with increased access to patient care data.

- A CHIN is an electronic highway providing access to data that are collected and stored in the central data repository. This provides information for healthcare delivery, outcome data, and clinical quality assessment.
- The Internet is a worldwide network of computer networks that fosters communication, collaboration, resource sharing, and information access. It is a multicultural library that is open all day, every day to ordinary computer users. The main uses of the Internet are sending and receiving electronic mail (e-mail) and browsing the World Wide Web (WWW).
- Telehealth is the process of using modern telecommunication and information technologies to provide healthcare.

TIPS FOR MANAGING INFORMATION AND TECHNOLOGY

- Create a vision for the future.
- Tie your vision to the institution's strategic plan.
- Learn what you need to know to fulfill the vision.
- Join committees that are moving in the direction of your vision.
- Be prepared to implement and support new technology.
- Never stop learning or you'll always be behind.

TERMS TO KNOW

biomedical technology
community health information networks (CHINs)
computerized patient record (CPR)
data
data processing
database
drug administration systems
ethics
expert system
informatics
information
information technology
integrated systems
knowledge
knowledge base

knowledge technology
mainframe computer
networked systems
nursing administration systems
nursing information systems (NIS)
nursing minimum data set (NMDS)
on-line interactive systems
physiological monitoring system
smart card
stand-alone systems
telehealth
therapeutic systems
voice technology
wireless messaging (WL)

REFERENCES

Bunschoten, B. (1996). What role will speech recognition play in health care? Health Data Management 4(1):38-43.
Daly, J., Maas, M., & Johnson, M. (1997). Nursing outcomes classification: An essential element in data sets for nursing and health care effectiveness. Computers in Nursing 15(2), 82-86.
Elliott, J. (1996). The smart card: Wising up on plastic money. Healthcare Informatics, 13(5), 29-32.
Furfaros, M., Muchoney, K., & Anania-Firouzan, P. (1996). CPR by the year 2000: A myth? Healthcare Informatics 13(5), 45-47.
Joint Commission on Accreditation of Healthcare Organizations (1994). Accreditation Manual. Chicago: The Commission.
Karpiuk, K., Delaney, C., & Ryan, P. (1997). South Dakota statewide nursing minimum data set project. J Prof Nurs 13(2):76-83.
Maas, M., Johnson, M., & Moorhead, S. (1996). Classifying nursing-sensitive patient outcomes. Image J Nurs Sch 28(4): 295-301.
McAlindon, M., Danz, S., & Theodoroff, R.C. (1987). Choosing the hospital information system: a nursing perspective. Journal of Nursing Administration, 17(19): 11-15.
Mills, M. (1995). Nursing participation in the selection of healthcare information systems. In Ball, M., Hannah, K., Newbold, S., and Douglas, J., eds. Nursing informatics: Where caring and technology meet. New York: Springer-Verlag.
Saba, V., & McCormick, K. (1996). Essentials of computers for nurses. New York: McGraw Hill.
Simpson, R. (1997). Take advantage of managed care opportunities. Nursing Management 29(3):24-25.
Tan, J. (1995). Health management information systems: Theories, methods, applications. Gaithersburg, Maryland: Aspen.
Warner-Matheron, A., & Hannah, K. (1995). Introducing nurse information systems in the clinical setting. In Ball, M., Hannah, K., Newbold, S., and Douglas, J., eds. Nursing informatics: Where caring and technology meet. New York: Springer-Verlag.
Werley, H., Ryan, P., Zorn, C., & Devine, E. (1994). Why the nursing minimum data set (NMDS)? In McCloskey, T. & Grace, H., eds. Current Issues in Nursing, St. Louis: Mosby.

SUGGESTED READINGS

Blewett, D., & Jones, K. (1996). Using elements of the nursing minimum data set for determining outcomes. J Nurs Admin 26(6), 48-56.
Bowles, K., & Naylor, M. (1996). Nursing intervention classification systems. Image J Nurs Sch 28(4), 303-308.
Aller, K., & Rosenstein, A. (1996). Outcomes measurement: Collecting data for payors, providers & patients. Infocare (Sep/Oct), 22-23.
Ball, M., Simborg, D., Albright, J., & Douglas, J. (1995). Healthcare information management systems, New York: Springer-Verlag.
Bunschoten, B. (1996). Measuring outcomes. Health Data Management 4(6), 40-48.
Goldstein, D., & Flory, J. (1997). Lasso the power of the Internet. Info Care (Jan/Feb), 37-42.
Hannah, K., Duggleby, W., Anderson, B., Mackenzie, W., Broad, L., Besner, J., Larsen, S., and Reyes, L. (1995). The development of essential data elements in Canada

(Health information: Nursing components. In Greenes, R., Peterson, H., & Protti, D., eds. *Proceedings of the Eighth World Congress on Medical Informatics*, Healthcare Computing and Communications Canada, Inc.: Edmonton, Alberta, Canada.

Lorenzi, N., & Riley, R. (1995). Informatics and organizational change. In Ball, M., Hannah, K., Newbold, S., and Douglas, J., eds. *Nursing informatics: Where caring and technology meet*. New York: Springer-Verlag.

Lorenzi, N., & Riley, R. (1995). *Organizational aspects of health informatics*. New York: Springer Verlag.

Marr, P., Duthie, E., Glassman, K., et al. (1995). Bedside terminals and quality of nursing documentation. In Saba, V., & McCormick, K., eds. *Essentials of computers for nurses*. New York: McGraw-Hill.

McAlindon, M. (1997). Nurse informaticists: Who are they, what do they do and what challenges do they face? In McCloskey, J., & Grace, H., eds. *Current Issues in Nursing*. New York: Mosby.

McAlindon, M. (1997). Choosing and installing an information system. In Ball, M., Simborg, D., Albright, J., & Douglas, J., eds. *Healthcare information management systems*. New York: Springer-Verlag.

Murphy, F., Karmali, K., McFarlane, G., & Agustin, K. (1996). Education strategy for the implementation of computerized nursing documentation. In Greenes, R., Peterson, H., & Protti, D., eds. *Proceedings of the Eighth World Congress on Medical Informatics*, Healthcare Computing and Communications Canada, Inc.: Edmonton, Alberta, Canada.

Petryshen, P., & Nagle, L. (1995). Establishing a meaningful relationship: Case costing and clinical practice. In Greenes, R., Peterson, H., & Protti, D., eds. *Proceedings of the Eighth World Congress on Medical Informatics*, Healthcare Computing and Communications Canada, Inc.: Edmonton, Alberta, Canada.

Simpson, R. (1996). Wireless communications: A new frontier in technology. *Nursing Management* 27(11), 20-21.

Simpson, R. (1997). The nursing management minimum data set needs YOU! *Nursing Management* 28(6), 20-21.

Tallon, R. (1996). Oximetry: State of the art. *Nursing Management* 27(11), 43-44.

Tallon, R. (1996). Infusion pumps. *Nursing Management* 27 (12), 44-46.

Tan, J. (1995). *Health management information systems*. Gaithersburg, MD: Aspen.

U.S. Congress, Office of Technology Assessment. (1995). *Bringing health care online: The role of information technologies*, OTA-ITC-624, Washington, DC: U.S. Government Printing Office, September.

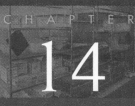

14

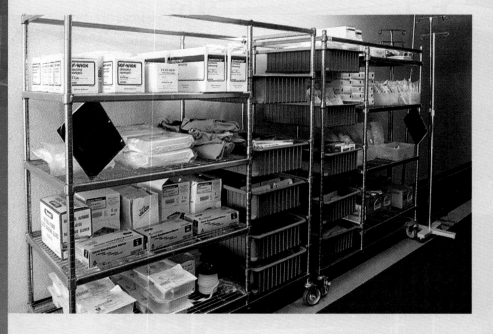

Managing Costs and Budgets

Donna Westmoreland
RN, PhD

This chapter focuses on methods of financing healthcare and specific strategies for managing costs and budgets in various patient care settings. It discusses the factors that escalate healthcare costs, sources of healthcare financing, reimbursement methods, cost-containment and healthcare reform strategies, and implications for nursing practice. It also explains the various types of budgets and outlines the budgeting process. An understanding of the cost and quality issues that drive changes in healthcare and the ethical implications of all financial decisions is crucial to achieving cost-conscious nursing practice.

Objectives

- Explain several major factors that are escalating the costs of healthcare.
- Compare and contrast different reimbursement methods and their incentives to control costs.
- Differentiate costs, charges, and revenue in relation to a specified unit of service, such as a visit, hospital stay, or procedure.
- Demonstrate why all healthcare organizations must make a profit.
- Give examples of cost considerations for nurses working in managed care environments.
- Discuss the purpose of and relationship among the operating, cash, and capital budgets.
- Explain the budgeting process.
- Identify variances on monthly expense reports.

Questions to Consider

- How can you stay abreast of changes in the healthcare system and what they mean for the practice of nursing?
- What are the charges for typical nursing care activities that you perform and the supplies you use?
- Who are the major payers to your organizations? What is their method of payment or reimbursement?
- Does the organization recoup all of the charges? If not, what portion of the charges do they get for various patient groups?
- How is nursing reimbursed in your organization?
- How can you increase your cost-effectiveness as a nurse?
- Do the nursing practices in your organization add value for patients?

A Manager's Challenge

From the Nurse Manager of an Internal Medicine Clinic Located in a Midwestern University Medical Center

The Internal Medicine Clinic (IMC) consists of one Primary Care section and eight specialty sections. The IMC is one of many clinics owned and managed by a physician group. Professional fees are the sole source of revenue for the IMC and are pooled into one fund. Professional fees are received for physician services provided in the hospital, in special procedure laboratories, and in the ambulatory clinic.

For the past 3 years, the IMC has experienced a 15% to 18% increase in ambulatory visit volume. At the same time, IMC revenues have declined. Yet administrators want to stay budget neutral. As payers decrease payment in all areas, it is easy for administrators to assume that the areas of greatest activity are the areas losing money. The next logical step then is to require that variable expenses in that area be reduced. Because nursing personnel are the greatest variable expense in the clinic, such thinking often leads to demands to reduce nursing staff or to substitute lower-paid personnel. As nurse manager of the IMC, my goal is to maintain a high-quality, high-performance work team that adds value for patients. In this situation, what steps can be taken before reducing staff in the IMC ambulatory clinic? How can I justify that the amount spent currently for staff keeps the clinic functioning in the black?

What do you think you would do if you were this manager?

INTRODUCTION

Healthcare costs in the United States continue to rise at a rate greater than general inflation and consume more than 15% of the gross domestic product (GDP). In 1994, we spent nearly $950 billion for healthcare (U.S. DHHS, 1996). This equals $3,510 per person and surpasses the per capita expenditures of other nations by almost 50%. Yet, with 41 million people uninsured and millions of others underinsured, many Americans are going without basic healthcare. With the exception of South Africa, the United States is the only industrialized nation where healthcare is a privilege rather than a right.

Despite our huge expenditures, the major indicators of health in the United States reveal significant problems. For example, our infant mortality rate is among the poorest of all industrialized nations, with black infants dying at a higher rate than white infants.

Births to teenagers are increasing, and more women and children are living in poverty, the leading cause of death in children. Breast cancer now strikes one in eight women, and violence-related injuries as well as homicides are increasing. In other words, as a nation we are not getting a high value return for our healthcare dollar.

The large portion of GDP that is spent on healthcare poses problems to the economy in other ways, too. Funds are diverted from needed social programs such as child care, housing, education, transportation, and the environment. The price of goods and services is increased, so the country's ability to compete in the international marketplace is compromised. One illustration is that up to 10% of the cost of a new American car goes to pay for the healthcare costs of automobile workers.

WHAT ESCALATES HEALTHCARE COSTS?

Total healthcare **costs** are a function of the **prices** and the **utilization** rates of healthcare services (*Costs = Price × Utilization*) (see Table 14-1). Price is the rate that healthcare providers set for the services they deliver. Utilization refers to the quantity or volume of services provided. Administrative inefficiency and unnecessary medical care were estimated to account for $200 billion of total healthcare costs in 1993. That figure does not even consider the increased costs due to overpricing of physician services and technologic procedures or fraud (Consumers Union, 1992).

The administrative inefficiency is primarily a result of the large numbers of clerical personnel that organizations use to process reimbursement forms. Hospitals in the United States spend an average of 20% of their **budgets** on billing administration alone.

Table 14-1	RELATIONSHIP OF PRICE AND UTILIZATION RATES TO TOTAL HEALTHCARE COSTS		
Price ×	Utilization Rate =	Total Cost	% Change
$1.00	100	$100.00	0
$1.08*	100	$108.00	+ 8.0%
$1.08	105†	$113.40	+ 13.4%
$1.08	110‡	$118.80	+ 18.8%

*8% increase for inflation.
†5% more procedures done.
‡10% more procedures done.

These expenditures add to the price of healthcare services.

Several interrelated factors contribute to the overutilization of medical services. These include induced demand, the surplus of highly specialized physicians, the attitudes of consumers, and the way healthcare is financed. Increased utilization of healthcare services is also a function of changing population demographics and disease patterns.

Induced demand refers to "the creation of medical 'need' by those who then profit from it" (Consumers Union, 1992, p. 439). It exists because physicians rather than consumers make most of the decisions regarding what healthcare services are needed and where they will be performed. In a normal marketplace, consumers and **providers** are separate and distinct, and the amount of the service demanded is mediated by its price. Generally, as the price rises the amount of the service used decreases. When the distinction between providers and consumers is blurred and when providers benefit by increased demand, higher utilization and higher prices result (Cleland, 1990). Moreover, treatment patterns, and thus costs, for similar diagnoses are highly variable among physicians, even within the same region.

This situation is further compounded by the large number of physicians choosing to practice in high-tech specialties rather than primary care (Grace, 1994). Because physicians generate demand for their services, growing numbers of specialists increase utilization of high-cost, high-tech services. And as expensive technology is purchased to support these practices, more services must be provided to pay for the equipment.

As a nation, our attitudes and behaviors as consumers of healthcare also contribute to rising costs (Grace, 1994). In general, we are a nation of consumers who prefer to "be fixed" when something goes wrong rather than to practice prevention. When we need "fixing," expensive, high-tech services typically are perceived as the best care. Many of us still believe that the physician knows best, so we do not seek much information related to costs and effectiveness of different healthcare options. When we do seek information, it is not readily available or understandable. Also, we are not used to using other less costly healthcare providers such as nurse practitioners.

The way healthcare is financed contributes to rising costs. When healthcare is reimbursed by third-party **payers**, consumers are somewhat insulated from personally experiencing the direct effects of high healthcare costs. We do not have a lot of incentives to consider costs when choosing among providers or using services. In addition, the various methods for reimbursing healthcare providers have implications for how they price and use services.

Changing population demographics also are increasing the volume of health services needed. For example, chronic health problems increase with age, and the number of elderly Americans is increasing. By the end of the decade, there will be 36 million Americans 65 years of age or older. The fastest growing population are those aged 85 or older. Additionally, infectious diseases such as AIDS and tuberculosis, as well as the growing societal problems of homelessness, drug addiction, and violence, increase demands for health services.

HOW IS HEALTHCARE FINANCED?

Healthcare is paid for primarily from three sources: government (42%), private insurance companies (33%), and individuals (20%) (see Figure 14-1). Three-fourths of the government funding is at the federal level. Federal programs include Medicare and health services for members of the military, veterans, Native Americans, and federal prisoners. Medicare, the largest federal program, was established in 1965 and pays for care provided to the elderly and some disabled individuals. Medicaid, a state-level program financed by federal and state funds, pays for services provided to persons who are medically indigent, blind, or disabled, and to crippled children.

Insurance is the second major source of financing for the healthcare system. Most Americans have private health insurance, which usually is provided by employers, although it can be purchased by individuals. Individuals also pay directly for health services when they do not have health insurance or when insurance does not cover the service. Health insurance benefits often do not cover preventive care or things such as eyeglasses, nonprescription medications, cosmetic surgeries, or alternative healthcare therapies.

REIMBURSEMENT METHODS

Four major payment methods are used for reimbursing healthcare providers: charges, cost-based reimbursement, flat-rate reimbursement, and capitated payments (Neuman, Suver, and Zelman, 1988). These methods are summarized in Box 14-1.

Charges consist of the cost of providing a service plus a markup for profit. Third-party payers often put limitations on what they will pay by establishing usual and customary charges. These limits are established by surveying all providers in a certain area. Usual and customary charges rise over time as providers continually increase their prices.

All allowable costs are calculated and used as the basis for payment in **cost-based reimbursement.** Each payer (government or insurance company) determines what the allowable costs are for each procedure, visit, or service. These payment schedules vary from state to state. Cost-based reimbursement is a *retrospective* payment method because the costs are determined after services are delivered. When the reimbursed costs are less than the full charge for the service, a **contractual allowance** or discount exists. Cost-based reimbursement was the predominant payment method in the 1960s and 1970s and is still used by some payers.

Flat-rate reimbursement is a method in which the third-party payer decides in advance what will be paid for a service or episode of care. For this reason, it is a **prospective reimbursement** method. If the costs of care are greater than the payment, the provider absorbs the loss. If the costs are less than the payment, the provider makes a profit. In 1983

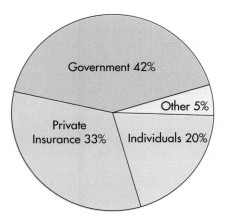

Figure 14-1 Sources of financing for healthcare.

Box 14-1
Major Reimbursement Methods
• Charges
• Cost-based (retrospective)
• Flat-rate (prospective)
• Capitated

Medicare implemented a prospective payment system (PPS) for hospital care that uses diagnosis-related groups (DRGs) as the basis for payment.

Exercise 14-1

What is the contractual allowance when a hospital charges $800/day to care for a ventilator-dependent patient and an insurance company reimburses the hospital $685/day? What is the impact on hospital income (revenue) if this is the reimbursement for 2500 patient days?

DRGs, a classification system that groups patients into categories based on the average number of days of hospitalization for specific medical diagnoses, considers factors such as the patient's age, complications, and other illnesses. Payment includes the expected costs for diagnostic tests, various therapies, surgery, and length of stay (LOS). The cost of nursing services is not explicitly calculated. With a few exceptions, DRGs do not adequately reflect the variability of patient intensity or acuity within the DRG. This is problematic for nursing because the amount of resources (nurses and supplies) used to care for patients is directly related to the patient acuity. Thus many nurses think that DRGs are not a good predictor of nursing care requirements.

In addition to Medicare, some state Medicaid programs and private insurance companies use a DRG payment system. Although DRGs are not currently used for specialty hospitals (pediatric, psychiatric, and oncology), they are a dominant force in hospital payment. The healthcare system radically changed with the implementation of PPS with DRGs as evidenced by increased patient acuity, decreased LOS in hospitals, and greater demand for home care and hospital and community-based nurses. Currently DRGs are being developed for ambulatory care and home care services.

Capitated payments are based on providing specified services to an individual over a period of time such as 1 year. Providers are paid a per person per year (or per month) fee. If the services cost more than the payment, the provider absorbs the loss. Likewise, if the services cost less than the payment, the provider makes a profit. **Capitation** is the mode of payment characteristic of health maintenance organizations (HMOs) and other managed care systems.

Health service researchers do not agree on the exact effects of these reimbursement methods on cost and quality. However, considering these effects is important because changes in payment systems have implications for how care is provided in healthcare organizations.

Exercise 14-2

A hospice is reimbursed $75/day by Medicare for home visits. For one particular group of patients, it costs the hospice an average of $98/day to provide care. What are the implications for the hospice? What options should the hospice nurse manager and nurses consider?

THE CHANGING HEALTHCARE ECONOMIC ENVIRONMENT

Healthcare is a major public concern, and rapid changes are occurring in order to reduce costs and to improve the health and wellness of the nation. As shown in Box 14-2, strategies shaping the evolving healthcare delivery system include managed care, organized delivery systems, and competition based on cost and quality. These strategies affect both the pricing and utilization of health services.

Exercise 14-3

For each reimbursement method, think about the incentives for healthcare providers (individuals and organizations) regarding their practice patterns. Are there incentives to change the *quantity of services* used per patient or the *number or types of patients* served? Are there incentives to be *efficient?* List the incentives. How might each method affect overall healthcare costs? (Think in terms of effect on utilization and price.) What do you think the effect on *quality of care* might be with each payment method?

Managed care is a system of care in which a designated person determines the services that the patient uses. A major goal of managed care is to decrease unnecessary services, thereby decreasing costs. Managed care also works to ensure timely and appropriate care. HMOs are a type of managed care system in which the primary physician serves as a gate keeper. Because HMOs are paid on a capitated basis, it is to their advantage to practice prevention and to use ambulatory care rather than more expensive hospital care. In other forms of managed care, a non-physician case manager arranges and authorizes the services provided. Many insurance companies have

---

Box 14-2
Healthcare Delivery Reform Strategies

- Managed care
- Organized delivery systems
- Competition based on price, patient outcomes, and service quality

used case managers for years. Nurses who work in home healthcare and in ambulatory settings often communicate with insurance company case managers to plan the care for specific patients.

Organized delivery systems (ODS) are composed of networks of healthcare organizations, providers, and payers. Typically, this means hospitals, physicians, and insurance companies. The aim of such joint ventures is to develop and market collectively a comprehensive package of healthcare services that will meet most needs of large numbers of consumers. The financial risks of the enterprise will be shared by hospitals, physicians, and payers. Although hospitals share some risk now with prospective payment, physicians have not generally shared the risk. This risk-sharing is expected to provide incentives to eliminate unnecessary services, utilize resources effectively, and improve quality of services.

Competition among healthcare providers increasingly is based on cost and quality outcomes. Decision making regarding price and utilization of services is shifting from physicians and hospitals to payers. Significant contractual discounts, that is, lower prices, are being demanded by payers. Scientific data that demonstrate positive health outcomes and high-quality services are required. Providers who are unable to compete on the basis of price, patient outcomes, and service quality will find it difficult to survive as the system evolves.

WHAT DOES THIS MEAN FOR NURSING PRACTICE?

What does the changing healthcare environment mean for the practicing professional nurse? We must value

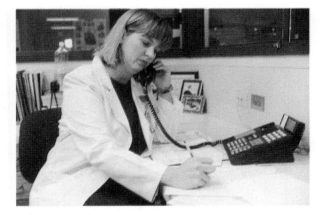

Nurses in ambulatory care settings often work directly with insurance companies to plan patient care.

ourselves as providers and think of our practice within a context of organizational viability and quality of care. To do this we must add "financial thinking" to our repertoire of nursing skills, and we must determine whether or not the services we provide add value for patients. Services that add value are of high quality, affect health outcomes positively, and minimize costs. The following sections help develop "financial thinking" skills and ways to consider how nursing practice adds value for patients through minimizing costs.

WHY IS PROFIT NECESSARY?

Private, nongovernmental healthcare organizations may be either for profit (FP) or not for profit (NFP). This refers to the tax status of the organization and designates how the profit can be used. **Profit** is the excess income left after all expenses have been paid (*Revenues* − *Expenses* = *Profit*). FP organizations pay taxes, and their profits can be distributed to owners and managers. NFP organizations, on the other hand, do not pay taxes and must reinvest all profits in the organization.

All private healthcare organizations must make a profit in order to survive. If expenses are greater than **revenues,** the organization experiences a loss. If revenues equal expenses, the organization breaks even. In both cases, nothing is left over to replace facilities and equipment, expand services, or pay for inflation costs. Some healthcare organizations are able to survive in the short run without making a profit because they use interest from investments to supplement revenues. The long-term viability of any private healthcare organization, however, is dependent on consistently making a profit. Box 14-3 presents an example of an income statement from a neighborhood nursing center.

Nurses and nurse managers directly affect an organization's ability to make a profit. Profits can be achieved or increased by decreasing costs or increasing revenues. In tight economic times, many managers think only in terms of cutting costs. Cost-cutting measures are important, especially to keep prices down so the organization will be competitive. But ways to increase revenues also need to be explored.

Exercise 14-4

Obtain a copy of an itemized patient bill from a healthcare organization and review the charges. What was the source and method of payment? How much of these charges was reimbursed? How much was charged for items you regularly use in clinical care?

Box 14-3

An Income Statement
Neighborhood Nursing Center Statement of Revenues and Expenses
FYE December 31, 1997

Revenues		
Patient revenues	$110,700	
Grant income	60,000	
Other operating revenues	5,300	
Total	$176,000	$176,000
Expenses		
Salary costs	$130,500	
Supplies	14,400	
Other operating expenses (rent, utilities, administrative services, etc.)	29,900	
Total	$174,800	174,800
Excess of revenues over expenses (profit)*		$ 1,200

FYE = Fiscal Year Ending.
*Loss would be shown in parentheses ( ) or brackets < >.

COST-CONSCIOUS NURSING PRACTICES

Understanding What Is Required to Remain Financially Sound

Understanding what is required for a department or agency to remain financially sound requires that nurses move beyond thinking about costs for individual patients to thinking about income and expenses and numbers of patients needed to make a profit. In a fee-for-service environment, revenue is earned for every service provided. So increasing the volume of services is desirable. In a capitated environment where one fee is paid for all services provided, increasing the overall number of patients served and decreasing the volume of services used is desirable. Many healthcare organizations function in a dual reimbursement environment, part capitated and part fee for service. Nurses need to understand their organization's reimbursement environment and strategy for realizing a profit in its specific circumstances.

Knowing Costs and Reimbursement Practices

As direct caregivers and case managers, nurses are constantly involved in determining the type and quantity of resources used for patients. This includes supplies, personnel, and time. Nurses need to know what costs are generated by their decisions and actions. And nurses need to know what things cost and how they are paid for in an organization so they can make cost-effective decisions. For example, nurses need to know per item costs for supplies so that they can appropriately evaluate lower-cost substitutes.

In ambulatory and home health settings, nurses must be familiar with the various insurance plans that reimburse the organization. Each plan has different contract rules regarding preauthorization, types of services covered, required vendors, and so on. Although nurses must develop and implement their plans of care with full knowledge of these reimbursement practices, the payer does not totally drive the care. Nurses still advocate for patients in important ways while also working within the cost and contractual constraints.

In hospitals, usually the cost of nursing care is not calculated or billed separately to patients but is part of the general per diem charge. One major problem with this method is the assumption that all patients consume the same amount of nursing care. Another problem with bundling the charges for nursing care with the room rate is that nursing as a clinical service is not perceived by management as generating revenue for the hospital. Rather, nursing is perceived predominantly as an expense to the organization. Although this perception may not matter in a capitated setting, accurate nursing cost data are needed to negotiate managed care contracts.

Exercise 14-5

How was nursing care charged on the bill you obtained? What are the implications for nursing in being perceived as an expense rather than being associated with the revenue stream? Why will this perception be less important in a capitated environment?

Capturing All Charges in a Timely Fashion

Nurses also help contain costs by making sure that all possible charges are captured. Several large hospitals report more than $1 million a year lost from supplies that were not charged. In hospitals, nurses must know which supplies are charged to patients and which ones are charged to the unit. Additionally, the procedures and equipment used need to be accurately documented. In ambulatory and community settings, nurses often need to keep abreast of the codes that are used to bill services. These codes change yearly, and sometimes items are bundled together under one charge and sometimes they are broken down into different charges. Turning in charges in a timely manner is also important because delayed billing negatively impacts cash flow by extending the time before an organization is paid for services provided. This is significant particularly in smaller organizations.

In home health and hospice organizations, billing is closely integrated with the clinical information system. For example, to ensure reimbursement the physician's plan of care and documentation that the patient meets the criteria for admission must be on the clinical record (Marrelli, 1997). Typically nurses are responsible for documenting this information.

Exercise 14-6

You used three IV catheters to do a particularly difficult venipuncture. Do you charge the patient for all three catheters? What if you accidentally contaminated one by touching the sheet? How is the catheter paid for if not charged to the patient? Who benefits/loses when patients are not charged for supplies?

Using Time Efficiently

The old adage that time is money is fitting in healthcare and refers to both the nurse's time and the patient's time. When nurses are organized and efficient in their care delivery and in scheduling and coordinating patients' care, the organization will save money. With capitation it is particularly important to do as much as possible during each episode of care in order to decrease repeat visits and unnecessary service utilization. Because LOS is the most important predictor of hospital costs (Finkler & Kovner, 1993), patients who stay extra days cost the hospital a considerable amount. Decreasing LOS also makes room for other patients, thereby potentially increasing patient volume and hospital revenues. Nurses can become more efficient and effective by evaluating their major work processes and eliminating areas of redundancy and rework.

Exercise 14-7

The Visiting Nurse Association (VNA) cannot file for reimbursement until all documentation of each visit has been completed. Typically, the paperwork is turned in a week after the visit. When the number of home visits increases rapidly, the paperwork often is not turned in for 2 weeks or more. What are the implications of this routine practice for the agency? Why would the VNA be very vulnerable financially during periods of heavy workload? What are some options for the nurse manager to consider to expedite the paperwork?

Discussing the Cost of Care with Patients

Talking with patients about the cost of care is important even though it may be uncomfortable. Discovering during a clinic visit that a patient cannot afford a specific medication or intervention is preferable to finding out several days later in a follow-up call that the patient has not taken the medication. Such information compels the clinical management team to explore optional treatment plans or to find resources to cover the costs. Talking with patients about costs is important in other ways, too. It involves the patients in the decision making and increases the likelihood that treatment plans will be followed. Patients also can make informed choices and better utilize the resources available to them if they have appropriate information about costs.

Exercise 14-8

A new patient visits the clinic and is given prescriptions for three medications that will cost about $120 per month. You check her chart and discover that she has Medicare and no supplemental insurance. How can you determine whether or not she has the resources to buy this medicine each month? If she cannot afford the medications, what are some options?

Meeting Patient Rather than Provider Needs

Developing an awareness of how feelings about patients' needs influence decisions can help nurses better manage costs. A nurse administrator in a home health agency recently related the story of a nurse who continued to visit a patient for weeks after the patient's health problems had resolved. When questioned, the nurse said she was uncomfortable terminating the visits because the patient continued to tell her he needed her help. Later the patient revealed that he had not needed nursing care for some time, although he had continued telling the nurse he did because he thought she wanted to keep visiting him. This story illustrates how nurses need to make sure whose needs are being met with nursing care.

Evaluating Cost-Effectiveness of New Technologies

The advent of new technologies is presenting dilemmas regarding managing costs. In the past, if a new piece of equipment was easier to use or benefited the patient in any way, nurses were apt to want to use it for everyone, no matter how much more it cost. Now they are forced to make decisions regarding which patients really need the new equipment and which ones will do fine with the current equipment. Essentially, nurses are analyzing the cost-effectiveness of the new equipment with regard to different types of patients. This is a new and sometimes difficult way to think about patient care, and at times it may not "feel fair."

Exercise 14-9

Last year a new positive pressure, needleless system for administering IV antibiotics was introduced. Because it was so easy and convenient for patients, the nurses in the home infusion company where you worked ordered them for everyone. Typically, patients get their IV antibiotics four times/day. The minibags and tubing for the regular procedure cost the agency $22/day. The new system costs $24/medication administration or $96/day. The agency receives the same per diem (daily) reimbursement for each patient. Discuss the financial implications for the agency if this practice is continued. Generate some optional courses of action for the nurses to consider. How should these options be evaluated?

Predicting and Using Nursing Resources Efficiently

Because healthcare organizations are service institutions, the largest part of their operating budget typically is for personnel. For hospitals in particular, nurses are the largest group of employees and often account for the majority of the personnel budget. Staffing is the major area nurse managers can impact with respect to managing costs, and supplies are the second area. To understand why this is so, it is helpful to understand the concepts of fixed and variable costs.

Fixed costs are costs that do not change in total as the volume of patients changes. Examples include rent, loan payments, administrative salaries, and salaries of the minimum amount of staff needed to keep a unit open. **Variable costs** are costs that vary in direct proportion to patient volume or acuity. Examples include nursing personnel, supplies, and medications.

In hospitals and community health agencies, patient classification systems are used to help managers predict nursing care requirements (see Chapter 23). These systems differentiate among patients based on their acuity of illness, functional status, and resource needs. Some nurses do not like these systems because they feel they do not adequately reflect the essence of nursing. However, we need to remember that they are tools to help managers predict resource needs. It is not necessary to describe all nursing activities and judgments in order for a tool to be a good predictor. Misguided efforts to sabotage classification systems, in the hope that better staffing will be achieved, work primarily to prevent developing tools to better manage practice. Used appropriately, patient classification systems can help evaluate changing practice patterns and patient acuity levels as well as help with budgeting processes.

Exercise 14-10

Given the definitions for fixed and variable costs, why do you think nurse managers make the greatest impact on costs through managing staffing and supplies?

The diagnostic services and treatment modalities ordered by physicians also impact the cost of patient care in hospitals. According to industry consultants, it takes several years for a hospital to see reductions in costs resulting from changes in physician practice patterns. The most immediate reductions in costs can be achieved by managing staffing and decreasing LOS.

Hospitals strive to lower costs so they will attract new contracts and be attractive as partners in provider networks. Thus staffing methodologies and patient care delivery models are being closely scrutinized. Work redesign, a process for changing the way to think about and structure the work of patient care, is the predominant strategy for developing systems that better utilize high-cost professionals and improve service quality and patient outcomes.

Exercise 14-11

What data are used to determine patients' needs in different healthcare agencies? What common nursing practices should be scrutinized carefully to determine whether they are meeting patient or provider needs?

Research Perspective

Petryshen, P., Stevens, B., Hawkins, J., & Stewart, M. (1997). Comparing nursing costs for pre-term infants receiving conventional vs. developmental care. Nursing Economics, 15(3), 138-145, 150.

The purpose of this study was to compare the nursing costs of two different approaches for treating very low birth weight (VLBW) infants. One group received conventional care, which included primary nursing, standardized care plans, and routine noise and lighting levels on the patient care unit. The other group received developmental care, which is a more individualized approach to caregiving that included coordinating clinical interventions to prevent frequent interruption during infant sleep and reducing the lighting and noise levels. In addition, developmental care included positioning and bundling infants in ways that prevent disorganization and promote self-regulation. Sixty infants were in each group.

Infants who received developmental care had improved physiological stability measures and fewer days in the neonatal intensive care unit (NICU) than infants receiving conventional care. The developmental care infants were moved from NICU to a transitional care unit earlier, and their nursing intensity needs were lower. The average cost savings for infants in the developmental group was $4,340 per infant during the first 35 days of life or less if they were discharged.

Implications for Practice

The findings from this economic evaluation support the implementation of developmental care for VLBW infants by demonstrating improved patient outcomes and lower costs.

Using Research to Evaluate Standard Nursing Practices

Another way nurses are restructuring their work to make sure they add value for patients is through research. For example, in the internal medicine clinics at the University of Nebraska Medical Center, nurses and physicians are developing a rule to predict which patients are at risk for orthostatic hypotension. This is significant because the mortality rates are high when orthostatic hypotension is present. Yet performing the sitting and standing blood pressure readings on all patients is costly in terms of nursing resources. After the rule has been developed and validated through research, the computerized patient record will automatically signal the nurse to take orthostatic blood pressures when needed. This chapter's "Research Perspective" illustrates cost savings from another practice alteration. Box 14-4 lists some cost-conscious strategies for nursing practice.

Box 14-4
Strategies for Cost-Conscious Nursing Practice

1. Understanding what is required to remain financially sound
2. Knowing costs and reimbursement practices
3. Capturing all possible charges in a timely fashion
4. Using time efficiently
5. Discussing the costs of care with patients
6. Meeting patient rather than provider needs
7. Evaluating cost-effectiveness of new technologies
8. Predicting and using nursing resources efficiently
9. Using research to evaluate standard nursing practices

▌ BUDGETS

The basic financial document in most healthcare organizations is the budget, a detailed financial plan for carrying out the activities an organization wants to accomplish for a certain period of time. An organizational budget is a formal plan that is stated in dollar terms and includes proposed income and expenditures. The budgeting process is an ongoing activity in which plans are made and revenues and expenses are managed in order to meet or exceed the goals of the plan. The management functions of planning and control are tied together through the budgeting process.

A budget requires managers to plan ahead and to establish explicit program goals and expectations. Changes in medical practices, reimbursement methods, competition, technology, demographics, and regulatory factors must be forecast in order to anticipate their effects on the organization. Planning encourages evaluation of different options and assists in more cost-effective use of resources.

Exercise 14-12

An average of 36 intermittent catheterizations are performed daily by a community nursing organization. A prepackaged catheterization kit is used that costs the organization $17. The four items in the kit when packaged individually cost the organization a total of $5. What factors should be considered in evaluating the cost-effectiveness of the two sources of supplies?

TYPES OF BUDGETS

Several types of interrelated budgets are used by well-managed organizations. Major budgets that will be discussed in this chapter include the operating budget, the capital budget, and the cash budget. The way these budgets complement and support one another is depicted in Figure 14-2. Many organizations also use program, product line, or special purpose budgets. Long-range budgets are used to help managers plan for the future. Often these are referred to as strategic plans (Finkler & Kovner, 1993).

Operating Budget

The **operating budget** is the financial plan for the day-to-day activities of the organization. The expected revenues and expenses generated from daily operations given a specified volume of patients is stated. Preparing and monitoring the operating budget, particularly the expense portion, is often the most time-consuming financial function of nurse managers.

The expense part of the operating budget consists of a personnel budget and a supply and expense budget for each cost center. A **cost center** is an organizational unit for which costs can be identified and managed. The personnel budget is the largest part of the operating budget for most nursing units.

Before the personnel budget can be established, the volume of work predicted for the budget period must be calculated. A **unit of service** measure appropriate to the work of the unit is used. Units of service may be patient days, clinic or home visits, hours of service, admissions, deliveries, treatments, and so on. Other factors needed to calculate the work load are the patient census and patient acuity mix. The formula for calculating the work load or the required patient care hours for inpatient units is: *Work Load Volume = Hours of Care Per Patient Day × Number of Patient Days* (see Table 14-2).

In some organizations, the work load is established by the financial office and given to the nurse manager. In others nurse managers forecast the volume. In both situations, nurse managers should inform administration about any factors that they know might affect the accuracy of the forecast.

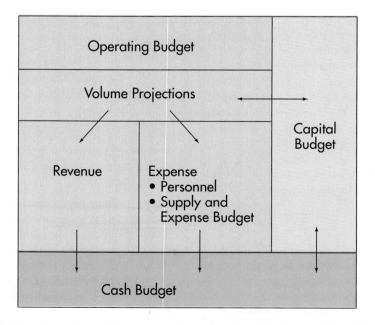

Figure 14-2   Interrelationships of the operating, capital, and cash budgets. (Adapted from Ward [1988].)

The next step in preparing the personnel budget is to determine how many staff members will be needed to provide the care. (This topic is discussed in more detail in Chapter 23.) Because some people work full-time and others work part-time, **full-time equivalents** (FTEs) are used in this step rather than positions. Generally, one FTE can be equated to working 40 hours per week, 52 weeks per year, for a total of 2080 hours of work paid per year. One-half of an FTE (0.5 FTE) equates to 20 hours per week. The number of hours per FTE may vary, so it is important to check.

The 2080 hours paid to an FTE in a year consist of both **productive** and **nonproductive hours.** Productive hours are paid time that is worked. Nonproductive hours are paid time that is not worked, such as vacation, holiday, and sick time. Before the number of FTEs needed for the work load can be calculated, the number of productive hours per FTE is determined. This is done by adding up the total number of nonproductive hours per FTE and subtracting from total paid hours. Or payroll reports can be reviewed to determine the percentage of paid hours that is productive for each FTE (Box 14-5). Finally, the total number of FTEs needed to provide the care is calculated by dividing the total patient care hours required by the number of productive hours per FTE (see Box 14-5).

Table 14-2	**WORK LOAD CALCULATION (TOTAL REQUIRED PATIENT CARE HOURS)**				
Patient Acuity Level*	Hours of Care Per Patient Day (hPPD)†	×	Patient Days‡	=	Workload§
1	3.0		900		2,700
2	5.2		3,100		16,120
3	8.8		4,000		35,200
4	13.0		1,600		20,800
5	19.0		400		7,600
TOTAL			10,000		82,420

*1 low; 5, high.
†HPPD = number of hours of care on average for a given acuity level.
‡1 patient per 1 day = 1 patient day.
§Total number of hours of care needed based on acuity levels and numbers of patient days.

Box 14-5
Productive Hours Calculation

Method 1: Add all nonproductive hours/FTE and subtract from paid hours/FTE

Example:	Vacation	15 days
	Holiday	7 days
	Average sick time	4 days
	Total	26 days

26 × 8 hours = 208 nonproductive hours/FTE
2080 − 208 = 1872 productive hours/FTE

Method 2: Multiply paid hours/FTE by percentage of productive hours/FTE
   Example: productive hours = 90%/FTE
            (1872 productive hours of total 2080 = 90%)
            2080 × 0.90 = 1872 productive hours/FTE

Total FTE Calculation

Required Patient Care Hours	÷	Productive Hours Per FTE	=	Total FTEs Needed
82,420	÷	1872	=	44 FTEs

The total number of FTEs calculated by this method represents the number needed to provide care each day of the year. It does not reflect the number of positions or the number of people working each day. In fact, the number of positions may be significantly higher, particularly if many part-time nurses are employed. And on any given day, some nurses will be off, on vacation, or ill. Also, some positions that do not provide direct patient care, such as nurse managers or unit secretaries, may not be replaced during nonproductive time. Only one FTE is budgeted for any position that is not covered with other staff when the employee is off.

Exercise 14-13

Change the number of patients at each acuity level listed in the box entitled "Work Load Calculation," but keep the total *number of patients the same.* Recalculate the required total work load. Discuss how changes in patient acuity affect nursing resource requirements.

The next step is to prepare a daily staffing plan and to establish positions (see Chapter 23). Once the positions are established, the labor costs that make up the personnel budget can be calculated. Factors that must be addressed include straight-time hours, overtime hours, differentials and premium pay, raises, and benefits (Finkler & Kovner, 1993). Differentials and premiums are extra pay for working specific times such as evening or night shifts and holidays. Benefits usually include health and life insurance, Social Security payments, and retirement plans. Benefits often cost an additional 20% to 25% of a full-time employee's salary.

Exercise 14-14

If the percentage of productive hours per FTE is 80%, how many worked or productive hours are there per FTE? If total patient care hours are 82,420, how many FTEs will be needed?

The supply and expense budget is often called the other-than-personnel services expense budget (OTPS). It includes a wide variety of items that are used in daily unit activities such as medical and office supplies, minor equipment, books and journals, orientation and training, and travel. Although different ways are used to calculate the supply and expense budget, the prior year often is used as a baseline. This baseline is adjusted for projected patient volume and specific circumstances known to affect expenses, such as predictable personnel turnover, which increases orientation and training expenses. And finally, a percentage factor is added to adjust for inflation.

The final component of the operating budget is the revenue budget. The revenue budget projects the income the organization will receive for providing patient care. Historically nurses have not been directly involved with developing the revenue budget, although this is beginning to change. In hospitals the revenue budget is established by the financial office and given to nurse managers. The anticipated revenues are calculated according to the price per patient day. Data about the volume and types of patients and reimbursement sources, that is, the **case mix** and the **payer mix**, are necessary to project revenues in any healthcare organization. Even when nurse managers do not participate in developing the revenue budget, learning about the organization's revenue base is essential.

Capital Expenditure Budget

The **capital expenditure budget** reflects expenses related to the purchase of major capital items such as equipment and physical plant. A capital expenditure must have a useful life of more than 1 year and must exceed a cost level specified by the organization. The minimum cost requirement for capital items in healthcare organizations is usually from $300 to $1000. Anything below that is considered routine operating costs.

Capital items are kept separate from the operating budget because their high cost would make the costs of providing patient care appear too high during the year of purchase. Each year, over the useful life of the equipment, a portion of its cost is allocated to the operating budget as an expense. Therefore capital expenditure costs do get subtracted from revenues and in turn affect profits.

Organizations usually set aside a fixed amount of money for capital expenditures each year. The competition is stiff, so complete, well-documented justifications are needed. Justifications should include amount of use; duplication of services; safety replacement; need for space, personnel, or renovation; impact on operational revenues and expenses; and impact on the strategic plan.

Cash Budget

The **cash budget** is the operating plan for monthly cash receipts and disbursements. Organizational survival depends on an organization paying bills on time. Yet organizations can be making a profit and still run out of cash. In fact, a profitable trend, such as a rapidly growing census, can induce a cash shortage because of increased expenses in the short run. Major capital expenditures can also cause a temporary cash crisis. Because cash is "the lifeblood of any organization" (Finkler & Kovner, 1993, p. 298), the cash budget is as important as the operating and capital budget.

The financial officer prepares the cash budget in large organizations. Understanding the cash budget and how it is developed helps nurse managers discern when constraints on spending are necessary even though the expenditures are budgeted.

THE BUDGETING PROCESS

The steps in the **budgeting process** are similar in most healthcare organizations, although the budgeting period, budget timetable, and level of manager and employee participation vary. Budgeting is done on an annual basis and in relation to the organization's fiscal year. A fiscal year exists for financial purposes and can begin at any point on the calendar. In the title of some financial reports, something like "FYE June 30, 1993," appears and means that this report is for the fiscal year ending on the date stated.

Major steps in the budgeting process include gathering information and planning, developing unit budgets, developing the cash budget, negotiating and revising, and using feedback to control budget results and to improve future plans (Finkler & Kovner, 1993). A timetable with specific dates for implementing the budgeting process is developed by each organization. The timetable may be anywhere from 3 to 9 months. The widespread use of computers for budgeting is reducing the time spread for budgeting in many organizations. Box 14-6 outlines the budgeting process.

The information gathering and planning phase provides nurse managers with data essential for developing their individual budgets. This step begins with an environmental assessment that helps the organization understand its position in relation to the entire community. The assessment includes the changing healthcare needs of the population, significant economic factors like inflation and unemployment, differences in reimbursement patterns, patient satisfaction, and so on.

Next, the organization's long-term goals and objectives are reassessed in light of the organization's mission and the environmental analysis. This helps all managers situate the budgeting process for their individual units in relation to the whole organization. At this point, programs are prioritized so that resources can be allocated to programs that best help the organization achieve its long-term goals.

Specific, measurable objectives are then established that the budgets must meet. The financial ob-

---

> **Box 14-6**
> ## Outline of Budgeting Process
>
> 1. Gathering information and planning
>   - environmental assessment
>   - mission, goals, and objectives
>   - program priorities
>   - financial objectives
>   - assumptions (employee raises, inflation, volume projections)
> 2. Developing unit and departmental budgets
>   - operating budgets
>   - capital budgets
> 3. Developing cash budgets
> 4. Negotiating and revising
> 5. Evaluating
>   - analysis of variance
>   - critical performance reports
>
> Adapted from Finkler & Kovner (1993).

---

jectives might be something like limiting expenditure increases to 3% or making 4% reductions in personnel costs. Nurse managers also set operational objectives for their units that are in concert with the rest of the organization. This is where units or departments interpret what effect the changes in operational activities will have on them. For instance, what will be the impact of using case managers and care maps for selected patients? Establishing the unit level objectives is also a good place for involving staff nurses in setting the future direction of the unit.

Along with the specific organization and unit level operating objectives, managers need the organization-wide assumptions that underpin the budgeting process. Explicit assumptions regarding salary increases, inflation factors, and volume projections for the next fiscal year are essential. With this information in hand, nurse managers can develop the operating and capital budgets for their units. These are usually developed in tandem because each affects the other. For instance, the purchase of a new monitoring system will have implications for the supplies used, staffing, and staff training.

The cash budget is developed after unit and department operating and capital budgets. Then the negotiation and revision process begins in earnest. This is a complex process because changes in one budget usually require changes in others. Learning to defend and negotiate budgets is an important skill for nurse managers. Nurse managers who successfully negotiate budgets know how costs are allocated and are comfortable speaking to what resources are contained in each budget category. They also can clearly and specifically depict what the impact of not having that resource will be on patient, nurse, or organizational outcomes.

Exercise 14-15

If you can interview a nurse manager, ask to review the budgeting process. Ask specifically about the budget timetable, operating objectives, and organizational assumptions. What was the level of involvement for nurse managers and nurses in each step of budget preparation? Is there a budget manual?

The final and ongoing phase of the budgeting process relates to the control function of management. Feedback is obtained regularly so that organizational activities can be adjusted to maintain efficient operations. **Variance analysis** is the major control process used. A **variance** is the difference between the projected budget and the actual performance for a particular account. For expenses, a favorable or positive variance means that the budgeted amount was greater than the actual amount spent. An unfavorable or negative variance means that the budgeted amount was less than the actual amount spent. Positive and negative variances cannot be interpreted as good or bad without further investigation. For example, if fewer supplies were used than were budgeted, this would show up as a positive variance and the unit would save money. This would be good news if it means that supplies were used more efficiently and patient outcomes remained the same or improved. A problem might be suggested, though, if using fewer or cheaper supplies led to poorer patient outcomes. Or it might mean that exactly the right amount of supplies were used but the patient census was less than budgeted.

Exercise 14-16

Review Box 14-7 and identify significant budget variances for the current month. Are they favorable or unfavorable? What additional information would help you explain the variances? What are some possible causes for each variance? Are the causes you identified controllable by the nurse manager? Why or why not? Is a favorable variance on expenses always desirable? Why or why not?

MANAGING THE UNIT LEVEL BUDGET

How is a unit-based budget managed? At a minimum, nurse managers are responsible for meeting the fiscal goals related to the personnel and the supply and expense part of the operations budget. Typically, monthly reports of operations (see Box 14-7) are sent

to nurse managers who then investigate and explain the underlying cause of variances greater than 5%. Many factors can cause budget variances, including patient census, patient acuity, vacation and benefit time, illness, orientation, staff meetings, workshops, employee mix, salaries, and staffing levels. To accurately interpret budget variances, nurse managers need reliable data about patient census, acuity, and length of stay; payroll reports; and unit productivity reports.

Nurse managers can control some of the factors that cause variances and not others. After the causes are determined and if they are controllable by the nurse manager, steps are taken to prevent the variance from occurring in the future. But even uncontrollable variances that increase expenses might require actions of nurse managers. For example, if supply costs rise drastically because a new technology is being used, the nurse manager might have to look for other areas where the budget can be cut. Information learned from analyzing variances also is used in future budget preparations and management activities.

Additionally, nurse managers monitor the **productivity** of their unit. Productivity is the ratio of outputs to inputs; that is, productivity = output/input (Finkler & Kovner, 1993). In nursing, outputs are nursing services and are measured by hours of care, number of home visits, etc. The inputs are the resources used to provide the services such as personnel hours and supplies. Productivity can be increased only by decreasing the inputs or increasing the outputs. Hospitals often use HPPD as one measure of productivity. For example, if the standard of care in a critical care unit is 12 HPPD, then 360 hours of care are required for 30 patients for 1 day. When 320 hours of care are provided, the productivity rating is 113% (360/320 = 1.13), meaning productivity was increased. In home health agencies, productivity is measured by the number of visits per day per RN. If the standard is 5 visits per day, but the weekly average was 4.8 visits, then productivity was decreased. Variances in productivity are not inherently favorable or unfavorable and thus also require investigation and explanation before judgments can be made about them.

Staff nurses play an important role in meeting budget expectations even though they do not have a direct accountability for the budget. Many nurse managers find that routinely sharing the budget and budget monitoring activities with the staff has enhanced the staff's ability to appreciate the relationship between cost and quality and to develop the cost-conscious nursing practices discussed previously.

Box 14-7

Statement of Operations
Neighborhood Nursing Center Profit and Loss Statement
March 31, 1998

Budget	Current Month Actual	Variance	REVENUES	Budget	Year-to-Date Actual	Variance
			Patient Revenues			
11,500	12,050	550	Routine	34,500	35,750	1,250
1,500	1,550	(50)	Contractual allowances	4,500	4,750	(250)
10,000	10,500	500	Net Patient Revenues	30,000	31,000	1,000
			Non-Patient Revenues			
5,000	5,000	0	Grant income (#138-FG)	15,000	15,000	0
500	500	0	Rent income	1,500	1,500	0
5,500	5,500	0	Net Non-Patient Revenues	16,500	16,500	0
15,500	16,000	500	Net Revenues	46,500	47,500	1,000
			EXPENSES			
			Personnel services			
7,750	8,500	(750)	Managerial/professional	23,250	24,400	(1,150)
2,000	1,800	200	Clerical/technical	6,000	5,800	200
9,750	10,300	(550)	Net salaries & wages	29,250	30,200	(950)
1,200	1,400	(200)	Benefits	3,600	4,000	(400)
10,950	11,700	(750)	Net Personnel Services	32,850	34,200	(1,350)
			Other than personnel services (OTPS)			
2,500	2,500	0	Operating expenses	7,500	7,500	0
1,000	1,100	(100)	Supplies & materials	3,000	3,050	(50)
300	450	(150)	Travel expenses	900	450	450
3,800	4,050	(250)	Net OTPS	11,400	11,000	400
14,750	15,750	(1,000)	Net Expenses	44,250	45,200	50
			REVENUES OVER/UNDER			
750	250	(500)	**EXPENSES**	2,250	2,300	50

A Manager's Solution

[?] I began by investigating the assumption that the IMC ambulatory clinic was losing money. Because expenses were reported as a whole for the IMC, they had to be broken down by section and by location where services were provided. A spreadsheet was used, and expenses were determined either by the hours of utilization or by the percentage of visit volume for that section. Once the expenses were known, the revenue needed to break even was determined for each section.

Next revenues were predicted. This was challenging because of the complexity of the payer mix. The Medicare Resource-Based Relative Value Scale (RBRVS) was used to calculate all predicted payments. In this system, each physician service is assigned a "relative value" based on the time, skill, and intensity it takes to provide the service. Then relative values are adjusted for geographic variations and multiplied by a national conversion factor to determine the dollar amount of payment. This system was selected because it was the minimum payment expected for all categories of payers, including managed care contracts. Thus using this system provided a conservative estimate of revenues. Once the payment for a specific service was calculated, it was multiplied by the number of times that service was provided in the ambulatory setting. The result was the potential revenue for that service in that section. The potential revenues for each service were added to provide a total predicted revenue for the section.

Predicted revenue for each section was compared to the revenue required to break even. In every instance, the predicted revenue exceeded the break-even revenue. As a result of this work, the administrators changed their view of the IMC ambulatory service as a "loss leader" and staff reductions were not required. In addition, a performance strategy for physicians based on Relative Value Units was developed and some fees were increased because they were found to be lower than allowed by the RBRVS system.

[?] *Would this be a suitable approach for you? Why?*

▮ CHAPTER CHECKLIST

Financial thinking skills are the cornerstone of cost-conscious nursing practice and are essential for all nurses. Also, nurses must determine whether or not the services they provide add value for patients. Services that add value are of high quality, positively affect health outcomes, and minimize costs.

Understanding what constitutes profit and why organizations must make a profit to survive is basic to financial thinking. Knowing what is included in operating, capital, and cash budgets; how they interrelate; and how they are developed, monitored, and controlled is also important. And finally, considering the ethical implications of all financial decisions is imperative for cost-conscious nursing practice.

■ U.S. health indicators suggest that as a nation we are not getting a high value return on our healthcare dollar.
  • Infant mortality and births to teenager rates are two critical examples.
■ Total healthcare costs are a function of price and utilization of services.
  • Most use of service is physician driven rather than consumer driven.
  • High-tech specialties also drive up costs.
■ The government and insurance companies are the major payers for healthcare services. Individuals are the third major payer.
  • Payments may be based on cost reimbursement, flat rates, or capitated payments.
■ Healthcare is moving toward managed care, organized delivery systems, and competition based on cost and quality outcomes.
■ All private healthcare organizations must make a profit in order to survive.
■ Nurse and nurse managers directly impact an organization's ability to make a profit.
■ Cost-conscious nursing practices include
  • understanding what is required to remain financially sound
  • knowing costs and reimbursement practices
  • capturing all possible charges in a timely fashion
  • using time efficiently
  • discussing the costs of care with patients
  • meeting patient rather than provider needs
  • evaluating cost-effectiveness of new technologies
  • predicting and using nursing resources efficiently
  • using research to evaluate standard nursing practices.

- Nurse managers have the most impact on costs in relation to managing personnel and supplies.
- Variance analysis is the major control process in relation to budgeting.

TIPS ON MANAGING COSTS AND BUDGETS

- Know the cost and charges (if applicable) of the top 20 most frequently used supplies on your unit
- Evaluate what each of your patients would find most helpful during the time you will be caring for them
- Decide which of your actions create costs for the patient or the organization
- Be aware of how changes in patient acuity and patient census affect staffing requirements and the unit budget
- Know how charges are generated and how the documentation systems relate to billing

TERMS TO KNOW

budget	organized delivery system (ODS)
budgeting process	payer mix
capital expenditure budget	payers
capitation	price
case mix	productive hours
cash budget	productivity
charges	profit
contractual allowance	prospective reimbursement
cost	providers
cost-based reimbursement	revenue
cost center	unit of service
fixed costs	utilization
full-time equivalent (FTE)	variable costs
managed care	variance
nonproductive hours	variance analysis
operating budget	

REFERENCES

Cleland, V. (1990). *The Economics of Nursing.* Norwalk, CT: Appleton & Lange.

Consumers Union (1992, July). Wasted health care dollars: Part I. *Consumer Reports,* pp. 435-448.

Finkler, S., & Kovner, C. (1993). *Financial Management for Nurse Managers and Executives.* Philadelphia: Saunders.

Grace, H. (1994). Debate: Can health care costs be contained? In McCloskey, J., & Grace, H., eds. *Current Issues in Nursing,* 4th ed. St. Louis: Mosby.

Marrelli, T. (1997). *The Nurse Manager's Survival Guide,* 2nd ed. St. Louis: Mosby.

Petryshen, P., Stevens, B., Hawkins, J., & Stewart, M. (1997). Comparing nursing costs for pre-term infants receiving conventional vs. developmental care. *Nursing Economics,* 15(3), 138-145, 150.

U.S. Department of Health and Human Services (1996). *Health United States 1995.* Hyattsville, MD: Author. DHHS Pub. No. (PHS) 96-1232.

SUGGESTED READINGS

Bailey, D. (1996, January 31) Budgeting skills. *Nursing Standard,* 10(19), 45-48.

Baker, M. (1992). Cost-effective management of the hospital-based hospice program. *Journal of Nursing Administration,* 22(1), 40-45.

Caroselli, C. (1996). Economic awareness of nurses: Relationship to budgetary control. *Nursing Economics,* 14(5), 292-298.

Cavouras, C., & McKinley, J. (1997). Variable budgeting for staffing: Analysis and evaluation. *Nursing Management,* 28(5), pp. 34, 36, 38.

Corley, M., & Satterwhite, B. (1993). Forecasting ambulatory clinic workload to facilitate budgeting. *Nursing Economics,* 11(2), 77-81, 114.

Folland, S., Goodman, A., & Stano, M. (1997). *The Economics of Health and Health Care,* 2nd ed. Upper Saddle River, NJ: Prentice-Hall.

Hall, M., & Anderson, F. (1997). Maintaining quality care while decreasing hospice costs. *Nursing Economics,* 15(3), 157-159, 163.

Moss, M., & Shelver, S. (1993). Practical budgeting for the operating room administrator. *Nursing Economics,* 11(1), 7-13.

Neuman, B., Suver, J., & Zelman, W. (1988). *Financial Management: Concepts and Applications for Health Care Providers,* 2nd ed. Owings Mills, MD: National Health Publishing.

Pelfry, S. (1991). Financial techniques for evaluating equipment acquisitions. *Journal of Nursing Administration,* 21(3), 15-20.

White, S., Bartug, B., & Bride, W. (1995). Supporting nursing innovations in a cost-conscious environment. *Critical Care Nursing Clinics of North America,* 7(2), 399-406.

Wyld, D. (1996). The capitation revolution in health care: Implications for the field of nursing. *Nursing Administration Quarterly* 20(2), 1-12.

Leading and Managing People

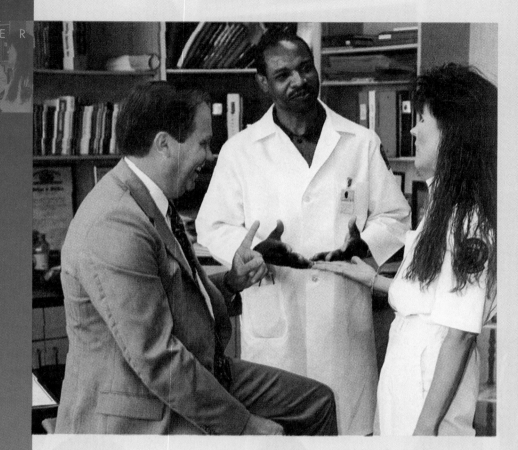

Communication and Partnership

Joe Brannan Hurst
PhD, EdD

This chapter describes ways to lead and manage more effectively by communicating and partnering with others, whether they are colleagues, patients, patients' family members, or suppliers. The principles and ways of communicating and partnering are useful in a wide range of settings, including patient care, leading a team, managing staff and resources, and sharing needed information. Paradoxically, communication can be both simple and complex, but either way, it is vital to leading, managing, teaming, and serving.

Objectives

- Examine a new paradigm of communication.
- Examine and practice effective communication processes.
- Identify key roles in and stages of effective teams.
- Determine personal patterns of communication.
- Define collaboration as effective partnering.

Questions to Consider

- What is communication and how can it be improved?
- How can supportiveness be increased?
- How can people observe, listen, speak, and act consistently with their intended results?
- How well do you communicate and partner with others?
- What ethical and professional principles guide nurse managers' communication?

Manager's Challenge
From a Clinical Manager at a Midwestern Health Center

My challenge involved two separate teams and their supervisors. We called these teams the "front office" and the "back office." The front handled patient sign-in procedures and scheduling, primarily. The back dealt with medical records and providing medical service. Whenever a patient became loud and demanding, the office at which it occurred tended to put the responsibility for not being able to meet the patient's request with the other office. For example, "We can't schedule you now as a walk-in because the back office can't do it," or "The front office was wrong to send you back here." Each team had regular meetings, led by their respective supervisors, to handle their concerns. Nothing was ever said to me or the other supervisor

about the growing defensiveness between the teams, the talking behind others' backs, and the lack of partnership. Later we found out that there was an underlying fear of "rocking of the boat" and making the supervisors, other team members, physicians, and administrators angry. In addition, the interrelationships between the two teams had been ignored for a very long time, even to the point that the large group's common goals and cohesiveness were overshadowed by the growing competitiveness and avoidance of confronting aggressive clients.

What do you think you would do if you were this manager?

INTRODUCTION

Communication is both simple and complex. Most simply, communication is the mutual creation of shared meaning between people. It is *not* merely a complex model involving senders, receivers, encoding, decoding, channels, and feedback. It is *not* merely information sharing either. It does, however, involve "simultaneous" speaking (verbally and nonverbally), listening, and acting between two or more people. Effective communication requires commitment, effort, focus, cooperation, and skill, which can be very complex at times, especially with difficult issues and people with diverse perspectives. Many communication situations in clinical settings require basic "communication for results." Being able to communicate effectively about client care, staff performance and scheduling, and team effectiveness is an important aspect of being a

nurse leaders/managers and will often involve paradoxically being very clear and direct and being somewhat open-ended and flexible (Johnson, 1992) and focusing on individuals and on the team (Johnson, 1992; Hurst, 1996).

COMMUNICATION AND PARTNERING DISTINCTIONS

This chapter takes an entirely new approach to managing, leading, and partnering communication. The new paradigm underlying this approach is that *human life occurs in conversation*, especially in the automatic interpretations of their environments that people constantly make. Traditionally, words like "leadership," "communication," "nurse," "patient," and "care" are considered mirrors to a real, objective world and, when clearly defined, aid understanding and application of knowledge. In this paradigm, such terms as "leadership," "communication," "nurse," "patient," and "care" are linguistic distinctions invented by human beings in conversation to specify and open up real-life arenas for coordinating actions to produce desired results.

Thus, if life occurs in conversation, it is being effective in conversation that can have the biggest impact on how people interpret their worlds and act accordingly. People who effectively lead, manage, and partner converse and listen differently than those who do not. They can also observe and listen to others' conversations, assess the conversations' effectiveness, and intervene (enter the conversations) with appropriate timing, focus, intention, professionalism, and skill.

Feedback is a common term referring to "sending some response or message back to someone." In the perspective that communication is a conversation (or series of conversations) for creating shared meaning, then speaking and listening naturally occur over and over again (or back and forth if you like) until people are clear that they have mutual meaning. Unfortunately, too often people assume that they know what everyone else knows until they all find out they really miscommunicated (or had different meanings). Most importantly, feedback could be viewed as information about how close any conversation's consequences come to the desired/intended results it set out to produce. It is this "results-focused" perspective that is critical to what follows in this chapter.

Partnership is built upon *common* goals, concerns, intentions, aspirations, and/or problems. If communication is shared meaning and coordination of action, then the people involved in the situation must cooperate or, as seen in the next chapter, collaborate in order to communicate. The major conversations resulting in partnering are (1) identify common concerns, goals, etc.; (2) create possibilities together to handle those commonalities in number (1); (3) take coordinated action to make the possibilities occur; (4) develop trust and mutual respect; and (5) share follow-along support for the actions needed to reach their goals.

Exercise 15-1

Before you read any further, complete the questionnaire in Box 15-1. Reflect on just how often you tend to do each of the behaviors listed in the survey and mark the appropriate number that represents your typical patterns of communication. What do you notice about your responses before you read about effective communication? Then look at these patterns after you've read the chapter and see how you could improve.

Box 15-1
Self-Examination Activity

Place a check mark in the appropriate column at the right-hand side indicating how often you see each statement applying to your behavior.

	ALMOST ALWAYS				
		QUITE OFTEN			
			OCCASIONALLY		
				ALMOST NEVER	
	NEVER 1	2	3	4	5
1. Ask for others' support					
2. Complain without taking or requesting action					
3. Promise action/results by a certain deadline					
4. Avoid committing to taking action					
5. Say "I hope or wish" when discussing results					
6. Acknowledge others for keeping agreements					
7. Provide excuses for lack of action/results					
8. Create exciting new possibilities					
9. Compliment others for action/results					
10. Do not hold others to their word					
11. Do as promised					
12. Make vague requests					
13. Dramatize own and/or others' problems					
14. Gossip about others					
15. Provide grounding for assertions					
16. Renegotiate "uncompleted" agreements					
17. Do not listen to others' gossip					
18. Create and discuss a future vision					
19. Declare possibilities for breakthroughs					
20. Refer to most situations as "problems"					

DISTINGUISHING FIVE BASIC TYPES OF CONVERSATIONS

Now let's look at five basic types of conversations in terms of their importance and form. The nurse leaders/managers who can initiate, effectively continue, assess the quality of, and influence the following types of conversations can make the needed difference in various settings and situations. These "conversations for results" include:

1. Conversations for being related to people and situations
2. Conversations for creating possibilities
3. Conversations for developing a structure (making possibilities into reality)
4. Conversations for action
5. Conversations for resolving breakdowns and creating breakthroughs (using 1 through 4 effectively to produce unprecedented results)

Conversations for Relatedness

Looking underneath the surface of relationships, there is a certain logic that binds people together in their interactions. This means that the two (or more) individuals communicating and having relationships together create for themselves a set of expectations of what they mean to each other at any moment in the exchange. Thus, whenever we first come together with others, there is some way, whether planned or not, in which both people become clear (or think they are) about the purpose that each one has come to fulfill and the "rules" by which they will relate (Johnson, 1996; McConnell, 1996). A closer look at this "connection" or set of expectations reveals that it consists of three basic issues:

1. Who do you "say" you will be in the relationship, situation, conversation, and/or group?
2. What do you think other people are like (i.e., your assumptions of their intentions, commitment, skills, knowledge, interests, etc.) in a conversation, relationship, and/or group?
3. How do the people involved view the situation, important goals, valued priorities and norms, etc.?

Exercise 15-2

Select a partner and practice communication that ensures all three elements are included.

In a direct conversation with a stranger, it might sound like this:

"Hello, I'm going to be your (1) *new head nurse, and I came down to* (1) *introduce myself and be friendly,* (2) *(assumes you want to be*

friendly, too), (3) *get clear what the procedures for rotation are, and* (3) *see how some of my ideas sound to you."*

Notice how this simple introduction addresses the three issues of the underlying conversation for **relatedness.** Without being overly complicated or drawn out, it sets the stage for a discussion that will either demonstrate that both sides of the relatedness are in fact as stated, or will show that one or the other of the speakers does not see the current conversation in this way. If not, then the relationship will be off to a rocky start and will be in need of a different relatedness (without clarifying the difference there will be rocky times later!).

For example, during their master's program, two young nurses started their relationship by saying "Let's be friends and not be committed" [(1) & (2) & (3); both will be uncommitted friends, will assume the other is, and will maintain this priority]. This was fine until one fell in love and wanted to alter the "rules." The three aspects of such conversations may take many different interactions over the period of time the relationship develops and lasts and may change greatly. In this case there were many ups and downs until a recent marriage clarified the total change in how they decided to relate. In a group conversation, it might sound like this:

"(1) You have nominated me chairperson of this committee. I want you to know how I see this job. (2) I assume we'll continue to meet regularly. (3) First, the group was established to plan the awards banquet. I think we ought to create the most exciting and special banquet ever. Second, I run tight meetings. I mean everyone gets to share and no dominating the discussion or rehashing of issues. Let's stay focused and get the job done in the least amount of time. Most importantly, I expect us all to participate and share the load. What do you all think?"

"(2) Well, you sound pretty gung ho to me. (1) I'm here because my chairperson said to come, but I'm far too busy to give this group much time or energy outside of attending the meetings whenever I can. (3) The banquet doesn't mean much to me or my department anyway."

There would have to be much more discussion and decisions regarding how these team members will actually relate to each other and the priorities for which the group was formed.

Conversations for being related to patients need to demonstrate to them that they are respected, their care is a valued service, and they have rights. These elements may need to be communicated loudly and clearly to angry clients, terrified family members, busy nurses and physicians, and disgruntled staff. These conversations must involve courtesy, unoffensive language, consideration, sensitivity, and concern. Although their stay may be short, relationships with

Research Perspective

Lee, J., & Jablin, F. (1995). Maintenance communication in superior-subordinate work relationships. Human Communication Research, 22(2), 220-257.

In this two-study research there was an examination of (1) strategic situations in which superiors and subordinates felt the need to maintain their relationships, (2) communication tactics and strategies that supervisors and subordinates consciously enacted to maintain them, and (3) how superiors and subordinates in different types of relationship exchanges employed maintenance behaviors and activities. This research focused on the conscious selection of relationship conversations.

The research questions sought to delineate in what strategic situations supervisors (sups) and subordinates (subs) consciously see the need to maintain their relationships, what types of maintenance activities are used by both, and how maintenance activities vary by both depending on how they view the relationship's quality. The sample included over 244 people, some students, and some employees of organizations. Focus groups, individual interviews, and questionnaires were used.

Sups and subs tended to classify their need for maintenance as "deteriorating" (50%), "escalating" (25%), and "routine" (25%). Additionally, some (1) routine situations could become deteriorating ones, including sups' unpredictable behavior and sups asking subs to do work-producing favors and some (2) escalating situations could wind up being deteriorating ones (e.g., close relationship between a sup and sub that is not perceived well by other subs). The perceived quality of the relationship had very interesting effects on maintenance behavior. Sups' perceptions had no effect; subs with higher quality perceptions ("in-group") tended to use less avoidance and indirect conversational refocus behaviors; and "out-group" (negative perceptions of quality) engaged in more direct/open authoritative or rule-bound and deceptive/distorting communications.

Implications for Practice

Nurse leaders/managers should be aware of these maintenance situations that, if not addressed effectively in the routine or escalating stages, will become deteriorating ones. In addition, they need to be aware of just how different in-group and out-group employees may feel, communicate, and act. Too often the only perceived opportunity for an out-group employee to communicate with a supervisor may have to do with deviations from their role expectations and the norms of their relationships. It was the supervisors in this study who did not vary their maintenance strategies according to a perceived quality of the relationship, which may reflect an overemphasis of task and directive focus.

---

patients must be as trusting, understanding, honest, and thoughtful as possible. Similarly, nurse managers should model these same conversations for relatedness with patients and staff, especially when it comes to confidentiality (Dowd & Dowd, 1996). Good leaders treat their peers and staff as well as they treat their most valued customers.

Being related to situations, too

Conversations for being related can define any situation by describing the details and "declaring" it a "problem," "crisis," "celebration," "breakdown," "breakthrough," or whatever. But people must be effectively related to what *is* happening, what needs to happen, and what will block and support future efforts. This could sound like:

"We are in big trouble! We are behind schedule and way off budget."

This interpretation judgmentally describes the situation as a problem.

This also could be said as follows:

"We have a situation to act on as soon as possible. We are 5 days behind schedule and $2,000 over budget."

Notice how these two different ways of describing this situation articulate a way of relating to the situation and to the people involved—one negatively and one in a more matter-of-fact manner. It is often the nurse leaders/managers who can (has to) assist others in being more rationally and accurately (have the "facts," so to speak) related to some very important, even emotion-laden situations.

Norms as conversations for relatedness

A nurse leaders/managers might say:

"I've worked on some very poor teams in the past. I ask that we set some ground rules for how we have meetings and work together so we can avoid wasting time, harsh feelings, miscommunication, and poor planning."

The conversation(s) that would follow in the group would establish ways to be related in the group, probably including norms, guidelines, or codes of conduct similar to those that follow. Below are suggested **norms** that you entertain using in groups and in one-on-one relationships now and in the future:

1. Be early or on time to be centered when actions start and be available to assist with getting started. B*e early/on time!*
2. Describe situations, breakdowns, difficulties, lack of results, negative surprises, etc. in factual, descriptive terms with some suggested time frame for action/completion instead of using words like "problem" or "crisis." S*top having problems!*
3. Work out difficulties among people and support others rather than gossip and listen to others gossip. *Stop gossip!*
4. Accept things that can't be changed and/or aren't important enough to worry about, or make requests of others who can take action, rather than complain. S*top inactive complaining!*
5. Get others to create and act on their own suggestions and possibilities. Encourage others to make choices and promises, act responsibly on their own, and ask for feedback and coaching. S*top giving and asking for advice!*
6. Be the kind of member and leader (everybody has to do both) who promotes high productivity and consideration for others.

Conversations for being related are vital to promoting one-on-one and team relationships. Establishing norms and sticking to them are a major aspect of this. Box 15-2 gives other suggestions for group norms.

Conversations for Possibility

Almost everyone has heard of and engaged in brainstorming. This is a specific technique for creating new ideas, techniques, etc. Technically, **possibilities** are more than this. They are new futures that are beyond the predictable extension of what already exists. When people have effective conversations for possibility, they are open to speculate, dream, freewheel, experiment, and create visions of the future that probably will not occur without a stretch, some risk, and unpre-

---

Box 15-2
Suggestion for Group Norms

- Getting members to agree to a set of rules for their behavior and being held accountable for when they break these rules.
- Speaking supportively without swearing; making others and policies, procedures, institutions, etc. wrong; invalidating others and their feelings or ideas; etc.
- Correcting the accuracy of others' information, etc. in a supportive way.
- Making promises that members intend to keep and communicate immediately to those accountable when a promise will be broken.
- Listening to the speaker without interruption.
- Starting and stopping meetings on time.
- Participating fully without dominating.
- Sharing the work load and leadership.
- Practicing patience and restraint.
- Having decisions made be "team decisions."
- Considering all ideas as belonging to the group.
- Being honest without criticizing people.
- Communicating when one has to be absent and taking the initiative to "catch up" and maintain one's team responsibilities.

---

dictable actions and results occurring. Too often people restrict their conversations for possibility because they think that saying something means it requires commitment to do it right away or deep analysis and evaluation. It will be your job to encourage this type of conversation when necessary.

An important aspect of one-on-one and group communication for accomplishment early in the process is envisioning the endpoints (desired outcomes) in the future that the group's commitment, actions, and resources are driving toward. Possibilities are an essential aspect of group and relationship success because they introduce challenge, stretch, uncertainty, and excitement—*risk*. Without risk there is little development of *motivation*, trust, cooperation, creativity, and *breakthrough*.

A conversation for possibility could start like this:

"We've been stuck in a rut about money and administrative support for our future plans. Let's take about 20 minutes right now to develop some really new ideas of how financial issues could be handled and how our relationship with the administration could be entirely different than ever before."

Or, one might be started like this:

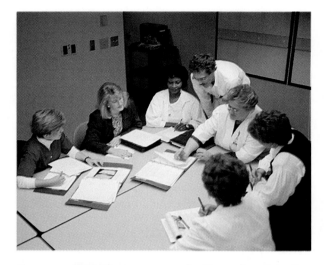

Encouragement of group communication and participation achieves desired outcomes.

"We have been complaining and gossiping for several meetings now. I am clear that we do not like how priorities are being set around here. We also know who is in charge. I request that we set up a meeting to create a whole new vision of what we want and then present that vision to the administration within one month."

Any new team must raise the question, "What are our purposes for being and staying together?" The answers usually involve a number of conversations for possibility.

Conversations for Structure

Once possibilities are determined, groups must create a "structure for fulfillment." A structure for fulfillment is a plan that matches resources, action, and a network of committed people with desired results and deadlines. So often people do not accomplish what they set out to do because they have an inadequate plan, one that fails to commit people and resources to *what it will take* to reach their goals. This plan may need revision because circumstances change, but it must exist clearly and firmly for the people involved in carrying it out.

This structure would include a description of the intended outcomes (results and ways to measure them). For example, some samples are listed here:

Example 1 The amount of funds raised will be 25% higher than any preceding year as shown in the net receipts of the committee tallied every month until the end of the fund raisers on July 15th.

Example 2 The group's productivity as measured by our output (cases completed) per week will increase by at least 50 over the same 6-month period last year.

Another aspect of the structure for fulfillment would be "tools" for measuring the accomplishment of the results and some "chart" or visual that describes the actions to be taken, desired consequences of the actions, deadlines for completion, and people responsible. In this way the group can follow the plan's direction and note progress. For each of these goals, a different way to assess and chart the results would be needed. For example, the first could use a chart of net receipts while the third would chart cases completed. The second might use a diary of observations.

Conversations for Action

Too often groups get off track and their actions and results do not match what they set out to accomplish. Also, groups get so task-oriented or off task-oriented that they do not consider process goals (e.g., becoming a closer team, improving decision-making processes, empowering members, being more efficient). There are six forms of statements that produce action the moment they are communicated. These include promises, requests, declarations, assertions, complaints for results, and compliments for results.

Promises

Promising one's word is pledging to do something. It reflects a high commitment to action and stakes one's word on getting it done. Effective promising includes (1) a concrete statement, (2) the conditions for fulfillment, and (3) the time frame. In the following sequence, Mary's statement is vague and noncommittal:

Mary: "Tom, I'll try to get the car so I can drive you."

She can be much clearer and state her commitment much more completely and accurately, as in the following statement:

Mary: "Tom. I will drive you to work tomorrow at 8:00 AM."

Notice the specific detail and the total commitment to doing it in the second example. Here are some other examples of promises:

1. I promise that I'll clean up my office by Sunday at 5:00 PM.
2. I will have the completed, spell-checked report to you by Friday noon.
3. You will receive a letter and a check from me by the end of the month.
4. I agree to get three volunteers and have their names for you tomorrow night at the meeting.

Promising makes action happen by committing oneself to specific results and communicating the commitment and the intended action concretely to others. In a complete event of promising, a fascinating aspect of communication occurs. There is a trust in the committed word of the promiser(s), an accountability to those listeners committed to the action and results, and the support that those committed listeners provide to the process. Too often, listeners are not listening. They "hope" that promisers are committed, but sense they are not. In these cases, they should not expect the promise to be kept. Committed listeners provide follow-along support and hold the promisers to their word. For example, teammates often nod their heads and agree to do things between meetings, but no one writes anything down! At this moment, someone must say, "These are important things we are saying we will have done in a week. Let's all please write our promises in our planners. I'll jot down the overall set and support the team in getting them done." Those blank stares and "uh huhs" need a similar follow-up when you hear that someone is hollowly agreeing.

Human dignity could be distinguished as the degree to which a person acts consistently with her or his word, values, principles, and aspirations. Important feelings of dignity and effectiveness are attached by the degree to which people keep their word. In addition, strong feelings are attached by those promised to people who break their promises, including distrust. Being *indignant* (angry) with those who do not act consistently with their word or principles may assist them in reclaiming their dignity.

Sometimes promises are not kept because the conditions of satisfaction were not clear originally; that is, Joellyn says she will submit a rough draft of the department's strategic plan by Thursday at noon. However, Jo does not share her department supervisor's idea about what goes in such a report and the criteria that make one excellent. So what she turns in is not what she promised, nor thought she was promising. Effective promises are best forged with the clearest statements of these conditions up front. This is a vital type of communication for nurse leaders/managers.

Requests

Making **requests** is asking others to take action for themselves and/or to become active in doing things you ask. Petitioning or requesting is the process of asking others to *promise* that they will get something done. Effective requests are specific in the action requested and include the necessary conditions to be satisfied and the time frame. In the following example, Mary's request is vague and indirect.

Mary: "Tom, I'm not able to move the big items of furniture in the department by myself. I'm looking for help."

Mary needs to state her request more clearly and directly.

Mary: "Tom, would you promise to move three big items of furniture in my department Friday afternoon before 4:30 PM?" (Or she could say: "Tom, I need some help moving heavy furniture. Could you come over with Jack on Friday afternoon for 1 hour before 4:30 PM to move two filing cabinets, a desk, and a bookshelf?") She also needs to hear a promise in return. Anything less may be a setup for miscommunication and incompletion.

Again notice the clarity and thoroughness of communication about what the speaker is requesting. This need not always be in one clear statement, but throughout a requesting dialogue the petitioner must be concrete about the action(s), condition(s), and time frame(s).

Effectiveness in making requests often involves matching intent with the words and ways one speaks them so that the others are clear about what one wants and, most importantly, what the relationship really is. Specifically, are you asking for a partner or invoking your status as official manager? All too often one wants to order or demand and actually begs or pleads, or vice versa. Many people are too unassertive to make specific direct requests because they are afraid they will be refused or impose on others. Leading might be best defined as the timely making of unreasonable requests of others that then lead to powerful results. Sometimes people order when they do not have a recognized superior status and power to order people around, or when they are unaware of the costs of developing such a relationship. These dominator types will be discussed later.

Possible responses to a request

Whenever people make a request of others, the listeners have many possible reactions that they may make. Most directly, they may promise to fulfill the request. They may also make a *counteroffer* to the request and thereby make a promise that has different conditions of satisfaction and/or time frame than originally asked. For example, Janet might say, "I can't do it all by 5:00 PM but I can do the first half by then and then the rest by 10:00." A third option is that they promise to promise at a later time. Janet could say, "Give me an hour and I'll let you know if I can do it all by 5:00 PM." Another option is to decline the request (an honest promise not to do it that should be honored). Finally, there is the common response that is not clear enough to know what the other will do about the request. People all too often hear such things as the following:

"I'll think about it."
"Maybe!"
"I'll try to be there on time."
"I'll do my best!" (*the best way to sound committed when one is not*)

In each instance, there is no promise. By carefully listening to others, people can train themselves to be very aware of where they stand and in so doing avoid the disappointment that comes from having their expectations left unmet and important actions and results left incomplete.

Declarations

Declarations are statements that create and describe a new set of possibilities. In regular conversation, people often "declare into existence" new opportunities. For example, the following statements illustrate declarations:

1. "I want to be your friend."
2. "You and I are the Workshop Project Team from now on."
3. "This is going to be a real challenge."
4. "The time is now!"

Each of these statements proclaims a new set of possibilities and opens up the range of optional actions and relationships speakers have with other people, their circumstances, and/or the universe.

An interesting aspect of declarations is that they have no "facts" supporting their truth. They are quite literally "made up" by the speaker. They are incredibly powerful in providing the direction that future actions can take for the individual and/or team making them. Nurse leaders/managers must create empowering declarations that they can fulfill.

A new committee might declare that it "stands for" the highest level of patient care. Out of the declaration, they now have the opportunity to choose future actions that transform a promising past into an effective future, as does any new team and its "declared" goals.

Important declarations include, "I forgive you," "We will reach our new target," "I trust you no matter what," "I love you," "I am lovable and capable," and "Patient care is our number one priority." "I am a recovering alcoholic" declares a whole new set of rela-

tionships and possibilities into reality. And, in reality, everything that is said about what is, was, and might be could be viewed as both a declaration and an assertion.

Assertions

Webster's Dictionary defines to assert as: "to set down as fact; assume; postulate." Since people's realities are reflected in their own interpretations of events and people, circumstances, etc., **assertions** or statements about the truth of any matter are most often assumptions, postulations, or points of view. The commitment reflected in asserting anything (describing what is true) is that one will supply further information, clarification, and evidence (grounding) for what one says, if asked to do so, or if needed.

Often, people make assertions that they have no way of backing up. In other words, they say things that "overstate the facts" or have no basis in fact or relevant evidence. Sometimes people make vague or very absolute assertions that serve to limit the times when they will have to supply further information and evidence. A commitment to concrete, open communication is what is most effective for bringing individuals to a deeply meaningful set of relationships. The dialogue below illustrates how people can back up their statements.

Sample Dialogue
Martina: "This is a good department."
Frank: "I'm not sure what you mean by 'good'."
Martina: "I have confidence that I contribute to the group and I know what is expected of me. Right now I'm pleased with my accomplishments."
Frank: "Right now I feel great, too. I'm feeling challenged and very unsure of how well I'll do! I know what I want to accomplish and have finally realized it is all right to do that. I am also looking forward to using what I learn outside of this group next month when I start my new job."
Martina: "I really like the other people in the group and trust them."
Frank: "I do trust and like them, although I'm not sure why! I feel pleased that I've been able to share things that others have found helpful."
Martina: "Me, too!"

Paying careful attention to the dialogue, one finds an asserting of two people's personal meaning of "good thoughts" about their group. Together they have trust, are helping others, and demonstrate cohesiveness in their relationship. Rather than arguing over meaning or just taking it for granted, they share, listen, accept, and agree (when meaning is shared). The short conversation above communicates, unlike the one below:

> Martina: "I feel good in this group."
> Frank: "Me, too! It's great."
> Martina: "Yes. Neat. I know just how you feel."

A simple question may determine a speaker's ability and willingness to supply evidence for any assertion: What grounds do you have for saying that? Similar requests might be, "How do you know?" or "Can you back that up with some evidence?" These simple questions at just the right time are part of a nurse leader's/manager's role. Another important form of asserting is the documentation nurses, other professionals, and nurse leaders/managers do regarding patients' care and progress as well as professional performance.

Active complaining

One nurse leader/manager discovered she had a great supply of time and energy for action when she stopped complaining inactively. She realized that she had spent a large amount of her work and relaxation time and energy stating **complaints** that were not (or could not be!) aimed at taking action and producing results. Now that she complains for action when it is appropriate, she saves time and energy and makes her complaints lead to positive action. Active complaining combines the skills of promising, asserting, and requesting. The form for effective complaining is as follows:

1. The statement of a prior promise that has been broken.
2. The assertion that the promise has been broken.
3. The request that a new promise be made to complete the prior promise.

The following statement is an example of complaining. Here, Erlinda states an inactive complaint. In other words, she gripes or groans about the current circumstances with little commitment to act.

"I am so angry at you changing our plans just like that. You can't work for me this weekend, you say! Why do you do this to me all the time? I hate it when you act this way!"

Most complaints reflect people's unstated requests, lack of commitment, and/or desire for agreement with their discontent. Without a prior agreement, there is virtually no basis for effective complaining (see why promises are so important?).

In the following example Valerie could complain for action and results. She (1) refers to a prior agree-

ment (promise), (2) points to actions and/or results that have not been completed by the specified deadline, and (3) requests compensatory action and/or "damages":

"You (1) promised that you would collect exemplary teaching exercises from all the teams, copy them, and bring them to tomorrow's meeting. You say that (2) you have only two examples now. I request that (3) you either get some other members to assist you in having this done for tomorrow, or contact all the group and reschedule the meeting to a time when they can meet and you can have all the exercises available."

Notice how this concise, orderly form for complaints focuses on accomplishing what was originally agreed. Nurse leaders/managers will have to make effective complaints on a regular basis and assist their peers and staff to make them as well.

Compliments for action

The same form for active complaining can be used to **compliment** others for keeping their agreements and doing and producing what they promise. Suppose Valerie wants to show her appreciation to Althea for doing what she said she would. She would (1) refer to their prior agreement, (2) point to the actions and/or results completed, and (3) express genuine appreciation, gratitude, thanks, etc. for what was accomplished. It would sound like this:

"You promised that you would collect exemplary teaching exercises from all the teams, copy them, and bring them to today's meeting. Not only did you do all that, but also you brought additional references and materials and very obviously got the group excited about working together. I really appreciate all that you accomplished, and thank you for keeping your word with me and the group. I know I can always count on you."

Such conversations focus on the vital aspects of active, committed communication: action, results, and being true to one's word. Powerful leverage and communication come from anyone's ability, courage, and timing with these four basic conversations for relatedness, possibility, structure, and action/results.

Breakdowns and Breakthroughs

To resolve breakdowns and create breakthroughs, it is important to synthesize the previous four strategies. For example, being clear about relatedness while intending to create possibilities potentiates effective communication. This synthesis is especially important when conversations occur between people in unequal work relationships. The Research Perspective provides implications for leaders/managers.

SUPPORTIVE AND DEFENSIVE COMMUNICATION

Leading, managing, and providing healthcare involve supportive communication and the avoidance of defensive communication (Gibb, 1961) as much as possible. The accuracy and cooperativeness of communication decrease rapidly when people feel threatened and act defensively. The categories of communication shown here describe how to communicate support.

Supportive Categories

1. **Description:** Communication that details others' behavior and accepts it, or communicates concrete fact, feelings, and opinion, is descriptive. Descriptions that refrain from judgments while sharing needed information are supportive. ("We got seven cases completed in today's team meeting," instead of "We sure were more productive this week without Phil.")
2. **Problem orientation:** Communication aimed at mutual collaboration and a willingness to be partners is supportive. Common goals, priorities, concerns, etc. become the focus. ("I am not sure how to proceed; let's do this together," rather than "I know exactly what to do; just listen to this.")
3. **Spontaneity:** Open and honest behavior communicates that there are no hidden motives. Straightforward communication builds supportiveness. ("I feel angry at the team's resistance, Sue, not with your nursing plan.")
4. **Empathy:** Empathy is a powerful interpersonal communication. One must be supportive of others when making efforts to understand them. ("Sounds like you are frustrated," rather than "You shouldn't get so upset with patients like that.")
5. **Equality:** Putting little importance on differences in status, ability, appearance, power, and worth communicates a sense of mutual trust, respect, and teamwork. ("We'll need all of our talents and effort; we are in the same boat" instead of "I am in charge here and I'll get us out of this.")
6. **Flexibility:** People who are open minded and willing to listen to and try out others' ideas are supportive. Supportive behavior includes exploring, trying new things, investigating, and reserving judgment. ("What are the advantages and disadvantages of both ways of doing it?")

Increases in these behaviors tend to lead to more personal backing and less perception of threat.

Another way to change a group interaction is to replace the defensive messages, as outlined below, with the supportive ones listed above. The purpose for defining them is to help you identify these message types, to consider them as cues to others' feelings of threat and defense, and to assist you in promoting support while decreasing defensiveness.

Defensive Categories

1. **Evaluative:** Continuous judgment places others in threatening situations. Behavior that emphasizes the negative and positive aspects of another establishes a judgmental tone and a defensive feeling. ("Oh, she's a wonderful worker, while he is a lazy slob.")
2. **Control:** Domination, persuasion, limitation, and planning for others often result in resistance and defending oneself. Doing it your way is not supportive of others' feelings, ideas, behavior, etc. ("You will do it this way, or else.")
3. **Strategizing:** Manipulating, tricking, and deceiving create defensiveness. Most often, the strategic game-playing person works to manipulate others and winds up being manipulated. Gibb (1961) found that everyone except the strategist knows she has been found out. ("If I tell them that they can choose, they'll have to choose what I want anyway because. . . .")
4. **Neutrality:** When people communicate that they do not care about others, they indirectly say, "You're not important enough for my help and attention." This neutrality leads to feelings of defense. ("I do not have time for your problem now, Maggie.")
5. **Superiority:** Superior messages communicate that one person believes she is better than someone else in terms of ability, status, position, power, and worth. ("I've much more experience here than you have.")
6. **Certainty:** Certainty communicates one's inflexibility and dogmatism. Being absolutely sure about complex problems, or other people, results in resistance. ("I'm sure that she's right.")

Exercise 15-3

Convert each of the above to a supportive statement.

By consciously trying to avoid these defensive messages, we all can contribute to the building of positive interpersonal relationships and a supportive group climate. If we can begin today to practice acting more supportively (i.e., empathic, problem oriented, equal, spontaneous, flexible, and descriptive) instead of threateningly (i.e., superior, certain, evaluative, neutral, controlling, and strategic), then we will have a positive effect on the groups of which we are a part.

Supportive and Defensive Cycles

People who feel supported and unthreatened will have more energy to work on a task, add ideas to a group, fulfill needed roles, and communicate with others. People who feel defensive use cognitive, emotional, and physical energy to protect themselves and in so doing detract from what they can accomplish individually and in the group. One important thing Gibb (1961) found from his research was that supportive behavior tends to lead to more supportive behavior and defensiveness tends to result in more defensiveness. Defensive listeners distort what they hear because they are arguing mentally, reacting to the speaker, listening through personal biases and prejudices, and/or hearing what they "wish" to hear. In such a situation, listeners are less able to use their mental advantage or empathize with the speaker.

Suppose you want to show support through empathy and say, "I know how you feel." However, the response you get is, "How could you know! Mind your own business." This is a clue that your intended support was not perceived that way. This might be because other people are involved, because there are other unknown factors in the situation, or because the listener "heard" strategy or neutrality rather than empathy.

If such an instance happens (e.g., you try to support someone else and receive a defensive message in response), then you have an obvious cue that your original intent or meaning was misunderstood. It may have been "misheard" or "misspoken" or *both*. So you could use perception checks, feeling descriptions, paraphrases, clarifying questions, etc. to create the meaning intended and impact ongoing conversations for relatedness, possibility, structure, and action.

▌ LISTENING FOR MEANING

Meaningful relationships are exciting and fulfilling because they involve deep communication, risk taking, trust, accomplishment, and personal growth. Most of us have experienced the exciting and touching closeness of at least one relationship where the communication was open, honest, clear, and emphatic. Effective listening is the process of working toward being fully heard. When people communicate at this level, they are bonded by empathy and their human commonalities. There are no strangers at this human-to-human level because people are all in the same condition. The distinctions of this section are basic to this type of communication and relationship. Paraphrasing is a powerful tool for stimulating interpersonal understanding, acceptance, clear communication, and accurate empathy (Johnson, 1996). Effective paraphrasing requires physical and mental attention and "active" listening. Too often interpersonal communication is marked by inattention, passive listening, and misunderstanding. The goal of this section is to examine paraphrasing and clarification.

Paraphrasing

Sometimes in normal conversation, people naturally use paraphrasing to check the accuracy of their understanding of the speaker's message. For instance, when people give their phone number and address, listeners often restate the numbers so they arrive at the right place for a party or avoid dialing the wrong number. This same concern for the accuracy of a phone number is important and useful when simple or complicated statements, important feelings, or vital directions are involved. The question is, how can people make sure that another person's understanding of intended meaning is the same meaning they got? How can they check their understanding of other persons' statements?

They could "invite" or encourage the speaker to say more, and they could ask for specific details. For instance, they could say, "Tell me more, please!" or ask, "What do you mean by that?" Unfortunately, as the speaker adds more detail and/or elaborates on what she or he means, the listeners' understanding is not guaranteed to get closer to what is meant. It could get further away from the original meaning, and they could become more confused. If you state in your own way what the speaker's remark conveys to you, the other can begin to determine whether the message is coming through as intended. Then, if the person thinks you misunderstand, you both can speak to the specific misunderstanding you have revealed.

Paraphrasing provides an important communication tool for (1) checking out the meaning, (2) comparing it to the meaning intended, (3) providing speakers with a clue about how they are coming across, and (4) providing a way for speakers to clear up any obvious misunderstandings.

The distinction paraphrase refers to any means used to show other people what their messages mean to those listening. This may be done orally, nonverbally, or as a written restatement of the original message. Most often, it is done verbally. A **paraphrase** is an oral rephrasing of the original communication in *one's own words*, with the intent of having the original speaker indicate whether this is what is meant.

Paraphrasing is not mind reading, but it does require careful attention and rephrasing of the meaning heard. For instance, Dave, in the dialogue below, pays careful attention to John and paraphrases effectively.

> John: "I'm able to work for you on the 3 to 11 shift this weekend."
>
> Dave: "So you are saying that you can fill in for me on Saturday from 3:00 PM to 11:00 PM. right?"
>
> John: "I cannot get there right at 3:00 and I have to leave early."
>
> Dave: "So you can only cover part of the work hours that I'll be gone, you mean?"
>
> John: "Yes, I can be there from about 3:20 to 9:45, if that helps."

Dave paraphrases John's statement, John adds the time constraints he is under, then Dave paraphrases again, which results in a very clear, concrete message between the two of them—enough for John to get someone else.

Paraphrases can come in many forms. Either statements or questions can be used to paraphrase the meaning of others' messages. They can be short or long. In the fullest sense, a paraphrase consists of three parts: (1) a lead-in that ensures the listener knows that the following statement is a restatement of what was originally said, such phrases as "What I heard you say . . ." or "So what you're saying is . . ." or "You mean . . ."; (2) a restatement of what was said; and (3) a tag question that asks the original speaker to confirm that the paraphrase captures the essential meaning. This simple tool is the most powerful one nurse leaders/managers have in getting themselves and others communicating (creating mutual meaning).

Clarifying Questions

Closely related to paraphrasing is the process of asking clarifying questions. A clarifying question is similar to a paraphrase in that it draws out from the other additional information about the topic at hand. It differs from paraphrasing in that the question is something on the mind of the listener and is not a restatement of what the original speaker said. Because of this, the focus of the conversation shifts from the original speaker to the person asking the clarifying question, since answering the question fills in information that the asker wishes to know. For example, in the

earlier example written below, Miles shares a paraphrase, while Mike asks a clarifying question:

> Pat: "I'd like you to use more analysis and evaluation in your monthly reports. I'd really. . . ."
>
> Miles: "Excuse me, but I'm not sure if I get what you mean. You'd like me to write more about what is happening and include my judgment of our progress, yes?"
>
> Mike: "What do you mean by analysis in this case, then? Or. . . ."
>
> Mike: "How can I build in an evaluation section in my monthly reports, since there is only one page on the form?"

Clarifying questions can be a powerful way to further the agenda on which you are working and can provide a lot of valuable information. What they do not do is have the original speakers know that listeners care about what they are thinking and what they want to pursue next in the conversation.

Exercise 15-4

Select a partner. Hold a conversation about a current societal topic (for example, a city council action, taxes, or voting). Demonstrate paraphrasing and clarifying.

FUNCTIONAL LEADERSHIP

There are many theories of group leadership. One of the dominant ones is highlighted in the theory box. Another theory, called **functional leadership,** is based on the task and maintenance behaviors already listed. The name *functional* comes from the view that everyone in the group who contributes (communicates verbally and/or nonverbally) one or more task and/or maintenance behavior to the group at a particular time "serves a function" for the group—he or she plays a "productive role" or "exerts leadership." In other words, members who demonstrate task and maintenance behaviors when they are needed provide "leadership" because they are assisting the group to reach higher goal achievement, stronger cohesiveness, and higher member morale (Johnson & Johnson, 1997).

One implication of this theory is that the responsibility for group effectiveness or lack of effectiveness rests with each and every member, not just with the group's official leaders. For example, is a member who sees the need for a particular behavior (orienting, for example) and does nothing about it more responsible for the resulting group ineffectiveness than the leader who honestly does not realize

Group Leadership Theories		
THEORY/KEY CONTRIBUTOR	**KEY IDEAS**	**APPLICATION TO PRACTICE**
Stages of Group Development and Situational Leadership Blanchard et al (1990) developed a theory of team leadership.	All teams develop by growing through four stages: (1) orientation, (2) dissatisfaction, (3) resolution, and (4) production. Leaders of the team display various leadership styles that match the stages above: (1) direction, (2) coaching, (3) participation, and (4) delegation.	Nurse managers can identify the stages of team development and either display necessary leadership or request that other members do it.

that the behavior is needed? This theory does not answer this question or raise blame. It does seek to have each member ask such questions about responsibility and the ability to have positive impact in any group. Another way to describe what effective leaders do is through this paradigm of functional leadership. Groups are positively influenced by people who are concerned about increasing task and maintenance while reducing individualistic behaviors.

OBSERVING AND USING TASK, MAINTENANCE, AND INDIVIDUALISTIC BEHAVIORS

A commonly used method of observing group behaviors is in terms of task, maintenance, and individualistic behaviors. The following sections list a set of task, maintenance, and individualistic behaviors and ways to use them in a group. One approach to viewing positive group membership is to avoid an "underuse" and an "overuse" of each behavior.

Exercise 15-5

Read the description of the task, maintenance, and individualistic behaviors on pages 259 to 262. Then reflect on and write out at least three task, three maintenance, and two individualistic behaviors you tend to demonstrate at present on at least one team.

Task Behaviors	Maintenance Behaviors	Individualistic Behaviors
1 _____	_____	_____
2 _____	_____	_____
3 _____	_____	_____

Task behaviors

The following behaviors help us to get the group started and stimulate sharing information, ideas, and opinions. Under each section is a description concerning how the underuse or overuse of a particular type of behavior may affect the group.

Task Behaviors: Starting and Sharing

1. **INITIATORS:** "The first item on our agenda is . . ."
   a. **Use:** Getting the group started.
   b. **Underuse:** Not initiating when the group needs to get started.
   c. **Overuse:** Initiating when the group needs maintenance or another task direction.
2. **INFORMATION SEEKERS:** "How many people have sent in their registrations?"
   a. **Use:** Increasing data and idea sharing.
   b. **Underuse:** Withholding key questions, letting the group "bog down."
   c. **Overuse:** Seeking more information when enough is available; seeking irrelevant data.
3. **INFORMATION GIVERS:** "Sixty percent of our clients said needs improvement"
   a. **Use:** Providing needed data.
   b. **Underuse:** Not sharing relevant data.
   c. **Overuse:** Supplying irrelevant information, giving biased details, fogging the issue.
4. **OPINION SEEKERS:** "What are our feelings about this idea?"
   a. **Use:** Increasing sharing of opinions, values, and goals.
   b. **Underuse:** Not responding to others' opinions.
   c. **Overuse:** Seeking opinions when facts are needed.

5. **OPINION GIVERS:** "I disagree that it might help us."
   a. **Use:** Letting the group know where members stand on issues.
   b. **Underuse:** Withholding key opinions when needed for group task or maintenance.
   c. **Overuse:** Providing opinions when facts are needed, interjecting irrelevant ideas.

6. **PROCEDURAL FACILITATORS:** "Could we try consensus decision making here?"
   a. **Use:** Helping move group to productive processes of action.
   b. **Underuse:** Resisting change, not moving quickly to new ways of acting.
   c. **Overuse:** Proposing irrelevant or cumbersome procedures.

7. **DOERS:** "I'll be glad to take notes."
   a. **Use:** Completing needed tasks.
   b. **Underuse:** Bogging group down while looking for someone to do the needed actions.
   c. **Overuse:** Trying to do everything at once, doing irrelevant tasks.

8. **RECORDERS:** "Here's what I've written. Is it accurate?"
   a. **Use:** Keeping accurate records of actions taken.
   b. **Underuse:** Losing track of group's past accomplishments, limiting responses when no one volunteers to record or when others view recording as a woman's job.
   c. **Overuse:** Noting irrelevant details, having one person do all the recording.

These task behaviors are important to getting the group started and to sharing needed ideas, opinions, information, and routine tasks. The ones below initiate an even deeper level of problem solving and commitment.

Task Behaviors: Accomplishment and Commitment

1. **ORIENTERS:** "We've been talking about the wealthy for 10 minutes. Let's get back to the report."
   a. **Use:** Keeping the group on task.
   b. **Underuse:** Ignoring the task behavior. Keeping the group off task.
   c. **Overuse:** Restricting the group to narrow limits or to one's own way of doing things.

2. **ELABORATORS:** "It sounds like we are talking about product quality instead of. . . ."
   a. **Use:** Providing deeper insights and complexity.

   b. **Underuse:** Maintaining a vague or superficial level when depth is needed.
   c. **Overuse:** Providing depth and complexity too quickly.

3. **COORDINATORS:** "The committee needs to meet tomorrow and share their ideas."
   a. **Use:** Encouraging cooperation and combining of ideas.
   b. **Underuse:** Ignoring the needs for scheduling and planning, and fostering competition.
   c. **Overuse:** Overplanning or building illogical relationships. Planning for others rather than with them.

4. **EVALUATORS:** "So far we have accomplished the following. . . ."
   a. **Use:** Measuring and judging group progress.
   b. **Underuse:** Providing little or no evaluation of group progress.
   c. **Overuse:** Constantly evaluating the group and restricting the freedom to act. Using unrelated standards.

5. **ENERGIZERS:** "I know we can get most of it done in 1 more hour."
   a. **Use:** Motivating groups to task accomplishments.
   b. **Underuse:** Accepting apathy. Providing little or no motivation.
   c. **Overuse:** Stimulating unproductive activity. Stimulating competition.

These behaviors promote added depth, cooperation, checks on progress, and motivation. Combined with the first eight task behaviors, these actions focus group energy on goal accomplishment and cooperation.

Any member can behave in various task areas during a particular session and over the life of the group. Sometimes all members are involved in one or more of these behaviors (e.g., opinion giving and evaluation) because it is vital to the group's success at that time. These behaviors may involve questions, statements, requests, nonverbal signals, and other behaviors needed for efficient group functioning. One basic question may serve several task functions at the same time (e.g., clarifying, orienting, and opinion seeking). Unfortunately, the same question said in a joking manner might result in individualistic behavior also (e.g., blocking or avoiding).

Maintenance Behaviors

Maintenance behaviors facilitate group process and stimulate positive feelings and interpersonal relationships. Group maintenance is just as important as task behaviors, but is often overlooked by group members. Outlined below are the effects of the use, underuse, and overuse maintenance behaviors.

1. **ENCOURAGERS:** "I really appreciate your efforts to get this done. Thanks!"
   a. **Use:** Accepting others and showing appreciation for their efforts.
   b. **Underuse:** Discouraging others or failing to encourage them.
   c. **Overuse:** Agreeing dishonestly or superficially

2. **GATEKEEPERS:** "Let's hear from our silent members; what do you think, Steve?"
   a. **Use:** Seeing that communication is open to all members.
   b. **Underuse:** Remaining quiet and allowing others to dominate or remain out of the discussions.
   c. **Overuse:** Dominating communication and controlling other's messages.

3. **HARMONIZERS:** "I'm sure we can find a solution that meets both your criticisms."
   a. **Use:** Relieving tension and building positive relationships.
   b. **Underuse:** Allowing unproductive conflict to continue.
   c. **Overuse:** Avoiding needed conflict or covering over issues with humor and light remarks.

4. **CONFLICT MANAGERS:** "Perhaps we can work out a compromise to resolve this."
   a. **Use:** Helping resolve group disagreements.
   b. **Underuse:** Refusing to compromise, accommodate, cooperate, etc. when needed.
   c. **Overuse:** Competing or yielding when inappropriate.

5. **STANDARD SETTER:** "To help us work together better, let's get to know each other better."
   a. **Use:** Motivating the group toward improved relationships.
   b. **Underuse:** Ignoring interpersonal needs and people's feelings.
   c. **Overuse:** Overemphasizing feelings while avoiding tasks.

6. **WELCOMERS:** "We've missed you. I'm glad you're back!"
   a. **Use:** Motivating the group toward improved relationships.
   b. **Underuse:** Ignoring other people's presence.
   c. **Overuse:** Welcoming superficially and ignoring tasks. Welcoming others while interrupting the group activity.

7. **LEVELERS:** "How do you feel about this? Be honest now!"
   a. **Use:** Promoting honest exchanges.
   b. **Underuse:** Withholding honest, relevant comments or requests for openness.
   c. **Overuse:** Pushing for openness prematurely or as avoidance of tasks.

Exercise 15-6

List at least three task and three maintenance behaviors you could add (with some stretch and risk) to your typical group behaviors above (especially use as replacements for any individualistic behaviors you identified).

Task Behaviors	Maintenance Behaviors	Individualistic Behaviors
1 _____	_____	_____
2 _____	_____	_____
3 _____	_____	_____

8. **FOLLOWERS:** "I like what Susan just selected."
   a. **Use:** Listening and participating actively.
   b. **Underuse:** Failing to follow the group's procedures or being totally inactive.
   c. **Overuse:** Forcing conformity through the silent majority or apathetic following.

9. **OBSERVERS:** "I've noticed that we've always used voting to decide things."
   a. **Use:** Noting and reporting on group progress.
   b. **Underuse:** Ignoring the group process.
   c. **Overuse:** Using observations to manipulate the group. Giving a report that is inaccurate or too detailed.

Maintenance refers to group building and cohesiveness. It is very productive for each member to view maintenance as an important group goal, no matter what the group task. Sometimes groups overemphasize tasks and get very little done, due to the lack of good feelings needed and the desire to spend the energy and time needed. Other groups underemphasize tasks, thus getting little accomplished while feeling very good about being together.

Individualistic Behaviors

Individualistic behaviors place member needs above group needs and interfere with task and maintenance. These behaviors may be caused by a low level of interpersonal skill, lack of interest, defensiveness, competition, ill-defined group goals, and unproductive conflict.

Below is an example of each of the individualistic behaviors, together with the task and maintenance behaviors that could replace individualistic needs with productive behaviors, and the maintenance behaviors that would help the group and the individual cope with the strong individual needs.

Reducing Unhelpful Behaviors

1. **BLOCKERS:** "I don't think it will work. I won't support it."
   a. **Helpful task/maintenance replacement roles:** Sharing reasons for blocking and the disadvantages that you see in the issue.
   b. **Helpful maintenance behaviors to cope with the individual needs:** Leveling about feelings and asking group to help deal with them.
2. **AGGRESSORS:** "John, that is a dumb, dumb way to look at this!"
   a. **Helpful maintenance replacement roles:** Expressing aggressive energy as encourager, standard setter, evaluator, or orienter.
   b. **Helpful maintenance behaviors to cope with the individual needs:** Describing aggressive feelings, leveling, setting standards, and working for cooperation.
3. **RECOGNITION SEEKERS:** "Here's a great idea I've used in the past."
   a. **Helpful task/maintenance replacement roles:** Getting attention to serve the necessary tasks, then giving attention to others through welcoming, encouraging, gate keeping, etc.
   b. **Helpful maintenance behaviors to cope with the individual needs:** Sharing feelings and facilitating the process regarding one's own needs and the needs of others.
4. **DOMINATORS:** "That'll never fly, Orville!"
   a. **Helpful task/maintenance replacement roles:** Energizing, evaluating, coordinating, standard setting, process facilitating, conflict managing.
   b. **Helpful maintenance behaviors to cope with the individual needs:** Leveling your own needs and feelings of certainty and uncertainty.
5. **AVOIDERS:** "I don't want to talk about this now. Can't we talk about it at the next meeting?"
   a. **Helpful task/maintenance replacement roles:** Relieving tension, orienting, coordinating, sharing opinions.

   b. **Helpful maintenance behaviors to cope with the individual needs:** Confronting group with the conflict stemming from the task and maintenance issues and one's resistance to change.
6. **SPECIAL INTEREST PLEADER:** "I think the group can do it this way and it sure would help me in my work if we do."
   a. **Helpful task/maintenance replacement roles:** Leveling, encouraging, cooperating, facilitating the group process.
   b. **Helpful maintenance behaviors to cope with the individual needs:** Sharing one's own interests and how the group can help meet them and other's interests. This can be done during the group meeting and outside of the formal setting.

Each of us can try to be as positive a member as possible by replacing individualistic needs and behaviors with task and maintenance behaviors that are group oriented. Sometimes one's own needs and feelings are very important and pull us toward individualistic action in one or more groups. When others in these groups can help us channel our behaviors into productive directions, all group members benefit. In this way, groups can grow and try to help all members to meet important personal and "group" needs. Remember, we all have similar needs; so working together we "all" can benefit.

Exercise 15-7

Return to Box 15-1. Would you assess yourself differently now that you have read this chapter?

▎ SUMMARY

Managing and leading demand effective communication for action and results, situational leadership, supportive communication, and functional leadership. The traditional term *follower* can be found in such functional behaviors as doer, recorder, observer, welcomer, information/opinion giver, and information/opinion seeker. Most importantly, committed speaking and listening, especially promises, requests, and active listening, produce a partnership aimed toward desired results.

A Manager's Solution

❓ What we did was to initiate combined team meetings once a month in which people could honestly address any issue. So we established norms for the group emphasizing honesty, full participation, cohesive teamwork, sharing the same information with any patient, and adhering to agency policy. Therefore when an aggressive patient tried to force someone to go beyond policy or tried to pit one office against the other, any staff person could assert the policy and get a supervisor if the patient persisted. An important aspect of what we did was to focus on commonalities between the team and the needs each had for cooperation with the other. The interaction of the supervisors enhanced and modeled that the high priority was to trust one another to maintain policy and support each other, rather than to blame, avoid responsibility, and talk behind each others' backs.

❓ *Would this be a suitable approach for you? Why?*

◼ CHAPTER CHECKLIST

Effective communication and leadership depend on continual efforts to attend to the details of the five basic types of conversations and set forms of communication for action. Nurse leaders/managers must be able to communicate clearly within the profession and within the broader, interdisciplinary healthcare context.

- Communication is a means of enhancing understanding; its basic principles include the following:
  - Communication is a means, not an end, but produces results.
  - The purpose of communication is to create mutual meaning.
  - Context and feedback affect communication.
- Collaborating to solve complex problems requires effective communication for action.

- Relationships are based on:
  - Who are you in the relationship?
  - What do you think others are like?
  - How does everyone involved view the situations, priorities, norms, etc.?
- Lack of commitment and committed speaking and listening for action interferes with effective communication.
  - Effective requests and promises are critical to leading and teamwork.
- Behavior conveys meaning more clearly than words.
  - Positive behaviors are desired actions that clearly convey their own importance.
  - Norms need to be clearly stated and adhered to.
  - Negative behaviors are undesired actions or actions that lack the desired results.
  - Negative behaviors can include gestures, facial expressions, and other forms of body language.
- Complaining and complimenting are important skills in leading and following.
- There must be an increase in supportive and a decrease in defensive communication.
- Active listening demands paraphrasing, clarifying questions, and commitment.

◼ TIPS ON COMMUNICATION AND PARTNERSHIP

- The life of a nurse leader/manager occurs in conversations for relatedness, possibility, structure, and action. The necessary focus should be on the (a) relationships needed to build and sustain partnerships and (b) results intended.
- Clear promises and results (and the ability to listen for them) is vital to leading and managing. Too often people do not get what they need or desire because they neither ask effectively nor listen for the real commitment of the person asked.
- Effective complaining and complimenting must be based on clear, committed agreements (promises) and aimed at specific action and results.
- As often as you have read and heard that paraphrasing is a vital tool for listening and communicating meaning effectively, it is rarely ever used enough.
- Defensive communication is a cue to you that people are feeling threatened, communication is likely to be distorted, and your support (in the six categories discussed above) is needed.

- Functional leadership requires task- and people-oriented behaviors from everybody, not just the nurse leader/manager. You cannot do everything, so see who naturally contributes which of the needed roles, request that others act in certain ways, and add what is needed regardless of whether you are comfortable doing it or not.
- Effective leadership often involves keen attention to the stage a group is in (and the nagging issues from earlier stages left unresolved) and a well-timed conversation with those who can assist the team and you in moving forward.
- Effective communication, leadership, and partnership require focused followership and behavior aimed at accomplishing the mission, goals, and objectives of the institution and team.

■ TERMS TO KNOW

assertions	paraphrase
complaints	partnership
compliments	possibilities
declarations	promises
functional leadership	relatedness
norms	requests

■ REFERENCES

Blanchard, K., Carew, D., & Parisi-Carew, E. (1990). *The One Minute Manager Builds High Performing Teams*. New York: William Morrow & Co.

Dowd, S., & Dowd. L. (1996). Maintaining confidentiality: Health care's ongoing dilemma. *The Health Care Supervisor,* 15(1), 24-31.

Gibb, J. (1961). Defensive communication. *Journal of Communication,* 11, 141-148.

Hurst, J. (1996). Building hospital TQM teams. *The Health Care Supervisor,* 15(1), 66-75.

Johnson, B. (1992). *Managing Polarities*. Amherst, MA: HRD Press.

Johnson, D. (1996). *Reaching Out*. Boston: Allyn & Bacon.

Johnson, D., & Johnson, F. (1997). *Joining Together*. Boston: Allyn & Bacon.

Lee, J. & Jablin, F. (1995). Maintenance communication in superior-subordinate work relationships. *Human Communication Research,* 22(2), 220-257.

McConnell, C. (1996). The evolving role of the health care supervisor. *The Health Care Supervisor,* 15(1), 1-11.

■ SUGGESTED READINGS

Adler, R., & Towne, N. (1995). *Looking Out, Looking In*. Orlando, FL: Holt, Rinehart & Winston.

Beebe, S. (1995). *Communicating in Small Groups*. New York: Harper Collins.

Corcoran, M. (1995). Collaboration: An ethical approach to effective therapeutic relationships. *Topics in Geriatric Rehabilitation,* 9(1), 21-29.

Fujishin, R. (1997). *Discovering the Leader Within*. San Francisco, CA: Acada Books.

Galanes, G., & Brilhart, J. (1997). *Communicating in Groups: Applications and Skills*. Dubuque, IA: Brown & Benchmark.

Sabey, M., & Gafner, G. (1996). Boundaries in the workplace. *The Health Care Supervisor,* 15(1), 36-40.

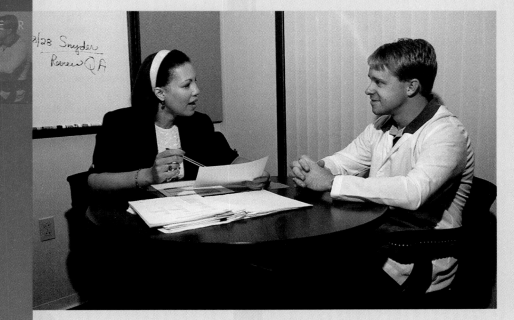

Selecting, Developing, and Evaluating Staff

**Cindy Whittig
Roach**
RN, DSN

This chapter illustrates the importance of selecting the right person for the organization as well as ensuring that the individual understands clearly what is expected of him or her. Emphasis is placed on the selection interview and the importance of the orientation process for new staff. **Role theory** is a useful organizing framework for the manager as well as for the employee to follow throughout all aspects of role performance. Effective communication of roles and role expectations among all members can facilitate improved performance, increased worker satisfaction, and, most importantly, improved quality of care delivered. The role of the manager as a coach who empowers employees to grow in a learning environment is explored.

Objectives

- Apply current philosophies of performance appraisal to a variety of situations.
- Relate concepts of role theory to performance.
- Differentiate five appraisal strategies.
- Examine specific guidelines for performance feedback.
- Distinguish key points for the appraisal interview.

Questions to Consider

- How does a manager hire and select the right people for a position?
- How does a manager develop new staff?
- How does a manager coach staff and create a learning environment?
- How does a manager empower staff members?
- What is your role at work? At home? At school?
- How do you deal with conflict in these roles?
- What are some of your assumptions about performance appraisals?
- What type of appraisal methods are you familiar with?
- How would you improve performance appraisals?
- What do you believe empowers you to improve your performance?

 A Manager's Challenge

From a Clinical Nurse Specialist at a Western Hospital Emergency Department

The emergency department was tasked with improving orientation for new nurses. The staff believes that we should be more responsive to individual learning needs. It is a challenge to retain and recruit qualified nursing staff, in part because of the high-stress environment, as well as a general lack of experienced emergency nurses. Successful completion of the orientation process has signifi-cance for the nurse, for the emergency department, and for the delivery of quality care. As a clinical nurse specialist, I was challenged to develop an improved orientation method that would be responsive to the wide variations in skill levels of newly hired emergency nurses.

What do you think you would do if you were this manager?

INTRODUCTION

Healthcare delivery systems are businesses that are economically driven. Whether the setting is inpatient or outpatient, the emphasis is on the provision of the highest quality care at an affordable price. The nurse manager is a key individual whose leadership can have a direct influence on many environmental functions. These factors begin with the selection of the right person for the right position as well as having the manager function in the role of coach. As a coach, the nurse manager can assist and encourage employees to perform at their highest levels with an empowered and self-directed manner. The nurse manager also functions to clarify the organization's mission and expectations. Professional healthcare providers must clearly understand what is expected of their performance as well as the ramifications if they do not meet those expectations. This can only be achieved when all members of the organization have clearly defined roles and overall objectives. Ambiguous roles are more detrimental to role performance and employee work satisfaction than conflict within the role.

Role ambiguity in the work place creates an environment for misunderstanding and hinders effective communication. In this situation, individuals do not have a clear understanding of what is expected of their performance or how they will be evaluated. **Role conflict,** in contrast, is easier to recognize. Employees know what is expected of them; they are either unwilling or unable to meet the requirements.

Human beings create the work environment. Clear expectations and positive attitudes by all individuals are essential if quality patient care is to be delivered. Employees who are empowered by a supportive leader and manager have unlimited potential to provide the best care possible.

SELECTING STAFF

The selection of staff would seem to be a relatively simple process. The manager wants the most qualified individual for the position. Choosing the right individual is the challenge! This individual must "fit" within the organization as well as within the specific work group. The employee and the manager must agree on what defines quality care and the manner in which it should be delivered. The manager must also decide if members of the existing staff are to be included in the screening and interview process for new employees. The following guidelines are suggestions for the manager and staff as well as for the prospective employee.

The manager's focus before and during the interview is to be prepared and have well-thought-out questions. The environment should be comfortable and provide privacy without interruptions. The interview questions can be related to the applicant's prior experience as well as directed to evaluate values and critical thinking skills. There may be technical skills that are important for the work environment that also must be discussed. Questions for the applicant should be answered honestly. Staff members may also be included in the interview and can provide information to the applicant as appropriate. After the interview is complete, it is important for the nurse manager to thank the person for the interview and inform him or her when the decision will be made. The manager should also inform the applicant if the decision will be made in writing or by telephone.

The applicant also has responsibilities in preparation for the employment interview. It is important to be on time and appropriately dressed. Conservative dress is always acceptable. A uniform is not necessary and usually not even preferable. First impressions may be lasting impressions. A review of the organization's goals and mission statement, as well as a review of the position description for which the interview is being conducted, is also appropriate. Be prepared to answer each question honestly and thoughtfully. It is equally important to the prospective employee to make the right decisions. The manager and the applicant must have a clear understanding of each other for there to be a good fit within the role. The applicant should keep to the subject at hand and avoid nonrelevant conversations. The individual must prepare in advance for any questions that might need to be discussed. At the end of the interview, the interviewee should thank the manager for his or her time and verify when the selection will be made. It is also appropriate to send the manager a brief note of appreciation for the interview.

DEVELOPING STAFF

Once the interview is completed and the applicant is offered the position, it is time to plan for orientation. Orientation to the organization is usually a structured program that is generally applicable to all new employees. It may include outlining the mission, benefits, safety programs, and other specific topics. Orientation to the work area usually depends on the specialty area involved, the skills that need to be verified, and the environment itself. Every individual brings to a new position various experiences and skills. It is imperative that the orientation period be used efficiently for both the employee and the organization. This is a very expensive endeavor, and everyone should use the time wisely.

As noted in the "Research Perspective" box, orientation can accomplish various things. It is a time for the new employee to learn the work environment and the staff therein. Many institutions provide a preceptor who is considered an expert clinician and resource. In fact, the Kolb (1985) Learning Style Inventory (LSI) may be administered to the new employee, with the information then shared with the preceptor. If the preceptor understands the new employee's learning style, he or she can provide a better focus for implementation of the orientation goals. After the learning style has been identified, the new employee works with the clinical nurse specialist to establish an orientation pathway that is designed to specifically address the individualized needs of the employee (see Figure 16-1).

Continued development of the staff is a unique role of the nurse manager. It is a challenge to merge a group of individuals with varying levels of expertise and experience. If the focus is centered around professional socialization and development, a common thread will "weave" itself throughout all employees. That common thread may be a particular philosophy of care delivery, further development of critical thinking skills for a specific specialty, or political activities in which members are involved. Some units encourage a monthly journal club or a brief presentation by employees to summarize information learned from a conference. One nursing unit sends a staff member to the monthly open meeting of the State Board of Nursing. This staff member then gives a summary of the report of the meeting. What an exciting way to keep informed!

Research Perspective

Kidd, P, & Sturt, P. (1995). Developing and evaluating an emergency nursing orientation pathway. Journal of Emergency Nursing, 21(6), 521-530.

This is an excellent example of how clinical research can be implemented into practice. Orientation procedures in the emergency department (ED) were first evaluated by the completion of a content analysis of exit interviews and expert clinician input from established preceptors. A pilot project pathway was then developed and tested using a convenience sample of seven ED orientee-preceptor pairs. A longitudinal descriptive correlational design was used to identify characteristics that might be associated with orientee success. Results were very positive about the usefulness of the orientation pathway. This pathway also provided one method to measure actual length of orientation necessary. Additional results of the study included the finding that experienced preceptors in the ED needed to be retained and an assessment of the learning style of the preceptor and the orientee that might contribute to teaching methods used to orient new employees.

Implications for Practice

Using data from exit interviews is one way to refocus on orientations. Assessing learning styles may enhance preceptor relationships.

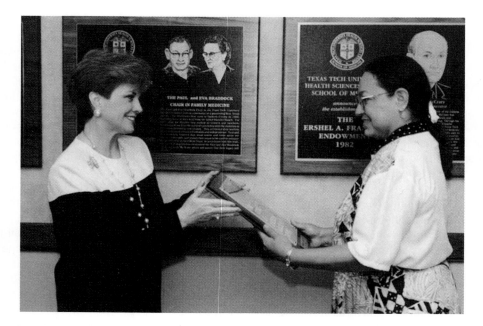

Acknowledging, rewarding, and reorganizing staff members' contributions is an effective way to empower the work force.

Empowerment strategies are also useful for staff development. **Empowerment** is a ". . . helping process; a partnership valuing self and other; mutual decision making; and freedom to make choices and accept responsibility" (Rodwell, 1996, p. 305). Kanter's (1993) theory of structural power in organizations is useful to understand how management can release control to groups so that they might perform work more effectively. This theory describes how power in organizations is not defined by personal characteristics but is defined by structural conditions. Employee attitudes, feelings of empowerment, and performance within roles can be influenced by specific environmental challenges and situations. These challenges

MEMORIAL HOSPITAL EMERGENCY DEPARTMENT
Orientation Critical Pathway Week #1
Excerpts from 9 day Pathway

Day 1	Day 4	Day 5
• Pyxsis Code Pick up in Pharmacy. If transfer within Memorial fill in new form @ pharmacy • Meet with CNS; complete Hazmat & TB Fit test.	• Video; Codemaster Defibrillator • Competency - Defibrillation	Orientee/Preceptor design this day based on individual needs.
Room Assignment : medical beds Date: _____ *Preceptor/orientee work as team.*	Chest Pain Center *Orientee with partial - full assignment. Uses preceptor as resource.*	Room Assignment *Orientee with partial - full assignment. Uses preceptor as resource.*
DAILY OBJECTIVES: • Introduction to staff, physical layout, equipment locations and patient flow. • Demonstrate basic knowledge of EmStat usage: Log on, Sign up for pt, Pt ready for physician evaluation, Shift change sign up. Discharge from EmStat. • Introduction to Documentation. Review Charting criteria for triage assessment. Identify location of references for same; Narrative charting; Discharge form; Food/Drug Interactions. • Observe assessment, interventions, evaluation and discharge of pt to home completed by preceptor.	DAILY OBJECTIVES: • Demonstrate use of EmStat for Chest Pain Alert Criteria. May simulate using created pt if have not had appropriate pt to this point • Locate and review equipment for Pacemaker Insertion (temporary), sternotomy tray, central lines and arterial lines. • Demonstrate assessment of Patient presenting for c/o chest pain, evidencing critical thinking process in history taking. • Utilize pain scale in assessing and tracking pain and responses to interventions.	DAILY OBJECTIVES: _____ _____ _____ _____ _____ _____
DAILY GOALS: • Identify learning needs to meet above objectives. • Communicate concerns r/t orientation to preceptor &/or CNS. • Other:_____ _____ _____	DAILY GOALS: • Identify learning needs to meet above objectives. • Communicate concerns r/t orientation to preceptor &/or CNS. • Other:_____	DAILY GOALS: • Identify learning needs to meet above objectives. • Communicate concerns r/t orientation to preceptor &/or CNS. • Other:_____
Goals/Objectives: Met__ Not Met__ • Explain Variances - Page Two	Goals/Objectives: Met__ Not Met__	Goals/Objectives: Met__ Not Met__

Figure 16-1 Orientation pathway.

can affect commitment to the organization as well as individual empowerment. Positive feedback, achievement recognition, and support for new ideas may enhance the employee's feeling of empowerment and his or her ability to perform effectively (Laschinger, 1996; McDermott, Laschinger, & Shamian, 1996).

One strategy for staff empowerment includes providing timely feedback for performance contributions, not simply during the annual performance appraisal. Support for implementation of innovative ideas and provision of opportunities for mentoring relationships are also valuable approaches for the manager and staff (Beaulieu et al, 1997). Many organizations use shared governance as a guide for accountability. A premise of shared governance is that power, control, and decision making can empower staff and enhance individual and group accountability. Empowerment has also been related to specific leadership styles. Morrison, Jones, and Fuller (1997) found a positive relationship between transformational leadership style, job satisfaction, and staff empowerment.

Implementation of empowerment strategies can enhance performance and provide an atmosphere that promotes work satisfaction. Employees must have clear role expectations and perceive that their contributions are valued. They should have a sense of empowerment and control for certain aspects of their environment. They are then more likely to be committed to the organization as well as to provide a higher level of patient care. These principles are applicable to both managers and staff members.

ROLE CONCEPTS AND THE POSITION DESCRIPTION

The acquisition of a role requires an individual to assume the personal, as well as the formal, expectations of a specified role or position. Many individuals function within multiple roles. As discussed in the theory box, role theory provides an appreciable framework for the development and evaluation of staff. Today's professional nurse is often a parent, spouse, and community volunteer and maintains full-time employment outside the home. There are many skills necessary for each role. There are also specified performance objectives for the role-taker (the individual actually performing the role) within the social context in which the role is acted out. The social context includes the physical and social environment. Acquisition of the role is time dependent; individuals apply their life experiences to each role and interpret the role within their own value system. As roles become more complex, the individual may take longer to assimilate the components of each particular role. Nursing graduates enter the profession with various levels of educational experiences as well as life experiences. The nurse manager plays an integral role in assisting these individuals in the development and acquisition of the complex role of the professional nurse. The important thing to remember is that role development evolves over time and with consideration to individual needs. Coaching is a technique that the manager can use to facilitate individual development and will be discussed later in this chapter within the context of performance appraisal.

What does all of this have to do with a position description? Everything! The **position description** provides written guidelines describing the roles and responsibilities of a specific position within the organizational context. The position description reflects functions and obligations of a specific work position. It is a contract for the individual that describes responsibilities of the work assignment as well as to whom the individual reports. The position description should reflect current practice guidelines for individuals and may have competency-based requirements. As paradigms of nursing delivery systems shift to the home and community, professional nurses must have a clear understanding of the performance that is expected. The nurse is also responsible for clearly understanding the position descriptions of the paraprofessionals to whom care is delegated. Clear and concise position descriptions for all employees are extremely important; they provide the basis for roles within the organization. An example of an abbreviated position description for a staff nurse in the emergency department appears in Box 16-1.

Exercise 16-1

Obtain a position description for a registered nurse from a community nursing service and a hospital. Compare them. Analyze the general categories (for example, communication) and the specific behaviors. What competencies do you have already? How will you develop other competencies?

PERFORMANCE APPRAISALS

Providing feedback to employees regarding their performance is one of the strongest rewards that an organization can provide. **Performance appraisals** are individual evaluations of work performance. Evaluations are usually done on an annual basis but may be required after a scheduled orientation period for

Role Theory

THEORY/KEY CONTRIBUTOR(S)	KEY IDEAS	APPLICATION TO PRACTICE
Role Theory and Role Dynamics in Organizations Kahn et al. (1964) developed this theory.	Roles within organizations affect an individual's interactions with others. Acquisition of these roles are time dependent and vary based on individual experiences and value systems. Role expectations for performance must be understood by all individuals involved for effective communication to take place.	The role of the professional nurse is complex. Role acquisition, role clarity, and role performance are enhanced by the use of clear position descriptions and evaluation standards.

Box 16-1

Excerpts From A Position Description

- Responsible for the provision of direct patient care to all age groups.
- Must have current certification in advanced cardiac life support (ACLS) and pediatric advanced life support (PALS).
- Required to accurately assess and prioritize patient care needs and delegate care appropriately to parapersonnel, including LPNs/LVNs and EMTs (emergency medical technicians).
- Responsible to the clinical nurse manager of the emergency department.

new employees. Ideally, evaluations are conducted on an ongoing basis, not at the conclusion of a predetermined period of time. This chapter's "Research Perspective", p. 268, illustrates a positive management intervention.

The process of providing feedback, for either above-average or below-average performance, is best received at a time closest to the incident(s) being evaluated. The actual appraisal is sometimes viewed as a negative experience. Many nurse managers perceive the appraisal as a time-consuming process of endless paperwork. Instead, the emphasis should be placed on role clarification (if necessary), evaluation of performance outcomes, and the contributions the employee has made to the organization. Performance appraisals provide the basis for many administrative decisions, including promotions, salary increases, and disciplinary actions. Appraisals should be de-

signed so that they can be supported in court. Court decisions can be made based on the evidence, or lack of evidence, presented in the evaluation instrument. Consider, for example, the individual who has been fired for reasons of poor work performance. The employee must be provided written notice that performance is unsatisfactory and that notice must specify what the employee must accomplish for satisfactory performance. This simple condition can make the difference for either the employee or the employer to justify the fairness for termination.

Performance appraisals can be either formal or informal. An informal appraisal might be as simple as immediately praising the individual for performance recognized. A compliment from a family member or patient might be conveyed. Some units have a specific bulletin board for thank-you notes from patients and their families. Sometimes a simple "Thank you for all your hard work today!" can be extended from the manager to the staff. In addition, staff members also have a responsibility to show the manager their appreciation and give positive feedback.

The formal performance appraisal involves written documentation according to specific organization guidelines. Whether the evaluation is informal or formal, it does not preclude interim evaluations. The key is that the praise or corrections be made as close in time to the episode as possible.

Brief *anecdotal notes* entered into the employee's file on a regular basis are important. These anecdotal notes, when accumulated over time, provide a more accurate cumulative appraisal. The anecdotal note describes an occurrence, either favorable or unfavorable, in a brief and concise manner. The purpose is to assist the manager with information throughout an entire rating period. An example of a brief anecdotal note appears here:

Example of an Anecdotal Note: Nurse "Smith"

> 2/14/94: Patient and family (Samuel Karruthers) stated how much they appreciated Ms. Smith's nursing care during this hospitalization. Her coordination of services and competent and caring manner decreased their anxiety and assisted them in learning what they needed to know for care in the home. She made the patient feel "special," not just another number, etc. Compliment relayed to employee.

These notes, combined with variance reporting, are another means of documenting employee performance that provide a more conclusive appraisal that reflects the entire rating period. Variance reporting identifies specific occurrences, based on benchmarks or specific standards. As an example, "The employee will have CPR certification by January 1." If the employee does not meet this deadline, a variance is recorded along with the specific circumstances or discipline planned. This topic is explored further in Chapter 20, Managing Personal and Personnel Problems.

The overall evaluative process can be enhanced if the manager employs the technique of coaching. **Coaching** is a process that involves the development of individuals within an organization. This coaching process is a personal approach in which the manager and the employee interact on a frequent and regular basis with the ultimate outcome that the employee performs at an optimum level. Coaching can be individual or may involve a team approach; when implemented in a planned and organized manner, it can promote team building as well as optimum performance of the employees. Coaching is a learned behavior for the nurse manager and takes time and effort to be developed. The rewards for both the employee and the nurse manager are significant; communication is enhanced and the performance appraisal process is an active one between the employee and the manager. Coaching is a management technique that can facilitate continual development as well as promote team building.

Exercise 16-2

> Select a partner. Observe some behavior and prepare an anecdotal note. Ask your partner for feedback about the content.

The formal performance appraisal usually involves some type of predetermined evaluation tool or instrument. The tool may be a simple one or may involve the integration of a variety of measuring methods. The instrument(s) should reflect the philos-

ophy of the organization and be as objective and specific regarding the employee's performance as possible. There are numerous instruments in use along with a variety of simple to complex scoring methods for each instrument. It is important for the new employee to have a clear understanding of timing as well as the content of the appraisal tool. The following example (Box 16-2) illustrates a type of peer appraisal method in which a staff nurse could evaluate another staff nurse within the area-specific content of assessment documentation.

Exercise 16-3

> Think back to your last performance appraisal, either in the clinical situation as a professional nurse or in the role of nursing student. Did you feel you were fairly and adequately evaluated? Were the comments reflective of your current practice and made by someone who had directly observed the care that you provided? What was the environment like for the interview? Were you comfortable with the evaluator? Was feedback given, both positive and negative? How did you feel at the conclusion of the interview? Taking the time to think about the answers to these questions might provide you insight and direction before your next performance appraisal interview.

The scoring procedures for the example shown in Box 16-2 can be as simple as satisfactory/unsatisfactory. A more complex scoring system, including a numerical rating scheme (using a range of 1 to 4, with 1 meaning "rarely meets standards," to 4 meaning "always exceeds standards") appears in Box 16-2. The results

---

Box 16-2

Peer Performance Appraisal, Staff Nurse

Area of Responsibility:

Assessment/Diagnosis: Provides continuous holistic assessment to include physical, psychosocial, spiritual, and educational needs. Directs outcome criteria so that discharge plans are timely and optimum quality care is delivered.

a. Data base (history/physical assessment) completed within 12 hours of admission. (Score 4)

b. Documentation reflective of continuous assessment per unit guidelines. (Example: neurovascular assessment of extremity following cardiac catheterization)   (Score 3)

c. Initiates plan of care according to critical path guidelines within 12 hours of admission. (Score 4)

d. Provides for safe environment.   (Score 4)

from the peer review process are then summarized and incorporated into the manager's formal performance appraisal.

PERFORMANCE APPRAISAL TOOLS

The type of appraisal tool used is not as important as *how* it is used. A formal written tool may have specific guidelines or a more open-ended format. General topics may be addressed in an anecdotal or "incident"-type format. The tool or evaluation form should facilitate accurate appraisal of the individual's performance as well as provide an opportunity to identify personal goals of the individual and goals of the organization.

There are primarily two categories of *performance appraisal tools*: structured and flexible. Table 16-1 summarizes examples of structured and flexible tools.

STRUCTURED (TRADITIONAL) METHODS

The *forced distribution scale* is a norm-referenced tool that prevents the evaluator from rating all individuals in the same manner. The evaluator is provided a

Table 16-1	STRUCTURED AND FLEXIBLE PERFORMANCE APPRAISAL TOOLS	
Structured (Traditional Method)	**Flexible (Collaborative Method)**	
Forced distribution scale	Behaviorally anchored rating scales (BARS)	
Graphic rating scale	Management by objectives	
	Peer review	

schematic diagram (see Figure 16-2) and asked to rate the individual according to all individuals the manager evaluates. As depicted in the figure, the evaluator has indicated that the individual rated is in the top 10% of employees but is not the best employee. This scale also provides the employee with a brief visual picture of how this evaluator has ranked performance in reference to others. This type of scale can undermine group cohesion and communication effectiveness by its very nature of rank-ordering individual performance. What this scale does provide, however, is a summary of the evaluator's overall ranking methods. For example, does the evaluator rank everyone in the middle 50% or below? Does the evaluator rank everyone as the best? A summary of the evaluation "track record" or history can be of value for the evaluator's performance appraisal!

This example illustrates that this individual is considered to be in the top 10% of all employees evaluated. It also illustrates that this particular evaluator has an even distribution of scores for the evaluation summary of all employees. This employee should feel positive about the evaluation. In reality, however, the employee is likely to feel just the opposite. The employee can see how many other employees, above him or her on the scale, are perceived as being better. In this way the forced distribution scale can undermine morale and group cohesion.

Graphic rating scales are another example of a structured approach to evaluation. They comprise a numbering system that indicates low and high values for evaluating performance. The rating scale is popular because it is easy to construct and easy to use. Problems with this type of scale are that it lacks specificity and may promote a **halo** or **recency effect.** The halo effect describes an evaluation based on isolated positive incident(s). The recency effect describes performance closer to the rating session as better remembered than that from previous months. For

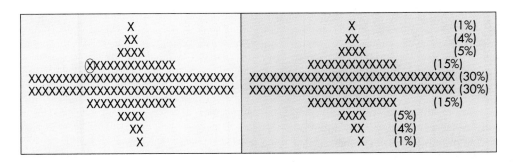

Figure 16-2 Forced distribution scale. *X,* Employee; ⊗, individual whom the employer is rating (evaluation history).

example, the employee performs in a satisfactory or less than satisfactory manner up until the month before the evaluation is due and then becomes "superemployee." If the evaluation is done with the majority of the information collected during the last month of the rating period, it may not accurately reflect the total performance. The evaluation then reflects the "best" behavior rather than behavior that occurred during the majority of time in the rating period. Supervisors tend to rate people the same from one rating period to the next. Thus, there is the potential for overinflation of the evaluation if the recent performance is all that is included. Anecdotal notes compiled consistently over the entire rating period are a much more equitable method for providing an accurate summary of the employee's performance. Some managers use small notes with adhesive backs to place inside an employee's file to document behaviors quickly as situations warrant. An empty sheet of paper placed in the front of each file would also serve the same purpose. Electronically the manager might also keep secured data files for the same purpose. Security of the files to maintain confidentiality is important.

As you can see from the example in Box 16-3, rating scales are relatively easy to construct and easy to complete. The problem is that they usually comprise generalizations, not specific behaviors, and that the rating is relatively subjective in nature. Some managers never give a "5" with the rationale that no employee "always does everything perfect" or that "no one is perfect."

Flexible (Collaborative) Method

The evaluation focus can also be conducted with a collaborative approach. How can the manager assist the individual to develop professionally? One method that has been used for many years is *management by objectives* (MBO). This method is also termed the establishment of learning goals, which are *mutually* established between the employee and the manager. Progress is documented throughout the rating period regarding the accomplishment of these goals. The MBO method is similar but more rigid in structure. An MBO approach requires that the employee establish clear and measurable objectives at the beginning of each rating period. These objectives are then addressed individually and in writing by both the employee and the manager during the performance appraisal evaluation. Learning goals are more difficult to define for both individuals. The approach can be simplified if it is performance based and outcome or results oriented. Then, in effect, the employee has created a "performance contract" as well as having defined definite goals for future professional performance. Box 16-4 illustrates goals and accomplishments.

Box 16-3
Example of a Rating Scale

CRITERIA	ALMOST NEVER			ALWAYS EXCEEDS	
1. Completes nursing care in a professional and competent manner	1	2	3	4	5
2. Is reliable; comes to work on time	1	2	3	4	5
3. Provides patient teaching as appropriate	1	2	3	4	5

Box 16-4
Learning Goals and Accomplishments

Learning Goals:
1. Prepare for and take ACLS certification examination.
2. Participate in shared governance committee as unit representative.

Accomplishments (12 months later—summary):
1. Successfully passed certification examination!
2. Participated in monthly meetings, chaired task force for development and implementation of new delivery system. Presented inservice class to staff on several units.

Behaviorally anchored rating scales (BARS) can also be implemented as a collaborative or flexible approach. The focus is on behavior and should include employees in the development. BARS combine ratings with critical incidents (specific examples that have occurred) or criterion references (examples usually based on standards of practice or competency-based standards). The criteria used for this scale are specific to the specialty of nursing delivered and outcomes that are preestablished. This scale is also considered more advantageous in terms of litigation. BARS describes the employee's performance quantitatively as well as qualitatively. Staff who are involved in the development of these instruments are more likely to understand the importance of evaluation for each criterion selected, as well as to have an understanding of their performance expectations. This is another example of clarification of roles and role expectations within the organization. The primary drawback of this scale is that it is expensive to develop and time-consuming to implement; it must be designed for each specific position description or standard of practice. However, it provides the manager with concrete information regarding an employee's performance, with minimal subjective interference. Box 16-5 provides an example.

This box illustrates, in part, how established nursing standards of practice, or protocols for practice, can be incorporated into the appraisal process using peer review. The data might also be used in an outcome review process as a component of a continuous quality improvement program. The final result would be summarized by the manager and incorporated into the employee's performance appraisal.

Peer review is also a flexible or contemporary strategy. If the guidelines are developed collaboratively, peer review may also be considered a developmental method of evaluation. That is, employees are involved in the development and implementation process. This method has increased in popularity. Nurses tend to function in their normal patterns in the presence of peers, and this can be a very solid rating method. However, it is important to obtain objective ratings based on performance, not subjective ratings based on personal friendships. This method should not be used if the manager is attempting to institute team-building strategies. The employees must trust and respect each other to willingly participate in the peer appraisal process.

Summary of Appraisal Instruments

Which instrument/method of appraisal is best? The objectives of the organization determine the tool(s) used. A combination of several tools is most likely superior to any one method. The primary success of any performance appraisal lies in the skills and communication abilities of the manager. Role ambiguity and uncertainty of standards of practice and methods for evaluation are significant contributors to decreased work satisfaction. The best-designed instrument will fail if the manager is ineffective and unable to communicate with the employee.

Exercise 16-4

Obtain a performance appraisal tool from the local health-care organization where you obtained a position description. Based on the descriptions provided, how would you characterize it? Is it structured or flexible? Is it quantitatively based, qualitatively based, or both? How does the tool reflect the position description?

Appraisal Interview Environment

The appraisal instrument is not the only factor in the evaluation process. The *environment* in which the appraisal is conducted is as important as the actual interview. The interview should be conducted professionally and in a positive manner. It is an ideal time for communication between the employee and the manager. There should be no interruptions if at all

---

Box 16-5

Example of a Behaviorally Anchored Rating Scale

Emergency staff nurse responsibilities for patient admitted with chest pain: (ER records evaluated per protocol; minimum 10/rating period). Met/Unmet
1. Vital signs recorded within 5 min of admission _____
2. Cardiac monitor, IV, Lab, and EKG done within 15 min _____
3. If sublingual nitroglycerin given, vital signs recorded every 5 min for 30 min _____
   a. Chest pain changes evaluated per protocol _____
   b. Post–chest pain 12-lead ECG documented _____

possible. This time is important for clarification of employee and organizational goals. Evaluation of employee performance in an objective and nonemotional manner should be conducted. The evaluation instruments should be clearly completed and time allowed for discussion. Future goals may be established. The manager and the employee should sign the appraisal form(s) and each be provided a copy. The effectiveness of the entire appraisal method relies on the manner in which the manager uses the tools and the feedback that the employee receives. Effective communication between the manager and employees can prevent potential performance problems on a unit. Specific behaviors by the manager enhance the actual appraisal process (see Box 16-6).

Exercise 16-5

Find a partner. Using an audiotape recorder, or a videotape recorder (preferred), conduct a performance appraisal. Seek feedback using the key behaviors in Box 16-6.

Box 16-6

Key Behaviors for the Performance Appraisal Session

- Provide a quiet, controlled environment, without interruptions.
- Maintain a relaxed but professional atmosphere.
- Put the employee at ease; the overall objective is for the best job to be done.
- Review specific examples for both positive and negative behavior (keep an anecdotal file for each employee).
- Allow the employee to express opinions, orally and in writing.
- Write future plans and goals, training needs, etc. (a "performance contract" for the future).
- Set follow-up date as necessary to monitor improvements, if cited.
- Show the employee confidence in his or her performance.
- Be sincere and constructive both in praise and in criticism.

A Manager's Solution

❓ I decided to apply patient care critical pathway principles to the orientation process for emergency department nurses. The clinical pathway represents a strategy to manage and achieve quality outcomes. The planning and implementation of the clinical orientation pathway (COP) included (1) analysis of existing orientation program for viable components; (2) current literature review; (3) collaboration of preceptor committee, professional development committee, and clinical nurse specialist for pathway development; (4) integration of previous department-specific orientation components (i.e., skills matrix and clinical competencies); (5) clinical trial of pathway; and (6) "fine tuning" with input from preceptors and orientees using the pathway during a 6-month trial period.

The staff and I believed that individual learners have unique learning styles that may affect the ability of the preceptor to enhance the orientation experience. For this reason we used the Kolb Learning Style Inventory (LSI) (1985). This tool allows the preceptor to focus and integrate the orientees' particular learning styles into the orientation experience.

The format for the COP (see Figure 16-1) allows for variances and variability in progression. The orientee and preceptor follow the progress on a daily basis, setting individual goals and objects.

The outcome of a COP model has demonstrated effectiveness in the following ways: (1) establishes time frames and desired outcomes in a concise, easy-to-follow format; (2) allows for self-paced flexibility based on Benner's (1984) "novice-to-expert" approach from previous relative nursing experience; (3) identifies positive and negative variances from the orientation pathway that may influence time frame parameters; and (4) identifies clearly the orientees' responsibilities and resources for outcome achievement. This pathway has been positively received by the preceptors and the orientees. It has also provided a more cost-effective method for the orientation process.

❓ *Would this be a suitable approach for you? Why?*

■ CHAPTER CHECKLIST

The manager plays a key role in the selection and development of staff. As a role model, the manager is also key in the establishment of the type of work environment that exists. Managers must be supportive and develop their staff to their highest potential. They must have accurate position descriptions and tools for evaluation of employee performance. These are integral to role development and professional socialization. Managers must also use various communication methods to empower their employees. Coaching and implementation of empowerment strategies positively contribute to overall staff performance as well.

■ The interview should include the following:
  • Screen the applicants.
  • Prepare questions in advance.
  • Control the environment.
  • Give explanations and role clarification.
  • Be a good listener.
  • Give honest answers to questions.
  • Provide closure.
  • Inform the applicant when he or she will be notified.
■ The role of the applicant includes:
  • Being on time and dressed appropriately.
  • Reviewing the organization's mission.
  • Preparing questions.
  • Answering questions honestly and completely.
  • Noting appreciation for the interview.
■ Development of the staff includes:
  • Organized and efficient orientation
  • Plans for education, team-building, and professional socialization
  • Active coaching
  • Implementation of empowerment strategies

Development of accurate position descriptions and tools for evaluation of employee is integral to role development and professional socialization. Nurse managers should use various communication methods to include coaching techniques.

■ Role theory describes how individuals perceive their position in an organization.
  • Distinction and clarity among the various positions are imperative if partnerships in quality patient care are to exist.
■ The position description serves several purposes:
  • Provides written guidelines that describe roles and responsibilities.
  • Reflects the position's overall function and obligations.
  • Serves as a contract between manager and employee.
  • Reflects current practice guidelines for the position.
■ Performance appraisals are a method of providing feedback to the employee in relation to individual performance.
  • Types of structured (traditional) performance appraisals include:
    – Graphic rating scales
    – Forced distribution method
  • Types of flexible (collaborative) performance appraisals include:
    – Behaviorally anchored rating scales (BARS)
    – Learning goals/management by objective (MBO)
    – Peer review

■ TIPS FOR CONDUCTING AN INTERVIEW

■ Screen the application and schedule a time for the interview.
■ Prepare questions in advance. Be concise but thorough.
■ Control the environment for noise and interruptions.
■ Explain and clarify the role for which the applicant is interviewing.
■ Be a good listener.
■ Answer questions honestly.
■ Inform the applicant when he or she will be informed of the decision.

■ TERMS TO KNOW

coaching	position description
empowerment	role ambiguity
halo or recency effect	role conflict
performance appraisal	role theory

■ REFERENCES

Beaulieu, R., Sharnian, J., Donner, G., & Pringle, D. (1997). Empowerment and commitment of nurses in long-term care. *Nursing Economics*, 15(1), 32-40.

Benner, P. (1984). *From Novice to Expert: Power and Excellence in Nursing Practice*. Menlo Park, CA: Addison-Wesley.

Bray, D. (1997). *Orientation Critical Pathway. Excerpts from 9-day Pathway*. Colorado Springs, CO: Memorial Hospital Emergency Department.

Kahn, R.L., Wolfe, D.M., Quinn, R.P., Snoek, J.D., & Rosenthal, R.A. (1964). *Occupational Stress: Studies in Role Conflict and Ambiguity.* New York: Wiley.

Kanter, R.M. (1993). *Men and Women of the Corporation,* 2nd ed., New York: Basic Books.

Kidd, P., & Sturt, P. (1995). Developing and evaluating an emergency nursing orientation pathway. *Journal of Emergency Nursing,* 21(6), 521-530.

Kolb, D.A (1985). *Learning-Style Inventory,* Boston: McBer & Co.

Laschinger, H.K.S. (1996). A theoretical approach to studying work empowerment in nursing; A review of studies testing Kanter's theory of structural power in organizations. *Nursing Administration Quarterly,* 20(2), 25-41.

McDermott, K., Laschinger, H.K.S., & Shamian, J. (1996). Work empowerment and organizational commitment. *Nursing Management,* 27(5), 44-47.

Morrison, R.S., Jones, L., & Fuller, B. (1997). The relation between leadership style and empowerment on job satisfaction of nurses. *Journal of Nursing Administration,* 27(5), 27-34.

Rodwell, C.M. (1996). An analysis of the concept of empowerment. *Journal of Advanced Nursing,* 23, 305-313.

SUGGESTED READINGS

Ashton, J.T., & Wilkerson, J. (1996). Establishing a team-based coaching process. *Nursing Management,* 27(3), 48N,48Q.

Biddle, B.J. (1979). *Role Theory: Expectations, Identities, and Behaviors.* New York: Academic Press.

Jackson, B.S., ed. (1996). The job that didn't fit. *Journal of Nursing Administration,* 26(1), 9-10, 30.

Prince, S.B. (1997). Shared governance. Sharing power and opportunity. *Journal of Nursing Administration,* 27(3), 28-35.

Shera, W., & Page, J. (1995). Creating more effective service organizations through strategies of empowerment. *Administration in Social Work,* 19(4), 1-15.

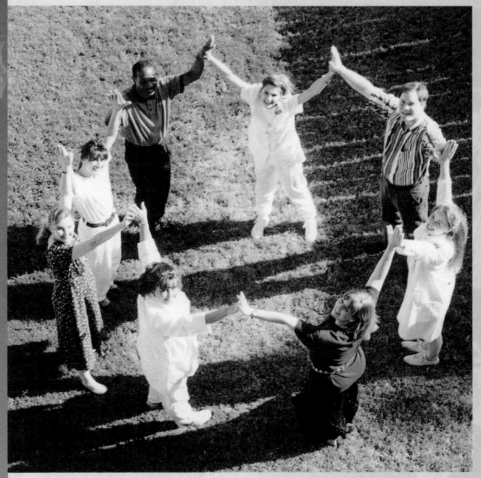

Team Building

Karren Kowalski
RN, PhD, FAAN

This chapter explains major concepts and presents tools with which to create and maintain a smoothly functioning team. Many areas of our lives require that we work together in a smooth and efficient manner; not the least of these is the team in the work setting. Such teams often include members with various backgrounds and educational preparation. A healthcare team often includes physicians, nurses, administrators, allied health professionals, and support staff such as housekeeping and dietary. Each team member has something valuable to contribute and deserves to be treated honorably and with respect. When teams are not working, all team members must change how they interact within the team.

Objectives

- Distinguish between a group and a team.
- Identify four key concepts of teams.
- Discuss the three personal questions each team member struggles to answer.
- Apply the guidelines for acknowledgment to a situation in your clinical setting.
- Compare a setting that uses the rules of the game with your current clinical setting.
- Develop an example of a team that functions synergistically, including the results such a team would produce.

Questions to Consider

- What differentiates a team from a group?
- How does one create a team?
- What are key aspects of a well-functioning team?
- What are the key issues or questions team members want to know?
- What role do agreements or guidelines play in a well-functioning team?
- How do some teams function like well-oiled machines and achieve extraordinary results?
- What are the behaviors and attitudes that destroy teams?
- Do teams go through stages of development?

A Manager's Challenge
From the Unit Director of a Neonatal ICU at a Midwestern Hospital

An extensive "team" of people work together to care for the neonate in a neonatal intensive care unit (NICU). They include MDs, RNs, respiratory therapists, physical therapists, social workers, neonatal nurse practitioners, and ancillary staff. Occasionally, specialists are consulted for specific cardiac, neurological, or gastrointestinal problems. These are intermittent "team" members who play a crucial role in the baby's care.

Recently, a new group of specialists joined our team. They were identified as a top-notch group who would, by virtue of the expertise and reputation, increase the census and revenues for the hospital. Our team was excited to have this opportunity to grow in an area where we had infrequent experience. However, things did not go smoothly. There were clinical disagreements and interpersonal conflicts. The experience evolved into mutual distrust and control issues.

As disagreements, insults, and complaints escalated on both sides, the situation came to a defin-

ing moment when the director of the specialty said, "I'm never bringing any of our patients here. I'm sending them to the PICU." The response from the NICU team was, "Fine with us; we don't need you, your patients, or the hassle." It seemed reasonable to not work together because in fact, functionally, we were already not working together. This response was in direct conflict with our belief that we could provide a valuable service and make a difference for both the patients and their families. This posed a dilemma for the staff, but everyone felt the situation was hopeless.

No one believed we could function as a team and, therefore, further efforts to work together were futile. We had tried and failed. Let's just cut our losses and move on. How does one create a team when no one believes it is possible and some believe it's not even necessary?

What do you think you would do if you were this manager?

INTRODUCTION

As we experience changes such as cost cutting and downsizing within healthcare, teamwork becomes an important concept. The old adage "If we do not all hang together we will all hang separately" was never more true than now as we move through the rapidly changing times in healthcare and into the twenty-first century. In our society, where so much emphasis is placed on the individual and individual achievement, teamwork is the quintessential contradiction. In other words, with all the focus on individuals, we still need individuals to work together in groups to accomplish goals. Everybody knows and understands this, particularly the rugged individuals who spend their Sundays watching football or basketball. These team sports are premier models of cooperation and competition. They are the model of **team** for business today and they represent a group of persons with their respective leader or "coach."

GROUPS AND TEAMS

The dictionary definition of **group** is a number of individuals assembled together or having some unifying relationship. Groups could be all the parents in an elementary school, all the members of a specific church, or all the students in a school of nursing because the members of these various groups are related in some way to one another by definition of their involvement in a certain endeavor. A team, on the other hand, is a number of persons associated together in specific work or activity. But not every group is a team and not every team is effective.

Parker (1990) says a group of people is not a team. From his perspective, a team is a group of people with a high degree of interdependence geared toward the achievement of a goal or a task. Often we can recognize intuitively when the so-called team is not functioning effectively. We say things like, "We need to be more like a team" or "I'd like to see more team players around here." Consequently, in the process of defining *team*, it is important to consider effective versus ineffective teams. Teams are groups that have defined goals, objectives, and ongoing relationships and are focused on accomplishing a task. Teams are essential in providing cost-effective high-quality healthcare. As resources are expended more prudently, patient care teams must develop clearly defined goals, use creative problem solving, and demonstrate mutual respect and support. Facilities with ineffective teams will find themselves out of business.

Exercise 17-1

Think of the last team or group of which you were a part. Think about what went on in that team or group. Specifically think about what worked for you and what didn't work. Use the "Team Assessment Questionnaire" in Box 17-1 to evaluate more specifically those things that worked or did not work for you on the team in which you participated. When you have finished answering the 22 questions, use the scoring mechanism at the bottom to discover how well your team or group functioned in terms of roles, activities, relationships, and general environment.

When a team functions effectively, there is a significant difference in the entire work atmosphere, the way in which discussions progress, the level of understanding of the team-specific goals and tasks, the willingness of members to listen, the manner in which disagreements are handled, the use of consensus, and the way in which feedback is given and received. The original work done by McGregor (1960) sheds light on some of these significant differences, which are summarized in Table 17-1.

In general, ineffective teams are often dominated by a few members, leaving others bored, resentful, or uninvolved. Leadership tends to be autocratic and rigid, and the team's communication style may be overly stiff and formal. Members tend to be uncomfortable with conflict or disagreement, avoiding and suppressing it rather than using it as a catalyst for change. When criticism is offered, it may be destructive, personal, and hurtful rather than constructive and problem-centered. Team members may begin to "stuff" their feelings of resentment or disagreement, sensing that they are "dangerous." This creates the potential for later eruptions and discord. Similarly, the team avoids examining its own inner workings, or members may wait until after meetings to voice their thoughts and feelings about what went wrong and why.

In contrast, the effective team is characterized by its clarity of purpose, informality and congeniality, commitment, and high level of participation. The members' ability to listen respectfully to each other and communicate openly helps them handle disagreements in a civilized manner and work through them rather than suppress them. Through ample discussion of issues, they reach decisions by consensus. Roles and work assignments are clear, but members share the leadership role, recognizing that each person brings his or her own unique strengths to the group effort. This diversity of styles helps the team adapt to changes and challenges, as does the team's ability and willingness to assess its own strengths and weaknesses and respond to them appropriately.

The challenges encountered in today's healthcare systems are prodigious. There are ongoing rounds of downsizing budget cuts, declining patient days, reduced payments, and staff layoffs. Effective teams participate in effective problem solving, increased creativity, and improved healthcare.

KEY CONCEPTS OF TEAMS

In very rare instances, a team may produce teamwork spontaneously, like kids in a school yard at recess. However, most management teams learn about teamwork because they need and want to work together.

Box 17-1

Team Assessment Questionnaire

Circle the appropriate number using the scale below.
(1 = not at all; 2 = limited extent; 3 = some extent; 4 = considerable extent)

1. People are clear about goals for the group.	1 2 3 4
2. Unnecessary procedures, policies, and formality are minimized.	1 2 3 4
3. Team members feel free to develop and experiment with new ideas and approaches.	1 2 3 4
4. The allocation of rewards is perceived to be based on excellent performance.	1 2 3 4
5. Recognition and praise outweigh threats and criticism.	1 2 3 4
6. Calculated risk taking is encouraged.	1 2 3 4
7. People are clear about their responsibilities and expectations for performance.	1 2 3 4
8. People are clear about how their roles/responsibilities interrelate with those of others.	1 2 3 4
9. People perceive others in the work group to be high performers.	1 2 3 4
10. People are clear about what personal characteristics/competencies are necessary for superior performance in their jobs.	1 2 3 4
11. The team produces high-quality decisions, products, and/or services.	1 2 3 4
12. The team is able to conduct effective meetings.	1 2 3 4
13. The team achieves its goals.	1 2 3 4
14. The team and its individual members are able to interact effectively with others outside the team.	1 2 3 4
15. The team makes decisions and produces output in a timely fashion.	1 2 3 4
16. The team members truly support each other in carrying out their respective responsibilities.	1 2 3 4
17. Team members are open in their communications with each other.	1 2 3 4
18. Team members follow through on commitments.	1 2 3 4
19. Team members trust each other.	1 2 3 4
20. All team members are equal contributors to the team process.	1 2 3 4
21. The group often evaluates how effectively it is functioning.	1 2 3 4
22. Individual members feel committed to the team.	1 2 3 4

If you'd like to score your team assessment questionnaire, enter the score you selected for each question. Next, take the scores for each area, then calculate the average score.

Roles	Activities	Relationships	Environment
Item/Score	Item/Score	Item/Score	Item/Score
7 _____	2 _____	5 _____	1 _____
8 _____	3 _____	14 _____	2 _____
9 _____	11 _____	16 _____	3 _____
10 _____	12 _____	17 _____	4 _____
18 _____	13 _____	19 _____	5 _____
20 _____	15 _____	22 _____	6 _____
21 _____			
Total Score _____	Total Score _____	Total Score _____	Total Score _____
Average Score = _____	Average Score = _____	Average Score = _____	Average Score = _____
(Total Score ÷ by 7)	(Total Score ÷ by 6)	(Total Score ÷ by 6)	(Total Score ÷ by 6)

If the average for a column (e.g., Activities) was 3.5, it means the group is fairly productive in its activity, falling halfway between "some extent" and "considerable extent." If the average for the relationships column was 1.5, it would indicate the respondent believes that team members have not been effective in developing relationships with one another that are clearly defined, effective, or respectful of one another.

Used with permission from Dubnicki (1991).

Table 17-1	ATTRIBUTES OF EFFECTIVE AND INEFFECTIVE TEAMS	
Attribute	**Effective Team**	**Ineffective Team**
Working environment	• Informal, comfortable, relaxed	• Indifferent, bored; tense, stiff
Discussion	• Focused • Shared by almost everyone	• Frequently unfocused • Dominated by a few
Objectives	• Well understood and accepted	• Unclear, or many personal agendas
Listening	• Respectful—encourages participation	• Judgmental—much interruption and "grandstanding"
Ability to handle conflict	• Comfortable with disagreement • Open discussion of conflicts	• Uncomfortable with disagreement • Disagreement usually suppressed, or one group aggressively dominates
Decision making	• Usually reached by consensus • Formal voting kept to a minimum • General agreement is necessary for action; dissenters are free to voice opinions	• Often occurs prematurely • Formal voting occurs frequently • Simple majority is sufficient for action; minority is expected to go along
Criticism	• Frequent, frank, relatively comfortable, constructive • Directed toward removing obstacles	• Embarrassing and tension-producing; destructive • Directed personally at others
Leadership	• Shared; shifts from time to time	• Autocratic; remains clearly with committee chairperson
Assignments	• Clearly stated • Accepted by all despite disagreements	• Unclear • Resented by dissenting members
Feelings	• Freely expressed, open for discussion	• Hidden, considered "explosive" and inappropriate for discussion
Self-regulation	• Frequent and ongoing, focused on solutions	• Infrequent, or occurs outside meetings

Adapted from McGregor (1960).

This kind of working together requires that they observe how they are together in a group and that they unlearn ingrained self-limiting assumptions about the glory of individual effort and authority that are contrary to cooperation and teamwork. Keys to the concept of team are:

- communication
- singleness of mission
- willingness to cooperate
- commitment

Communication

The word *team* is most frequently reserved for a very special type of working together. This working together requires communication in which the members understand how to conduct interpersonal relationships with their peers in thoughtful, supportive, and meaningful ways. It requires that team members be able to resolve conflicts among themselves and do so in ways that enhance rather than inhibit their working together. In addition, team members must be able to trust that they will receive what they need while being able to count on one another to complete tasks related to team functioning and outcomes. To communicate effectively, people must be willing to confront issues and to openly express their ideas and feelings—to use interactive skills to accomplish tasks. In nursing, constructive confrontation has not been a well-used skill. Consequently, if communication patterns are to improve, the onus is on each of us as individuals to change communication patterns. In essence, for things to change, each of us must change.

Mission

Each and every team must have a purpose—that is, a plan, aim, or intention. However, the most successful teams have a mission—some special work or service to which the team is 100% committed. The sense of mission and purpose must be clearly understood by all and agreed to by all (Fisher & Thomas, 1996). The more powerful and visionary the mission is, the more enrolling it will be to the team. The more energy and excitement engendered, the more motivated all members will be to do the necessary work.

Willingness

Just because a group of people has a regular reporting relationship within an organizational chart does not mean the members are a team. Boxes and arrows are not in any way related to the technical and interpersonal coordination, nor the emotional investment, required of a true team. Most of us have been involved in organizations where people could accomplish assigned tasks but were not successful in their interpersonal relationships. In essence, these employees received a salary for not getting along with a certain person or persons. Some of these employees haven't worked cooperatively for years! Organizations can no longer afford to pay people to not work together. Personal friendship or socialization is not required. Cooperation is a necessity.

Commitment

Commitment is a state of being emotionally impelled and is demonstrated when there is a sense of passion and dedication to a project or event—a mission. Frequently this passion looks a little crazy. In other words, people go the extra mile because of their commitment. They do whatever it takes to accomplish the goals or see the project through to completion. An example of commitment is discussed by Charles Garfield when he talks about being a part of the team that created the lunar landing module for the first man to walk on the moon. People did all kinds of

things that looked crazy, including working extended hours and shifts, calling in to see how the project was progressing, sleeping over at their work station so as not to be separated from the project—and all because each and every individual knew they were a part of something that was much bigger than themselves. They were a part of sending a man to the moon, something that human beings had been dreaming about for thousands of years. In other words, it was a historical moment and people were intensely committed to making it happen.

Many people go through their entire lives hating every single day of work. Needless to say, most of them are not committed. Since we spend an extensive amount of time in the work setting, it is critically important to both physical and mental well-being that people enjoy what they do. If this is not the case for you, then try to find a different job or profession—one you might love. Life is too short to do something that you hate doing every single day. While you are moving into whatever you decide you love doing, commit to yourself to do your best at whatever you are now doing. Be 100% present wherever you are. Do the best work you are capable of doing. This honors you as a human being and it honors your co-workers and patients.

Exercise 17-2

Box 17-2 contains eight questions. In a quiet place, spend at least 20 minutes thinking about and writing answers to these eight questions. Pay particular notice to question 7.

There are many examples of commitment, such as that of Jan Skaggs, the Vietnam veteran who was the driving force behind the building of the Vietnam War Memorial. He was a clerk in the Washington, D.C. bureaucracy who attended a veterans' meeting and decided there needed to be a memorial to those who lost their lives in Vietnam, a memorial that had all 58,000 names inscribed. He had a high school diploma and didn't even own a suit, but 5 years and 7 million dollars later the wall was dedicated (Lopes, 1987). This is a demonstration that one does not have to have a college degree in order to be committed. Sometimes a college degree can inhibit people from accomplishing their goals because they become diverted from a purpose, from a mission, or from life goals by things like good grades and a high IQ. Rather than understanding grades and IQ as tools of measurement, they see them as an end in themselves.

It is possible to teach almost anyone the technical aspects of what needs to be done in most patient care settings. It is far more difficult to teach people to

Box 17-2
Exploring Commitment

The key to finding your compelling mission/passion that will lead you to success and peak performance is to ask yourself the right questions. Your answers to these questions will tell you what you need to know about yourself. Read each question, then stop and think for a few minutes and answer each question honestly. Don't censor or edit out anything even if it seems impossible or unrealistic— allow yourself to be surprised. Let your imagination soar.

1. Am I deriving any satisfaction out of the work I am now doing?
2. If they didn't reward (praise or pay) me to do what I now do, would I still do it?
3. What is it that I really love to do?
4. What do I want to pursue with my time and energy that is worthwhile?
5. What motivates me to reach out and do my very best, to excel?
6. What is it that only I can say to the world? What needs to be done that can best be done only by me?
7. If I won $10,000,000 in the lottery tomorrow, how would I live? What would I do each day and for the rest of my life?
8. If I were to write my own obituary right now, what would be my most significant accomplishment? Is that enough?

Repeating this exercise often will give you additional insights and information about what you really want and love to do. If taken seriously, the exercise should help you to have an understanding of why you selected this profession and whether or not you have the stamina to do whatever it takes to make a contribution and to make a difference in the practice of nursing.

love what they do or to care about patients and their families—even the most difficult and unique patients and families.

■ TOOLS AND ISSUES THAT SUPPORT TEAMS

When individuals come together in a group, they spend a fair amount of their time in group process or social dynamics, which allows the group to advance toward becoming a team and getting a goal accomplished. Each person within the group struggles with three key questions that must continually be reevaluated and renegotiated. These three questions according to Weisburg (1988) are:

1. Am I in or out?
2. Do I have any power or control?
3. Can I use, develop, and be appreciated for my skills and resources?

This chapter's "Literature Perspective" focuses on Weisburg's work.

"In" Groups and "Out" Groups

Most of us want to be valued and recognized by others as a part of the group, one who "knows" or understands. Most people want to be at the core of decision-making power and influence. In other words, they want to be part of the "in" group, and researchers have demonstrated that those who feel "in" cooperate more, work harder and more effectively, and bring enthusiasm to the group. The more we feel not a part of the key group, the more "out" we feel, the more we withdraw, work alone, daydream, and engage in self-defeating behaviors. Often intergroup conflict results when individuals who feel they are "out" and want to be "in" create a schism or a division that prohibits the team from accomplishing its goals.

Power and Control

Everybody wants at least some power and everybody wants to feel they are in control. When faced with changes that we are unable to influence, we feel impotent and experience a loss of self-esteem. Consequently, all of us want to feel we are in control of our immediate environment and that we have enough power and influence to get our needs met. When a situation or an event arises that we are unable to handle, we attempt to compensate for it in some way; most of these ways are not productive to smoothly functioning teams.

Exercise 17-3

Think about a time when you or a small group of your classmates wanted to change a class, an assignment, or the grading curve or a test. The faculty or the school administration adamantly refused. How did you feel? What was the response? Did you engage in gossip and making the faculty or the administration wrong? You may have been "right," but the sense of a loss of control or power is very uncomfortable, sometimes fear-producing. Very mature behavior is required to maintain a positive, problem-solving approach.

Literature Box

Weisburg, M.R. (1988). Team work. Building productive relationships. In Reddy, W.B., & Jamison, K., eds. Team Building Blueprints for Productivity and Satisfaction. Alexandria, VA: NTL Institute for Applied Behavioral Sciences, San Diego, CA: University Associates, pp. 62-71.

Building productive relationships in the workplace is critical to team success. Increasing productivity requires observing team members at work and unlearning deeply ingrained, self-limiting assumptions about individual effort and authority that work against cooperation. In some respects this is an ongoing process of renewal that cannot occur without some disarray and confusion.

Implications for Practice

Every team member must deal with three key issues: (1) Am I in or out? (2) Do I have any power and control? (3) Can I use, develop, and be appreciated for my skills and resources? These issues must be addressed periodically if trust, motivation, and commitment are to be maintained in the team. Differences of opinion must be expressed constructively with honor and respect for each other.

Appreciation for Individual Skills

It is important for all to feel as though their skills and tools and contributions are needed and valued and that they are respected for what they have to offer to the work place/team/group. Everyone has weaknesses, and there is no need to emphasize these or to spend time in ongoing correction. Rather, focus should be placed on people's strengths, specifically, acknowledging and emphasizing what people do well.

Part of focusing on people's strengths is being willing to acknowledge peers, faculty, and the other significant people in one's life. In contrast, many role models focus on correction. Consequently, many of us spend a large portion of our time correcting others rather than appreciating people for all the wonderful things they are. It is almost as though we believe there is a finite number of available acknowledgments and we must not give out too many of them as they must be held in reserve for very important events. In addition, we do not always give acknowledgments in a way they can be received and valued. Box 17-3 can serve as a guide for giving **acknowledgment.**

To deal with the three personal issues discussed in this section, it is critically important that team members learn how to state openly what is on their minds and that they be responsive and respectful as other members of the team do the same. In other words, give and receive feedback constructively. There are essential elements that must be in place for people to be able to give and receive feedback in constructive ways.

Box 17-3
Guidelines for Acknowledgment

1. Acknowledgments must be specific. The specific behavior or action that is appreciated must be identified in the acknowledgment. For example, "Thank you for taking notes for me when I had to go to the dentist. You identified three key points that appeared on the test."
2. Acknowledgments must be "eye to eye" or personal. Look the person in the eye when you thank them. Do not run down the hall and say "Thanks" over your shoulder. Written appreciation also qualifies as "eye to eye."
3. Acknowledgments must be sincere, from the heart. Each of us recognizes insincerity. If you do not truly appreciate a behavior or action, do not say anything. Insincerity often makes people angry or upset, thus defeating the goal.
4. Acknowledgments are more powerful when they are given in public. Most people receive pleasure from public acknowledgment and remember these occasions for a long time. For people who are shy and believe they would prefer no public acknowledgment, there is an opportunity to work on a personal growth issue with them. Public acknowledgment is an opportunity to communicate what is valued.
5. Acknowledgments need to be timely. The less time that elapses between the event and the acknowledgment, the more powerful and effective it is and the more the acknowledgment is appreciated by the recipient.

Exercise 17-4

Within the next 3 days find three opportunities to acknowledge a peer or acquaintance using the five "Guidelines for Acknowledgment" shown in Box 17-3. In addition, do at least one self-acknowledgment using the guidelines.

Group Agreements

One of the most helpful tools available is to have the team come to an agreement about the ground rules concerning how they will be in relationship to one another (Mears, 1997). There are various ways that this can take place. There are even multiple kinds of guidelines or rules that can be used to set the context for how people will be. One example of a set of guidelines can be found in Box 17-4. These are called "The Rules of the Game." They have gone through multiple transitions and redesign, but the basic tenets are pretty much the same. People must agree on the goals and mission in which they are involved. In addition, they have to reach some understanding of how they will be together. Such tenets or rules as "We will speak supportively" go a long way to avoid gossip, backbiting, bickering, and misinterpreting other people. As you review these group agreements, keep in mind that a part of this process is the willingness of members of the team to be accountable for upholding the agreements and to give feedback when the agreements have been violated. When there are no rules, people have implicit permission to behave in any manner they choose toward one another, including angry, hurtful acting-out behavior.

Trust

Trust is the basis by which leaders/managers facilitate the activities and the progress of the team. Hogan defines leadership as "the ability to persuade a group to set aside individual preoccupations in order to pursue a common goal, and leadership should be evaluated in terms of how a group performs vis a vis the other groups with which it competes" (1997, p. 1). Hogan concludes that the essential task of leadership is to build high-performance teams. Thus the key sign that leaders/managers are performing poorly is the degree to which their team members don't trust them.

Trust is also a major issue among group members, and one of the first questions to come up in the group is who can one trust or not trust. In the early days of organizational development, McGregor (1967) defined trust in the following way:

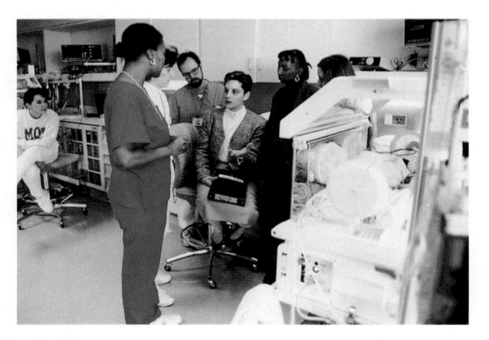

Working cooperatively, an effective team produces extraordinary results that no one team member could have achieved alone.

Box 17-4

"Rules of the Game" for Women's and Children's Hospital, Rush-Presbyterian–St. Luke's Medical Center

These "Rules of the Game" were adapted from a San Francisco real estate broker who was the founder and president of Hawthorn-Stone. Dr. Karren Kowalski proposes that we use them, not only among ourselves, but with each new person who joins the organization, asking if we/they are willing and able to do the very best we/they can to support the rules.

1. BE WILLING TO SUPPORT RUSH'S PURPOSE, GAMES, RULES, AND GOALS
   By first asking if people will support the rules, we have their agreement that they can be held accountable for times when they violate the "rules of the game."
2. SPEAK SUPPORTIVELY
   This means no swearing; if it doesn't serve, don't say it; if it doesn't support, don't say it; don't make other people wrong; you may choose *not* to say negative things. Language either empowers or limits people in terms of achieving their potential. How we speak about a colleague, the institution, our job, the work place, etc., does make a difference.
3. CORRECT SUPPORTIVELY
   Dr. Kowalski says, "Make corrections *without* invalidation or correct without crucifixion."
4. ACKNOWLEDGE THAT WHATEVER IS BEING COMMUNICATED IS TRUE FOR THE SPEAKER AT THAT MOMENT
   Most of the time people make comments because they truly believe them. Therefore it is important not to judge what is being said and misinterpret it, but to listen so that we can understand what is being said. Emphasis is on active listening.
5. COMPLETE YOUR AGREEMENT
   Only make agreements that you intend to and are willing to keep. This is especially important for those who (a) procrastinate and (b) say "yes" to everything. If one must break an agreement, communicate this information ASAP.
6. IF A PROBLEM ARISES, FIRST USE THE SYSTEM FOR CORRECTIONS, THEN COMMUNICATE THE PROBLEM WITH OPTIONAL SOLUTIONS TO THE PERSON WHO CAN DO SOMETHING ABOUT THE PROBLEM
   This is another way to eliminate gossip, judgment, and self-righteousness.
7. BE EFFECTIVE AND EFFICIENT
8. OPTIMIZE EVERY EVENT—CREATE MORE WITH LESS
   Items 7 and 8 go together. Look for value in every event. Focus on what *can* be learned or done; use "lateral thinking" to create effective options.
9. HAVE THE WILLINGNESS TO WIN AND TO ALLOW OTHERS TO WIN
   "Win/lose" is a "zero sum game." Effective problem solving allows everyone to win—to get their needs met.
10. FOCUS ON WHAT WORKS
    The converse is, get beyond what's not working. Be willing to try something new. When it's broke, fix it!
11. WHEN IN DOUBT, CHECK OUT FEELINGS
    When there seem to be blocks to communication or progress, it is often related to how people are feeling. Check this out, ask the person/people in question. Get the feelings out in the open where they can be checked out, tested, responded to.
12. AGREE TO DISAGREE UNTIL REACHING CONSENSUS
    Commit to working together toward mutually agreeable solutions. This keeps things in a forward motion without judgment. It keeps things hopeful.
13. TELL THE TRUTH FROM THE POINT OF VIEW OF PERSONAL RESPONSIBILITY
    Always begin with the assumption that you are willing to assume 50% of the responsibility. This eliminates "you, you, you" messages and allows you to work with others toward a solution, not toward blame.

Adapted from Thurber.

Trust means: "I know that you will not—deliberately or accidently, consciously or unconsciously—take unfair advantage of me." It means, "I can put my situation at the moment, my status and self esteem in this group, relationship, my job, my career, even my life, in your hands with complete confidence." (p. 163)

One can see from this description how critical trust is within a team. The leader role-models trust through behaviors such as setting the ground rules by which the team will function and holding team members accountable for adhering to the rules. It is also important to remember that trust is probably the most delicate aspect within relationships and is influenced far more by actions than by words. In other words, what people do is more powerful than what they say. Trust is a fragile thread that can be severed by one "act." Once destroyed, trust is more difficult to reestablish than its initial creation. What you *do* is more powerful than what you say.

▌ CREATING SYNERGY

Teams function with varying levels of effectiveness. The interesting part of this is that effectiveness can be systematically created. Truly effective teams are ones in which people work together to produce extraordinary results that could not have been achieved by any one individual (Mears, 1997). This phenomenon is often described as **synergy.** In the physical sciences, synergy is found in metal alloys. Bronze, the first alloy, was a combination of copper and tin and was found to be much harder and stronger than either copper or tin separately. Neither could the tensile strength of bronze be predicted by merely adding the tensile strength of tin and of copper.

We see the same properties of synergy in human endeavors, for example, in the 1980 United States hockey team. Many people can remember this hockey game, in which the United States defeated the Russians. The team consisted of a bunch of kids, none of whom could establish a successful career in the National Hockey League. However, for 2 weeks they were the best hockey team in the world. That was because they knew how to work together to produce extraordinary results. Likewise, Jackson (1995) describes the creation of this same synergistic kind of team in his book about coaching the Chicago Bulls basketball team.

To consistently create synergy, one must follow some basic rules:

- Establish a clear purpose.
- Listen actively.

- Be compassionate.
- Tell the truth.
- Be flexible.
- Commit to resolution.

Establish a Clear Purpose

Creative synergy requires a clear purpose. Each member of the team must understand the reason they are together, determine what he or she wishes to accomplish (as delineated by defined goals and objectives), and express his or her belief in both the value and feasibility of the goals and tasks. Teams function best when the members can not only tell others about their purpose but also define and operationalize succinctly the meaning and value of this purpose.

Listen Actively

Listening actively means that one is completely focused and tuned into the individual who is speaking. It means listening without judgment. It means listening to the essence of the conversation so that you can actually repeat to the speaker most of the speaker's intended meaning. It means being 100% present in the communication. It does *not* mean developing a defensive response or argument in your head while the other person is still speaking. To listen actively, a person must be absolutely focused on the speaker, absorbing words, posture, tone of voice, and all the clues accompanying the message, so that the intent of the communication can be received. Specific principles used in **active listening**, including examples, are found in Table 17-2.

Be Compassionate

To be compassionate means to have a sympathetic consciousness of another's distress and a desire to alleviate the distress. Consequently, it is inappropriate to focus time and energy on making the other person wrong, especially when your perspective differs from his or hers. It means listening from a caring perspective—one that is focused on understanding the viewpoint of the other person rather than insisting on the "rightness" of one's own point of view.

Tell the Truth

To tell the truth means to speak clearly to personal points and perspectives while acknowledging that they are, merely, a personal perspective. If an observation is made about the tone or behavior of a speaker that has an impact on the ability of others to hear the message, feedback can be provided in a way that does

Table 17-2	ACTIVE LISTENING
Use of Active Listening	**Examples**
To convey interest in what the other person is saying	I see! I get it. I hear what you're saying.
To encourage the individual to expand further on his or her thinking	Yes, go on. Tell us more.
To help the individual clarify the problem in his or her own thinking	Then the problem as you see it is . . .
To get the individual to hear what he or she has said in the way it sounded to others	This is your decision, then, and the reasons are . . . If I understand you correctly, you are saying that we should . . .
To pull out the key ideas from a long statement or discussion	Your major point is . . . You feel that we should . . .
To respond to a person's feelings more than to his or her words	You feel strongly that . . . You do not believe that . . .
To summarize specific points of agreement and disagreement as a basis for further discussion	We seem to be agreed on the following points . . . But we seem to need further clarification on these points . . .
To express a consensus of group feeling	As a result of this discussion, we as a group seem to feel that . . .

not make the speaker wrong. This is accomplished in an objective rather than subjective manner using neither a cynical nor a critical tone of voice. To be effective, it is important to own—be responsible for—personal opinions and attitudes.

Be Flexible

Flexibility and openness to another person's viewpoint are critical for a team to work together well. No single person has all the right answers. It is, therefore, important to acknowledge that each person has something to contribute and must be heard. Flexibility reflects a willingness to hear another team member's point of view rather than being committed to the "rightness" of a personal point of view.

Commit to Resolution

To commit to resolution means that one can agree to disagree with someone even when that perspective is different. Rather than assuming the person is wrong, this is a commitment to hear his or her perspective, listen to the real message, identify differences, and creatively seek solutions to resolve the areas of differences so that there can be a common understanding and shared commitment to the issue. Both parties need to then agree that they feel heard and agree to

the resolution. This differs greatly from compromise and majority vote as seen in the democratic process. When compromise exists, there is acquiescence or relinquishing of a significant portion of what was desired. This generally leaves both parties feeling negative about themselves or the agreement. Consequently, most compromises must be reworked at some future date. Working on conflict and its resolution (Table 17-3) is time-consuming yet essential to effectively functioning teams (Ersenhardt, Kahwajy, & Bourgeois, 1997).

Synergy cannot occur when one team member becomes a self-proclaimed expert who has the "right" answer. Synergy also cannot occur when people refuse to speak. Each team member has good ideas. These need to be shared. They are not shared, however, when someone feels uncomfortable in the team. It is a stretch to speak up and appear wrong or inadequate. The challenge each person faces is to push through discomfort levels and become a full participant in problem identification and resolution for the overall benefit of the team.

Our society tends to be dualistic in nature. **Dualism** means that most situations are viewed as right or wrong, black or white. Answers to questions are often reduced to yes or no. As a result, we some-

Table 17-3	ASPECTS OF CONFLICT	
Destructive	**Constructive**
Diverts energy from more important activities and issues	Opens up issues of importance, resulting in their clarification
Destroys the morale of people or reinforces poor self-concepts	Results in the solution of problems
Polarizes groups so they increase internal cohesiveness and reduce intergroup cooperation	Increases the involvement of individuals in issues of importance to them
Deepens differences in values	Causes authentic communication to occur
Produces irresponsible and regrettable behavior such as name-calling and fighting	Serves as a release for pent-up emotion, anxiety, and stress
	Helps build cohesiveness among people sharing the conflict, celebrating in its settlement, and learning more about each other
	Helps individuals grow personally and apply what they learn to future situations

Adapted from Hart (1980).

times forget there is a broad spectrum of possibilities. It is important to exercise creativity and explore numerous possibilities. This will allow the team to operate at its optimum level.

We have all known people who were self-proclaimed experts, to whom it was critically important that they be right and acknowledged as right, who become judgmental of others whose perspective and opinions differ from theirs. Consequently, it is important when creating a synergistic team to be able to tell the truth to these individuals and to encourage them to stretch and look at different ways of functioning. This requires good negotiation skills and conflict resolution skills, something for which few of us have been trained. If self-proclaimed experts think we are judging them, they will not hear the questions, the observations, or the "truth" because the message is delivered by making them wrong rather than originating from compassion. The most valuable contribution an individual can make to an organization is a passionate commitment to the creation of synergistic teams.

THE VALUE OF TEAM BUILDING

The value of team building is to enhance functioning in any one or all of the processes identified by Dyer (1987):

- the setting of goals or priorities
- the allocation of the way work is performed
- the manner in which a group works: its processes, norms, decision making, and communications
- the relationships among the people doing the work

When things are not going well in an organization and there are problems that need to be resolved, the first intervention people think of is "team building." Naturally, for teams (a collection of people relying on each other) to be effective, they must function smoothly. The difficulty is that when organizations are feeling stress and facing difficulties, they generally do not have teams whose members function well together. Team building can address any one of the activities identified above, depending on the available time and other resources. A team-building consultant can teach a team how to set goals and priorities; help a team analyze the distribution of the work load using various team members' strengths; examine a team's process, norms, decision-making, and communication patterns; and promote resolution of interpersonal conflicts or problems within the team.

Regardless of which areas are problematic, appropriate assessment of the team is essential. The problems may be in priority or goal setting, allocation of the work, team decision-making, or interpersonal relationships among the members. The success of the team depends on its members and its leadership.

Team building has grown out of an area of social psychology that focused on group dynamics. In the late 1950s and early 1960s group dynamics centered on an entity called training groups or "T" groups. As is often the case with new technology, some people did not have positive experiences with "T" groups and, as a result, such groups acquired a questionable reputation. The notoriety focused on the confrontational style and lack of sensitivity in sharing observations and information. People within the groups felt they were considered to be wrong about various behaviors, attitudes, and activities. As a result, distrust often predominated.

In examining group dynamics, Dyer (1987) found two major problems with "T" groups: (1) Much of the research was done with strangers who had no history with one another and could focus only on what was happening in the present. In contrast, work groups within corporations are not made up of strangers but rather of people who have a long history with each other. The "T" group trainers were not clear about what areas to explore and what areas to leave alone. (2) "T" groups were done with strangers who then dispersed and never met again. Consequently, there was safety in anonymity. In contrast, work units that continued intact after the sessions contained people who had to be responsible for interpersonal relationship issues raised in the "T" group meeting.

With all this heavy baggage about "T" groups, it is understandable that anxiety exists concerning the safety of being vulnerable and exposed if personal issues are revealed. That's why it is helpful for the team-building facilitator to make a thorough assessment of major issues and the willingness on the part of members to work on issues. Frequently, trainers or facilitators will interview members of the team individually to discover what the critical issues are. The kinds of questions that might be asked are found in Box 17-5.

This kind of tool enables the leader of the team to understand what the issues are before going into the team-building exercise so that he or she is not surprised nor becomes defensive. It also gives the facilitator some sense of what the major issues are within the group so that he or she has a better understanding of how to work with the group.

Box 17-5
Interview Questions for Team Building

1. What do you see as the problems currently facing your team?
2. What are the current strengths of your institution or work group? What are you currently doing well?
3. Does your boss do anything that prevents you from being as effective as you would like to be?
4. Does anybody else in this group do anything that prevents you from being as effective as you would like to be?
5. What would you like to accomplish at your upcoming team-building session? What changes would you be willing to make that would facilitate a smoother-functioning team and accomplishment of the team goals?

MANAGING EMOTIONS

Probably one of the greatest fears in team-building exercises is that people will become emotional, that they will lose control of themselves or the environment or they will appear weakened or vulnerable. Men have a particularly difficult time with this fear, but many women also want to appear in a good light and are hesitant to be open and vulnerable. When one is considering Bocialetti's (1988) maxim that "the whole person comes to work," the team and its leadership must define how this will be developed for them. Although many people acknowledge that we are all thinking and feeling persons, management/leadership is usually more willing to deal with the "thinking" side than the "feeling" side of individuals within the team.

Because people spend such a large percentage of their time in the work setting, it would be unrealistic to believe that they always and continually appear in an unemotional and controlled state. Human beings simply do not function that way. What is observed is people's aspirations, their achievements, their hopes, and their social consciousness; they are observed falling in love, falling in hate and anger, winning and losing, and being excited, sad, fearful, anxious, and jealous. Consequently, these "feelings" are important components of organizational life and do much to undermine work effectiveness. Most of us know of situations where, because of an emotional disagreement, two individuals have avoided each other for years. Because of the power of emotions and the inevitability of their presence, their impact on interpersonal relationships, and their influence on productivity and the quality of work, emotions should be a high priority when examining the functioning of the team.

According to Bocialetti (1988), people are sensitive to what happens when emotions are revealed. When people yell or get angry or upset, and when goals, objectives, and tasks are disputed, employees see the following:

- a member intimidating and frightening others within the group
- embarrassment
- a member overstating or exaggerating one's view in order to appear right
- provocation of defensive and hostile responses
- overconcern with one's self—self-absorption
- gossip
- loss of control
- a member distracting others from "real work"
- disruption or termination of relationships within a group

These are behaviors that destroy any hope of creating a smoothly functioning team, one that supports its members to grow and learn and provide quality patient care. On the other hand, the cost of suppressing emotions or "feelings" includes:

- physical and psychological stress
- withdrawal from participation
- loss of energy and depression
- reduction of learning
- hiding of important data because of fear
- festering problems and emotions
- preventing others from being acknowledged
- decreasing motivation
- weakening the ability to receive constructive feedback
- the loss of one's influence

These kinds of outcomes lead to the conclusion that suppressing emotions at work is neither healthy nor constructive for team members.

When emotions are handled appropriately within the team, there are several positive outcomes that have impact on the work setting. One creates a sense of internal comfort with the workings of the team and the organization. When stress is lowered and kept at lower levels on the average, problems are much more easily resolved. It is similar to releasing steam slowly with a steam valve rather than having the gasket blow. Interpersonal relationships on the team are more stable and people have a sense of closer ties and collegiality when emotions are handled. There are fewer negative relationships or interactions, which results in more effective and pleasant working relationships all around.

Work group effectiveness improves when the team is functioning smoothly and emotions and "feelings" are being handled on a routine basis rather than waiting for a volcanic eruption. Problems of withdrawal, boredom, and frustration are much less likely to overwhelm the team and lead to its breakdown. The skills and tools previously discussed (e.g., speaking supportively) are the basic tools one needs to handle the emotional aspects of the team. Choosing to cope with emotional upset must be a conscious choice, one that requires practice to improve the skill.

THE ROLE OF LEADERSHIP

Teams usually have a leader. In addition, teams function within large organizations that have leaders. Without the approval and the support of the leader, team building, which can be a costly endeavor in terms of consultation fees as well as work time and resources of the team, is difficult to undertake and of questionable effectiveness. Although very strong teams may be able to educate themselves regarding some of the issues, such as establishing goals and priorities or clarifying their own team process, it is exceedingly difficult to address any kind of relationship issue among team members without a more objective outside party facilitating the process.

Because leadership is such a pivotal part of smoothly functioning teams, it is illuminating to examine leaders more carefully. Truly progressive leaders understand that leadership and followership are not necessarily a set of skills; rather, these are qualities of character, a manifestation of a person's own being. On speaking specifically to leadership, we are not talking about "putting on a role." In actuality, leaders realize more fully their capacity for influence, risk taking, and decision making. Leadership, and to some degree followership, is as much about character and development as it is about education. According to Peter Vaill (1989), leadership is concerned with bringing out the very best in people. For leaders who truly believe this, team building is a natural outgrowth of this value. This type of leader understands that the very best in a person is tied intimately to the individual's deepest sense of himself or herself, to one's spirit. The efforts of leaders must touch the spiritual aspect in themselves and others. Warren Bennis (1989) once said that leaders simply care about more people. Consequently, this caring manifests itself in doing whatever it takes to improve team functioning. This may imply involving oneself in team building with the team. The risk in such an endeavor is that the team leader is open to being vulnerable, to being judged by others, and to being wrong. However, if the leader has role modeled the "rules of the game" and has held people to account for these rules as well as holding himself or herself to account, the team-building exercise will not degenerate into judging and laying blame.

If true leadership is about character development as much as anything, then character development is also beneficial for "followers"—that is, members of the team. The areas of character development often addressed include communication, particularly those aspects of speaking supportively that avoid laying blame and justifying and enhance understanding the other person's message. Box 17-6 highlights an example of character development, which the chapter author relates from her own Vietnam experience.

Leaders understand the multiple aspects of the issue of control. They take control of their lives rather than being at the mercy of others—victims. They have clarity regarding their own control issues. They focus time and energy primarily and almost exclusively on those issues, events, and behaviors over which they have control. Their activities are thus primarily focused on areas relating directly to them—not on world events or other happenings over which they have neither influence nor control.

Confidence, which loosely translates as faith or belief that one will act in a correct and effective way, is a key aspect of character. Thus it follows that confidence in oneself can be closely tied to self-esteem, which is satisfaction with oneself. The greatest deterrent to self-esteem and self-confidence is fear. Fear is described by some as "false evidence appearing real" (see box at right). Susan Jeffers (1987) believes the core fear—the one that rules our lives—is one of "I can't handle it." So the core of our fears is "I can't handle it," and it is exactly the opposite of being confident or holding oneself in high esteem. Working on self-confidence requires an attitude of belief, of confidence, of I "CAN DO" whatever is required (see Box 17-6) (Fisher & Thomas, 1996).

False Evidence Appearing Real

Simply caring about more people translates into a willingness to focus time and energy on members of the team. From one perspective, caring is risking being with someone and sharing both suffering and joy. Healing often emerges from caring. Behaviors that demonstrate caring include giving of oneself in terms of warmth and love and particularly giving one's time. The second aspect of caring is truly listening to team members and hearing and understanding them. The third aspect includes being 100% present for them. The fourth is to honor the other person—to see their wholeness, their possibilities, their hope.

It becomes clear that leading the team is not the easiest thing to do. But neither is being an active, fully participating member of the team. Both require taking risks, including being in a relationship. Being in a team-building experience and hearing those things that have not worked for people about their interactions with peers as well as with the leader can be scary but worthwhile. It requires a focus on personal and professional growth. It requires building character.

Box 17-6

The "Can Do" Brigade: An Army Nurse's Study in Character Development

As life events are reviewed, important or pivotal learning can be identified. One life event that significantly impacted me was the year I spent as an Army Nurse Corps officer in South Vietnam. This was the first time I remember an awareness and understanding of confidence in the face of incredible obstacles. I had spent the first 10 months of my nursing career in labor and delivery at Indiana University before volunteering for a guaranteed assignment to Vietnam. I went to Fort Sam Houston for 6 weeks of basic training where they taught me really important things like how to salute, how to march, and how many men in a battalion. No one ever asked me if I could start an IV or draw a tube of blood. This was important because Indiana University had the largest medical school class in the United States at that time and nurses did nothing that interfered with medical education. Therefore I had never started an IV or drawn blood. When I arrived in Saigon, they put me in a sedan with another nurse and sent me up to the Third Surgical Hospital, one not unlike the one in MASH. We even had a Major Burns—that was not his name but it was his function. Surgical hospitals receive only battle casualties; their purpose is to stabilize and to transport.

The Third Surgical Hospital was located in the middle of the 173rd Airborne Brigade whose job it was to defend the Bein Hoi Air Base, where all the sorties in the south were flown during the war. We were stopped at the gate by an MP who stepped up and saluted very snappily. He knew that a staff car must contain either a very high ranking officer or, if it was his lucky day, females.

While I was in Vietnam, 500 American women and 500,000 American men were there. He looked in the window, saluted snappily, and said "Afternoon, ma'am!" He wanted to know where we were going; he talked to us for a few minutes and assured us if there was anything he could do for us we should just give him a call. He saluted us and said, "CAN DO." I didn't understand because I didn't know that there are units with very high esprit de corps who attach snappy little sayings at the end of things like salutes, phone conversations, memos, and so forth.

The 173rd was the "CAN DO" brigade. When we got to the hospital and met the chief nurse, she took us down to the mess hall and introduced us to all the doctors and nurses. We were sitting and having coffee when the field phone rang in the kitchen and the mess sergeant yelled out, "Incoming wounded." Everybody got up and started to leave for the Preop area. I just sat there until the chief nurse said, "Come on." I said, "You don't understand, I deliver babies." She was not impressed! She took me by the arm and led me to Preop.

When we got there we discovered there weren't just a few incoming wounded, there were more than 30 and some were very seriously injured. She immediately told the sergeant to call headquarters battalion of the 173rd Airborne and tell them that the Third Surg needed blood. She turned to me and said, "Lieutenant, you are responsible for drawing 50 units of fresh whole blood." I was shocked! I had never drawn a tube of blood, but I found in the back section of "Preop" a Specialist 4th class who was already setting up "saw horses" and stretchers, putting up IV poles, and hanging plastic blood sets. I started to help and soon I heard trucks out back. I opened the door and looked outside. There were two huge Army trucks and out of the back of these were jumping kids, 17, 18, 19, and 20 years old. They were covered with red mud from the bottom of their boots to the tops of their helmets. I looked at them and I looked at the clean cement floor and in an instant my mother came to me. I put my hand on my hip and said, "Where have you boys been?" One PFC stepped forward and saluted me very snappily and said, "Ma'am, we just came in this afternoon from 30 days in the field, we have been out in the rice paddies chasing the Viet Cong, we have not had a hot meal, and we've not had a shower but Sergeant Major said the Third Surg needs blood!" He saluted smartly and said, "CAN DO!" They were very clear. After 30 days of chasing and being chased by the Viet Cong, giving a unit of blood was easy. "CAN DO!" They were confident. They were kids who had looked into the face of death. At that moment, I knew if they CAN DO, I Can Do! Life requires confidence; with confidence, you can make your dreams come true!

Exercise 17-5

The "Gordian Knot": A Team-Building Game

Gordian knot is a term sometimes used to describe a problem that cannot be solved. However, teamwork can sometimes solve seemingly impossible problems, as this game will illustrate.

In a group of 8 to 10 people, form a tight circle with your shoulders touching and your hands placed in the center. Take the hand of two other people across the circle from you. The goal is to unwind the knot until the entire circle is holding hands side by side. You *may not* let go of hands to unwind the knot unless your instructor gives you special permission to do so!

Debriefing

After your group has unwound its knot, together choose one or two categories of questions from Part I of the "Team-Building Discussion" outline that follows. Discuss these questions, writing down your answers as you go so that you can report to the class later. Be sure to support your answers with examples from your group's experience with the game. Then, complete all questions in Part II.

PART I

LEADERSHIP AND BUILDING TEAMWORK

What did it feel like not to have a designated leader? _____
Who became the leader? _____
How? _____
Did the leadership process work? _____
How did you feel about it? _____
Who came up with new ideas? _____
Did the team support this process? _____
How were conflicts resolved and problems solved? _____
How did you build a sense of teamwork? _____

TEAM MEMBERSHIP

Did you feel a part of the team? _____
Why or why not? _____
Did your team have a good mix of skills and abilities? _____
Did you adapt to the needs of others or to the needs of the team? _____
Did you meet your objectives without wasting time and energy? _____
What role did you play as a team member? _____

TRUST AND OPENNESS

What was the team's level of trust and open communication? _____
Great Deal = 10   Much = 7   Some = 5   Little = 3   None = 0
What contributed to this level of trust? _____
Did you deal with issues candidly and honestly? _____
What was your level of trust? _____
What would have increased the team's level of trust and openness? _____

CONTRIBUTION TO THE TEAM-DEVELOPING RELATIONSHIPS

Did you all know and agree to the mission of the team? _____
How were decisions made? _____
Who participated in making them? _____
When did you need to make decisions? _____
Were they primarily about what to do (tasks) or how to do it (process)? _____
Did you use each other as resources? _____
Did you work well together? _____
How did your relationships develop and strengthen? _____
How do you feel about each other now? _____

CULTIVATING A FEELING OF SATISFACTION ABOUT YOUR TEAM

Do you feel proud of your team? _____
How do/did you feel rewarded by being a member of this team? _____
Did you have fun? _____

Exercise 17-5—cont'd

Did the challenge cease to be fun? _____

How did the team handle this? _____

Are you satisfied with your results? _____

DEVELOPING THE TEAM THROUGH RISK TAKING

Did you, individually or as a team, try out any new or uncomfortable communications or behavior? Give examples.

_____

Did that feel safe? _____

Did you support each other in your risk taking? _____

PART II

EVALUATE AND SHARE WITH THE REST OF THE TEAM HOW YOU FEEL YOU DID AS A PARTICIPANT

Consider the following:

Was I active or passive? _____

Did I communicate clearly? _____

Did I take risks? _____

Did I support others? _____

Did I ask for help or support from others? _____

Was my behavior typical for me? _____

How would I do it differently? _____

Give each other honest and helpful feedback on the congruency of self-perception versus the perception of other team members.

Debriefing exercise courtesy of: Walter Kowalski
BreakThroughs, Inc., Englewood, CO

A Manager's Solution

❓ The first question that needed to be asked was "Were we committed to providing the most optimal care for the neonate?" In other words, why would teamwork be important in this situation? What's the vision or mission? After getting agreement among the NICU team, we strategized on how to create a "team" with the specialists. Getting clear on your intent is very important. A meeting with the director of the specialty, the NICU medical director, and nursing leadership was arranged. We discovered that we shared a common goal that was the best care possible for the baby. Keeping that goal as the focus, we then identified areas of mutual respect. From there, both sides were willing to listen to each other's concerns. Care guidelines could be identified as well as areas of responsibility. Ideas on how to improve the communication process were also discussed. A plan based on patient needs complete with agreements was implemented.

Were we a team yet? The answer is no. There was still a little skepticism and reserve. Everyone seemed to have a "wait-and-see" attitude. The first big chance was identified when the specialty group insisted a patient of theirs be admitted to NICU because they believed it was the best place for the baby to be. Another measurable outcome was having the agreements honored. This reinforced to everyone that their concerns had been heard and respected. Mutual trust was building, and a collegial relationship began. A year later, it is hard to imagine that this situation ever occurred. There is enthusiasm for this specialty's physicians and their patients. It is certainly a change in attitude.

There are many components to team building, but the most important component is to be clear about your mission and intention when working with potential team members. The intention to provide the best care possible assisted each one of us to be more open, creative, and trusting. These are all necessary components of team building. Remember, teams are made up of individuals. Ask yourself if you are willing to accept responsibility for your response and actions. Be the change that you want to see.

❓ *Would this be a suitable approach for you? Why?*

CHAPTER CHECKLIST

Nurse managers must help build teams. Although the manager does not have to lead the team, the manager must ensure that the group can function effectively as a team. The team members must be able to communicate with each other effectively, share a single mission, be willing to cooperate with each other, and be committed to achieving their objectives. Successful teamwork requires leadership, trust, and willingness to take risks.

■ A team is a highly interdependent group of people that:
  • Has defined goals and objectives
  • Has an ongoing relationship
  • Is focused on accomplishing a task
■ Attributes of effective teams include:
  • Clarity of purpose
  • Informality
  • Participation
  • Listening
  • Civilized disagreement
  • Consensus decisions
  • Clear roles and work assignments
  • Shared leadership
  • Diversity of styles
  • Self-assessment and self-regulation
■ Each team member deals continually with three questions:
  • Am I in the "in" group or the "out" group?
  • Do I have any power or control?
  • Can I use, develop, and be appreciated for my skills and resources?
■ Focusing on team members' strengths and acknowledging what they do well are two of the keys to team building.
  • To be effective, acknowledgments must be:
    – Specific
    – Personal
    – Sincere
    – Timely
    – Public
■ One of the most helpful tools for teams is a set of ground rules that govern how members will interact with each other.
■ Trust is essential for successful teamwork.
■ Synergy allows a team to produce results that could not have been achieved by any one individual. Creating it requires:
  • Active listening
  • Compassion

  • Honesty
  • Flexibility
  • Commitment to resolution of conflicts
■ Managing emotions is a key strategy in team building.
■ Leadership is a pivotal part of a smoothly functioning team.
  • Leadership relies on personal character development as much as on education.
  • Confidence is a key aspect of the leader's character.
    – A "can do" attitude is one of the most important confidence-building strategies a leader can adopt.
■ Taking a risk and experimenting with a new behavior is the most effective way to change behavior.

TERMS TO KNOW

acknowledgment	group
active listening	synergy
commitment	team
dualism	

TIPS FOR TEAM BUILDING

■ Commit to the purpose of the team.
■ Develop team relationships of mutual respect.
■ Create and adhere to team agreements concerning function and process.
■ Build trust.

REFERENCES

Bennis, W. (1989). *On Becoming a Leader.* Reading, MA: Addison-Wesley.

Bocialetti, G. (1988). Teams and management of emotion. In Reddy, W.B., & Jamison, K., eds. *Team Building Blueprints for Productivity and Satisfaction.* Alexandria, VA: NTL Institute for Applied Behavioral Sciences. San Diego, CA: University Associates, pp. 62-71.

Dubnicki, C. (May-June, 1991). Building high-performance management teams. *Healthcare Forum Journal,* pp. 19-24.

Dyer, W. (1987). *Team Building Issues and Alternatives.* Reading, MA: Addison-Wesley.

Ersenhardt, K., Kahwajy, J., & Bourgeois, L. (1997). How management teams can have a good fight. *Harvard Business Review,* July-Aug, 77-85.

Fisher, B., & Thomas, B. (1996). *Real Dream Teams: Seven Practices Used by World Class Team Leaders to Achieve Extra Ordinary Results.* Delray Beach, FL: St. Lucia Press.

Hart, L.B., (1980). *Learning from Conflict.* Reading, MA: Addison-Wesley.

Hogan, R. (1997). What we know about leadership. *Academic Leader,* 13 (12), 1.

Jackson, P. (1995). *Sacred Hoops: Spiritual Lessons of a Hardwood Warrior.* New York: Hyperion.

Jeffers, S. (1987). *Feel the FEAR and DO IT Anyway.* Columbia, NY: Fawcett.

Lopes, S. (1987). *The Wall.* New York: Collins.

McGregor, D. (1960). *The Human Side of Enterprise.* New York: McGraw-Hill.

McGregor, D. (1967). *The Professional Manager.* New York: McGraw-Hill.

Mears, P. (1997). *Healthcare Teams: Building Continuous Quality Improvement.* Boca Raton, FL: St. Lucia Press.

Parker, G.M. (1990). *Team Players and Teamwork.* San Francisco, CA: Jossey-Bass.

Thurber, M. *Hawthorne-Stone Real Estate:* San Francisco, CA.

Vaill, P. (1989). *Managing as a Performing Art.* San Francisco, CA: Jossey-Bass.

Weisburg, M. (1988). Team work: Building productive relationships. In Reddy, W.B., & Jamison, K., eds. *Team Building Blueprints for Productivity and Satisfaction.* Alexandria, VA: NTL

Institute for Applied Behavioral Sciences. San Diego, CA: University Associates.

■ SUGGESTED READINGS

Barr, O. (1993). Reap the benefits of a cooperative approach. *Professional Nurses,* 473-474.

Dubnicki, C. (May-June, 1991). Tuning up your team. *Healthcare Forum Journal,* 34, 25-28.

Francis, D., & Young, D. (1979). *Improving Work Groups: A Practical Manual for Team Building.* San Diego, CA: University Associates.

Jeffers, S. (1992). *Dare to Connect: Reading Out in Romance, Friendship and the Workplace:* Columbia, NY: Fawcett.

Nanus, B. (1992). *Visionary Leadership.* San Francisco, CA: Jossey-Bass.

Schmieding, N.J. (1993). Nurse empowerment through context structure and process. *Journal of Professional Nursing,* 9, 239-245.

Sibbet, D., & O'Hara-Devereaux, M. (1991). The language of teamwork. *Healthcare Forum Journal,* 34, 27-30.

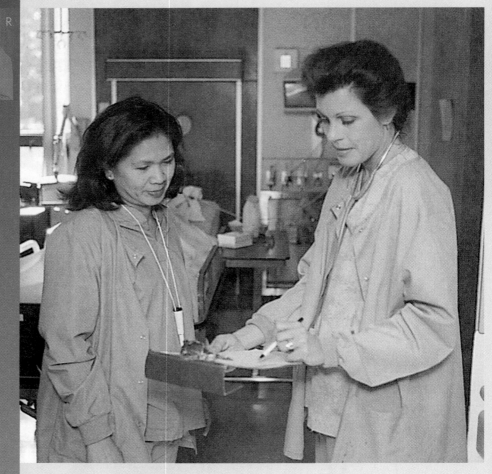

Delegation: An Art of Professional Practice

**Patricia S.
Yoder-Wise**
RN, C, EdD,
CNAA, FAAN

Delegation is a complex process that can be quite effective in accomplishing work. This chapter defines various aspects of delegation, including legal perspectives and how to make delegation decisions. The emphasis is on the role of the nurse as delegator, irrespective of the formal position an individual may hold.

Objectives

- Define delegation and its component parts.
- Describe how tasks and relationships influence delegation to a specific individual.
- Value the legal authority for a registered nurse to delegate.
- Value the complexity of decision making.

Questions to Consider

- How does a registered nurse make delegation decisions?
- How complex is delegation?
- When is it appropriate to delegate?
- To whom can tasks be delegated?
- What can be delegated?

A Manager's Challenge

From the Director of Nursing of a Mental Health and Mental Retardation Hospital Located in the Southwestern United States

One evening, while working as the charge nurse on a mental health unit, I assigned the admission of a patient well known to me to a registered nurse new to our unit. I knew the patient being admitted had an extensive history of self-mutilation; in fact, several months earlier she had self-mutilated during hospitalization with a razor hidden in the sole of her tennis shoe. I communicated to the admitting nurse to "be careful" with the admission. A couple of hours after the admission was complete, the patient was found by staff to have engaged in self-mutilating behavior. When I questioned the patient, she stated she had hidden a small razor under an adhesive bandage she had secured to her arm.

What do you think you would do if you were this manager?

INTRODUCTION

Delegation is a complex, loophole-ridden, work-enhancing strategy. It can make the difference between caring for a group of patients and experiencing great anxiety and caring for that same group with a controlled expectation of what can be achieved. Used properly, it can enlarge the impact you have on patient care; used improperly, it can be frustrating and scary. Delegation is an art and a skill, which can be developed and honed into one of the most effective professional management strategies. Each of the following sections is designed to foster the best of delegation.

HISTORICAL PERSPECTIVE

Until the early 1970s, registered nurses were quite familiar with the art of delegation. Most care occurred in acute care hospitals, which were staffed by registered nurses (RNs) (mostly diploma graduates, frequently prepared in the hospital in which they worked), licensed practical/vocational nurses (LP[V]Ns), and nurse aides (commonly called unlicensed assistive personnel today). Staffing ratios were such that it was not uncommon for relatively few registered nurses to be present on a nursing unit. Direct care was provided primarily by LP(V)Ns and the aides. Of course, while there were a few complex procedures, the direct care provided was related primarily to physical comfort and to what today would be termed "simple treatments."

As care became far more intricate and the monitoring demands and expectations placed on nursing increased, it was logical to move to a higher ratio of RNs. Thus, during the two decades of the 1970s and 1980s, many nurses entered the profession with relatively limited experience or knowledge about the details of delegation—there was no one in the clinical area to whom one could delegate anything related to patient care except the basic physical care. Sometimes even that was dealt with by the professional staff.

In the mid-1990s a dramatic shift from primary nursing (an all-professional staff concept) to a multi-level nursing staff occurred. As a result, it has become critical to address the topic of delegation in some detail again. This, however, is not a return to delegation as it was known earlier. In part, the difference today is based on the sophisticated demand for cost containment and reduction and the new complexities

301

that are present in healthcare today. As the healthcare industry emphasizes community-based care, the challenge of delegation, and the resultant supervision, becomes even more difficult. The increase, especially in unlicensed assistive personnel, has in the past related to a shortage of nurses. Today's use of such staff relates to lowering costs. However, when Krapohl and Larson (1996) reviewed the literature from 1988 to 1994 about support personnel in nursing, they concluded, "No empirically strong evidence was found to confirm that nursing support personnel improved quality or increased nurse and patient satisfaction" (p. 108). Furthermore, these studies could not demonstrate cost impact.

Barnum (1994) summarizes this historical flow using three sets of variables: "1. a *patient*-orientation versus a *task* orientation, 2. the number of caregivers assigned to each patient (a continuum from one, to a few, to many), and 3. the total quantity of resources available to the nursing organization" (p. 403). In essence, Barnum says we change from the ideal of one-to-one care when resources are plentiful and with equal facility embrace a group of caregivers when that is the better resource approach to use. So our flexibility to alter how we function based on the changes we find has allowed nursing to survive and sometimes thrive.

▌ DEFINITION

Delegate, or **delegation**, is defined as follows:

- To transfer the work to your subordinates (Marrelli, 1997, p. 146)
- Getting work done through others or as directing the performance of one or more people to accomplish organizational goals (Marquis & Huston, 1992, pp. 254-255)
- To assign responsibility and authority for performing tasks (functions, activities, or decisions) to individuals (Sullivan & Decker, 1992, p. 216)
- "Turning over authority and responsibility for doing a job to a subordinate; and explaining the 'what' and 'why' of a selected problem or job, while leaving the 'how' to the subordinate" (Coburn & Sturdevant, 1992, p. 32)
- "To transfer responsibility for the performance of an activity from one individual to another, with the former retaining accountability for the outcomes" (American Nurses' Association, 1994, p. 11)

Each of these definitions contains at least two people (a **delegator** and a **delegatee**), work, and

some kind of transfer of authority to perform some work. None of these definitions suggests it is an abdication of responsibility for the overall outcomes or performance or the abdication of the need to be involved. This is an important point, since it is sometimes difficult to remain in touch with others who are completing work on behalf of a manager of care.

A definition of delegation then might be as follows: *achieving performance of care outcomes for which you are accountable and responsible by sharing activities with other individuals who have the appropriate authority to accomplish the work.* Acceptance of the delegated work must occur, either passively (that is, no protest occurs) or actively (that is, communication indicates acceptance). Thus delegation only can occur when two people are involved in a mutual work situation, and one of the persons has accountability and the other has some authority for performing specific tasks. As an example, when two RNs work together sharing activities, delegation does not occur. On the other hand, if one RN has specific accountability for an outcome and that nurse asks another RN to perform a specific component of the overall function, that is delegation. Delegation also occurs when an RN assigns a licensed practical (vocational) nurse (LP[V]N) or unlicensed assistive personnel (UAP) (defined by the American Nurses' Association [1994, p. 2] as unlicensed people "trained to function in an assistive role to the registered professional nurse in the patient/client activities as delegated by and under the supervision of the registered professional nurse") to perform a specific function or aspect of care. Authority is a critical component. It may be designated by law, such as the nursing practice act, or it may be designated by educational preparation/certification. Typically, a position description further defines what the nature of the authority is for a specific position.

Achieving Performance Outcomes

Achieving performance outcomes is the driving force of all healthcare. If what anyone does has little or no benefit to improving the delivery of care, it is, of course, ineffective. Therefore all care is based on attaining expected outcomes, whether that care is provided directly by an individual or group of professionals or whether that care was shared between professionals and assistants. Performance of care outcomes relates to the profession's keeping its trust with the public, that is, to perform safely and competently. In ever-changing healthcare settings, it is critical to know that you must delegate in order to achieve all that is expected of you. In essence, this means that if you cannot trust others or if you are frustrated because you cannot do it all yourself, the way in which healthcare is delivered will be very frustrating or your career opportunities will be fairly limited.

Accountability and Responsibility

The terms "accountability" and "responsibility" refer to the legal expectation the state has vested in persons with the designation of RN. **Accountability** means that someone must be able to explain actions and results. Legally the RN is accountable for nursing care. **Responsibility** refers to reliability, dependability, and obligation to accomplish work. Responsibility also refers to each person's obligation to perform at an acceptable level. Thus the assistant, whether a UAP or an LP(V)N, is obligated to perform at acceptable levels that which the assistant can perform. That person is also responsible for informing the delegator what limitations, if any, would prevent the accomplishment of expected outcomes.

Sharing Activities

Sharing activities may sound simplistic; however, when someone with the legal accountability for a role shares elements, that individual is not giving away role elements. That individual is sharing activities or functions to ensure total outcomes. Therefore the delegation definition here emphasizes that care itself is not delegated; only elements (activities) are. Sharing may consist of many strategies ranging from asking an assistant to perform a specific task, to expecting the same performance as the day before. For delegation to be effective, the RN must accept that sharing activities is important and that there are benefits to patient care.

The professional, technical, and amenity (PTA) model (Hansten & Washburn, 1994) is a useful framework for determining which activities may be shared. Amenity (hotel-like service factors) may almost always be delegated. Certain technical tasks may be delegated if the delegatee is appropriately qualified and the circumstances don't warrant a different approach. Professional aspects may never be delegated. Each aspect is important in the total care; and each can be measured. For example, patient surveys often address amenity factors, flow sheets frequently document technical factors (or specific reports note deviations), and broader responses such as patient behavior are reflective of the professional aspects.

Other Individuals

Other individuals may include persons with no formal preparation or recognition (for example, UAPs), those with dependent status (such as LP(V)Ns who function under the direction of a physician or RN) or others who are designated as being accountable to the delegator (for example, other RNs or healthcare providers who report to a designated delegator such as a nurse manager).

Span of control is an important concept to keep in mind when interacting with others to achieve care. This term refers to how many people you have responsibility for. For example, if a nurse has responsibility for five staff, each of whom cares for 10 patients, the nurse has responsibility for five staff and 50 patients. This may not be as overwhelming as it may seem at first if the patients are in stable condition and their needs predictable; if the staff are well prepared, experienced providers of routine care; or if the geographic area is restricted. On the other hand, if each of these factors is not true of a situation, this responsibility may be overwhelming. Thus, if elements of care are rendered by others, it is important to assess each of these factors to know how manageable the situation is.

Appropriate Authority

Appropriate authority to perform certain functions stems from various sources. For example, the practice of LP(V)Ns is defined by state titling or practice acts as well as institutional policies. UAPs, such as certified nursing assistants, are prepared to meet a specific set of functions. That, coupled with institutional policies, defines what UAPs may do. Position descriptions may provide more specific insight about the authority designated in certain positions. In essence, the term *appropriate authority*, as used in the definition above, refers to a baseline indicator that some other individual is expected to be able to perform certain aspects of care and therefore may receive an assignment to execute those aspects.

It is probably important to note that the American Nurses' Association (ANA) differentiates between direct and indirect delegation (1995). The difference relates to whether the RN is actively deciding what to delegate (direct) or whether the decision is based on organizational protocols that designate certain tasks as appropriate for others to perform (indirect). Even when organizational protocols indicate someone else may perform a task on behalf of the RN, it is still important to know if the employee is competent to perform the tasks. This expectation suggests that the delegator will make initial and ongoing assessments related to the delegatees' performance.

Three elements of nursing may not be delegated (ANA, 1995). They are initial nursing assessment, and subsequent ones, requiring professional judgment; determination of nursing diagnosis, care goals, plan, and progress; and interventions that require professional knowledge and skill.

A FRAMEWORK FOR DELEGATION

One way to consider the concept of delegation can be found in Hersey and Blanchard's original work about leadership styles (1988). (See the theory box below.) These researchers explained leadership behavior in the context of two factors: ability and willingness. In essence, the greater the ability and willingness of the delegatees, the more likely it is that the delegator could use delegation as the strategy for interacting with that person in a specific situation. In other words, both the amount of guidance (task behavior) and the amount of support (relationship behavior) would be relatively low. This seems logical for established work relationships. But not all situations are established. For example, it is possible that a delegatee has limited knowledge and ability to perform a task. Such a situation would require more guidance. If the relationship is limited, that is, these two people are unlikely to work together again, it is likely that the delegator would simply tell the individual what to do and how to perform. Hershey and Blanchard call this "tell." In another instance, however, there may be only a new task, that is, the relationship is an ongoing one or the relationship will become such. Then the researchers found that the best strategy is to explain what to do and how to do it. This option is labeled "sell." Logically, if producing outcomes in a given situation is the driving force, delegators are much less likely to expend additional time and effort investing in a casual, limited relationship than they are in one that will be repeated. A final behavior described by these researchers is called "participate." This behavior is appropriate for situations when the delegatee has abilities and willingness, but the relationship is relatively new (Figure 18-1). In other words, in such situations it is important for both the delegator and the delegatee to determine mutual expectations and conditions of performance.

Each of these behavior styles is evident in real work situations. Davis and Farrell (1995) say effective delegation has a foundation on a personal relationship of mutual trust. For example, when a new team begins to work together, the first thing the delegator needs to evaluate is the ability and willingness of the delegatee, and this must be based on trust. If those factors are low, the delegator has two ways to interact with the delegatee: tell or sell. If the nature of the relationship is limited, for example, the delegatee has been reassigned from one service to another for this day only, telling is the appropriate strategy. Little, if any, time is lost on interaction, and a fair amount of guidance is provided. On the other hand, if the relationship is an ongoing or developing one, it will be important for the delegatee to gain the necessary ability and/or comprehend the motivation related to the situation. Thus selling or explaining is the appropriate strategy. While this strategy is more time consuming, the interaction leads to a more supportive relationship.

When the delegatee has a high degree of ability and willingness and the expected task is familiar,

Situational Theory		
THEORY/KEY CONTRIBUTORS	**KEY IDEAS**	**APPLICATION TO PRACTICE**
Hersey and Blanchard (1988) created this theory to explain how leader/managers need to behave differently.	A wise leader analyzes how an individual interacts in a specific situation. The analysis consists of the sophistication of the employee and the task itself and the need for interaction. A leader then responds differently based on this analysis.	Treating people equally is unfair. Before delegating, an RN must know what a specific employee needs in a specific situation.

little guidance is needed. If the relationship is new or developing, more support is needed, so the delegator and delegatee need to interact in a participating mode. This approach helps each learn more about the other and contributes to advancing to the most developed situation where true delegation is possible; that is, the delegatee is willing and able, needs little guidance, and needs relatively little support to accomplish work. Such behavior is evident in cases where people have worked together in the same situations for some time. The delegatee knows what needs to be done, what needs to be reported, how to prioritize, and when to ask for help.

Delegation can be viewed as a spectrum of behaviors based on the context and needs in a specific situation. Knowing how to interact with a given delegatee is one of the key challenges of a delegator if effective outcomes are desired. The Research Perspective, page 306, describes one study of nurses' indirect care intervention that includes the task of delegation.

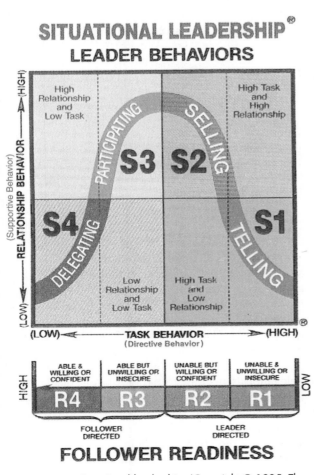

Figure 18-1   Situational leadership. (Copyright © 1985. The Situational Leadership model is the registered trademark of The Center for Leadership Studies, Escondido, CA. All rights reserved. Used with permission.)

ASSIGNMENT VERSUS DELEGATION

Assignment transfers both responsibility and accountability. This strategy is most common when one registered nurse assigns a patient/client to another. While nurses typically refer to the way work is distributed as an assignment, in reality, some portions of the work distribution are delegated care not assigned. Thus UAPs receive delegated activities while RNs receive assigned care/assignments. Table 18-1 depicts the differences.

IMPORTANCE OF DELEGATING

"We accomplish all we do through delegation—either to time or to other people. If we delegate to time, we think efficiency. If we delegate to other people, we think effectiveness." (Covey's *The 7 Habits of Highly Effective People Calendar*—September 29, 1995)

To accomplish care in a timely manner, delegation is a critical skill. It clearly saves time in the long run and, when effective, is very cost-effective. At its worst, however, it is exceedingly costly. Therefore making the best decisions about care is imperative. One of the misperceptions about the profession of nursing that has been a plague is to think of nursing care in terms of psychomotor tasks. It is important, therefore, for professional nurses to convey the consistent message that doing a task is one component of care. Even though the performance of a psychomotor task is critical, the critical analyses "behind the scenes" are clearly the precipitator of the actions.

"Nobody can do everything. Everybody knows this. But many people, especially women, don't like

Table 18-1	DELEGATION VERSUS ASSIGNMENT	
Aspect	**Responsibility**	**Accountability**
Delegation	yes	no
Assignment	yes	yes

Research Perspective

McCloskey, J.C., Bulechek, G.M., Moorhead, S., and Daly, J. (1996). Nurses' use and delegation of indirect care interventions. Nursing Economics, 14, 22-33.

As the Nursing Interventions Classification (NIC) continues to develop, these researchers chose to study what has been termed the "glue role" of nurses, that is, making healthcare work. It isn't only the caregiver role of nurses that makes them invaluable in healthcare; it is also the integrator role. As changes in healthcare occur, the result is that the nurse's role as integrator is actually expanding.

Nurses (n = 171) were surveyed about indirect care interventions (n = 26). Respondents derived from 500 randomly selected members of the Academy of Medical-Surgical Nurses. The majority, as might be expected, worked in hospitals (95%). Delegation (80%) was exceeded only by documentation (97%) as a task respondents said they performed several times a day. Nurses who worked the night shift were found to spend significantly more time in these two tasks than nurses who worked other shifts.

"Overall, the nurses reported that they would *not* delegate the majority of the indirect care interventions" (p. 31). Additionally, the LP(V)N was viewed as the most useful assistant.

Implications for Practice
The more nurses know about how much time interventions consume, the better staffing needs can be predicted.

The indirect care interventions nurses perform enhance the success of direct care by all providers. This glue role provides for achieving quality outcomes. Whether a nurse is in a leader or a follower role, the glue role is an expectation of the nursing profession.

to delegate" (Reardon, 1995, p. 146). Why is this? (Of course this is important to nursing, a profession that is composed of over 90% women.) According to Reardon, "A preference for relational equity makes it difficult for them to use status as a reason for assigning others projects they themselves do not want to do or have no time to do" (p. 146). So, while delegating is important, it may be more of a challenge for women than for men.

Hansten and Washburn (1994) identify five advantages of delegating. Patients receive more attention because there are more staff. Because all of the RN's time is not consumed with direct care activities, there is more time for what might be viewed as the professional component, such as managing and teaching. There is an increased sense of belonging. Overtime is reduced because the team is efficient and productive. Finally, nurses report that they feel less pressure because they don't have to do everything alone. Those advantages suggest that delegation has direct patient and professional benefits.

Seldom should a decision to delegate be based on time-saving considerations alone, but the truth is that in an effective team, delegation can be an effective time conservation technique.

Exercise 18-1

Ask a staff nurse and a nurse manager about their individual perspectives of the pros and cons of delegation. Do they fit with the themes at the end of the chapter? Now ask a UAP employee the same questions.

LEGAL AUTHORITY TO DELEGATE

Most state practice acts address the concept of delegation; some explicate rules and regulations governing what may be delegated and when. State boards of nursing are vested with protecting the public; therefore they regulate practice and the educational preparation required to practice nursing. It is this expectation that specific knowledge about nursing and delegation is needed to perform safely that makes the nurse legally accountable, and thus liable. As Huston (1996) points out, this new role increases the scope of liability for the registered nurse.

Legally the concept of delegation is a complex one. First, the individual doing the delegation is personally responsible for prudent action. If delegation is not performed within acceptable standards, malpractice may be the outcome. Additionally, according to Guido (1995, p. 45), "failure to delegate and supervise within acceptable standards may extend to direct corporate liability for the institution." Furthermore, "whenever care is provided by other than a registered nurse, the accountability for care remains with the manager [of care]/delegator even though others provide various aspects of care" (Yoder-Wise, 1995, p. 219). This view of professional liability is consistent with the fact that state licensure conveys both privilege and expectations.

Exercise 18-2

Review your state nursing practice act, rules, and regulations. Discuss with two or more classmates what your state provides as direction about delegation. What conclusions can you reach?

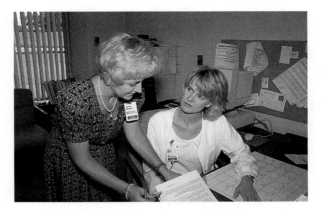

Nursing managers face complex decisions involving patients and staff.

SELECTING THE DELEGATE

In many settings, you are one of several professional staff members who have the authority to delegate; therefore you probably will not be able to select the person who will work with you. On the other hand, a few opportunities may occur in your career when you have this chance to select your own assistant. If you do, consider three factors that Marquis and Huston (1992) identify: "Select someone with a similar philosophy; choose an assistant with different strengths and weaknesses than your own; and select an assistant who can be a good follower" (p. 259). While those factors were described for an assistant manager, they make sense in terms of an assistant for an RN who manages the care of a group of patients. For example, an assistant who does not concur with you about the goals of hospice might actually work at counter purposes to the organizational philosophy. Additionally, if the assistant is like you in terms of strengths and weaknesses, you will both want to do the same things and to avoid the same things. Finally, if an assistant is not a good follower, you may spend more time than necessary in attempting to control delegated work. For example, an LP(V)N who has functioned in a physician's office for some time may not be used to working under the directions of an RN or having nursing care supervised.

SUPERVISING THE DELEGATEE

"Because the registered nurse is always accountable for assessment, diagnosis, planning, and evaluation, it is important that UAPs understand what elements of implementation they may carry out and why the registered nurse is responsible for analyzing data gathered" (Yoder-Wise, 1995, p. 219) "Supervision in its broadest context is the active process of directing, guiding, and influencing the outcome of an in-dividual's performance of an activity or task" (ANA, 1994, p. 9). Supervision consists of the initial direction (the delegation) and periodic inspection (reassessment and evaluation) (Hansten & Washburn, 1994). Both elements must be present to ensure effectiveness in entrusting an element of care to someone else.

DELEGATION DECISION MAKING

"Many people refuse to delegate to other people because they feel it takes too much time and effort and they could do the job better themselves. But effectively delegating to others is perhaps the single most powerful high-leverage activity there is" (Covey's *The 7 Habits of Highly Effective People Calendar*—September 30/October 1, 1995).

Considering how much information must be processed to make a sound decision about delegation, it is logical that a specific matrix has been devised to make the process consistent. Although the original work was performed in critical care settings, it is easy to see why several factors can drive all decisions. Deciding to delegate, what to delegate, and to whom requires an active decision-making process.

In 1990 the American Association of Critical Care Nurses (AACN) identified the factors in the list below as ones that require active decision making before delegating a component of care:

- Potential for harm
- Complexity of task
- Need for problem solving and innovation
- Unpredictability of outcome
- Level of interaction with patient

These factors are accompanied by a rating scale of 0 (better outcome of delegation) to 3 (less desirable outcome). In essence, when no risks are likely, each of the above five factors would be rated with zeros. When risks are great, however, a score approaching 15 would be likely. Realistically, the experienced RN may take only a few minutes or less to reach a conclusion about what can be delegated. On the other hand, RNs in beginning competence levels may need to carry a reminder to be sure to consider all factors, and that decision may take longer. When new staff are incorporated, or when the RN changes practice settings, the thought process may be more deliberate.

Potential for Harm

Potential for harm refers to the possibility that in the performance of a task or function something might negatively affect the patient. Thus the more unstable the patient's condition is, the more potential there is for harm. As a result, when there is greater potential for harm, either there is less desirability to delegate care elements or the amount of close supervision is increased.

Complexity of Care

Complexity of care is a similar factor; that is, if care is less complex, it is more likely that someone with less preparation can safely provide care. If, on the other hand, the care is complex, there is greater risk in delegation. As a result, an RN may want to delegate only a few elements of care—those that are the least complex. Additionally, the delegation may be more specific; the delegatee would have less individual determination of how to perform the delegated care. An example might be when several tasks need to occur in sequence and some of them are very detailed and others are relatively simple. The RN might specify exactly when some task must be done and how.

Need for Problem Solving and Innovation

Need for problem solving and innovation relates to whether the delegatee will need to figure out how to modify care or find new strategies for performing the func-

tions. This factor is important in any situation, but it is critical when supervision is less direct. Such is the case with most community-based care. If being able to establish (invent) individualized care is important, the RN may determine that only a professional staff member may deliver care until the care pattern is established. The more experienced the assistant, the more likely that individual also has significant experience in innovating aspects of care.

Unpredictability of Outcome

Unpredictability of outcome refers to how like the "textbook picture" this particular care situation is. When predictable outcomes are fairly certain, for example, with established treatments with a given patient population, it is more likely that it is safe to delegate care elements. On the other hand, new treatments may mean that nursing is yet in the stage of determining what the outcomes are likely to be. Therefore delegation may not be the best option.

Level of Interaction

Level of interaction with the patient refers to such aspects as the need for psychosocial interactions and educational strategies. Again, while many delegatees can provide both, it may be necessary to establish the expected interactions or it may be possible to delegate only a component of the interaction.

Exercise 18-3

Select three clients from a clinical facility where you have been assigned recently. Use the AACN decision-making approach to determine a rating for those clients. Based on your rating, would you delegate care for any of the clients? What is your rationale?

Integrating Factors

Combining these factors into an integrated whole for making decisions is valuable. It is possible that one factor may be the overriding element. For example, when the potential for harm is great, the other factors may be relatively less influential. Thus reaching decisions about what to delegate, when, and to whom is a complex process.

Sullivan and Decker (1992) describe a five-stage delegation process. Briefly, the five stages involve (1) determining what could be delegated; (2) evaluating the delegatee's fit with tasks to be performed; (3) deciding what to delegate and what level of supervision is needed; (4) delegating; and (5) providing feedback. Each of these stages depends on the preceding one. Each is necessary to ensure safe, accountable delegation.

Providing *specific feedback* about performance is the best strategy for shaping future behavior. Therefore statements such as "you performed that procedure with ease" are more effective than saying "nice job." Equally important is the feedback from the person performing the tasks. Was the work completed? How did the patient respond? What changes were noted? These are examples of what the RN must know from the person who performed the delegated portion of care.

Whenever possible, provide positive feedback; however, it undermines your credibility to convey satisfaction when the performance is less than desirable. Therefore *being honest* about feedback is the best strategy. Goleman (1995) suggests using the "artful critique," which "focuses on what a person has done and can do rather than reading a mark of character into a job poorly done" (p. 153). In other words, being honest about the circumstances and performance and what we can do to change them helps the person develop for the future.

Finally, it is important to remember that some individuals occupy positions for which they are not qualified. One strategy for dealing with this is to lower your expectations so that the individual can be successful. Before doing that, however, it will be critical to think about the effect on others. For example, why is one employee held to the standard and another is not? Who becomes responsible for accomplishing the work the one person cannot achieve? Is it fair to compensate for someone who cannot meet performance expectations? What are the potential liabilities of altering the standards of performance? Reaching decisions about delegating elements of care is a complex process. One model includes identifying the required nursing tasks and the patient's problems and evaluating the abilities of various staff to make an appropriate decision (Conger, 1993). When the professional nurse knows the individual is incapable of appropriate performance and does not intervene, the potential for liability increases. Even eliminating the legal questions, ethical considerations should influence the nurse (ANA, 1976).

The National Council of State Boards of Nursing (1995) proposed five rights of delegation as (1) the right task, (2) the right circumstances, (3) the right person, (4) the right direction/communication, and (5) the right supervision. Keeping these in mind enhances success when delegation occurs.

DELEGATION PROCESS

Unless you are well established at delegation or unless you work consistently with only persons you know well, you will need to plan how to delegate in order to be effective. Table 18-2 provides a decision tree for delegation. The first step involves professional accountability. If an RN has not assessed the patient, delegation should not occur. This step ensures that an RN has determined baseline data and needs. Only if the delegatee is properly prepared to accept a specific delegation should the RN proceed to delegate.

Exercise 18-4

Think about what you could delegate, then use the delegation communication template found in Box 18-1 to practice with a classmate the transfer of specific responsibilities for care.

In settings other than those of confined geography, such as hospitals, long-term care facilities, and clinics, one of the greatest challenges of delegation relates to supervision. In such situations, it is especially important to be very clear about what is expected of the delegatee. Box 18-1 presents a communication template to use when delegating. The more that is understood between the delegator and the delegatee about a particular delegation situation, the greater the chances are of being effective in patient care.

Box 18-1
Delegation Communication Template

- State exactly what is being delegated and what the expected outcome is.
- Convey recognition of the authority to perform what is expected.
- Identify priorities.
- Acknowledge monitoring activities you may perform.
- Specify any performance limitations, such as time limits on performing a procedure.
- Specify deadline, including exact timing if that is important.
- Specify report time lines and data expected.
- Specify parameter deviations, including when immediate action must be taken.
- Identify appropriate resources, including people who may be consulted.
- Be clear about what may not be delegated.

Table 18-2 ┃ BOARD OF NURSE EXAMINERS DELEGATORY DECISION-MAKING TREE

Has the RN made an assessment of the patient's nursing care needs prior to delegation?
Yes ↓   No → Perform assessment

Is the unlicensed person identified and properly trained?
Yes ↓   No → Provide and document training

Does the reasonable and prudent RN believe the task is appropriate to delegate and can be performed safely by this unlicensed person?
Yes ↓   No → Do not delegate

Does the task require the unlicensed person to exercise nursing judgment?
No ↓   Yes → Do not delegate

Is the responsible RN available to provide adequate supervision?
Yes ↓   No → Do not delegate

Is the task appropriate for *routine* delegation to an unlicensed person according to Rule 218.9?
Yes → May delegate   No ↓

If the task is one that should not be *routinely* delegated, but may be delegated, are the additional criteria met as defined in 218.10(b)?
No → Do not delegate   Yes → May delegate

Is the task prohibited by Rule 218.7?
Yes → Do not delegate   No ↓

Is the task medication administration?
No → May delegate   Yes → Do not delegate unless exemption applies (Rule 218.8)

Is the task patient teaching or counseling?
No → May delegate   Yes → Do not delegate

a. Provide and document training for the specific task
b. Evaluate competency to perform task
c. Develop policies and procedures

Unlicensed person has no authority to perform task

Delegating practitioner supervises

RN must notify delegating practitioner

Tasks Delegated by Others
Has the task been delegated by another licensed practitioner?
Yes ↓   No → Unlicensed person has no authority to perform task

Is RN responsible for supervision?
Yes ↓   No → Delegating practitioner supervises

Has the unlicensed person been appropriately trained?
Yes ↓   No → RN must notify delegating practitioner

Rules Sections References
218.7   Nursing tasks that may not be delegated
218.8   Administration of medication
218.9   Specific nursing tasks that may be delegated
218.10   Nursing tasks that may not be routinely delegated

From Board of Nurse Examiners for the State of Texas, August 1993. Reproduced with permission.

PRACTICALITIES OF DELEGATION

Delegation clearly is a complex process, but there are some ways to simplify the process. For example, when it is possible, selecting the delegatee whose talents match the task is better than merely selecting a competent individual. In large organizations, this approach is possible; it is less likely to be so in smaller facilities.

Letting the delegatee implement the task in his or her own way can be a challenge. It is unlikely that someone else will do a task just as the delegator would. However, if no safety or ethical discrepancies are likely, delegation really is a matter of trust. If the delegator intervenes, the delegatee loses confidence or becomes frustrated and the delegator has lost the benefits of delegating.

Having deadlines helps keep the delegatee on target without oversupervising. Being clear about the need to check quality and effectiveness ensures that there will be ongoing monitoring.

Exercise 18-5

Using the assignments made by a nurse manager where you have a clinical experience, answer the following questions:

- Is it clear *what* is delegated? Why do you respond as you did?
- Were delegation decisions logical? Why do you respond as you did?
- From what you know about your nursing practice act and professional standards, do the assignments make sense legally and ethically? What is your rationale?

INTEGRATED CARE

In the late 1990s, care has moved from multidisciplinary, coordinated care to an integrated approach. Again, this provides an impetus for a multiskilled worker. Having someone who performs "what is needed now" for the patient or the professional staff is the focus rather than the "me and my assistants" approach. However, as McCloskey et al (1996) suggest, it is the nurse who will continue to provide the important "glue role" so that care achieves positive outcomes.

CHAPTER CHECKLIST

Delegation obviously is a complex issue. It has many facets, each of which by itself is complex. One of the critical roles of RNs is that of the "glue factor," where the RN coordinates care across the spectrum of providers and affects the quality of care. Current research suggests that many indirect care interventions would not be delegated by RNs because of these complexities and quality implications.

- Delegation involves achieving outcomes and sharing activities with other individuals who have the authority to accomplish work for which the delegator is accountable and responsible.
- The ways in which delegation can actually be enacted can be based on a situational leadership model.
- Nursing practice acts, rules, and regulations provide the legal structure for delegation; the *Code for Nurses* provides the ethical structure.
- Knowing the skills and abilities of the delegatees is critical to feeling comfortable and confident in delegation.
- The AACN framework for making decisions about delegation is comprehensive.

TIPS FOR DELEGATING

- Be familiar with your nursing practice act and the corresponding rules and regulations.

A Manager's Solution

❓ The nurse to whom I had assigned the admission was very upset; she felt that the self-mutilating behavior might have been prevented if she had "been more careful." My responsibility for the incident was apparent. Instructing someone to "be careful" was not adequate instruction, especially since I was aware of the patient's history for self-mutilation. I met with the admitting nurse to discuss this with her and my intent to communicate more thoroughly when I assigned future work. This incident improved my delegation skills and strategies. Now when I delegate or assign, I indicate not only what is being delegated but the information needed to do the job correctly. Delegation that results in positive patient outcomes depends on good communication; talk to your staff!

❓ *Would this be a suitable approach for you? Why?*

- Ascertain the skills of unlicensed assistive personnel to whom you may delegate tasks.
- Assess your patients with the perspective that some of their care will be provided by others.
- Use the communication template to enhance successful delegating.
- Use a decision-making screen, such as the one developed by AACN for critical care patients, to determine what can be delegated to unlicensed assistive personnel.
- Evaluate on a regular basis your effectiveness in delegating to others.

■ TERMS TO KNOW

accountability   delegator
delegatee   responsibility
delegation

■ REFERENCES

American Association of Critical Care Nurses (1990). *Delegation of Nursing and Non-Nursing Activities in Critical Care: A Framework for Decision Making.* Laguna Viquel, CA: American Association of Critical Care Nurses.

American Nurses Association. (1976). *Code for Nurses.* Kansas City, MO: American Nurses Association.

American Nurses Association. (1994). *Registered Professional Nurses and Unlicensed Assistive Personnel.* Washington, D.C.: American Nurses Association.

American Nurses Association. (1995). *The ANA Basic Guide to Safe Delegation.* Washington, D.C.: American Nurses Association.

Barnum, B.S. (1994). Realities in nursing practice: A strategic view. *Nursing & Health Care,* 15, 400-405.

Coburn, J.M., & Sturdevant, N.J. (1992). The acquisition of delegation skills: Collaboration between education and service. *Nurse Educator,* 17(6), 32-34.

Conger, M.M. (1993). Delegation decision making: development of a teaching strategy. *Journal of Nursing Staff Development,* 9, 131-135.

Covey, S. (1995). The Covey Calendar.

Davis, J.M., & Farrell, M. (1995). Factors affecting the delegation of tasks by the Registered Nurse to patient care assistants in acute care settings: A selected review of the literature. *Journal of Nursing Staff Development,* 11, 301-306.

Goleman, D. (1995). *Emotional Intelligence.* New York: Bantam Books.

Guido, G.W. (1995). Legal and ethical issues. In Yoder-Wise, P., ed. *Leading and Managing in Nursing.* St Louis: Mosby.

Hansten, R.I., & Washburn, M.J. (1994). *Clinical Delegation Skills: A Handbook for Nurses.* Gaithersburg, MD: Aspen Publishers, Inc.

Hersey, P., & Blanchard, K.H. (1988). *Management Organizational Behavior,* 5th ed, Englewood Cliffs, NJ: Prentice Hall.

Huston, C.L. (1996). Unlicensed assistive personnel: A solution to dwindling health care resources or the precursor to the apocalypse of Registered Nursing? *Nursing Outlook,* 44(2), 67-73.

Krapohl, G.L., & Larson, E. (1996). The impact of unlicensed assistive personnel on nursing care delivery. *Nursing Economics,* 14, 99-109.

Marquis, B.L., & Huston, C.J. (1992). *Leadership Roles and Management Functions in Nursing: Theory and Application.* Philadelphia: J.B. Lippincott.

Marrelli, T.M. (1997). *The Nurse Manager's Survival Guide: Practical Answers to Everyday Problems.* St Louis: Mosby.

McCloskey, J.C., Bulechek, G.M., Moorhead, S., & Daly, J. (1996). Nurses' use and delegation of indirect care interventions. *Nursing Economics,* 14, 22-33.

National Council of State Boards of Nursing (1995). Delegation: Concepts and decision-making process. *Issues,* 16(4), 1-4.

Reardon, K.K. (1995). *They Don't Get It, Do They?* Boston: Little, Brown, and Company.

Sullivan, E.J., & Decker, P.J. (1992). *Effective Management in Nursing.* 3rd ed. Redwood City, CA: Addison-Wesley.

Yoder-Wise, P. (1995). *Leading and Managing in Nursing.* St Louis: Mosby.

■ SUGGESTED READINGS

Barter, M., & Furmidge, M.L. (1994). Unlicensed assistive personnel: Issues relating to delegation and supervision. *JONA* 24(4), 36-40.

Barter, M., McLaughlin, F.E., & Thomas, S.A. (1997). Registered nurse role changes and satisfaction with unlicensed assistive personnel. *JONA,* 27(1), 29-38.

Bernreuter, M.E. & Cardona, S. (1997). Survey and critique of studies related to unlicensed assistive personnel from 1975-1997, Part 1. *Journal of Nursing Administration,* 27(6), 24-29.

Bernreuter, M.E. & Cardona, S. (1997). Survey and critique of studies related to unlicensed assistive personnel from 1975-1997, Part 2. *Journal of Nursing Administration,* 27(7/8), 49-55.

Hanston, R., & Washburn, M. (1996). Why don't nurses delegate? *JONA,* 26(12), 24-28.

Minnesota Nurses Association (1997). *Position Paper: Delegation and Supervision of Nursing Activities.* St Paul: The Association.

Parkman, C.A. (1996). Delegation: Are you doing it right? *American Journal of Nursing,* 96, 43-48.

■ APPENDIX

The Best and the Worst of Delegation

The following lists were derived from suggestions made by the participants in the North Carolina Center for Nursing's Leadership Seminar held in September, 1995 in Raleigh, NC.

Best

- The best of delegation is when the organization functions well with each person believing that his part is vital to the well-being of the whole (Sally Harris).

- Reasonable expectations; leader facilitates; the task/job/goal is completed satisfactorily; all of those working as a part of the team are instilled with a sense of ownership of the goals; the leader serves as a resource person to team members, and takes on part of the task but doesn't take on so much that they can't be there as that resource (Patricia Heatherley).
- May lose control; afraid to delegate; have time for more important things, not routine things; raise morale of staff; help staff to grow; help to motivate staff (Sharon Williams).
- Focus on people. Activity will happen with aims and goals. Delegate with planning process in mind—from need and opportunity to evaluation using knowledgeable input of groupings "to trial" and evaluation to establishing policy and teaching/communication to entire community with proper follow-up (Ruth-Marie Rosser).
- Delegate to another something you really want to do, but know they will do a better job (Candace Hughes).
- Delegate the primary nurse with the responsibility of telling her patient the "Chemo" treatments are completed and throwing a party to celebrate (Glenda George).
- Comment on the positive attributes a person has that are needed to get a job done and *then ask* for their assistance; "With you on this job, I know it will get done"—The person knows you have confidence in them; always be firm and direct in an emerging situation; use eye contact and facial expressions to relay the importance of a task or job that is needed; respect the person's responsibilities while realizing why *this* job is a priority. "I know you're busy but I really need your expertise and skills" (Susan D. Freeman).
- Prepare and know your task well—know the strengths and weaknesses of the people you work with and delegate the proper tasks to the people with the appropriate strengths for successful outcomes (Marsha Beard).
- Use all members of the team as participants in a well-directed way (Rebecca S. Pettit).
- When the outcome is . . . the delegated (doer) feels (as well as knows) his/her task was a definite contribution no matter how trivial the task is (Vanena Stewart).
- Realizing that others *can* do just as well as yourself and can add refreshing ideas. ("If you want it done right do it yourself" can produce burn out and exhaustion) (Laura Blackman).
- You can accomplish more; increase involvement of others (Cathy Gage).

- Treating people with respect and treating them as if they can handle the delegated job (Lynn Bryant).
- Accomplish many tasks; work together; have fun! (Debbie Hennessee).
- The person doing the delegating having confidence in the person being given a task—but also who remains as a resource for that person (Mary Ann Morgan).
- To have power and resources and knowledge and feedback needed to delegate. To have back-up for what I do from the person who delegated to me (Anna West).
- The task you have delegated has been accomplished to your satisfaction (Sheila Stewart).
- Work completed on time with more and new ideas (Bessie Yates).
- Promote a team atmosphere in all things—delegate to those willing to do the task and who are capable (Juanita S. Bethune).
- To delegate something and everyone involved does what is expected of them (Candi Hinson).
- Know what can be delegated; know the person I am delegating to; know with (little doubt/no doubt) that delegated task/job will be done and done correctly (Frankie Raleigh).
- Delegating a task to a new person and having that person do a beautiful job. A person who states he/she knows what to do (Montie E. Pakowski).
- Delegate to someone who really wants to do the task. She may not know exactly how or what to do but if she wants to do it she will seek out the appropriate resources or find help to complete the task (Valarie Gatlin-Best).
- Delegate a task—the person being delegated to does not feel demeaned; be consistent—delegate certain tasks to certain people; stimulate personnel by encouraging others; be open, honest; when looking at the picture as a whole . . . look for positives/not negatives (Debbie Kenedy).
- Seeing others succeed (Tracey Weeks).
- Delegate a task—accept the way that a group or individual completes that task/decisions made even if you feel it could be done "BETTER"—or you could do it a different way. This fosters a sense of accomplishment, personal/professional growth for that individual or group (Linda Rankin).
- Saves time for the delegator and allows more time for higher functions (Janet Reaves).
- What was delegated has been completed and done well (Frances P. Gullyes).
- Always telling personnel how to perform delegated task (Jewell Mabery).

• After gardening (i.e., watering, weeding, fertilizing, pruning, nurturing) a staff member to grow him/her to a ripe level of ownership and sense of responsibility, delegation takes place from within that individual. A flower seed will germinate without being told if given the proper environment (Dawn A. Wascoe).

• Having a leader who will actually do the task if necessary, not just expect it to be done (Karen W. Lineberry).

• You acknowledge to someone that you respect them enough to share in responsibility, trust enough to give someone the "glory" (David N. Currin).

• Be truthful, let others participate; give task—allow others to design how; allow freedom (JoPierce Schuchardt).

• Encouragement and listening; being a role model; don't be negative; be self-oriented and open-minded; be excited! (Mary Ann Turner).

• Things that were delegated and done (Helen D. Flowe).

• RNs can get to the jobs that only RNs can do (Kimberly E. Carr).

• Being able to accomplish more by delegating (Ella Bryant).

• Sharing the responsibility/work load/joys of the task involved (Edith Boland).

• You get another's input in getting the task done (Diane Yorke).

• Decide if it's best for you to take on some of the work load as well. Sometimes it is—sometimes it isn't. Time constraints may be an issue. The characteristics of the group you're working with are, too. Followers expect delegation out of a leader (Kimberly C. Calloway).

• Good news—a praise; giving a pat on the back (Joy Moss).

• Provides opportunities to increase others' skills and knowledge (learn from each other); provide opportunities to increase communication skills; get more done; instill encouragement, motivation in others (Kathy G. Clark).

• Delegate the *right* task to the *right* person at the *right* time using *right* communication techniques and giving positives (feedback) *right* back! (Andrea Novak).

Worst

• When that which is delegated is not what each person feels equipped to do and when the leader takes all the credit for everything that goes right and none of the responsibility when things go wrong (Sally Harris).

• Unreasonable expectations; leader dictates; goal(s) not attained; no one knows what they are doing or why; there are members on the team who feel they are doing much more of the work than others (Patricia Heatherley).

• Delegate and then "forget" the delegated activity and the person to whom it was assigned (Ruth-Marie Rosser).

• Delegate to another without explanation of expected outcome, goals—then finding fault with results (Candace Hughes).

• Having to delegate to a person the responsibility of telling the patient he can't go home but has to go to a nursing home (Glenda George).

• "Go do this now!" (Susan D. Freeman).

• A leader who embraces the "martyr syndrome" attitude is someone who feels "no one can do this task better than I," therefore this leader does not delegate, or when he or she does delegate it is poorly and sometimes even with resentment (Marsha Beard).

• Feel guilty putting the task off on others who already have too much to do (Rebecca S. Pettit).

• When the outcome is: the delegatee (doer) feels or perceives he/she has been forced to complete a task of little or no value with either too much direction or no direction (Vanena Stewart).

• Depending on someone else to do their part (Cathy Gage).

• Ordering people around, not asking (Lynn Bryant).

• Negative attitude; poor performance (Debbie Hennessee).

• Poor communication when delegating a task (Mary Ann Morgan).

• To be delegated with no power to get the resources that are needed. To be expected to delegate without enough information or power (Anna West).

• The person to whom the task was delegated was unable to accomplish the task due to lack of expertise (Sheila Stewart).

• Work not completed because persons stated did not understand instruction or what was needed. They did not return to clear up their misunderstanding of the project (Bessie Yates).

• *Assume anyone* can do every task (Juanita S. Bethune).

• When delegating—not having the support of your supervisor; nonverbal communication; tone of voice (Candi Hinson).

• To delegate a task to someone who could do the task, yet chooses not to do so nor to say he/she is not going to do the task (Frankie Raleigh).

• Delegating a task to a person who has qualifications but doesn't understand how to do it and tries to do it without asking for help (Montie E. Pakowski).

• Delegate to a friend for a task mainly because he/she is a friend, not because he/she has the credentials and/or experience (Valarie Gatlin-Best).

• "Hurry up! I want it now! So I'll just do it myself. . . ." Delegation goes down the drain (Bev Ellis).

• Delegating all tasks at or below person's level (job description)—not stimulating person's potential; not working as a team (Debbie Kenedy).

• Being responsible for wrong decisions or actions; not pleasing everyone (Tracey Weeks).

• Delegate a task—but end up doing it yourself because you thought that individual did not do it as you feel it should be done, or criticize decisions made or the way the task was done. Sometimes it is difficult to relinquish control—a good leader does not need to control (Linda Rankin).

• Poor attitude.

• Fear of rejection/being disliked (Janet Reaves).

• *What* was delegated was done poorly or not at all (Frances P. Gullyes).

• Not utilizing staff to maximum potential because always pulling the more educated staff members down (Jewell Mabery).

• Giving orders may get someone to do a "job" at that moment, but it will not get him/her to continue doing that "responsibility" when not being observed (Dawn A. Wascoe).

• A leader who is "talk" only. He/She does not have the experience to understand what does and does not work (Karen W. Lineberry).

• You ask yourself, can someone else do this as well as I? And will that reflect on me? (David N. Currin).

• One who must control all; one who never makes mistakes (JoPierce Schuchardt).

• Not being able to listen, discourage new ideas; not be enlightened by ideas. "It is not those we heal that make a difference, it is those we understand" (Mary Ann Turner).

• Things that were delegated and *not* done (Helen D. Flowe).

• Nurses who like to do total care for their patients no longer can because they are expected to "delegate" to others those tasks that do not require an RN. This decreases the opportunity for the RN to interact with the patient—opportunities that RNs can use for teaching and assessment (Kimberly E. Carr).

• Having to delegate to someone who is not very reliable but you find it necessary to include him/her (Ella Bryant).

• Trying to get everyone to do their "fair" share (Edith Boland).

• You get another's input in getting the task done! (Diane Yorke).

• Not delegating and doing it yourself—this makes others feel as if you don't trust them—plus it causes more stress and work for you (Kimberly C. Calloway).

• Not following up on a task you've delegated (whether it be to assess completion of the task and/or to express appreciation to the delegatee) is perhaps the worst (and most common) mistake in delegation. Just Not Doing It! (Christina Griffiths).

• Getting someone to do what even I don't want to do (Joy Moss).

• Tell someone exactly how to do the project; state "You will do this or else"; frequently interfere; do not allow self-expression—creativity; delegate in a negative manner; give impression it's something you are not interested in or don't want to do yourself; be unavailable when needed (Pamela R. Blue)

• If task is delegated inappropriately, may be viewed as "dumping" work; resistance to cooperation, more stress; person being delegated to may feel overwhelmed, unmotivated (Kathy G. Clark).

• Delegate a task, then follow that person around observing and/or making comments/suggestions while this person is performing the assigned task (Andrea Novak).

Top Tips for Delegation

1. If someone else can do as well as you can and wants to do it, by all means, let him (S. Harris).
2. Remember where the person you're delegating to is coming from, i.e., don't deliberately set someone up for failure and still provide an opportunity for challenge in the task you want them to accomplish. Most important: the reason we're not alone in the world is to get help from others! (D. Yorke)
3. Never ask someone to do something that you are *not* willing to do yourself; know the people that you are delegating to and match the tasks with their skills and talents; and *always, always, always* thank people for completing tasks and praise a job well done (K. Carr).
4. Provide clear communication (understanding each other's view) (S. Driver).
5. Ask in a pleasant manner and expect follow-through.
6. Listen!!!
7. Listen to what others say; and don't be afraid to trust.

8. Look for a person who is experienced in the area needed. Experience allows a person to be com-fortable, and a comfortable person is more cap-able of managing the expected and unexpected; encourage education—it's an ongoing process.

9. Asking is better than telling so gain the coop-eration of your colleagues through respect, fair treatment, and being available to educate when needed.

10. "Grow" your staff to a level of ownership and sense of responsibility that will encourage them to have an inner delegation voice.

11. Always treat people with respect and thank them (Janet Reaves).

12. Do not give an opportunity to say no by the wording of your request; give options (Janet Reaves).

13. Ask from someone; don't demand.

14. Delegate, then follow through to evaluation.

15. If you always do the right thing, everyone will respect you.

16. Be open-minded and flexible.

17. Respect others' feelings.

18. Be organized; be a thinker.

19. Be honest, direct, and to the point. Do not sugar-coat everything. For every negative thing, always say at least one positive thing.

20. When delegating a task, you need to make sure the person has the following qualities: enthusi-asm, credentials/qualifications, accountability, dependability, and open-mindedness.

21. Watch nonverbal communication; use proper tone of voice; know what it is you are delegating; and be resourceful (Candi Hinson).

22. Know what you can legally delegate, safely del-egate, and who you are delegating to (Frankie).

23. Gain cooperation of the individual to accept an assignment; provide training for the task dele-gated; assist as needed during the training period (be available); trust and give ownership of the task (Anne Vanderburg).

24. Be practical with your selection of a person to do skill or project; give concise instructions for com-pleting the task and allow adequate time; re-member we're only human and we can't do it all; we must delegate and use the team approach.

25. Give clear instruction with a date of completion.

26. Know the strengths and weaknesses of those you delegate to; delegate to develop weaknesses into strengths for the purpose of increasing self-esteem (Candace Hughes).

27. Comment on the positive attributes a person has that are needed to get a job done and then ask for their assistance; always be firm and direct in emergency situations; make that person feel needed to get a job done (Susan D. Freeman).

28. Do not delegate a disciplinary problem; do not delegate to one who is overworked.

29. Know the strengths and weaknesses of the person to whom you are delegating a task (S. Stewart).

30. Trust the person to perform the task assigned; praise generously for work well done (J. Mabery).

31. Teach by role model; no task is too small if *we learn the art of* delegation! (Bev Ellis)

32. Don't delegate something you would not do your-self; know the basics of what you are delegating; speak with confidence to the person you are del-egating to in order to plant the seed of success, not failure; delegate as a mentor only to the per-son you are delegating to because a leader is always eager to teach; follow through on your commitment to be available to the person should he/she need you to complete the task delegated; walk your talk; evaluate the task com-pleted and the person's performance and give positive feedback and praise; give clear instruc-tions and directions for completing the task del-egated and be receptive to questions; delegate with realistic expectations and goals; allow suffi-cient time for the task delegated to be completed and have a contingency plan if it's not; know the skill level and ability level of the person you are delegating to; "Don't get a shovel to do the work of a tractor" (Glenda George).

33. Include the other person in explanation of why the task delegated is needed (Anna West).

34. Clear communication of tasks and goals; knowl-edge of skills of person to whom you are delegat-ing; creating atmosphere so person being given a task can ask questions without fear; delegating in a positive way.

35. Approach with *"we can"* accomplish said goal/ task. Delegate pieces of task to volunteers or person *most interested* or capable of achieving task (Betty Zimmerman).

36. Choose appropriate task—match to the appro-priate person. The person who is honest, open, and willing to do the task to the best of his/her ability—he/she will be motivated and productive.

37. Employ accountability, responsibility, and em-powerment; clearly communicate task; give sup-port and encouragement.

38. Know people's strengths and weaknesses; use their strengths; give smaller/less important projects to help build a weakness up; pair someone with a strength with someone who has that as a weakness.

39. Empowerment of person to pass a task off to a capable individual to perform.

40. Ask employees—not order—to do task (Lynn Bryant).

41. The realization of others' strengths and gifts and using them to the fullest. Understanding their input is of value to the profession and is important to their self-worth.

42. Assess person's skill and delegate the task the person is more capable of doing.

43. Believe that your team members trust you and support you as you delegate to them.

44. Have the group/team meet in a comfortable, non-threatening setting and place the task before the group with these instructions: The following list is a group of tasks that must be completed by our group/team by X date. All will need to participate to make this successful. I need to know which task you will be completing by Y, with a follow up date by Z and completion date X.

45. Know skills/ability knowledge base about the person/people working with you—to delegate tasks safely and for them to be performed competently (Andrea Novak).

46. *Assess*: total work load, skills of staff, time needed for tasks, environmental factors, physical arrangements. *Plan*: what will be delegated, when task will be delegated, how (communication) task will be delegated. *Implement*: be specific, give encouragement, give rationale, allow for questions, clarification, give time frames and expectations, follow up in appropriate time frame. *Evaluate*: completion of task delegated, get feedback from coworker, outcomes of overall work, assess variances and process, make revisions, look for ways (methods) to improve (Kathy Clark).

47. Allow input into project; allow creativity; promote excitement about project before delegation; be a good listener; trust; praise; motivate; reward (Pamela Blue).

48. Feedback from staff about what they feel most qualified doing and/or leading (Joy Moss).

49. Above all, speak to others as you would like to be spoken to (Christina Griffiths).

50. Don't be afraid to delegate. Delegate to everyone involved. Start your delegation process as soon as there is a need for such—don't procrastinate. Delegate to your peers as well. Ask for input/ideas from those involved in the delegation process. Delegate appropriately—based on what another is able to do. Require time limits for completion. Follow up on what you delegated—only when necessary; show faith in the one you delegated to. A group expects a leader to delegate (Kim Calloway).

51. Know your people and their abilities (Edith Boland).

52. Keep in mind the right person for the task. Delegate in order to accomplish more (Ella Bryant).

53. Don't ask someone else to do something that you wouldn't do. Let them know no task is too little (Sheila Driver).

54. Be organized. Be a thinker. Use constructive criticism (Joan L. Faulkner).

55. Mentally define the job to be done. Assess abilities of team members. If teaching is needed, it should be done. Assess resources (non-labor). Set priorities with team. Assign individual responsibilities. Follow up. Evaluate.

56. Delegate responsibility. Clear, concise, and assure understanding of the task. Select individual who is motivated, capable, and willing.

57. Identify roles/jobs to be delegated. Define their scope/parameters. Define expectations. Be sure all know the final goal. When possible, include the group in dividing tasks by the team members' strengths, interests. Divide tasks/roles equitably.

58. If someone else can do it as well as you can and wants to do it, by all means, let him! (Sally Harris)

59. Must release control and ownership of project/task; must learn to rely on others; must learn to trust others; must learn to train others; must learn to reduce (give up) authority; must learn to emphasize strengths of others and help them strengthen their weak areas (Anne Vanderburg).

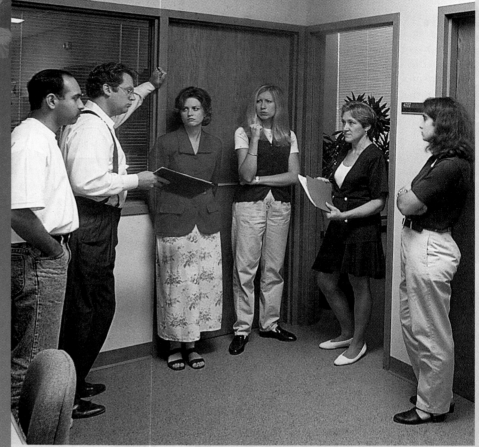

Conflict: The Cutting Edge of Change

Joe Brannan Hurst
PhD, EdD

Mary J. Keenan
RN, PhD

This chapter focuses on increasing the nurse manager's ability to deal with conflict by providing effective strategies for conflict resolution. To resolve conflicts, the nurse manager must be able to determine the nature of the particular conflicts, choose the most appropriate approach for each situation, and resolve the conflicts effectively. Since some conflicts are by nature unresolvable, an understanding of polarities and polarity management will also help the nurse manager recognize the upsides and downsides of an issue and capitalize on its positives.

Objectives

- Use a model of the conflict process to determine the nature and sources of hypothetical and actual conflict.
- Assess your preferred approaches to conflict and commit to new ways to be more effective in resolving future conflict.
- Determine which of the five optional approaches to conflict is the most appropriate approach in hypothetical and real situations.
- Diagram the structure and dynamics of important polarities (unresolvable conflicts) and identify ways to manage them.

Questions to Consider

- What situations, issues, and people trigger conflict for you? Why? How do you trigger conflict for others?
- How do you usually determine why people are having conflict? How do you usually react to and resolve conflict?
- What typical consequences occur from conflicts in which you are involved?
- How have you tended to handle unresolvable or recurring conflicts in the past? How could you handle them in the future?

 A Manager's Challenge

From a Clinical Manager at a Midwestern Health Center

In our small agency we had four physicians who were on call for their own patients from Monday through Friday (except when they were on vacation). On the weekends and holidays the physicians rotated on call every fourth weekend or holiday. This worked just fine until two of the physicians left and the first replacement did not want any call time, even though it was paid time. The two physicians who had been on call every fourth week had conflicts about covering regular call, vacation time, and sick call. One of them tended to use a more assertive, competing style in making requests of the other, who tended to be more accommodating. The latter began to be "burned out" and take more sick time off. Actually, our conflict resolution strategies were making the situation worse. I was avoiding and they were competing, compromising, and accommodating.

What do you think you would do if you were this manager?

INTRODUCTION

Much has been written and said about how to solve problems and how to resolve conflicts rationally, logically, and effectively. The trap in all this is the assumption that such rational processes lead to solutions and resolutions in all situations. For instance, Scott (1990) demonstrates this trap when she suggests:

The basic way to use the rational-intuitive approach to managing conflict is to look on any conflict situation as a problem or potential problem to be solved. Then, you select the appropriate problem-solving techniques from a supply of possible strategies for dealing with conflict. (p. 3)

Conflict arises from a perception of incompatibility. In other words, conflict primarily stems from differences in beliefs, values, attitudes, goals, priorities, methods, information, commitments, ideas, interpre-tations of reality, personalities, backgrounds, needs, interests, and/or motives (Scott, 1990).

Conflicts are more than just debates or negotiations. They represent an escalation of everyday competition and discussion into an arena of hostile or emotion-provoking encounters that strain personal or interpersonal tranquility, or both. (Scott, 1990, p. 1)

Controversy can be defined as a situation in which opinions, ideas, information, theories, and conclusions are perceived as incompatible with those of another person or group (Johnson & Johnson, 1997). Controversy, however, is very important for high-quality group decision making and individual relationships because, if managed well, it can stimulate creativity, agreement, increased commitment, cohesiveness, and collaboration. Conflicts can be based on differences in needs, values, and goals; on scarcities of particular resources; or on rivalry (Johnson & Johnson, 1997).

TYPES OF CONFLICT

Conflict occurs in all areas of our lives and in three broad categories. Conflict can be intrapersonal, interpersonal, and organizational in nature.

Intrapersonal conflict occurs within a person. Questions often arise that create a conflict over priorities, ethical standards, and different ways to act. When a nurse manager decides what to do about the future (e.g., "Do I really want to study for a higher degree or start our family now?"), there are conflicts between personal and professional priorities. Some issues present a conflict over comfortably maintaining the status quo (e.g., "My relationship with the experienced nurses on the unit is so very smooth and I want it to stay that way."), or taking risks in order to make suggestions and confront people when needed (e.g., "Would telling them their technique is way out of date and suggesting new ones like I learned jeopardize my rapport with them?").

Interpersonal conflict occurs when we realize that everybody does not see the world exactly the same way. There are conflicts among patients, nurses, care teams, family members, physicians, and other staff. A manager may be called on to assist two nurses in resolving a scheduling conflict, or determining whether sharing particular information would, or would not, be a violation of confidentiality. Patients resist suggestions for changing their diet, exercise, and health habits. Members of healthcare teams often have disputes over the best way to treat particular cases. Interpersonal conflict is common and can create the energy to build important relationships and teams.

Organizational conflict occurs when confronting the policies and procedures in patient care and personnel management, as well as the accepted norms of behavior and communication within any organization. Some organizational conflict is related to hierarchical structure and role differentiation among employees, such as labor and management negotiations and financial administrators' and department chairs' arguments over cost cutting. Nurse managers can become enmeshed in institution-wide conflict concerning cost reductions and quality of care, advances in technology and research versus expansion of access to care, and increasing profitable services while reducing unprofitable ones.

A major source of organizational conflict stems from new systems to promote more participation and autonomy in staff nurses. The trend is to charge nurses with determining and carrying out both direct patient care and unit goals for quality patient care. Increasing autonomy in staff nurses simultaneously changes their role and relationships with nurse managers (Keenan, Hurst, & Olnhausen, 1993). As staff nurses assume more autonomy and accountability for identifying areas for quality improvement in patient care, they may desire more shared responsibility with their managers. While managers' span of control continues to increase, previously clear roles become blurred and subsequently need to be redefined for staff and managers. All such changes involve organizational conflict mixed with intrapersonal and interpersonal conflict and management of change *and* stability.

THE CONFLICT PROCESS

Conflict proceeds through four stages: frustration, conceptualization, action, and outcomes (Kinney & Hurst, 1989). The ability to resolve conflicts productively depends on understanding this process (see Figure 19-1) and on developing creative ways to deal with conflict. Notice how the arrows in Figure 19-1 flow both ways between stages. This illustrates that moving into a subsequent stage may lead to a return to and change in a previous stage. For instance, two nurses view the conflict (conceptualize it) as a fight to control, while a third thinks it's about professional standards. A nurse manager gets them all to talk. They have expressed much frustration and mistrust. All agree that the real conflict comes from a difference in goals, which leads to less negative emotion and a much clearer understanding of all the issues.

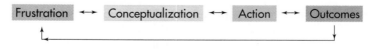

Figure 19-1   Stages of the conflict process.

Frustration

When people or groups perceive that their goals may be blocked, they feel frustrated. This frustration may escalate into stronger emotions, such as anger and deep resignation. This frustration comes from what people believe to be true, even though there may not be a real conflict at all! For example, a nurse may perceive that a patient is uncooperative when in reality the patient is afraid or has another set of priorities than the nurse. At the same time, the patient may view the nurse as controlling and insensitive. When such frustrations occur, it is a cue to stop and clarify the nature of major differences.

Conceptualization

Everyone involved develops an idea or picture of what the conflict is about. This may be an instantaneous "snapshot," or it may develop over a period of time. This concept of the conflict may be very clear in people's minds, or it may be very fuzzy. Everyone involved has an individual interpretation of what the conflict is and why it is occurring. Most often these interpretations are different and involve the person's own perspective.

Regardless of its clarity or accuracy, however, the conceptualization forms the basis for everyone's reactions to the frustration. The way the individuals perceive and define the conflict has a great deal of influence on the creative resolution and productive outcomes to follow. For example, within the same conflict situation, some individuals may see the conflict as insubordination and become angry, while others view it as trivial bickering and withdraw. Such differences in conceptualizing the issue could block its resolution. Thus it is important for each person to clarify "the conflict as I see it" and "how it makes me feel" before all the people involved can define the conflict (i.e., develop an accurate conceptualization together) and proceed to resolve their differences.

People are not likely to reach outcomes that truly resolve the conflict and satisfy them unless they have a clear understanding of the differences among them. During the conceptualization process, we can ask two very powerful questions:

1. What is the nature of our differences?
2. What are the reasons for those differences?

People may differ on four aspects of a conflict: (1) facts, (2) goals, (3) methods to achieve goals, and (4) the values or standards used to select goals, priorities, and methods.

It is usually easier to provide accurate information than to work out differences in values, priorities, methodology, and standards. Disagreements over facts may uncover conflicts over goals, means, and values, which may lead to the conflict expanding or even escalating out of control. Values, opinions, and beliefs are more personal, thus generating disagreements that can be threatening and adversarial. The more accurately any conflict is defined, the more likely it will be resolved.

Action

Intentions, strategies, plans, and behavior "flow" out of the conceptualization. A pattern of interaction among the individuals involved is set in motion (e.g., "Let's work together" or "We're not getting any place this way"). As actions are taken to resolve the conflict, the way that some or all parties conceptualize the conflict may change. The important point is that people are always taking some action regarding the conflict, even if that action is avoiding it or deciding to do nothing.

There are five distinct action-oriented approaches to resolving conflict (see page 324). The longer ineffective actions continue, the more likely people will experience frustration, resistance, or even hostility. The more the actions appropriately match the nature of the conflict, the more likely it will be resolved with desirable results.

Outcomes

As a result of the actions taken, there are tangible and intangible consequences, or "outcomes." The conflict may be resolved with a new plan that incorporates the goals of two or more people, so no one loses. Productivity and efficiency may increase, decrease, or stay the same. Emotions may be high with anger and resistance left over, so further conflicts arise. Relationships may be strengthened, weakened, or ended. Such outcomes have very important consequences in the work setting. Assessing the degree of conflict resolution (see Box 19-1) is useful for improving individual and group skills in resolutions.

Exercise 19-1

Observe (or recall) a situation in which conflict is apparent. Note arguments each person/side makes and how each responds to the other's comments. What was the outcome? Was the conflict resolved? Was anything left unresolved?

When assessing the degree to which a conflict has been resolved, there are two general outcomes to assess: the degree to which important goals were achieved and the nature of the subsequent

<table>
<tr><td>

Box 19-1

Assessing the Degree of Conflict Resolution

I. Quality of decisions
    A. How creative are resulting plans?
    B. How practical and realistic are they?
    C. How well were intended goals achieved?
    D. What surprising results were achieved?
II. Quality of relationships
    A. How much understanding has been created?
    B. How willing are people to work together?
    C. How much mutual respect, empathy, concern, and cooperation has been generated?

(Adapted with permission from Hurst & Kinney, 1989.)

</td></tr>
</table>

relationships among those involved (see Boxes 19-2 and 19-3). There are four questions you could ask about the nature of the subsequent relationships (Johnson & Johnson, 1997): (1) Are the relationships stronger and are people better able to interact? (2) Do the members like and trust each other more? (3) Are all the members satisfied with the results of the conflict? (4) Have group members become more able to resolve future conflicts with one another?

Exercise 19-2

It's time to assess your tendencies to approach conflict. As you read and answer the thirty-item conflict survey on p. 323, think of how you face and respond to conflict in professional situations. After completing the survey, tally, total, and reflect on your scores for each of the five approaches. Consider the following questions:

Box 19-2

Snapshot of Two Conflicts

Unproductive	**Productive**
Suppose I perceive a conflict between you and me because you disagree with my ideas about how to motivate others to accomplish quality improvement projects. Looking at the four stages in the process of conflict, we might find the following in an unproductive conflict:	The same conflict could present itself and evolve through the same process with different outcomes.
1. **I** am **frustrated** working together on the quality improvement committee because you usually put down my ideas for change. **You** are frustrated because you perceive that I do not support your goals for improved patient care.	1. **I feel frustrated** that we have to work on the same committee together because I believe that you tend to resist and disagree with my ideas for change. **You** seem to think that what the organization is doing now works just fine.
2. **I** see **(conceptualize)** the conflict as your ignorance of new concepts and research findings. Besides you want things pretty much your way. **You** see it as my eagerness to "shake up" people, promote myself as a leader, and increase my power.	2. As **we talk** we realize **(conceptualize)** that we want the same thing: incentives to support quality improvement projects.
3. **My** view leads to my being forceful **(action)** with you and sharing new research studies and articles that I have found to prove my point, which confirms your judgment of me. **You** resist me with your considerations about why the new techniques will not work and by refusing to read the articles.	3. Our commitment to getting these incentives spurs us to identify critical areas for study. At the same time, **we decide (action)** that we need to look at new plans and research to suggest improvements and additions for our quality improvement endeavors. I say, "If you look at current and new plans, I will work on securing supporting research." We agree and others on the committee agree to do other necessary tasks.
4. The **outcome** is that **we** have created a **defensive climate** and a lack of desire to work together. We have clouded the real issue and generated hostility among all of the group. The committee submits a compromise plan to which no one is committed and it then disbands. **The project essentially has failed.**	4. The committee then prioritizes areas for study and develops a time frame **(outcomes)**. It creates an incentive program **combining the strengths** of our plan with some new ideas to promote internal motivation and productivity and recommends it to the personnel committee. The committee continues and the **project is successful.**

Box 19-3
Conflict Self-Assessment

Directions: Read each of the statements below. Assess yourself in terms of how frequently you tend to act that way during conflict at work. Place the number of the most appropriate response in the blank in front of each statement. Put 1 if the behavior is never typical of how you act during a conflict; 2 if it is seldom typical; 3 if it is occasionally typical; 4 if it is frequently typical; or 5 if it is very typical of how you act during conflict. Please complete all items.

_____ 1. Create new possibilities to address all important concerns.

_____ 2. Persuade others to see it and/or do it my way.

_____ 3. Work out some sort of give-and-take agreement.

_____ 4. Let other people have their way.

_____ 5. Wait and let the conflict take care of itself.

_____ 6. Find ways that everyone can win.

_____ 7. Use whatever power I have to get what I want.

_____ 8. Find an agreeable compromise among people involved.

_____ 9. Give in so others get what they think is important.

_____ 10. Withdraw from the situation.

_____ 11. Assertively cooperate, until everyone's needs are met.

_____ 12. Compete until I either win or lose.

_____ 13. Engage in "give a little and get a little" bargaining.

_____ 14. Make others' needs met over my own needs.

_____ 15. Avoid taking any action for as long as I can.

_____ 16. Partner with others to find the most inclusive solution.

_____ 17. Put my foot down assertively for a quick solution.

_____ 18. Negotiate for what all sides value and can live without.

_____ 19. Agree to what others want to create harmony.

_____ 20. Keep as far away from others involved as possible.

_____ 21. Stick with it to get everyone's highest priorities.

_____ 22. Argue and debate over the best way.

_____ 23. Create some middle position everyone agrees to.

_____ 24. Put my priorities below those of other people.

_____ 25. Hope the issue does not come up.

_____ 26. Collaborate with others to achieve our goals together.

_____ 27. Compete with others for scarce resources.

_____ 28. Emphasize compromise and trade-offs.

_____ 29. Cool things down by letting others do it their way.

_____ 30. Change the subject to avoid the fighting.

Conflict Self-Assessment Scoring

Look at the numbers you placed in the blanks on the conflict assessment on the previous page. Write the number you placed in each blank on the appropriate line below. Add up your total for each column, and enter that total on the appropriate line. The greater your total for each approach, the more frequently you tend to use that approach to conflict at work. The lower the score, the less frequently you tend to use that approach to conflict at work.

Collaborating	Competing	Compromising	Accommodating	Avoiding
1. _____	2. _____	3. _____	4. _____	5. _____
6. _____	7. _____	8. _____	9. _____	10. _____
11. _____	12. _____	13. _____	14. _____	15. _____
16. _____	17. _____	18. _____	19. _____	20. _____
21. _____	22. _____	23. _____	24. _____	25. _____
26. _____	27. _____	28. _____	29. _____	30. _____
Total _____	Total _____	Total _____	Total _____	Total _____

Throughout the rest of this section, there are descriptions of each approach and related self-assessment and commitment to action activities. Use these totals to stimulate your thinking about how you do and could handle conflict at work. Most importantly, consider if your pattern of frequency tends to be consistent, or inconsistent, with the types of conflicts you face. That is, does your way of dealing with conflict tend to match the situations in which that approach is most useful?

From Hurst (1993). Used with permission.

Exercise 19-2—cont'd

- Which approach(es) do you prefer? Which do you use least?
- Why do you think you tend to act that way?
- Considering the types of conflicts you tend to have, what are the strengths and weaknesses of your pattern?

As you read the rest of this section use this pattern of scores and your reflections to examine the appropriate uses of each approach, assess your use of each approach more extensively, and commit to new behaviors to increase your future effectiveness.

MODES OF CONFLICT RESOLUTION

There are five general, distinct approaches to conflict resolution: (1) avoiding, (2) accommodating, (3) competing, (4) compromising, and (5) collaborating (Johnson & Johnson, 1997; Thomas & Kilmann, 1973). These approaches can be viewed along two different continua: (1) from uncooperative to highly cooperative and (2) from unassertive to highly assertive (Thomas, 1975). (See the Conflict Self-Assessment on page 323.)

On the cooperative continuum actions can range from complete competition to total cooperation. Two nurses might compete for a manager position on the one extreme while teaming cooperatively to institute the expansion of their unit. On the assertiveness continuum actions range from ignoring one's own goals (highly unassertive) to doing what it takes to get what one intends (highly assertive). A nurse manager might forgo asking for time off (unassertive) at a time when the clinical manager predicts the unit will be short-staffed and overly busy (assertive).

It is unlikely that anyone would select any one approach to the exclusion of the others. In fact, as we will examine later in the discussion of polarity management, people tend to move up and down or back and forth between these continua in some combined action that is appropriately assertive and cooperative, depending on the nature of the conflict situation.

Avoiding

Avoiding or withdrawing is very unassertive and un-cooperative because avoiders neither pursue their own needs, goals, and concerns immediately nor as-sist others to pursue theirs. The positive side of with-drawing may take the form of diplomatically side-stepping or postponing an issue until a better time or simply walking away from a "no-win" situation (see Box 19-4). The self-assessment that follows Box 19-5

Box 19-4

Positive Uses for the Avoiding Approach

1. When facing trivial and/or temporary issues, or when other far more important issues are pressing (e.g., tangential issues are only symptoms of deeper conflicts).
2. When there is no chance to obtain what one wants or needs, or when others could resolve the conflict more efficiently and effectively.
3. When the potential negative results of initi-ating and acting on a conflict are much greater than the benefits of its resolution.
4. When people need to "cool down," distance themselves, or gather more information, perhaps gaining a hindsight or meaningful view.

Box 19-5

Avoidance: Self-Assessment and Commitment to Action

If you tend to use avoidance frequently, ask:

1. Do people have difficulty getting my input into and understanding my view of conflicts?
2. Do I block cooperative efforts to resolve issues?
3. Am I distancing myself from significant others?
4. Are important issues being left unidentified and unresolved?

If you do not use avoidance very often, ask yourself:

1. Do I find myself overwhelmed by a large number of conflicts and need to say "no"?
2. Do I assert myself even when things do not matter that much? Do others view me as an aggressor?
3. Do I lack a clear view of what my priorities are?
4. Do I stir up conflicts and fights for some reason?

Commitment to Action

Reflecting on my assessment of myself, what two new behaviors would increase my effective use of avoidance at work?

1.
2.

will help you recognize your own avoidance behaviors and use them more effectively.

Accommodating/Smoothing

When accommodating, people neglect their own needs, goals, and concerns (unassertive) while trying to satisfy those of others (cooperative). This approach has an element about it of being self-sacrificing, obeying orders, or serving other people. For example, sometimes we don't care where we eat, and others do. So we say, "Fine, let's eat there! I like all kinds of food, I'm really hungry, so let's go." Box 19-6 lists some appropriate uses of **accommodation.**

Accommodators frequently feel disappointment and resentment because they "get nothing in return." This is a built-in by-product of the overuse of this approach. The self-assessment in Box 19-7 asks you to examine your present use of accommodation and challenges you to think of new ways to use it more effectively.

Competing/Coercing

During competition, people pursue their own needs and goals at the expense of others'. Sometimes people use whatever power, creativeness, or strategies are available to "win." **Competing** may also take the form of standing up for your rights, defending important principles, and contending for limited funds (see Box 19-8).

People who compete well frequently may not be able to hear the truth, have others disagree, or be challenged, even when they are wrong. They often

---

Box 19-6

Appropriate Uses of Accommodation

1. When other people's ideas and solutions appear to be better or when you have made a mistake.
2. When the issue is far more important to the other(s) than it is for you. (This is a natural, logical step to cooperation and collaboration.)
3. When you see that accommodating now "builds up some important credits" for later issues.
4. When you are outmatched and/or losing anyway; when continued competition would only damage the relationships and productivity of the group and jeopardize accomplishing major purpose(s) and maintaining credibility.
5. When preserving harmonious relationships and avoiding defensiveness and hostility are very important.
6. When letting others learn from their mistakes and/or increased responsibility is possible without severe damage (and you are able to avoid saying, "I told you so!").

Box 19-7

Accommodation: Self-Assessment and Commitment to Action

If you use accommodation frequently, ask yourself:

1. Do I feel that my needs, goals, concerns, and ideas are not being attended to by others?
2. Am I depriving myself of influence, recognition, and respect?
3. When I am in charge, is "discipline" lax?
4. Do I think people are using me?

Infrequent use of accommodation may result in your being viewed as unreasonable or insensitive.

If you seldom use accommodation, ask yourself:

1. Am I building goodwill with others during conflict?
2. Do I admit when I've made a mistake?
3. Do I recognize legitimate exceptions?
4. Do I know when to give in, or do I assert myself at all costs?

Commitment to Action

What two new behaviors would increase your effective use of accommodation?

1.
2.

Box 19-8

Appropriate Uses of Competing

1. When quick, decisive action is necessary.
2. When important, unpopular action needs to be taken. When trade-offs may result in long-range, continued conflict.
3. When people are right about issues that are vital to group welfare.
4. When people have had others take advantage of their noncompetitive behavior and now feel obliged to compete.

react by being threatened, defensive, and aggressive. Competition within work groups can generate ill will, a win-lose stance, and commitment to inaction. Use Box 19-9 to help you learn to use competing more effectively.

Box 19-9
Competing: Self-Assessment and Commitment to Action

If you use competing frequently, ask yourself:

1. Am I surrounded by people who agree with me all the time and who avoid confronting me?
2. Are others afraid to share themselves and their needs for growth with me?
3. Am I out to win at all costs? If so, what are the costs and benefits of competing?

If you tend not to compete, ask yourself:

1. How often do I avoid taking a strong stand and then feel a sense of powerlessness?
2. Do I avoid taking a stand so that I can escape risk?
3. Am I fearful and unassertive to the point that important decisions are delayed and people suffer?

Commitment to Action

What two new behaviors would increase your effective use of competition?

1.
2.

Negotiating/Compromising

Negotiating involves both assertiveness and cooperation on the part of everyone and requires skill. There is a give and take resulting in conflict resolution with people meeting their important priorities as much as possible. **Compromising** is often an exchange of concessions or creation of a middle position. This is the preferred means of conflict resolution during union negotiations, when each side is appeased to some degree. In this mode, nobody gets everything they think they need.

Negotiation and compromise are valued approaches. They are chosen when less accommodating or avoiding is appropriate (Box 19-10). Compromising is a blend of both assertive and cooperative behaviors, although it calls for less finely honed skills for each behavior than does collaboration. Negotiation is more like trading (e.g., "You can have this if I can have that."). Compromise is one of the most frequently

---

Box 19-10
Appropriate Uses of Compromise

1. Two powerful sides are committed strongly to perceived mutually exclusive goals.
2. Temporary solutions to complex issues need to be implemented.
3. Conflicting goals are "moderately important" and not worth a major confrontation (coercion/competing).
4. Time pressures people to expedite a workable solution.
5. When collaborating and competing fail.

Negotiating Theories

THEORY/KEY CONTRIBUTORS	KEY IDEA	APPLICATION TO PRACTICE
GETTING TO YES: **Negotiating Agreement, Principled Negotiation, or Negotiation on Merits** theories were developed by Fisher and Vry (1991).	Principled negotiation can produce mutually acceptable agreements in every type of conflict. The method to use is (1) separate the people from the problem; (2) focus on interests, not positions; (3) invent options for mutual gain; and (4) insist on using objective criteria.	Negotiation requires extra efforts to communicate: speak and listen for mutual understanding. Getting to yes comes from building a working relationship and creatively developing options with which those involved will benefit.

Fisher, RS, & Vry, W. (1991). *Getting to Yes: Negotiating Agreement Without Giving In.* New York: Penguin Books.

selected behaviors used by nurse managers because it supports a balance of power between themselves and others in the work setting. The self-assessment in Box 19-11 will help you become more aware of your own use of negotiation and compromise and improve it.

Collaborating

Collaborating, the opposite of both avoiding and competing, is the creative stance. It is both assertive and cooperative as people work creatively and openly to find the solution that most fully satisfies all important concerns and goals to be achieved. **Collaboration** involves analyzing situations and defining the conflict at a higher level where shared "superordinate" goals are identified and commitment to work together is generated (see Box 19-12). For example, when nurses and physicians work together, they can collaborate by replacing "Who's in charge?" with "What does the patient require?" and "Where does each of us fit into the plan?" This requires discussion about the plan (superordinate goals), how this will be accomplished, and who will make what contributions to achieving the plan.

The same scenario fits for patients and families as well. What is their superordinate goal? Who will do what so that they can reach this goal? The stakes are high (quality patient care) as all stakeholders (e.g., patient, nurse, family, and physician) agree to work together.

Trivial issues do not require collaboration and consensus seeking. Some people favor collaboration to reduce their risk taking and to spread responsibility. Use the self-assessment in Box 19-13 that follows to determine your own use of collaboration.

At the onset of conflict, people can carefully analyze situations to identify the nature and reasons for conflict and choose an appropriate approach promoting collaboration. In other words, we can collaborate on the decision to withdraw, compete, or negotiate. For

---

Box 19-11

Negotiation/Compromise Self-Assessment and Commitment to Action

If you tend to use negotiation frequently, consider:

1. Do I ignore large, important issues while trying to work out creative, practical compromises?
2. Is there a "gamesmanship" in my/our negotiations?
3. Am I sincerely committed to compromise or negotiated solutions?

If you tend to use negotiation infrequently, ask yourself:

1. Do I find it difficult to make concessions?
2. Am I often engaged in strong disagreements or do I withdraw when I see no way to get out?
3. Do I feel embarrassed, sensitive, self-conscious, or pressured to negotiate, compromise, and bargain?

Commitment to Action

What two new behaviors would increase your compromising effectiveness?

1.
2.

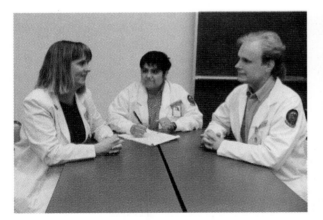

Compromise supports a balance of power between self and other in the workplace.

Box 19-12

Appropriate Uses for Collaboration

1. To seek creative, integrative solutions where both sides' goals and needs are important, thus developing group commitment and a consensual decision.
2. To learn and grow through cooperative problem solving, resulting in greater understanding and empathy.
3. To identify, share, and merge vastly different viewpoints.
4. To be honest about and work through difficult emotional issues interfering with morale, productivity, and growth.

If you tend to collaborate frequently, consider:

1. Do I spend valuable group time and energy on issues that do not warrant or deserve it?
2. Do I postpone needed action to get consensus and avoid making key decisions?
3. When I initiate collaboration, do others really respond that way? (Are there hidden agendas, unspoken hostility, and/or manipulation in the group?)

If you tend to collaborate infrequently, ask yourself:

1. Do I ignore opportunities to cooperate, risk, and creatively confront conflict?
2. Do I tend to be pessimistic, distrusting, withdrawing, and/or competitive?
3. Am I involving others in important decisions, eliciting commitment, and empowering them?

Commitment to Action

What two new behaviors would increase your collaboration effectiveness?

1.
2.

example, suppose you and I are disagreeing about the timing of procedures for patients under your care. At the point that we both agree that it's your responsibility and decision to make, we collaborate and agree. I say, "I see your point, so let's do it that way." Or we might talk and subsequently agree that you are too emotionally involved with a patient's problem and that it may be time for you to withdraw from providing the care and enlist the skills of another nurse. This discussion can result in collaborative efforts for you to withdraw. Another less desirable choice could be to compete and let the winner's position stand (e.g., "Do as I say" or "I'm in charge of this patient.") The decision to compete or collaborate depends on you and the other person.

The nature of the differences, underlying reasons, importance of the issue, strength of feelings, commitment, and goals involved all have to be considered when selecting an approach to resolving conflict. Preferred and previously effective approaches

can be considered, but they need to match the situation. Effective resolution may require switching to a more appropriate method.

MANAGING UNRESOLVABLE CONFLICTS

Not all of the conflicts confronting people are resolvable. In fact, most of our own present problems and conflicts, especially the continuing or reappearing ones, are probably unresolvable. Such conflicts cannot be resolved by the right amounts of money, time, resources, staff, support networks, state-of-the-art technology, diet, exercise, vacation time, teamwork, courage, training, rational thinking, and/or leadership (see Box 19-14). These conflicts are inherently unresolvable (Hurst, 1996; Johnson, 1992).

Many conflicts (and problems) are inherently unresolvable because they consist of two interdependent, dynamic polar opposites that require a shifting emphasis from pole to pole over time, rather than the selection of the one "best" option. Resolvable conflicts (and solvable problems) tend to be either/or choices that lead to some end. Unresolvable conflicts, or **polarities**, involve a both/and decision of when to emphasize one pole and then its opposite. For instance, a manager's need to give clear direction to a team automatically places less emphasis on the team's deciding on the direction themselves. But sooner or later, for the team to be successful, that manager will experience the need for the team to work on its own, setting its own direction. Johnson (1992) has identified several common polarities with which people deal continually. These include self and others, individual and team, individual and organizational responsibility, control and participatory management, specific and general communication, tasks and relationships, centralization and decentralization, and stability and change. Others you are probably confronting include "me and my department," personal life and professional life, stimulation (stress) and tranquility, conditional acceptance (love) and unconditional acceptance (love), cost and quality, management and leadership, and planning and acting.

Polarity Structure

Polarities have six important elements (Figure 19-2), including two neutral, interdependent poles; two sets of resulting positive consequences ("upsides"), one for each pole; and two sets of associated negative consequences ("downsides"). To determine the

Research Perspective

Volkema, R.E., & Bergmann, T.J. (1996). Conflict styles as indicators of behavioral patterns in interpersonal conflicts. Journal of Social Psychology, 135(1), 5-15.

This study was done to examine the relationships between the cooperativeness and assertiveness dimensions of the Thomas-Kilmann Conflict Mode instrument and a wide variety of conflict behaviors demonstrated in recent conflict situations. Both the strategic (large-scale, enduring) and the tactical (small-scale, episodic) intentional components of conflict were examined. The Thomas-Kilmann modes of conflict resolution (collaborating, competing, accommodating, avoiding, and compromising) were used to interpret the assertiveness and cooperativeness dimensions and their effects on behavior. Another survey was used to identify three levels of conflict behavior, including (1) "setting the tone for negotiations," (2) "falling back" in response to others' actions, and (3) "gaining advantage" or changing to the course of the conflict.

The sample included 202 graduate students in an organizational theory course. Approximately 58% were male; their mean time working in their present agency was 3 years and in their current job was 2 years.

The results suggested that the Thomas-Kilmann view of conflict does reflect the strategic large-scale, enduring intentions. At the tactical level, however, there tended to be a clear pattern for the three levels. Level one tended to be a "constructive engagement," while level two appeared to be a response to others' "good faith" negotiations, and level three tended to be a genuine "reaffirming" of the person's basic intentions and self (saving face).

Implications for Practice

Nurse leader/managers/followers will be involved in many conflicts. This study describes just how different people's intentions, values, and responses could be during conflict. This is especially important for any person's shift of intentions throughout the same conflict from setting a tone to preserving one's integrity and self. Noting such differences among people, and within the level one to level three sequence, will increase nurse leader/managers' abilities to facilitate conflict resolution while assisting them in empathizing and saving face with others.

Box 19-14
How to Tell If a Conflict May Be Unresolvable

PROBABLY IS UNRESOLVABLE	ASK THESE QUESTIONS ABOUT THE SITUATION	PROBABLY IS RESOLVABLE
Answer is yes	Is this difficulty ongoing?	Answer is no
Answer is yes	Are there two interdependent poles?	Answer is no
Answer is yes	Does choosing one need to incorporate the other to succeed?	Answer is no
Answer is yes	Is this really a both/and decision?	Answer is no

nature of the unresolvable conflicts, one has to ask five basic questions, as shown in Box 19-15.

By answering these basic questions, an individual or team can diagram the specifics of any polarity situation. Typically, people see only half the situation—the upside of their preferred pole and the downside of its opposite—and are therefore blind to the other two quadrants—their preferred pole's downside and its opposite's upside (Johnson, 1992). This blindness,

coupled with the need to be right, leads to much conflict with those who favor the opposite pole and see only the other two quadrants. Just the awareness that there are such things as polarities and diagramming important ones tend to increase collaboration and "win/win" thinking because people learn that fighting over one pole leads to experiencing its downside consequences (Hurst & Vander Veen, 1995; Johnson, 1992).

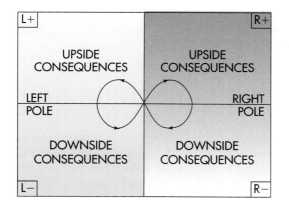

Figure 19-2 Generic structure and predictable flow of polarities.

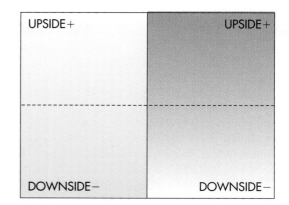

Figure 19-3 Polarity diagram.

Polarity Dynamics

Visually, a polarity diagram consists of the two polar opposites on a horizontal axis divided into four quadrants of results by a vertical line. Although simple in form, polarity diagrams clearly picture the consequences to be experienced and the nature of its historical and predictable flow.

Notice in Figure 19-2 that polarities naturally and predictably "flow" (arrows represent a plot of changes in results) from the downside of pole L toward the upside of pole R; then into the downside of pole R; then toward the upside of the first, pole L; and finally back to the downside of L where it all began. For example, a nurse manager was confronted by an angry team because they felt as they were being treated like children and told what to do all the time (control management's downside, L−). Working together they

initiated team meetings and decision-making procedures (actions emphasizing participatory management) that resulted in more ideas, ownership of the area, and self-direction from the team and its individual members (participatory upside, R+). However, after a few months of overemphasizing participation, the team began to lose its focus and cohesiveness (participatory downside, R−) and came to the manager for direction. The manager listened and provided clarification (action emphasizing control management) and the team regained its focus and efficiency (upside of control management, L+).

Polarities have this infinite-type swing to them as represented by the shape of the flow of the arrows in Figure 19-2. Although these swings reflect quite limited or unlimited changes in consequences with vastly differing lengths of time between them (or they may be skewed toward one pole), they will occur over time.

Wide, rapid, or very prolonged swings usually lead to disruptions in the smooth conduct of activity. When any polar opposites like change and stability are approached as separate independent problems or conflicts—as they generally are—the outcomes tend to reflect the greater amount of time and intensity of consequences in the downside "quadrants" (see Figure 19-3). Sometimes people hang onto one pole so long—usually for fear of the other pole's downside—that they either are forced to change their emphasis or do so very rapidly and extremely. This leads to a "flip" from the downside the original pole to the downside of the new pole, with almost no experiencing of the upside on the way! (Johnson, 1992). This hanging onto one pole in order to reap the benefits of its upside and avoid its opposite's downside,

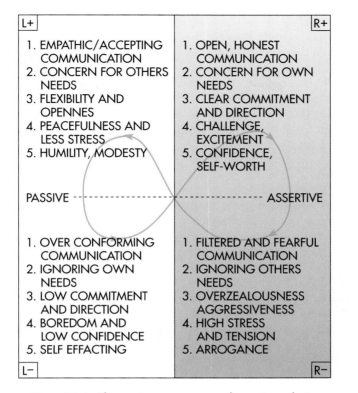

L+	R+
1. EMPATHIC/ACCEPTING COMMUNICATION 2. CONCERN FOR OTHERS NEEDS 3. FLEXIBILITY AND OPENNES 4. PEACEFULNESS AND LESS STRESS 5. HUMILITY, MODESTY	1. OPEN, HONEST COMMUNICATION 2. CONCERN FOR OWN NEEDS 3. CLEAR COMMITMENT AND DIRECTION 4. CHALLENGE, EXCITEMENT 5. CONFIDENCE, SELF-WORTH

PASSIVE - ASSERTIVE

1. OVER CONFORMING COMMUNICATION 2. IGNORING OWN NEEDS 3. LOW COMMITMENT AND DIRECTION 4. BOREDOM AND LOW CONFIDENCE 5. SELF EFFACTING	1. FILTERED AND FEARFUL COMMUNICATION 2. IGNORING OTHERS NEEDS 3. OVERZEALOUSNESS AGGRESSIVENESS 4. HIGH STRESS AND TENSION 5. ARROGANCE
L−	R−

Figure 19-4   The passive acceptance and assertive polarity.

is what Johnson (1992) calls, "the one pole myth," or being "stuck" (p. 156).

The polarity diagram in Figure 19-4 was generated by a team of college students working on assertiveness ("crusading" away from the passive downside toward the assertive upside). They drew this on a chart pad by asking these questions: (L−) With what negative results of passiveness are we dissatisfied?; (R+) To what positive outcomes of assertiveness are we committed?; (R−) What negative consequences would occur from overemphasizing assertiveness (excluding any passive acceptance)?; and (L+) What are the positive consequences of being passively accepting?

Exercise 19-3

After rereading the section on polarity dynamics, fill out the blank polarity diagram shown in Figure 19-3. First, answer the questions listed in Box 19-15. Be specific about the upside and downside consequences of each pole. Then draw a time line through the quadrants, starting in the lower left quadrant and moving through the upper right, down into the lower right, up toward the upper left, and finally back into the lower left. Shape the line to conform with how your orga-

Exercise 19-3—cont'd

nization has moved through this polarity over time. Talk to some people who have been around for a while to get their historical perspective on this issue. Then consider the following questions:

- Who tends to crusade for what pole? What are their positions and years of experience?
- How are resources, time, and personnel wasted on mismanaging this polarity?
- What blocks the effective managing of this polarity?
- What already aids in its management?
- What new things and actions would add to its management in the future?

By seeing the total picture, they could take steps to make changes flexibly without overemphasizing any one pole for too long. Most importantly, they would draw the results line (arrows) that best represented how this polarity usually flowed. They could see how stuck they had been, especially with almost every assertive act "feeling" negative and being resisted by others and almost every positive passive act lumped in with the negatives of "giving in." It is very important to draw such diagrams with input from as many people as possible.

Polarity Management

"The objective of polarity management is to get the best of both opposites while avoiding the limits of each" (Johnson, 1992, p. xii). In other words, once people determine their conflict is a polarity, they can act to maximize both poles' upsides and minimize both poles' downsides. This is called "polarity management," which requires a shifting focus from pole to pole when cues of approaching downside consequences are noted. The key to effective polarity management is to sense oncoming downside consequences, or be sensitive to feedback that there are negative consequences occurring, and take action toward the opposite pole. One nurse manager noticed that two teams had been functioning so long that individual members were complaining about being overlooked and their creativity stifled by the group. The manager scheduled a luncheon party, presented individual awards to each member, and initiated a creative suggestion box for staff to contribute individual and team ideas for improving quality and efficiency.

Polarity management involves two opposing groups that usually are in conflict. "Crusaders" are dissatisfied with the downsides of the present pole and advocate action toward its opposite. "Tradition bearers" prefer the present pole, citing its upsides, and point to the downsides of the crusaders' preferred pole as reasons to keep the emphasis where it is. Typically, the communication between crusaders and tradition bearers is argumentative, competitive, and defensive. Both sides know they are right and the other side is wrong. Polarity management alters this communication to a mood of cooperation, collaboration, and support because both sides realize that any decision to emphasize one pole results in everyone experiencing the downside of that pole, and if stuck at that pole long enough, experiencing the downsides of both poles at once! (Johnson, 1992).

There are several things a manager and an organization can do to begin managing polarities more collaboratively and effectively. Many of them are listed in Box 19-16.

As a rule, the more skilled people are at problem solving and conflict resolution, the more likely they will mismanage polarities. This happens when people treat both/and decisions like either/or ones, thus looking for the right choice. Yet no one right choice exists, at least in the long run. To manage polarities, it is important to partner with others and shift action to what is needed next in a timely manner.

Box 19-16
Actions for Managing a Polarity

The following list of actions exemplifies steps in the management of any polarity:

- Note that the situation involves at least one continuous both/and polarity.
- Diagram in writing the polarity's poles, upsides, and downsides.
- Draw a time line (arrows representing its past, present, and predictable future flow) with dates to identify the history of this particular polarity.
- Listen carefully to people with preferences for the opposite pole. Solicit their input regularly.
- Identify key individuals and groups who are "crusading" for the new pole and "traditionally supporting" staying at the present pole. Involve them in analyzing and managing this polarity.
- State major goals and objectives in terms of maximizing the upside consequences.
- Determine what present policies, procedures, committee structures, and typical actions (a) block the effective management of this polarity (shifting from pole to pole) and (b) exemplify and/or support managing this polarity effectively. Then create new ones that would facilitate managing this polarity in the future.
- Note which people are most accurately sensitive to any changes in results toward either downside and encourage and listen to their ongoing feedback.
- Identify and create flexible ways to shift resources to either pole and to monitor results.
- Continually diagram polarities and monitor their flow.
- Value crusaders' and tradition bearers' viewpoints, their ongoing collaboration, and healthy competition between them.

CHAPTER CHECKLIST

Conflicts may be resolvable or unresolvable, and they are common in healthcare and dealing with people. To resolve conflict, people need to identify their differences, priorities, and common goals; determine which approach to conflict is most appropriate; and act in that way to resolve it. When conflicts involve polarities, people need to analyze their structure and

A Manager's Solution

[?] The solution was created by the three physicians and me sitting down with a commitment to develop a plan that would work for everyone. This included a promise to find a fourth physician as soon as possible. Next, the reality of call was discussed. Once the actual numbers of calls taken, patients actually needing to be seen, and true emergencies were made clear, all three physicians agreed to share call more equitably. Third, the informal way of scheduling call was replaced by a formal 3-month one.

I developed a clearer definition of emergencies so that there would be fewer calls made to the physicians on weekends and holidays. I also established a procedure for scheduling the three of them ahead of time and putting it where everyone knew who would be on call. Then any changes they needed to make between themselves could be written on the posted schedule. The essence of this solution was collaboration among the four of us.

[?] *Would this be a suitable approach for you? Why?*

dynamics, identify ways to shift emphasis among opposite poles, and partner with others concerned.

- The three types of conflict are:
  - Intrapersonal
  - Interpersonal
  - Organizational
- The conflict process flows among four stages:
  - Frustration
    - Blocked goals lead to frustration.
    - Frustration is a cue to stop and clarify differences.
  - Conceptualization
    - The way a person perceives a conflict determines how he or she reacts to the frustration.
    - Differences in conceptualizing an issue can block resolution.
  - Action
    - Intentions, strategies, plans, and behavior flow out of conceptualization.

- Outcome (may be both tangible and intangible)
- When assessing how well a conflict has been resolved, one must consider:
  - The degree to which important goals were achieved.
  - The nature of subsequent relationships among those involved in the conflict.
- The five modes of conflict resolution are:
  - Avoiding
  - Accommodating
  - Competing
  - Compromising
  - Collaborating
- Each mode of conflict resolution can be viewed along two different continua:
  - From uncooperative to highly cooperative
  - From unassertive to highly assertive
- A conflict probably is unresolvable if:
  - The difficulty is ongoing.
  - There are two interdependent, polar opposite positions.
  - One pole needs to incorporate the other to succeed.
  - It is a "both/and" rather than "either/or" decision.
- Polarities are unresolvable conflicts.
  - Polarities have six important elements:
    - Two neutral, interdependent poles
    - Two sets of resulting positive consequences ("upsides")
    - Two sets of associated negative consequences ("downsides")
  - Polarity management requires a shifting focus from one pole to the other when cues of the approaching downside consequences become evident.

TIPS FOR ADDRESSING CONFLICT

- Communicate to yourself and others that conflict is a necessary and beneficial process typically marked by frustration, different conceptualizations, a variety of approaches to resolving it, and ongoing outcomes.
- In sorting out the different conceptualizations of a conflict situation, determine any similarities and differences in facts, goals, methods, and values.
- To assess the degree of conflict resolution, ask questions about the quality of decisions (i.e., creativity, practicality, achievement of goals and breakthrough results) and quality of the relationships

(i.e., understanding, willingness to work together, and mutual respect and cooperation).

■ Remind yourself of your preferences for perceiving and resolving conflict (e.g., which of the five approaches do you avoid and which do you overuse?) and assess each situation and match the best approach for that type of conflict regardless of which is your favorite approach.

■ Assist others around you in assessing conflict situations and seeing how they can best approach them.

■ Persistent and recurring problems and conflicts often are polarities that inherently are unresolvable. Approach them by mapping their upsides and downsides and creating ways to balance actions toward each pole when appropriate.

■ TERMS TO KNOW

accommodation	controversy
avoiding	interpersonal conflict
collaboration	intrapersonal conflict
competing	negotiating
compromising	organizational conflict
conflict	polarities

■ REFERENCES

Fisher, R.S., & Vry, W. (1991). *Getting to Yes: Negotiating Agreement Without Giving In.* New York: Penguin Books.

Hurst, J.B. (1993). Human Resource Development Center, University of Toledo, OH.

Hurst, J. (1996). Assisting clients to maximize polarities and stop trying to solve unsolvable problems. *Guidance & Counseling,* 11(4), 23-26.

Hurst, J.S., & VanderVeen, N. (1995). Polarity analysis and management: An alternative approach to unsolvable conflicts. *CACD Journal,* 15, 11-16.

Hurst, J., & Kinney, M. (1989). *Empowering Self and Others.* Toledo, OH: University of Toledo.

Johnson, B. (1992). *Polarity Management: Identifying and Managing Unsolvable Problems.* Amherst, MA: HRD Press.

Johnson, D.W., & Johnson, F.P. (1997). *Joining Together: Group Theory and Group Skills,* 6th ed. Englewood Cliffs, NJ: Prentice-Hall.

Keenan, M.J., Hurst, J.B., & Olnhausen, K. (1993). Polarity management for quality care: Self direction and manager direction. *Nursing Administration Quarterly,* 18(1), 23-29.

Kinney, M., & Hurst, J. (1989). *Group Process in Education.* Lexington, MA: Ginn Custom Publishers.

Scott, G.G. (1990). *Resolving Conflict with Others and Within Yourself.* Oakland, CA: New Harbinger.

Thomas, K. (1975). Conflict and conflict management. In Dunnette, M., ed. *The Handbook of Industrial Psychology.* Chicago, IL: Rand McNally.

Thomas, K.W., & Kilmann, R.H. (1973). Thomas-Kilmann conflict mode instrument. In Pfieffer, J.W., Heslin, R., & Jones, J.E. *Instrumentation in Human Relations Training.* San Diego, CA: University Associates, pp. 266-268.

Volkema, R.E. & Bergman, T.J. (1996). Conflict styles as indicators of behavioral patterns in interpersonal conflicts. *Journal of Social Psychology,* 135(1), 5-15.

■ SUGGESTED READINGS

Anderson, L. (1993). Teams, group process, success, and barriers. *Journal of Nursing Administration,* 23(9), 15-19.

Baker, K.M. (1995). Improving nurse conflict resolution skills. *Nursing Economies* 13(5), 295-298.

Castantino, C.A., &. Merchant, C.S. (1995). *Designing Conflict Management Systems.* San Francisco: Jossey-Bass.

Curtin, L. (1993). Empowerment: On eagle's wings. *Nursing Management,* 24(6), 7-9.

Dawson, R. (1993). *The Conflict Decision Maker: How To Make the Right Business and Personal Decisions Every Time.* New York: William Morrow.

Flarey, D.L. (1993). The social climate of work environments. *Journal of Nursing Administration,* 23(6), 9-15.

Hurst, J. (1996). Building hospital TQM teams. *The HealthCare Supervisor,* 15(1), 68-75.

Kusbell, E., & Rub, S. (1996). Dealing with conflict: the Margaret Chapman case. *Journal of Nursing Administration,* 26(2), 34-40.

Marcus, L.J. (1995). *Renegotiating Healthcare.* San Francisco: Jossey-Bass.

Martin, K., Wimberly, D., & O'Keefe, K. (1993). Resolving conflict in a multicultural nursing department. *Nursing Management,* 25(1), 49-51.

Ryan, D.K., Oestreich, D.K., & Orr, G.A. (1996). *The Courageous Messenger.* San Francisco: Jossey-Bass.

Valentine, P.E. (1995). Management of conflict: Do nurses/women handle it differently? *Journal of Advanced Nursing* 22, 142-199.

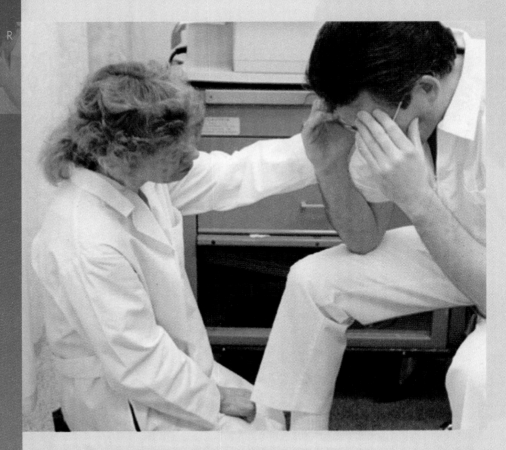

Managing Personal/ Personnel Problems

Arlene P. Stein
RN, PhD

Cindy Whittig Roach
RN, DSN

The purpose of this chapter is to discuss various personal and personnel problems that a manager must face in all nursing settings. Some specific tips and tools are provided as ways to intervene, coach, correct, and document problem behaviors. Emphasis is placed on effective communication, both written and verbal.

Objectives

- Differentiate common personnel/personal problems.
- Relate role concepts to clarification of personnel problems.
- Examine strategies useful for approaching specific personnel problems.
- Prepare specific guidelines for documenting performance problems.

Questions to Consider

- How do you react when you see that an employee is absent frequently and you or others seem to have a heavier work load as a result?
- Have you ever been in a position where you were not really sure what was expected of you? How did you feel?
- What would you do if you observed clinical incompetence in a coworker or student peer?
- What is the best approach to deal with someone you believe is chemically dependent or impaired at work?

?

A Manager's Challenge

From the Director of Maternal/Child Services at a Western Hospital

On the pediatric unit in an acute care hospital, new monitoring equipment was installed. This necessitated the instigation of some new standards of care. These new standards of care meant that everyone who worked in that area had to demonstrate competency in them.

The clinical manager and I determined that competency could be demonstrated through a basic ECG take-home test. Of the 42 nurses who took this test, seven failed with a score of less that 70%. These seven who failed were required to take an 8-hour class focusing on a review of pediatric dysrhythmias. This class consisted of a pre- and post-test along with hands-on didactics. Six of the seven failed the post-test and/or the didactic. These six people were then required to do a 6-week basic ECG class. We also provided a tutor who was a Clinical Nurse Specialist to help them with their homework when necessary. Three of these six failed the basic ECG class.

We thought perhaps these failures might result from test anxiety, and we wanted to be as fair as we possibly could with these individuals. We then permitted them to view the videotapes of all of the classes and review their tests along with the tutor. They were then retested; one person passed but two failed. Keep in mind that everyone was told at the beginning that it was a job requirement to pass this test, which indicated mastery of the standard of care for this pediatric unit.

How can a manager deal fairly with employees who fail to meet established standards of care despite numerous efforts on the manager's part to assist the employee meeting these standards?

? *What do you think you would do if you were this manager?*

INTRODUCTION

In managing nursing personnel, much of the satisfaction that a manager receives comes from working with people. On the other hand, working with people presents some of the greatest challenges with which a manager must cope. Problems such as absenteeism, uncooperative or unproductive employees, clinical incompetence, employees with emotional problems, and chemically dependent employees are only a few of the issues that challenge a manager. If a manager wants to be successful, these problems must be dealt with in ways to minimize their effects on patient care and on staff morale. Documentation of performance problems as well as documentation for termination is critical. Overall goals are to assist the employee in the improvement of performance, maintain the highest standards for the delivery of patient care, and provide a supportive environment in which all employees might deliver the best care and attain work satisfaction.

■ PERSONNEL/PERSONAL PROBLEMS

Absenteeism

One of the most vexing of these problems to the nurse manager is that of **absenteeism**, because inadequate staffing adversely affects patient care both directly and indirectly. When an absent caregiver is replaced by another one who is unfamiliar with the routines, employee morale suffers, and the care may be less than established standards. Working short-staffed or working overtime to cover for absent workers creates physical and mental stress (Taunton et al, 1995). Replacement personnel usually need more supervision, which not only is costly but also may decrease productivity and the quality of patient care. Indirectly, co-workers may become resentful from being forced to assume heavier work loads and/or be pressured to work extra hours. Chronic absenteeism may lead to increased staff conflicts and eventually to an increase in absenteeism among the entire staff.

Absenteeism also has a deleterious effect on the financial management of a nursing unit. Replacement of absent personnel by temporary personnel or overtime paid to other employees is very costly, and the cost of fringe benefits used by absent workers is very high. Managing absenteeism is important for all of the aforementioned factors. Also, as our care delivery systems become more complex and technologically oriented, the successful nurse manager must realize that technology is not a replacement for human caregivers. We cannot replace absent caregivers with machines.

Absenteeism cannot be totally eliminated. There are always unplanned illnesses, accidents, bad weather, sick family members, a death in the family, and even jury duty, which are legitimate reasons for missing work and cannot be controlled by management. However, most researchers believe that some portion of absenteeism is voluntary and preventable; thus there are many attempts to identify the cause and thereby instigate a cure.

Using role theory as a framework, absenteeism can be linked to **role stress** and **role strain** (see theory box). Absence from work is a way of withdrawing from an undesirable situation short of actually leaving, and many employees increase their absenteeism just prior to their resignation. If the healthcare worker is experiencing some form of role stress, leading to role strain, it might be manifested through absenteeism. Hardy and Conway (1988) state that role strain may be reflected by (1) withdrawal from interaction, (2) reduced involvement with colleagues and organizations, and (3) job dissatisfaction. All of these could be manifested through absenteeism. Using this framework, management of absenteeism is based on the belief that competent role performance requires interpersonal competence. "Role competence is the ability of a person in an interdependent position, which is ongoing in time, to carry out lines of action that are task and interpersonally effective" (Hardy &

Theory		
THEORY/KEY CONTRIBUTOR	**KEY IDEA**	**APPLICATION TO PRACTICE**
Role Theory is not considered a true scientific theory but more of a perspective or framework to understand individual behavior as it applies to specific roles. (Hardy & Conway, 1989).	Professional socialization is a learned behavior and clarifies specific role prescriptions or sets of rules that are inherent within a given profession.	Within each area of practice, or within each organization, there are specific rules, behaviors, and expectations that are prescribed and that will direct practice. It is the responsibility of each professional nurse to completely understand their role. When this does not occur, role ambiguity or role strain may result. Absence of role clarity can also lead to decreased work satisfaction.

Conway, 1988, p. 195). Hardy and Conway further explain that role competence is (1) learned through socialization processes, (2) necessary for adequate role performance, and (3) accountable for individual and social progress. In other words, to engage successfully in roles, people need role-specific skills; but they also need interpersonal competence to guide their behaviors. Role behavior occurs in a social context rather than in isolation. Therefore the nurse manager needs to know the existing situation, when it has changed, when it needs to be changed, and how to change it. Studies have shown an inverse relationship between job satisfaction and absenteeism, indicating that attention to enhancing nurses' job satisfaction may be an effective strategy toward reducing absenteeism. This chapter's "Research Perspective" highlights this study (Taunton et al, 1995).

An adaptation from Haddock's (1989) model of **nonpunitive discipline** is also useful in addressing absenteeism behavior, as the example in the next paragraph illustrates. Using absenteeism as an example, this model demonstrates how undesirable behaviors, such as absenteeism, can be successfully changed. Figure 20-1 illustrates how changing undesirable behaviors can be accomplished.

When an employee demonstrates an unacceptable level of absenteeism the manager can take the following steps to help clarify role expectations:

Step 1: Remind the employee of the employment standards of the agency. Sometimes an employee does not know, or has forgotten, the existing standards, and a reminder with no threats or discipline is all that is needed.

Step 2: When the oral reminder does not result in a behavior change, put the reminder in writing for the employee. These oral and written reminders are simply statements of the problem and the goals to which both the manager and the employee agree. The employee must voluntarily agree with the manager that the behavior in question is not acceptable and must agree to change.

Step 3: If the written reminder fails, only then grant the employee a day of decision, which is a day off with pay to arrive at a decision about future action. Pay is given for this day so that it is not interpreted as punishment. The employee must return to work with a written decision as to whether or not to accept the standards for work attendance. Remember that this is a voluntary decision on the employee's part. Emphasize to the employee that it is the employee's decision to adhere to the standards.

Step 4: If the employee decides not to adhere to standards, terminate him or her. On the other hand, if the employee agrees to adhere to the standards, and in the future does not, the employee in essence has terminated employment.

Research Perspective

Taunton, R.L., Hope, K., Woods, C.Q., & Bott, M.J. (1995). Predictors of absenteeism among hospital staff nurses. Nursing Economics, 13(4), 217-229.

This correlational prospective study examined absenteeism among nurses in four large acute care hospitals in a Midwestern metropolitan area. An organizational dynamics paradigm was used as a tool to measure effectiveness in predicting absenteeism among the nurses in these hospitals. The predictors of absenteeism differed by hospital. The role of the manager, organizational policies related to criteria for excessive absence, incentives for attendance, and deterrents to absence were correlated with absentee rates.

Implications for Practice

The findings in this study indicate that organizational policies are very important in managing absenteeism. Along with this it was found that consistency among managers in the application of policies increased their effectiveness in controlling absenteeism. The authors suggest that organizations provide clear expectations, incentives, and deterrents and promote leadership based on effective communication, consideration of individuals, and developing work group cohesion to minimize disruptive absenteeism.

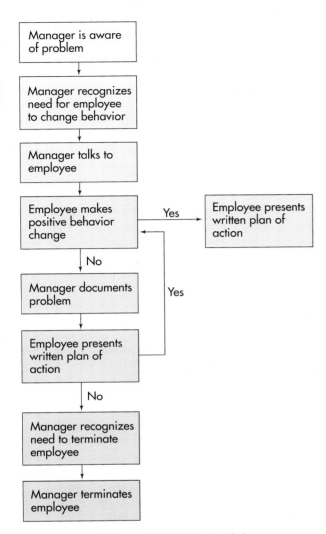

Figure 20-1 Model for behavioral change.

Hersey, Blanchard & Johnson (1996) identify two major dimensions of job performance—motivation and ability—that relate to this problem. The type and intensity of motivation vary among employees because of differing needs and goals that employees express. The manager can best handle employees with motivation problems by attempting to determine the cause of the problem and by trying to provide an environment that is conducive to increased motivation for the employee. If the employee is uncooperative or unproductive due to a lack of ability, education and training would be an appropriate intervention.

Exercise 20-1

Review the policy manual at a local healthcare organization. Determine what constitutes excessive absenteeism. What are the consequences?

The manager can determine lack of ability on the part of an employee in various ways. Frequent errors in judgment or techniques are often an indication of lack of knowledge, skill, or critical thinking. This illustrates the need for the nurse manager to carefully document all variances or untoward events. When the nurse manager does thorough documentation, trends may be discovered that in turn suggest a specific employee is having problems. The nurse manager can cite problem behaviors and perhaps even trends to the employee. Corrective action is easier to pursue and resolution is more effective in this manner. When the problem is determined to result from a need for more education or training, the manager can work with the education department, or the clinical specialist for the involved unit, to help the employee improve his or her skills. Most employees are extremely cooperative in situations such as this as they want to do a good job, but sometimes don't know how. Employees may deny they need help or may be too embarrassed to ask for help. When the manager can show an employee concrete evidence of a problem area, cooperation is enhanced.

Sometimes an unproductive employee simply lacks maturity. Immaturity in an employee may not be readily apparent to the manager but may be manifested in any of the following actions: defiance, testing of work place guidelines, passivity or hostility, or little appreciation for any management decisions. The challenge for the nurse manager is not to react in kind, but rather relate to this employee in a positive and mature manner. For example, if an employee states, "Administration is always making decisions to make our jobs harder," rather than making a hostile or

Keep a copy of the written agreements and also give the employee a copy (Rogers, Hutchins, & Johnson, 1990).

This model of nonpunitive discipline allows employees to free themselves from some role stress by clarification of role expectations. Employees can receive satisfaction from the realization that a problem is not inadequate performance attributed to personal faults, but rather a lack of clarification of role expectations within the organization.

Uncooperative or Unproductive Employees

The problem of *uncooperative or unproductive* employees is another area of frustration for the nurse manager.

defensive comment in reply, the manager could take the employee aside and say, "I notice that you seem to be angry about this new policy. Let's talk about it some more." Immature employees either act immaturely all of the time or regress to an immature level when stressed. The nurse manager must recognize immaturity in an employee and react calmly and without anger. The manager must keep in mind that this employee may be displaying dynamics rooted in unresolved areas of personality development and that the behavior is not a personal attack on the manager. The best way to deal with this behavior is to confront the employee with the specific problem and define realistic limits of acceptable behavior with consequences for nonadherence. Generally, employees comply with specific limits, but will test management in other areas. As this testing occurs, the manager must continue the same limit-setting technique. Remember that the immature employee usually has problems because of a lack of self-worth, power, and self-control. Praise and affirmation are valuable tools that the manager can use to help these employees feel better about themselves.

Exercise 20-2

A nurse comes to you, the nurse manager, and states that one of the other nurses is tying a knot in the airvent (pigtail) of nasogastric tubes. What would you do?

Clinical Incompetence

Clinical incompetence is possibly one of the most frustrating problems that the nurse manager faces, even though it may be entirely correctable. The problem may surface immediately in a new employee. At other times, clinical incompetence comes as a surprise to a nurse manager if co-workers "cover" for another employee. Some nurses are unwilling to report instances of clinical incompetence because they do not want to feel responsible for getting one of their peers in trouble. When other employees are engaged in enabling behavior by covering for the mistakes of one of their peers, the nurse manager may be surprised to discover that the employee does not know or cannot do what is expected of him or her in the job. Sadly, the employee in question has been able to cover incompetencies by hiding behind the performance of another employee. The nurse manager must remind employees that part of professional responsibility is to maintain quality care and thus they are obligated to report instances of clinical incompetence, even when it means reporting a co-worker. "Anytime you close your eyes to violations of a safety rule or a required practice, you are creating a dangerous workplace" (Curtin, 1996).

Most healthcare agencies use skills checklists to ascertain that their employees have and maintain essential skills for the job they're expected to do. A skills checklist is an excellent way to determine basic clinical competency (see Box 20-1). This list typically contains a number of basic skills along with ones that are essential for safe functioning in the area of employment. The employee may be asked to do a self-assessment of the listed skills and then have performance of the skills validated by a peer or co-worker. This is a very effective method for the manager to assess the skill level of employees and to determine where additional education and training may be necessary. Additionally, if the manager discovers that an employee is unable to adequately perform a skill, it is easy for the manager to check the skills list and see at what level this employee is functioning and recommend a specific plan for remediation. Sometimes an employee may be able to perform all of the tasks on a skills checklist, but is still unable to effectively manage overall patient care. If in questioning the employee, or in evaluating the employee's performance, the manager determines that there is a lack of knowledge or that there are problems with time management, formal education may be the proper course of action. In either event, the manager must establish a written contract containing a plan of action with time limits in which certain expectations must be achieved. This assures compliance on the part of the employee.

Emotional Problems

Emotional problems among nursing personnel may have an impact not only on the involved individual, but also on co-workers and ultimately on the delivery of patient care. The nurse manager must be aware that certain behaviors, such as poor judgment, increased errors, increased absenteeism, decreased productivity, and a negative attitude, may be manifestations of emotional problems in employees.

Example
A nurse manager began hearing complaints from patients about a nurse named Nancy. Patients were saying that Nancy was abrupt and uncaring with them. The manager had not received any complaints about Nancy before this time, so she questioned Nancy about why this was occurring. Nancy reported that her mother was very ill and she was so worried about her and was so upset that she couldn't sleep and was tired all of the time. She went on to say that she was having trouble being sympathetic with complaining patients when they didn't seem to be as sick as her mother.

Box 20-1

Example of a Skills Checklist

Purpose

1. The clinical skills inventory is a three-phase tool to enable the newly hired RN and the nurse manager to determine individual learning needs, verify competency, and plan performance goals.
2. The RN will complete the self-assessment of clinical skills during the first week of employment. The RN will use the appropriate scale to document current knowledge of clinical skills.
3. The nurse manager will document observed competency of the orientee or delegate this to a peer. All columns must be completed on the inventory level.
4. At the end of orientation, the new RN and the manager will use the inventory to identify performance goals on the plan sheet. The skills inventory will be in a specified place on the nursing unit so that it is available to the manager and other RNs. It should be updated at appropriate intervals as specified by the manager.

Scale for Self-Assessment

1 = Unfamiliar/never done
2 = Able to perform with assistance
3 = Can perform with minimal supervision
4 = Independent performance/proficient

Score for Validation of Competency

1 = Unable to perform at present
2 = Able to perform with assistance
3 = Progressing/repeat performance necessary
4 = Able to perform independently

CLINICAL SKILLS	SELF-ASSESSMENT		COMMENT	VALIDATION			COMMENT
	SCALE	DATE		SCORE	DATE	INITIALS	
Epidural catheter care							
NG/Dobbhoff							
Insertion							
Management							
Preoperative care/teaching							
Postoperative care/teaching							

Plan Sheet for Skills Inventory

Name _____

Date _____

GOALS	DATE TO BE COMPLETED
_____	_____
_____	_____
_____	_____
_____	_____
_____	_____
_____	_____
_____	_____
_____	_____
_____	_____

Orientee's signature _____

Manager's signature _____

Date _____

Skills Inventory adapted from one used at Memorial Hospital, Colorado Springs, CO.

When a trend of these behaviors is evident, a problem that an employee is unable to handle may be the cause. The nurse manager is not and should not be a therapist, but must intercede, not only to help the individual with problems but also to maintain proper functioning of the unit. In dealing with the employee who exhibits behaviors that indicate emotional problems, the manager, after identifying the problem, should assist the individual to get professional help to cope with the problem. The manager may have to make some adjustments in the individual's work setting and schedule if this is deemed necessary and does not have a negative effect on patient care. Even though the manager is aware that an employee is experiencing emotional difficulties, the standards of care and practice cannot be compromised in the hope of "going easy" on the individual. If standards are lowered to help an individual, the effect will be deleterious to all people involved. The most important approach that the manager can take with an emotionally troubled employee is to provide support and encouragement and to assist the individual to get appropriate help. Many agencies have some kind of employee assistance program (EAP) to which the manager should refer any troubled employee. During this process, the manager must remember to check with the human resources department about any implications that may occur because of the Americans with Disabilities Act (ADA). If an employee has a documented mental illness, the employing agency may be under certain legal constraints as specified in the ADA. The nurse manager should always remember that there are many resources available to assist with personnel problems. The manager should never feel required to know all of the legal implications regarding employment policies. Rather, the manager must know that help is available and how to access it.

Exercise 20-3

As a nurse manager in a community health agency, you have just had a meeting that was called by several of your staff nurses. They expressed concern regarding another nurse colleague who has come to work tearful several times during the past week. They state she frequently goes into the break room when she is in the agency and appears as if she's been crying when she comes out. She has refused to discuss her distress with her colleagues. These nurses express concern and want you to help her. What is your response? What would you do?

Chemical Dependency

Chemical dependency among nursing personnel places patients and the organization at risk. The **chemically dependent** employee adversely affects staff morale by increasing stress on other staff members when they have to assume heavier work loads to cover for the chemically dependent employee who is not performing at full capacity, or who is frequently absent. As a result, patient care may be jeopardized when staff are focusing more on the problems of a co-worker than on those of the patients they are assigned to care for.

The manager is responsible for early recognition of chemical dependency and referral for treatment when appropriate. State laws vary as to the reportability of chemical dependency. As is true of all nurses, a nurse manager is responsible for upholding the nurse practice act and should be familiar with the legal aspects of chemical dependency in the state in which he/she is employed. Here again, as with the employee with emotional problems, the nurse manager should be aware of ADA issues and check with the human resource department for help with how to handle the employment of a chemically dependent employee. Most states and agencies have reporting requirements regarding substance abuse. The state board of nursing is an excellent source of information for the nurse manager unfamiliar with the legal aspects of the nurse practice act. All nurse managers should familiarize themselves with the nurse practice act in the state in which they reside as well as the personnel policies relating to substance abuse in their employing agency. Furthermore they should make certain that staff also are familiar with legal requirements.

Identification of an employee with a chemical dependency is usually difficult, especially when one of the primary symptoms is denial. Blazer and Mansfield (1995) found that substance abuse is not higher among nurses than for any other group of working females. They further state that their study does not support previous findings of serious substance abuse among nurses. Despite the conflicts in research findings about the incidence of substance abuse among nurses, 65% of disciplinary actions against nurses involve drug abuse (Ellis, 1995). Because of this, it is highly probable that a manager is likely to encounter a chemically dependent person at some career point.

In the present social climate there is more interest in helping affected individuals than in punishing them, and there is also more empathy and understanding toward them.

The primary clue that a manager should be alert for when there is a suspicion of chemical dependency is any behavioral changes in an employee. This change could be any deviation from that which the employee normally exhibits. Some specific behaviors to note might be mood swings, a change from a tidy appearance to an untidy one, an unusual interest in patients' pain control, frequent changes in jobs and shifts, or an increase in absenteeism and tardiness.

When a manager suspects an employee may be chemically dependent, the manager must intervene as patient care may be jeopardized, as already described. A manager facing a problem with an impaired nurse must be compassionate yet therapeutic. Knowing that denial may be one of the primary signs of substance abuse, the manager must focus on performance problems that the nurse is exhibiting and urge the nurse to voluntarily seek counseling or treatment. Employee assistance programs always protect the employee's privacy and are usually available free or at a minimal charge to the employee. The manager should strive to refer any troubled employee to the employee assistance program whenever possible. This removes the manager from the counseling role and helps employees get the professional help they need without fear of a breach in confidentiality. If a nurse refuses to seek help voluntarily for a substance abuse problem, the manager is responsible for following the established policy for such employees. The manager must remember that if the substance-abusing employee is terminated and not reported, the manager not only may be violating a law, but also may be enabling this employee to get employment in

another agency and potentially be in a position to harm patients and co-workers.

Many states have rehabilitation programs for chemically impaired nurses, so that some may return to nursing if rehabilitated. Nurse managers are sometimes asked to assist with monitoring the progress of a chemically impaired nurse. Specific guidelines are established through the rehabilitation program with the cooperation of the employee, the agency, and the manager. The manager is typically asked to provide feedback about the employee's progress to the employee as well as to the state or rehabilitation program involved. These programs vary, but, for example, a nurse who has been an admitted abuser of meperidine may be allowed to work in a setting where this drug is never used, or the nurse may not be permitted to administer any controlled substances to patients. This, of course, puts an added burden on other staff members, but it can be a positive experience for all, as nurses face some of their professional responsibility by helping another nurse while upholding patient care. Often, as a part of their therapy, these nurses are required to openly share with other staff members what their problem is and what they are doing to control it. When handled in a positive, professional way, the nurse manager can turn a potentially destructive situation into a positive constructive one.

Exercise 20-4

Review your state's nurse practice act and rules and regulations. What are you required to do if you believe a nurse has a problem with chemical dependency?

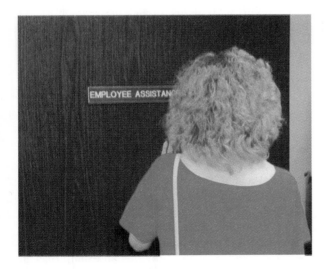

Many agencies have an employee assistance program to which the manager can refer the troubled employee.

DOCUMENTATION

Documentation of personnel problems is unquestionably one of the most important, but also one of the most onerous, aspects of the nurse manager's job. As much as some managers would wish, personnel problems probably will not "just go away by themselves," and so will have to be dealt with eventually. Through careful ongoing documentation of problems the manager makes the task of identifying and correcting problems much less burdensome.

Documentation cannot be left to memory! When an employee is involved in a problem occurrence, or if an employee receives a compliment or does something extremely well, a brief notation to this effect should be placed in the personnel file. This entry should include the date, time, and a brief description of the incident. It is helpful also to add

Box 20-2

Documentation of Problems

- Description of incident—an objective statement of the facts related to the incident.
- Actions—statement(s) describing all actions taken by the manager when the problem was discovered.
- Plan—statement(s) describing the plan to correct and/or prevent future problems.
- Follow-up—dates and times that the plan is to be carried out, including required meeting with the employee.

Example:

Several patients reported to the nurse manager that Becky, one of the night shift RNs, was "curt" and "gruff" and seemed uncaring with them. The manager called Becky into her office and reiterated the complaints that she had received. The nurse manager was specific as to times and incidents. The manager then reminded Becky about what her expectations were relating to patient care, emphasizing the importance of a caring attitude with all patients. She discussed with Becky what the possible cause of Becky's behavior might be, such as problems at home or lack of sleep. Becky denied being curt or gruff, but agreed that some of her mannerisms might be misinterpreted. The manager suggested to Becky that perhaps she needed to be particularly aware of her body language and to soften her tone of voice. After discussing this incident and reminding Becky of the importance of caring in nursing, the manager told Becky that this behavior would not be tolerated. The manager told Becky she wanted to meet with her every Friday morning at the end of Becky's shift to discuss how the week had gone and to determine how she was interacting with the patients assigned to her. The manager also told Becky that she would be checking with patients to see what they had thought of Becky. The manager routinely asked patients about their nursing care as she made rounds, so this was not an unusual thing for her to do. These weekly meetings were to be conducted for 6 weeks followed by monthly meetings for a 3-month period. If there was no recurrence of problems, the meetings would be discontinued after this time.

Box 20-3

Steps in Progressive Discipline

1. Counsel employee regarding the problem.
2. Reprimand employee. A verbal reprimand usually precedes a written one, but some organizations issue both a verbal and a written reprimand simultaneously. When the documentation is written, the employee must sign to verify that the problem was discussed. This does not mean that the employee agrees with the reprimand. It means only that the employee is aware of a written verbal reprimand that is to be placed in the employee's personnel file. The employee always receives a copy of a written reprimand.
3. Suspend employee if the problem persists. The employee will be suspended without pay for a period of time, usually several days or longer according to the agency policy. During this time the employee may realize the seriousness of the problem based on the resulting discipline.
4. Allow the employee to return to work with written stipulations regarding problem behavior.
5. Terminate employee if problem recurs.

a small notation as to what was done about a problem when it occurred. Along with this, the nurse manager should keep a log or summary sheet of all reported errors, unusual incidents, accidents, and any other untoward effects. These extremely important data should include the date, time, and names of involved individuals and should be tallied at monthly intervals for analysis by the manager. The few extra minutes each day that the manager spends tracking these data provides invaluable information to the manager about organizational and individual functioning. This tracking can then be used to pinpoint problem areas, areas of excellence in individual performance, and overall organizational problem areas. The manager who keeps careful records about organizational functioning has greater control in the management of personal and personnel problems. Box 20-2 describes content and format for such documentation and provides an example as an illustration.

PROGRESSIVE DISCIPLINE

When an employee's performance falls below the acceptable standard, despite corrective measures that have been taken, some form of discipline must be enacted. Most organizations use some form of progressive discipline to correct problem behaviors. **Progressive discipline** consists of evaluating performance and providing feedback with steps of increasing sanctions. These sanctions progress from least severe to most severe, as described in Box 20-3.

TERMINATION

At times, even though the manager has done everything possible to gain the cooperation of a problem employee, the problems may persist. Then there is no choice but to terminate the employee. Since *termination* is one of the most difficult things a manager does, it is best to follow certain guidelines. First, the manager must feel secure in the fact that everything possible has been done to help the employee correct the problem behaviors. Second, the manager recognizes that if employment continues, this employee will have a deleterious effect on overall organizational functioning and, more importantly, on nursing care. Third, the employee has been made fully aware of the problem performance and of the fact that all of the correct disciplinary steps have been followed. Finally, a nurse manager should check with the human resources and legal departments before proceeding to be certain termination is justifiable legally and that proper steps have been followed. It is extremely helpful to feel confident in the knowledge that all policies regarding termination have been followed before an actual termination meeting with the employee. It is always preferable to err on the side of caution when proceeding with termination of an employee. Remember that termination is something that the employee has caused as a result of persistent problem behaviors. Termination is not done at the whim of management; it results from failure on the part of the employee to change a problem behavior.

Example
Linda has gone through all of the steps in the progressive discipline process as a result of her abusive behavior toward her co-workers. She returned to work and seemed to be doing well until about 6 weeks later when she slammed down her clipboard during report and angrily accused the charge nurse of always giving her the worst assignments. The nurse manager was present and asked Linda to come into her office. At this point, she told Linda she was relieving her of her assignment that day and asked her to go home to cool off. The manager told her that she would call her the following day about what would be done. Linda went home and the manager reviewed the incident with her boss. They both agreed that Linda's behavior not only was intolerable but also violated the terms of her probation and therefore she should be terminated. The manager called Linda the following day as she had agreed to do and asked Linda to come and meet with her. The manager and her boss met with Linda and reviewed the incidents and the disciplinary measures leading up to this one. The nurse manager asked her boss to be present at the scheduled meeting as it is a good practice to have a witness in a confrontive situation such as termination. The manager stated to Linda that she regretted it had come to this, but pointed out to her that her behavior had violated all of the agreed upon stipulations and as a result she would be terminated immediately. Linda was tearful and had numerous excuses, but the manager remained firm and merely repeated that Linda, in not fulfilling the agreement, had chosen to end her employment.

CONCLUSION

All employees share a role along with managers to prevent and control personal/personnel problems in their work setting. Everyone must be willing to refuse to assist unethical behavior from co-workers and to speak out and act appropriately when problems occur.

A Manager's Solution

[?] As a final step, we met with the two individuals who had not passed, despite all of our efforts, and gave them the opportunity to transfer to another clinical area of their choosing, and where they would feel comfortable, if an opening was available. We made it clear to them that they could not work on the pediatric unit because they had not met the established standards of care. One of the individuals chose to resign from the organization and the other one transferred to another area.

[?] *Would this be a suitable approach for you? Why?*

CHAPTER CHECKLIST

To obtain satisfaction from working with people, a nurse manager must be knowledgeable about personal and personnel issues that are likely to occur in the work setting. The nurse manager must be able to detect, prevent, and correct problems that affect nursing care and staff morale in a nursing agency. Proper documentation and follow-up are key elements in the successful management of all personnel issues.

- Among absenteeism's detrimental effects are these:
  - Patient care may be below standard.
  - Replacement personnel require additional supervision.
  - Absenteeism may increase among the entire staff.
  - Financial management of the unit suffers adverse effects.
- Effective strategies to reduce absenteeism include:
  - Enhancing nurses' job satisfaction.
  - Using Haddock's model of nonpunitive discipline:
    - Remind the employee of the problem orally.
    - Follow up with a written reminder if the oral one fails.
    - Grant the employee a day of decision if the written reminder fails.
    - Terminate if the employee decides not to adhere to standards.
- Uncooperative or unproductive employees may lack motivation, ability, or maturity.
  - The nurse manager can try to provide an environment that is more conducive to motivation.
  - Education and training are appropriate interventions for lack of ability.
  - Praise and affirmation are often the most effective strategies for an employee who lacks maturity.
- Clinical incompetence is a highly correctable problem for nurse managers.
  - Clinical incompetence may be masked by co-workers' enabling behavior.
  - A skills checklist helps determine basic clinical competency and pinpoint the need for additional training and education.
- When emotional problems are evident, the nurse manager should assist the employee in getting professional help. The nurse manager is responsible for early recognition of chemical dependency and referral for treatment when appropriate.
  - The manager must:
    - Uphold the state's nurse practice act.
    - Be familiar with state laws on chemical dependency.
    - Know the healthcare organization's personnel policy on chemical dependency.
  - Some warning signs of possible chemical dependency are:
    - Behavioral changes such as mood swings
    - Sudden and unusual neglect for personal appearance
    - Unusual interest in patients' pain control
    - Increased absenteeism and tardiness
- Documentation of problems should include:
  - A description of the incident
  - A description of the manager's actions
  - A plan to correct/prevent future occurrences
  - Dates and times of follow-up measures
- Progressive discipline may be used when other corrective measures have failed. Steps in progressive discipline are:
  - Counsel the employee regarding the problem.
  - Reprimand the employee (first verbally, then in writing).
  - Suspend the employee if the problem persists.
  - Allow the employee to return to work, with written stipulations regarding problem behavior.
  - Terminate the employee if the problem recurs.

TIPS IN DOCUMENTATION OF PROBLEMS

- Identify the incident and related facts.
- Describe actions taken by the manager when the problem was identified.
- Develop an action plan for everyone involved.
- Schedule follow-up to evaluate progress of the action plan.
- Remember to document everything objectively and completely!

TERMS TO KNOW

absenteeism	progressive discipline
chemically dependent	role strain
nonpunitive discipline	role stress

■ REFERENCES

Blazer, L.K., & Mansfield, P.K. (1995). A comparison of substance use rates among female nurses, clerical workers, and blue collar workers. *Journal of Advanced Nursing*, 21, 305-313.

Curtin, L. (1996). Ethics, discipline and discharge. *Nursing Management*, 27(3), 51-52.

Ellis, P. (1995). Addressing chemical dependency. A need for consistent measures. *Nursing Management*, 26(8), 56-58.

Haddock, C. (1989). Transformation leadership and the employee discipline process. *Hospital Health Service Administration*, 34(2), 185-194.

Hardy, M.E., & Conway, M.E. (1989). *Role Theory: Perspectives for Health Professionals*, 2nd ed. Norwalk, CT: Appleton & Lange.

Hersey, P., Blanchard, K., & Johnson, D.E. (1996). *Management of Organizational Behavior: Utilizing Human Resources*, 7th ed. Englewood Cliffs, NJ: Prentice-Hall.

Rogers, J.E., Hutchins, S.G., & Johnson, B.J. (1990). Non-punitive discipline: a method of reducing absenteeism. *Journal of Nursing Administration*, 20(7/8), 41-43.

Taunton, R.L., Hope, K., Woods, C.Q., & Bott, J. (1995). Predictors of absenteeism among hospital staff nurses. *Nursing Economics*, 13(4), 217-229.

Taunton, R.L., Perkins, S., Oetker-Black, S. & Heaton, R. (1995). Absenteeism in acute care hospitals. *Nursing Management*, 26(9), 80-82.

■ SUGGESTED READINGS

Cabot, S.J. (1995). Easing the pain of separation. *Provider*, April, 57-59.

Hughes, T.L. (1995). Chief nurse executives' responses to chemically dependent nurses. *Nursing Management*, 26(3), 37-40.

Irvine, D.M., & Evans, M.G. (1995). Job satisfaction and turnover among nurses: Integrating research findings across studies. *Nursing Research*, 44(4), 246-253.

Mee, C.L., Cirone, N.R., & Levinger, C.V. (1996). MERG: Medication event rating grid. *Nursing Management*, 27(4), 34-38.

Yoder-Wise, L. (1995). Staff nurses' career development relationships and self-reports of professionalism, job satisfaction, and intent to stay. *Nursing Research*, 44(5), 290-297.

Managing Consumer Care

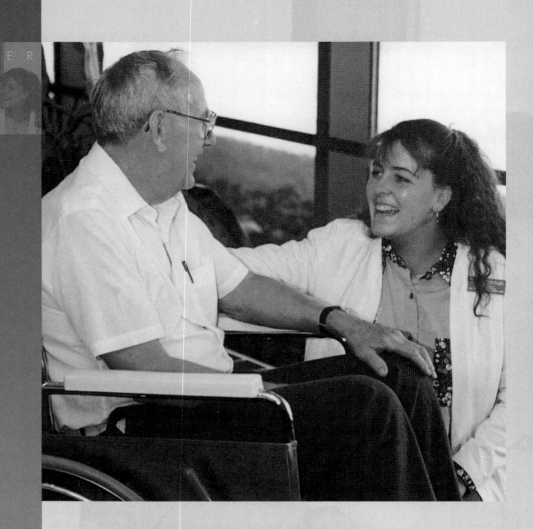

Consumer Relationships

Brenda L. Cleary
RN, PhD, CS, FAAN

This chapter explores the changes that have altered consumer relationships with healthcare providers and looks specifically at the nurse's responsibilities to the consumer. The nurse manager sets the tone for effective staff-patient interaction. Since nurses are the healthcare providers who spend the most time with the consumer, the chapter provides concepts and strategies to assist in developing effective nurse-consumer relationships.

Objectives

- Categorize health consumers' interactions into three relationship structures.
- Interpret the results of selected changes that have influenced consumer relationships in healthcare.
- Examine the importance of a service-oriented philosophy to the quality of the nurse/consumer relationship.
- Apply the four major responsibilities of nursing: service, advocacy, teaching, and leadership to the promotion of successful nurse/consumer relationships.

Questions to Consider

- Why is the consumer perspective so important to nursing leaders?
- What changes have taken place that have altered the relationships between consumers and providers of healthcare?
- What concepts must you apply in order to provide service-oriented nursing care to consumers?
- How do you take into consideration cultural diversity and individual differences when you practice nursing?
- What is consumer advocacy and who is responsible for it?

 A Manager's Challenge

From the Director of a Home Health Agency in the Southeastern United States

Consumer satisfaction is our primary goal at St. Joseph of the Pines Home Health. We respond promptly to any concern voiced by clients/caregivers, no matter how trivial they seem. It is their perception that is important, and we go to great lengths to ensure satisfaction.

A concern was telephoned to our agency by a client's spouse. She stated that during a home health visit the day before, the RN had written on a piece of paper that was the wrapper for a collectible she had purchased for her husband. She had paid a large price for the collectible in the wrapper, and now it was less valuable because of the defacement. The husband was reportedly upset about the matter and wanted something done about it.

The nurse manager and immediate supervisor initiated an inquiry with the RN, who said she did not remember anything of this nature happening. The nurse manager then made a visit to the home to further explore the incident with the family. As she examined the wrapper, she discovered that the writing did look like the RN's handwriting. The manager sincerely apologized on behalf of the agency, but explained that we did not reimburse for this type of incident. When the visit was completed, she thought the matter was resolved other than the leftover business of the other RN personally processing the situation with the family during her next visit. Both husband and wife seemed satisfied with the apology and the visit to discuss the matter.

Wrong! Approximately 10 days later, I received a call at the administrative office from the spouse of the client, reporting the entire incident again. Apparently, she had called the agency directly once more and perceived that our staff had been "curt" with her. I listened carefully to her explain the incident. When she completed her explanation, I thanked her for bringing her concern to my attention and let her know I would follow up.

What would you do if you were this manager?

INTRODUCTION

In the delivery of healthcare, *consumer relationships* refer to the multitude of encounters between the consumer (client/patient/customer) and the representatives of the healthcare system. Who are the consumers of healthcare and what do they expect from providers? What are their likes and dislikes and how do they evaluate the care they receive?

We all are consumers of healthcare—friends, neighbors, families, people like us, and people very different from us. Consumers are diverse culturally, ethnically, socially, physically, and psychologically. Consumers have to some degree become far better connoisseurs of healthcare than in the past. They have access to a limitless amount of information regarding health. Not all of what they read, hear, or see is valid, but they are better informed now than they ever have been. They question providers regarding the care they receive or don't receive and they ask, "Why are you doing that?"

The Consumer Focus

Consumer relationships are constantly changing and thus affect the providers of health services: primary care and public health services, managed care organizations, hospitals, home health agencies, and nursing homes, as well as individual providers such as physicians and nurses. As inpatient services shrink, outpatient services grow, and competition for patients becomes fierce, the focus has moved from **healthcare providers** to **healthcare consumers.** As noted in the "Manager's Challenge," *the consumer will drive what goes on in our healthcare settings.* The healthcare processes are being redefined with the consumer as the center of everything. How consumers view and value the care they receive becomes important data. In the "Manager's Challenge" there are distinct relationships that consumers enter into in meeting their healthcare needs, including the healthcare agency, the insurer or payer, the physician, the nurse, and allied health providers. Changes in physician practices, access to **service,** insurance coverage, and nurses' roles and responsibilities are a few of the significant factors that have influenced these relationships.

Physician/Consumer Relationships

Physician/consumer relationships changed as the physician's mode of practice moved from a single, private enterprise to the multigroup practice. The groups may even be incorporated into health maintenance organizations, managed care programs, or physician-hospital organizations. When consumers visit a group practice, they may be unable to select a specific physician. Patients no longer know their physicians as they did in the past, and physicians may be unfamiliar with their patients, resulting in decreased opportunity for the development of mutual respect and trust.

Rural consumers of healthcare have seen their local hospitals close and have had to seek care in regional health centers. They may not know the physicians from whom they are redirected to seek care, which often leads consumers to be more critical and less accepting of the care delivered. They often feel alienated and insecure in unfamiliar circumstances even though they may be receiving the best medical attention. The patient's perceptions are becoming an increasingly valued outcome of care.

Agency/Consumer Relationships

Consumers of health services are accustomed to receiving acute care in an inpatient setting. In many situations, this option is no longer available. Patients may be angry and frightened at the thought of being on their own or with service provided only periodically from home health agencies. When inpatient services are deemed appropriate, the specific hospital or health agency that the client must patronize most likely will be dictated by the type of insurance coverage and the insurance carrier. Managed care options require that the consumer use particular and specific health facilities or be responsible for all or a larger portion of the bill.

No longer is a trip to the emergency department an option for a sore throat at midnight. The price tag for that service is prohibitive. Consumers are seeing their options for seeking care shrinking and the costs increasing. The insurance plans available to most people include a co-payment or a deductible clause requiring the consumer to meet a certain dollar amount before the insurance companies will pay their 60% to 90% of the bill, resulting in a significant impact on the consumer.

Among the growing number of Americans without health insurance, there may be alienation from our healthcare system (or lack thereof). Medicare and Medicaid recipients also find themselves in the midst of changes in terms of how healthcare costs are managed.

Nurse/Consumer Relationships

Nurses are the healthcare providers who spend the most time with the consumer. These encounters are generally personal and intensely meaningful. Therefore the nurse is in a unique position to influence and promote dramatic and effective positive consumer relationships. The nurse manager sets the tone for effective staff/patient interactions, with exciting opportunities presented in patient-focused care.

Changes from hospital/nursing home care to outpatient care have particularly altered the nurse/consumer relationship. Nurses are taking leadership roles as primary providers (nurse practitioners, midwives), teachers and educators, and home healthcare managers and advocates, particularly in compensation and insurance arenas. Nurses may emerge as the **gatekeepers** of the healthcare system, the liaisons between the consumer and the complex healthcare market. The nurse in the role of gatekeeper can be an influential advocate for consumers who fall through the cracks of the complicated healthcare system. This group includes those who receive no care and need it most, such as the homeless, the uninsured or underinsured, the drug user, the alcoholic, children of poverty, the migrant worker, and the AIDS victim.

Henson (1997) presented an analysis of the concept of mutuality (i.e., mutual accountability) in relationships with clients. Mutuality balances power and respect and promotes productive communication.

Nurses are held in high regard by the consumer. The public views the nurse as knowledgeable, worthy of respect, concerned for others, honest, caring, confidential, friendly, hardworking, and as especially trustworthy (Blecher, 1997). Nurses, by virtue of this favorable status with the public, occupy positions of influence and can foster and promote successful consumer relationships across healthcare settings.

Four major responsibilities of nurses in promoting successful consumer relationships are developed in this chapter:

1. Service
2. Advocacy
3. Teaching
4. Leadership

Exercise 21-1

List as many ways as you can think of that the nurse might carry out the four responsibilities listed above. Compare your list with those of your peers.

SERVICE

A service orientation responds to the needs of the customer. In the "Manager's Challenge," activities were centered around the patient, including how nursing care and all other services were delivered so that patient care was a "whole" concept. As Box 21-1 illustrates, no matter where the services are delivered, the focus is the patient **(consumer focus).**

A service orientation is different from the concept of **service lines.** In this concept all related types of services are grouped into one functional unit of management. Typical service line units are women's services, cardiac services, orthopedic services, and oncology services.

Most healthcare facilities are not "customer friendly"; that is, they are built and organized in a manner that best serves the organization, not the consumer. They are departmentalized with each department having specialized functions. Patients are trans-

---

Box 21-1

Seven Primary Dimensions of Patient-Centered Care

- **Respect for patient's values, preferences, and expressed needs,** which includes attention to quality of life, involvement in decision making, preserving a patient's dignity, and recognizing patients' needs and autonomy.
- **Coordination and integration of care,** i.e., clinical care, ancillary and support services, and "front-line" patient care.
- **Information, communication, and education,** which includes information on clinical status, progress, and prognosis; information on processes of care; and information and education to facilitate autonomy, self-care, and health promotion.
- **Physical comfort,** which considers pain management, help with activities of daily living, and hospital environment.
- **Emotional support and alleviation of fear and anxiety,** which demands attention to anxiety over clinical status, treatment, and prognosis; anxiety over the impact of the illness on self and family; and anxiety over the financial impact of the illness.
- **Involvement of family and friends,** which recognizes the need to accommodate family and friends and involve family in decision making; to support the family as caregiver; and to recognize family needs.
- **Transition and continuity,** which addresses patient anxieties and concerns about information on medication, treatment regimens, follow up, danger signals after leaving the hospital, recovery, health promotion, and prevention of recurrence; coordination and planning for continuing care and treatment; and access to continuity of care and assistance.

Used with permission from Gerteis et al (1993).

---

ported from department to department to receive services. They risk loss of privacy, excessive exposure, and increased discomfort and fatigue during the transfer and waiting episodes. One vice president of nursing cited that on an average day a seriously ill patient in her facility would be exposed to about 50 different personnel in the course of receiving treatment and care. This approach is *not* "service oriented." A service mentality means bringing the services of the institution to the consumer in a manner that is least disruptive. Services, when possible, should come to the consumer and should be as easy, comfortable, pleasant, and effective as possible. In healthcare, components of customer service include such areas as technical competence, people skills, systems, and the environment (Leebov, 1988).

Exercise 21-2

List the things that you think are not consumer friendly in your nursing situation. (Example: Patients admitted to healthcare facilities are asked to repeat information several times to various people in the agency such as admitting staff, nursing, and x-ray technicians.)

Providing satisfying and meaningful service is not easy. Every consumer is different and every situation is different. How things are done and how needs are met vary in each situation. Service is not a prescribed set of rules and regulations and is not a one-dimensional concept. *Service* means placing a premium on the design, development, and delivery of care. For example, a home care patient needs IV antibiotic therapy. Inserting the IV catheter is the task-oriented, production piece of the care. The service piece is taking into consideration the special needs of the patient, such as placing the needle in the left arm so he can continue to use his cane with his right arm, or using some local anesthetic before needle insertion to reduce discomfort. Several characteristics are used to differentiate a service from a product. Some of these are shown in the example in Box 21-2.

In delivering nursing care, both service and product characteristics are present. Some of the actions in nursing require very prescribed rituals—the actual physical act of production, such as insertion of a Foley catheter. In performing this act, certain physical prop-

erties are apparent and the outcome predictable. At the same time, no two patients are alike; human interaction alters the situation, and unforeseen variables demand spontaneity. Caring, concern, and respect for the individual are intangible characteristics that affect the ultimate success or failure of the physical nursing act. As nurses we provide nursing care. Quality nursing care must be both clinically correct and satisfying to the customer. "Clinically correct" is the product piece and "satisfying to the consumer" is the service.

A service orientation is consumer driven and consumer focused, and places the emphasis on the quality of the nurse/patient relationship. The importance of relationships is reflected in current nursing theory in the caring philosophy. **Caring** has been described as the essence of nursing. It denotes a special concern, interest, or feeling capable of fostering a therapeutic nurse/patient relationship. Caring is important, but it is not enough to simply care. The ability to think and take appropriate, timely action must be a part of the therapeutic process. The nurse must do the right thing right and at the right time.

The concept of nursing as a caring service is seen in the reality of *"high tech–high touch."* **High tech** denotes a mechanistic perspective, whereas **high touch** denotes a caring, humanistic perspective. Caring for patients can be described as challenging in an environment driven by technology. At the same time, patients depend on nurses to deliver high tech care in a caring humanistic manner. The more high technology is used in healthcare, the more the patient wants and needs high touch—someone who is trusted and respected and who will add humanness to the experience. The quality of these human contacts becomes the measure by which the consumer forms perceptions and judgments about nursing and the health agency. Particularly in healthcare, consumers are frequently not able to judge or evaluate the quality of interventions, but they always have the ability to

Box 21-2 **Differentiating Characteristics Between a Service and a Product**	
SERVICE	**PRODUCT**
• Intangible (without physical boundaries)	• Tangible (possesses physical properties)
• Unpredictable	• Predictable
• Spontaneous	• Produced and stored
• Created and consumed simultaneously	• Created/can be consumed at a later time
• Heterogeneous (no two items are alike)	• Homogeneous
• Personal, human interaction	• Impersonal

evaluate the quality of the relationship with the person delivering the service.

Exercise 21-3

Make a "what-if" list of things that would enhance services to the consumers of healthcare. Example: What if nurses were referred to patients at the same time that physicians were referred to patients?

Each individual nurse is responsible for quality patient care. The nurse manager is accountable for quality management. A consulting firm of organizational strategists (Booz-Allen) generated the term *patient-focused care*. However, there is no clearly explicated model or one widely accepted definition for this concept. A common thread across healthcare systems employing patient-focused care strategies is refocusing on expected patient outcomes rather than on a multiplicity of tasks (Johnston & Cooper, 1997; Reisdorfer, 1996).

▌ADVOCACY

Nurses today practice in a healthcare environment dominated by unrest and insecurity. Some of these forces are shown in Box 21-3.

These forces bring about ethical and moral questions such as Who gets care?; Where do they get care?; How much care?; Who has the right to die?; Who has the right to live?; and Who makes the decisions? Differing values and beliefs, along with economic constraints and limited resources, affect decisions that are made.

Consumers have some basic rights that need to be protected—the right to individualized care; the

---

Box 21-3

Forces of Unrest and Insecurity in Today's Healthcare Environment

1. Increased costs
2. Shift to outpatient services
3. Complex social problems (AIDS, violence, poverty)
4. Decreased access to healthcare
5. Aging population (increasing lifespan)
6. Technological and genetic advances
7. Culturally and ethnically diverse work/consumer groups
8. Underrepresentation of women and ethnic groups in health-related research

---

right to their own values, beliefs, and cultural ways; and the right to know and participate in care decisions. Within the healthcare system remains the unresolved issue of two levels of care that are rationally based on economics, but tend to result in racial-cultural discrimination (Malone, 1993). Not only has care been on a two-tiered basis, but also minorities and women have been significantly underrepresented in health-related research.

Who in the healthcare system is in a position to be the guardian of these rights for the consumer? The nurse is! The nurse acts as the primary person to care about anything that might happen to prevent a successful outcome for the patient and to intervene on the patient's behalf. The nurse is in the position to address the issues of cultural, ethnic, and racial sensitivity.

Advocacy is a multidimensional concept and has many different meanings and applications. An advocate is one who (1) defends or promotes the rights of others; (2) changes systems to meet the needs of others; (3) empowers and promotes self-determination in others; (4) promotes autonomy of diverse cultures and social groups; (5) assures respect, equality, and dignity for others; and (6) cares for the humanness of all.

Nurses practice in a healthcare system that is culturally, economically, and socially diverse, just as consumers are. Nurses are responsible to consumers to assist them in successfully accessing and participating in these system. Some patients enter the healthcare system much like immigrants entering a foreign country. The result may be culture shock for such patients as they enter a system with a set of values, beliefs, behaviors, and language unlike their own. "The moral consequences of respecting differences within a multicultural society are complex, raising difficult questions for ethicists and policymakers as well as researchers and clinicians" (Davis and Koenig, 1996, p. 6).

Nurses need to recognize the culture of their work setting and realize it differs from the culture of the consumer who enters the system. The advocate role requires the nurse to perceive value conflict and then mediate, negotiate, clarify, explain, and intervene. The nurse can advocate by being a liaison between the consumer and the system. The nurse's role is to interpret the rules and customs of the agency to the consumer. It is also to negotiate changes when the consumer and agency differ in values and beliefs. An example is shown in Box 21-4.

To provide culturally appropriate care, the nurse must possess knowledge about various culturally

Box 21-4
Racial and Cultural Differences

SCENARIO: A young adult African-American male, shot while running from the police, had been hospitalized for over 3 weeks. A psychiatric clinical nurse specialist made the following assessment:

PERSPECTIVE OF NURSING STAFF

1. No one wants to take care of this patient. Avoiding him is common. His call light goes unanswered.

2. The patient is loud, rude, and uses vulgar language.
3. Nursing staff suspects that sexual activity is occurring between the man and his girlfriend in the hospital.
4. Nurses feel physically and sexually threatened when trying to provide care.

PERSPECTIVE OF PATIENT OF COLOR

1. Feels isolated and forgotten. Room is at the end of the hall. Infrequently sees nurses and physicians. Has little information about his gunshot wounds and fears he's never going to walk again. He fears he will die in his room and no one will know.
2. Speaks loudly and uses vulgar talk to emphasize his concerns.
3. Makes comments with sexual overtones and spends hours with girlfriend when she visits; . seeks comfort and affirmation through sexuality.
4. Family only comes on weekends and then in large numbers.

Summary: Stereotypes about African-American males were operational on the unit. The staff members avoided the patient because of the sexual overtones, and they withheld information regarding his condition. Overt and covert battles of will with the patient resulted in further patient isolation.

Adapted from Malone (1993), p. 26.

diverse groups (see Chapter 8). It takes time to develop cultural sensitivity and awareness. Some guidelines that are useful in learning to appreciate and value diversity are:

1. Avoid stereotyping.
2. Avoid making assumptions.
3. Learn by observing ethnic groups in interaction.
4. Adjust expectations to be culturally sensitive.
5. Create a more level playing field—modify your behavior to accommodate diversity.

Powerlessness or an imbalance in power between the consumer and the system results in value decisions being forced on the recipient of care. Consumers who lack economic means by being either uninsured or underinsured become powerless in the healthcare delivery system. They are at the mercy or will of those who control the power and the money. These consumers (described above) may be denied access to care, or if they receive access they may not receive equal care.

Less-privileged consumers have a right to healthcare and a right to know what services or care they are entitled to. The nurse must be willing to see that economic constraints do not prevent them from receiving

what they need. Some advocacy for the recipients of inequality in our healthcare system is done on the here-and-now level—initiating a referral to a social agency, appealing on behalf of the consumer to the ethics committee. On a broader scale it means becoming involved professionally and politically to change the systems and policies to provide equality and access to healthcare.

Exercise 21-4

Using the scenario in Box 21-4, determine how the nurse working as a **culture broker** can mediate the cultural differences between the staff and the patient.

Race/ethnicity as a factor in health and healthcare has been the subject of concern, yet minority health is often erroneously assumed to be a unitary phenomenon, when, in fact, there is extraordinary diversity. The interactions and relationships among race/ethnicity, social class, and health need further exploration (Nickens, 1995).

According to Dreher (1996), nursing can be described as a cultural phenomenon. Nursing, as a profession, has strived for greater diversity among its ranks with only very modest progress (Minnick et al, 1997). In the meantime, cultural diversity training and sensitivity have never been greater in importance. An urban teaching facility with nearly 3,000 employees and communication problems related to race, gender, and other cultural differences instituted mandatory training in cultural diversity and customer service. Through the process, the medical center significantly increased its patient base and improved its bottom line (Cater & Spence, 1996).

It is most useful to define diversity broadly, to include not only race and ethnicity, but also age, gender, class, religion, and sexual orientation. Cole (1995) reminds us that the disabled also should be considered in diversity programs.

Some of the keys to becoming a successful nurse advocate are (1) developing networking systems within work agencies and professional associations to assist in providing information and services to patients, (2) acquiring the knowledge needed to access systems, (3) learning about community resources and support networks, and (4) developing skill in referring and engaging clients.

A client/patient advocate's ultimate aim is to empower the patient or consumer of healthcare. Client empowerment is an emerging, fashionable trend in healthcare today. However, as VanderHenst (1997) points out, there is a lack of a clear, conceptual definition for the term. The nurse manager should keep in mind the most basic element of empowerment, i.e., helping people assert control. In the healthcare industry, control applies to factors that affect health. For example, the application of a "strengths" model of case management in a long-term care Medicaid waiver program helped people and communities identify and develop capacities, talents, skills, and interest, and connect with necessary resources (Fast & Chapin, 1996). According to a 1996 analysis by Doty, Kasper, and Litvak, Medicaid clients in three states were more satisfied with program elements that gave them more choice and control. Kelly-Powell (1997) used a grounded theory research approach to explore how patients with life-threatening conditions choose to personalize treatment decisions and thus exercise control over their health and healthcare.

In health facilities, nurses can evaluate the quality of care the consumer is receiving by comparing it to the quality indicators or critical pathways in the quality review process. If patient care standards cite that patients with a particular bronchial condition need a chest x-ray on day two and another on day five, all patients should receive this same level of care. In agencies using critical paths to prescribe the plan of care, patients should not be denied treatment, therapy, or tests because of ability to pay if the critical path requires specific action. Nurse managers

are in a unique position to access and assure that all patients receive appropriate care. The tone set by the manager signals staff to report and document discrepancies and omissions. Nurse managers must acknowledge and respect the legal, ethical, and moral responsibilities of the staff to advocate for patients.

The savvy manager knows that the way in which consumers define quality may not always be in sync with the way "experts" define it. Research suggests that in the area of subacute care, for example, healthcare providers need to focus greater attention on (1) access to services, (2) communication/coordination, and (3) values (Stahl, 1997).

Quality medical care and quality nursing care are not dependent on ability to pay or social acceptance. If it's good care, it's good care irrespective of the economic circumstance of the consumer. Nurses are the guardians of that right for consumers. Nurses have historically been the champions for the poor and the underserved. It is no different today.

TEACHING

Consumers of healthcare have a right to know and a need to know how to care for their own health needs. Nurses have an obligation to teach the consumer. This obligation is mandated in the states' nurse practice acts. The Joint Commission on Accreditation of Healthcare Organizations (JCAHO) also mandates patient teaching in its family and patient education standards. The American Nurses' Association has advocated patient teaching since the publication of its Model Nurse Practice Act in 1975. More and more, consumers are demanding knowledge about their health status and plan of care. Teaching is wonderful, fun, rewarding, and hard work. It is one of the most positive experiences nurses can have. Consumers are entitled to information regarding health concerns, to participate in caring for their health needs, and to contribute to finding solutions to their health problems. Education empowers consumers to exercise self-determination. It allows them to have greater control over what happens, to make informed decisions, and to choose wisely from options. An ancient proverb says that if you give a man a fish, you feed him for a day, but if you teach a man to fish, you feed him for a lifetime. Knowledge is power. Sharing knowledge means sharing power.

The changes in healthcare actively affect the way nurses teach consumers. Probably the most significant change is shorter hospital stays and thus more care in outpatient settings. This requires that patients be able to manage their own healthcare earlier and more independently. Hands-on, technical training is needed in many instances, such as self-catheterization. Research has shown that in patient teaching, nurses' perceptions of their patients' understanding of post-discharge treatment plans differ from the perception of patients themselves. Nurses perceived patients to be much more knowledgeable than their patients reported (Reiley et al, 1996). Teaching prevention and health promotion will increase the consumer's quality of life. Three "Ps" for a successful consumer education focus are shown in Box 21-5.

Teaching can be simple or complex. In teaching elemental, task-oriented behaviors, the nurse uses basic materials, simple relationships, guides, sequencing of steps, and cause-and-effect relationships. Teaching

directed more broadly toward changing health behaviors actually seeks to modify beliefs and attitudes through persuasive communication (Stubblefield, 1997). The nurse manager needs to assure teaching resources and to validate that teaching is documented as part of the plan of care. Teaching behaviors should be addressed in performance evaluations.

EXAMPLE: Teaching insulin administration

1.	Material	Demonstrate the use of the equipment. Return demonstration by trainee.
2.	Simple relationships	Interpret the significance of the blood sugar level to the amount and type of insulin given.

Box 21-5

Three "Ps" for a Successful Consumer Education Focus

1. Philosophy—Patient education is an investment with a significant positive return. Money invested in teaching is money well spent. Time and energy invested are time and energy well spent.
2. Priority—Education is important. Quality nursing care always has an educational component. Informed consumers want to participate and look to nurses to teach them.
3. Performance—Clinical teaching excellence is a required skill of nurses. They must possess a variety of techniques and methods in order to meet the needs of the diverse consumers served.

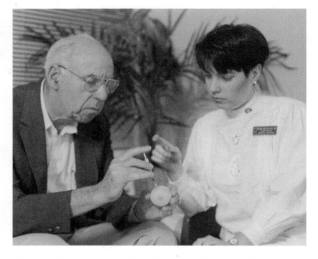

Successful consumer education requires excellent clinical teaching skills.

ASSESSING

Analyze the learner
Assess knowledge
 & skills
Analyze the task
Assess performance level
 needed

DIAGNOSING & PLANNING

Set the strategy
Plan the content
Develop the time frame
Assess readiness to
 learn
Establish expectations

IMPLEMENTING

Initiate planned strategies
Test for readiness
Sequence the tasks
Vary the learning aids
Adjust for cultural diversity

EVALUATING

Analyze achievements
Examine consumer
 skill level
Compare progress to
 plan strategy
Validate success
 or revise

Figure 21-1 Teaching model adapted to the nursing process.

3. Guides   Illustrate the rotation of injection sites with a chart.

4. Sequencing   Apply a step-by-step procedure to follow to encompass the task from start to finish.

5. Cause and effect   Explain the relationship of sterile technique to infection prevention—"If you contaminate the needle, infection can result."

As a step-by-step process, teaching can be adapted to the problem solving process model shown in Figure 21-1.

The following example uses the nursing process model in teaching a patient about diabetes.

Assess   Patient is a 16-year-old, Hispanic male with no prior knowledge of diabetes or skill in drug administration. English is a second language. He needs to give his own insulin, using sterile technique, by the time he is discharged from the hospital.

Plan   Begin with demonstration, return demonstration of basic subcutaneous injection. Progress step by step to basic understanding of diabetes, blood sugar, and insulin dosage by the time of discharge. Home health to continue training.

Implement   Set times, twice a day, to spend 1 hour in instruction with patient. Begin with demonstration, return demonstration, and repeat instructions. Adjust learning materials to accommodate language barrier.

Evaluate   Patient has met minimal skill level of subcutaneous technique. He can administer insulin safely but has limited disease and cause/effect understanding. To be followed per home health with continued teaching.

As a conceptual process, teaching fits into the general systems theory model as shown in Figure 21-2. The following example uses the general systems theory model in teaching a patient with diabetes:

Input   Present information on the disease, the procedures to be learned, the skills necessary for successful achievement, and the cause and effect relationships. Have materials in Spanish at the high school reading level. Demonstrate the drug administration technique.

Throughput   Language barrier eased with materials printed in Spanish. Fear threat to macho image typical of 16-year-old male. Allow time to practice techniques demonstrated.

Output   Return demonstration successful. Give posttest to assess knowledge (in Spanish).

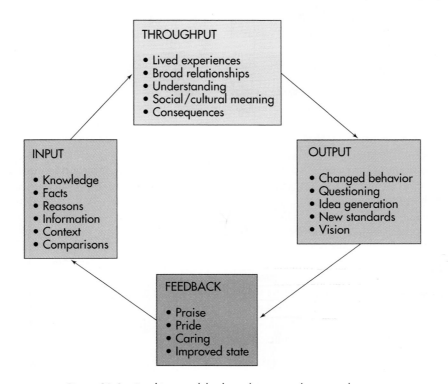

Figure 21-2   Teaching model adapted to general systems theory.

Feedback   Praise for successful return demonstration. Give example of sport/movie heroes with diabetes.

Nurses need to be prepared and skilled to teach. They must be able to adapt to the learning styles of the consumer by using a variety of styles and a flexible approach in meeting the educational goals. Selected learning preferences are shown in Box 21-6. Being knowledgeable in the subject and able to individualize the information to meet the consumer's ability to learn are critical to quality teaching (Babcock & Miller, 1994).

Exercise 21-5

Using one of the models presented, prepare a teaching plan based on your actual nursing experience.

Patient-specific information must also be shared with family caregivers. Bailey and Mion (1997) developed the Caregiver Satisfaction with Information Questionnaire (Box 21-7).

Box 21-6
Selected Learning Preferences

- Auditory (words)
- Visual (sight)
- Active (participate)
- Passive (contemplate)
- Linear (step by step)
- Circular (model, picture)
- Rational (reasoning)
- Abstract (global)

▌ LEADERSHIP

Awareness and understanding of major changes reflecting a paradigm shift in healthcare will equip nurse managers to participate in shaping healthcare organizations of the future. According to a 1996 publication by Issel and Anderson, there are six emerging areas of transformation in healthcare:

1. From person as customer to population as customer (i.e., population-focused care)
2. From illness care to wellness care
3. From revenue management to cost management
4. From autonomy to interdependence of professionals (i.e., interdisciplinary approaches to care)
5. From continuity of provider to continuity of information
6. From patient as nonconsumer to consumer of cost and quality information

Nurse managers are in a pivotal position to influence the cost and the quality of care delivered by the staff. They set the tone for the vision and mission of the unit and the focus for the staff. They must believe in and model the consumer-based service philosophy. One who truly believes in the need to provide service that is satisfying to the consumer knows that each and every consumer is different. What will satisfy one person will not satisfy another.

Box 21-7
Caregiver Satisfaction with Information Questionnaire

*1. In regard to ease of getting information, please rate the willingness of hospital staff to answer your questions.

*2. In regard to instructions, please rate how well the nurses and other staff explained about tests, treatments, and what to expect.

*3. In regard to informing family and friends, please rate how well family and friends were kept informed about the patient's condition and needs.

*4. In regard to information given by the nurses, please rate how well the nurses communicated with patients, families, and doctors.

†5. In regard to updates concerning the patient's condition, please rate how well the nurses informed you concerning the rest and comfort level of the patient.

†6. In regard to updates concerning the patient's condition, please rate how well the nurses informed you concerning the nutritional status of the patient.

†7. Please rate how well the nurses informed you of the results of tests done for ongoing monitoring of the patient's illness (e.g., temperature, blood pressure, blood glucose monitoring).

†8. In regard to the patient's daily schedule, please rate how well the nurses informed you about the patient's actual and anticipated schedule each day.

*Items from the survey, *Your Hospital Stay: The Patient's Viewpoint,*® produced and distributed by NCG Research, Inc.
†Items developed by the authors.

To be successful as leaders in nursing requires being open, flexible, and ready to change. Leadership requires (1) a belief that the intangibles have economic value, (2) a tolerance for ambiguity, (3) a relinquishing of direct control over every key process, (4) an appreciation that the organization is dependent on both people-related and production-related skills, and (5) a tolerance and excitement for sudden and sometimes dramatic change (Albrecht & Zemke, 1985).

Change is the modus operandi of the nursing environment no matter what the healthcare setting. What works today may not work 6 months from now. Given the rapidly changing environment, the pressure to control costs, and advances in technology, science, and information, nurse managers need a whole new set of beliefs, behaviors, and skills. Selected examples of these are as follows:

1. Keep the consumer as the center of focus.
2. Recognize that each staff member has a unique contribution to make to the success of the unit. Allow staff to be creative and flexible in their work, ask for suggestions and new approaches to old problems, and seek participation in decision making. Managers set the tone; staff deliver the service.
3. Promote dignity, worth, caring, individual contributions, and cultural sensitivity in the staff. Successful managers recognize individual accomplishments and support failures. They accept that human beings are not perfect at all times and that it is okay to take a risk, look foolish, and fail. They implement hiring practices that foster selection of qualified racially and culturally diverse applicants.
4. Understand the economic value of service. Managers must believe that service will pay real dollar dividends to justify the cost in terms of adequate quality and quantity of staff.
5. Evaluate patient outcomes and perceptions of care. It is imperative to ask patients about the services provided and how it felt to them, not after the fact but while they are receiving the service.

Patient outcomes or the notion of evidenced-based standards and measurement of care are attracting greater attention and achieving much greater emphasis in marketplace reform of healthcare. The focus of healthcare reform in the marketplace and of the movement toward managed care is the provision of quality care, but controlling costs is paramount. There is a growing collective voice among consumers which notes that healthcare institutions and professionals seem to be more focused on profits than on patient care (Grayson, 1997).

In the area of consumer relations, patient satisfaction with care is a particularly relevant measure. In the past, we have evaluated patient satisfaction with healthcare, with varying degrees of success. Current research efforts are aimed at developing valid and reliable patient outcome measures, including patient satisfaction. Nursing systems and nursing administration researchers are particularly interested in response to and satisfaction with nursing care. However, valid measurement of patient satisfaction is an evolving science, and nurses do not always accurately gauge what factors are most important to patients.

At a 387-bed geriatric hospital in Montreal, Canada, a cross-sectional satisfaction survey was administered to random samples of patients, families, and nursing staff. Findings revealed significant differences in the ranking and perception of quality indicators (Meister & Boyle, 1996).

Managers must be willing to give up direct control of every process. Staff must be given power and permission to be in control and to make decisions at the consumer-staff level of interaction. Some of our greatest successes come out of spontaneous actions. Giving up control involves being willing to take a risk and a belief in the other person's ability to perform. Leadership behaviors contributing to individual and personal excellence are (1) allowing professionals more influence over their practice, (2) giving staff opportunities to learn new and varied skills, (3) giving recognition and reward for success and support and consolation for lack of success, and (4) fostering motivation and belief in the importance of each individual and the value of his or her contribution. The leader's role is to create within the worker a passion to do and contribute to the work effort successfully.

We do best those things that we know how to do skillfully and those things about which we feel passionately. Fitting the right person to the right job is important. Maximum contribution is required from each staff member in today's healthcare agencies. Since the leader is the one who sets the standard for the success or failure of the staff's contributions, it is important to assess each staff member carefully—what is his or her skill level and commitment level, and what can be done to assist in making a maximum contribution? Figure 21-3 is an example of a completed staff assessment tool. Nurse managers can compile similar information for members of their staff. The information can be used to form staff development plans.

When staff know the leader is sincerely concerned about their welfare, they are better able to use their time, energy, and talents to serve the needs of the consumer. Staff that are nurtured and cared for will be better able to nurture and care for the consumer.

Exercise 21-6

Forming small groups, assess each member of the group using the headings shown in the staff assessment tool (Figure 21-3 below).

■ CHAPTER CHECKLIST

Times have changed and the role of the nurse manager has changed. The trend of healthcare moving into the community, home, clinic, and outpatient setting has placed a whole new perspective on how to provide quality, cost-effective nursing care. Patients must participate in their care and need service-oriented nurses to be teachers, advocates, and leaders in their behalf. Managing care delivery in these diverse settings requires the use of flexible and creative skills. The key

is to keep the patient as the center of focus and provide cultural and racially sensitive nursing care.

■ Consumer relationships in healthcare typically involve interactions between the consumer and:
- The physician
  - The physician-patient relationship is changing, due to changes in the way medical care is delivered.
- The nurse
  - Nurses, as the healthcare providers who spend the most time with the consumer, set the tone for effective staff-patient interactions.
- The healthcare agency
  - The agency's approach to care is determined by its mission and philosophy.
- The healthcare payers
  - Insurance coverage and carriers usually dictate the services patients receive and where they receive them.

■ Because of their favorable status with consumers, nurses are in a unique position to promote positive consumer relationships.

Staff Member	Skill Level	Commitment Level	Suggested Action
(1) S. Baker, RN	High technical competence Able to teach others Learns quickly Needs improved people skills	Appears bored Does only what is assigned No enthusiasm Critical of any change	Assign challenges to utilize technical strengths Provide situations where teaching others occurs Plan: Team assign with D. Carroll
(2) D. Carroll, RN	6 mos. post basic program Learns quickly Slow with technical skills Needs technical supervision Excellent people skills	Excited about work Asks for new experiences Accepting of new ideas Volunteers to help others	Improve technical skills Provide safe & successful learning experiences Plan: Team assign with S. Baker
(3) J. Ratke, RN	Moderate technical competence Works best alone Not interested in teaching co-worker Good people skills	Restless, distracted Looking for a change Accepts new ideas Self commitment - not group oriented	Set up an independent project of her choosing (e.g., unit research idea) Provide some special technical training to ↑ skills
(4) C. Thomas, RN	High level technical skills Enjoys helping others Excellent people skills Looks for challenges	Team player Interested in welfare of group Critical of poor performers Acts as cheerleader for change	Utilize willingness and group skills to plan and present a unit activity (e.g., inservice education production, unit open house)

Figure 21-3   Staff assessment tool.

A Manager's Solution

? Initially, I met with the manager and the RN involved to discuss the matter. The direct care RN had begun to piece together parts of the incident. We decided it would be appropriate for the RN and her manager to arrange another visit with the client and his wife for conflict resolution and to attempt to bring closure to the issue. The RN promptly arranged the visit.

During the follow-up visit, the events of the home health visit at issue were rehashed. The client (husband) suddenly remembered handing the wrapper to the RN to jot down the desired information for him. The RN recalled it was just a piece of paper he handed her, never having any idea of its value or significance.

Open and honest communication helped bring resolution to this situation. Several important points may be learned from this incident, such as:

- Effective communication involves active listening, not passive conversation.
- A nurse should refrain from writing on anything other than official documents.

- Always respect property of the client, even papers that look like nothing of value.
- Extra effort to resolve an issue pays off.
- It is important to try and understand a situation from the customer (consumer) perspective.
- Support involved staff, but don't isolate them from the situation. Allow them to be a part of the solution.
- Capitalize on the opportunity for critiquing an unpleasant incident, not only to decrease the likelihood of recurrence, but also to allow for professional growth in handling sensitive situations.
- Home health staff are at greater risk for consumer conflict and allegations than those working in a more structured environment.

? *Would this be a suitable approach for you? Why?*

- Four major responsibilities of nurses in promoting successful consumer relationships are:
  - Service
  - Advocacy
  - Teaching
  - Leadership
- A service orientation is consumer-driven and consumer-focused, emphasizing the quality of the nurse-patient relationship and the delivery of services in a caring atmosphere.
  - Services differ from products:
    - Services are intangible, unpredictable, created and consumed simultaneously, and personal.
    - Products are tangible, predictable, produced and stored, and impersonal.
- The nurse can advocate by serving as a liaison between the consumer and the healthcare system.
  - Nurses can interpret the agency's rules and customs for the consumer and negotiate if conflicts arise.
  - Nurses also help secure culturally appropriate care and mediate cultural differences.
- Teaching is the sharing of information and education to help consumers become independent, self-responsible, and self-determining.

- Nurses have an obligation to teach the consumer.
- The three "Ps" for successful consumer education are:
  - Philosophy: patient education is an investment with a significant positive return.
  - Priority: education is important.
  - Performance: clinical teaching excellence is a required skill for nurses.
- Teaching can follow the five-step nursing process model.
- Leadership fosters decision making at the consumer-staff level of interaction. Effective leadership strategies for the nurse manager include:
  - Keeping the central focus on the consumer; remember that the consumer may be a whole population.
  - Recognizing staff members' unique contributions and helping them maximize their personal excellence.
  - Promoting staff members' sense of dignity, worth, caring, cultural diversity, and sensitivity.
  - Understanding the economic value of service.
  - Valuing interdisciplinary approaches to care.
  - Evaluating patient outcomes and patients' perceptions of care.

TERMS TO KNOW

consumer focus

culture broker

gatekeeper

healthcare consumer

healthcare provider

high tech

high touch

service

service lines

TIPS FOR BEING CUSTOMER FOCUSED

- Ask yourself if this service/approach is one you would wish to receive.
- Remember that in the new pyramid of health services, it is the consumer who is the apex—the rest is there to support that person.
- Enter care relationships with the mindset of how to make care better from the receiver's perspective.
- Use the Service, Advocacy, Teaching, Leadership approach.

REFERENCES

Albrecht, K., & Zemke, R. (1985). *Service America! Doing Business in the New Economy*: Homewood, IL: Dow Jones-Irwin.

Babcock, D.E., & Miller, M.A. (1994). *Client Education, Theory and Practice*. St. Louis, MO: Mosby.

Bailey, D.A., & Mion, L.C. (1997). Improving care givers' satisfaction with information received during hospitalization. *Journal of Nursing Administration*, 27(1), 21-27.

Blecher, M.B. (1997, April 5). The nurse will see you now. *Hospitals & Health Networks*, 71, 96-99.

Cater, R., & Spence, M. (1996). Cultural diversity process improves organizational community in urban teaching medical center. *Journal of Cultural Diversity*, 3(2), 35-39.

Cole, R.S. (1995). Include the disabled in diversity programs—or else! *The Public Relations Strategist*, 1(2), 34-39.

Davis, A.J., & Koenig, B.A. (1996). A question of policy: Bioethics in a multicultural society. *Nursing Policy Forum*, 2(1), 6-11.

Doty, P., Kasper, J., & Litvak, S. (1996). Consumer-directed models of personal care: Lessons from Medicaid. *Milbank Quarterly*, 74(3), 377-409.

Dreher, M.C. (1996). Nursing: A cultural phenomenon. *Reflections*, 22(4), 4.

Fast, B., & Chapin, R. (1996). The strengths model in long-term care: Linking cost containment and consumer empowerment. *Journal of Case Management*, 5(2), 51-57.

Gerteis, M., Edgman-Levitan, S., Daley, J., & Delbanco, T.L. (1993). *Through the Patient's Eyes: Understanding and Promoting Patient-Centered Care*. San Francisco: Jossey Bass.

Grayson, M. (1997, February 20). Get the picture: Consumers sound off on health care. But you may not like what they tell you. *Hospitals & Health Networks*, 71, 30-32.

Henson, R.H. (1997) Analysis of the concept of mutuality. *Image*, 29, 77-81.

Issel, L.M., & Anderson, R.A. (1996). Take charge: Managing six transformations in health care delivery. *Nursing Economics*, 14(2), 78-85.

Johnston, C.L., & Cooper, P.K. (1997). Patient-focused care: What is it? *Holistic Nursing Practice*, 11(3), 1-7.

Kelly-Powell, M.L. (1997). Personalizing choices: Patients' experiences with making treatment decisions. *Research in Nursing & Health*, 20, 219-217.

Leebov, W.L. (1988). *Service excellence: The customer relations strategy for health care*. Chicago: American Hospital Publishing, Inc.

Malone, B.L. (1993). Caring for culturally diverse racial groups: An administrative matter. *Nursing Administration Quarterly*, 17(2), 21-29.

Meister, C., & Boyle, C. (1996). Perceptions of quality in long-term care: A satisfaction survey. *Journal of Nursing Care Quality*, 10(4), 40-47.

Minnick, A., Roberts, M.J., Young, W.B., Marcantonio, R., & Kleinpell, R.M. (1997). Ethnic diversity and staff nurse employment in hospitals. *Nursing Outlook*, 45, 35-40.

Nickens, H.W. (1995). The role of race/ethnicity and social class in minority health status. *Health Services Research*, 30(1), 151-162.

Reiley, P., Iezzoni, L.I., Phillips, R., Davis, R.B., Tuchin, L.I., & Calkins, D. (1996). Discharge planning: Comparison of patients' and nurses' perceptions of patients following hospital discharge. *Image, Journal of Nursing Scholarship*, 28(2), 143-147.

Reisdorfer, J.T. (1996). Building a patient-focused care unit. *Nursing Management*, 27(10), 38-44.

Stahl, D.A. (1997). Quality measures: Meeting consumer needs. *Nursing Management*, 28(8), 20-21.

Stubblefield, C. (1997). Persuasive communication: Marketing health promotion. *Nursing Outlook*, 45, 173-177.

VanderHenst, J.A. (1997). Client empowerment: A nursing challenge. *Clinical Nurse Specialist*, 11(3), 96-99.

SUGGESTED READINGS AND RESOURCES

Aspling, D.L., & Lagoe, R. (1996). Benchmarking for clinical pathways in hospitals: A summary of sources. *Nursing Economics*, 14(2), 92-97.

Chafey, K., Rhea, M., Shannon, A.M., & Spencer, S. (1998). Characterizations of advocacy by practicing nurses. *Journal of Professional Nursing*, 14, 43-52.

Lipson, J.G., Dibble, S.L., & Minarik, P.A. (1996). *Culture and Nursing Care: A Pocket Guide*. San Francisco: UCSF Press.

Living Longer and Better with Health Problems: A Nurse Advisor Handbook. (1996). Springhouse, PA: Springhouse Corporation.

Nursing World: The American Nurses Association (*http://www.nursingworld.org*).

Sigma Theta Tau International Honor Society of Nursing (*http://stti-web.iupui.edu*).

Taking Your Medications Safely: A Nurse Advisor Handbook. (1996). Springhouse, PA: Springhouse Corporation.

US Department of Health & Human Services (*http://www.dhhs.gov*).

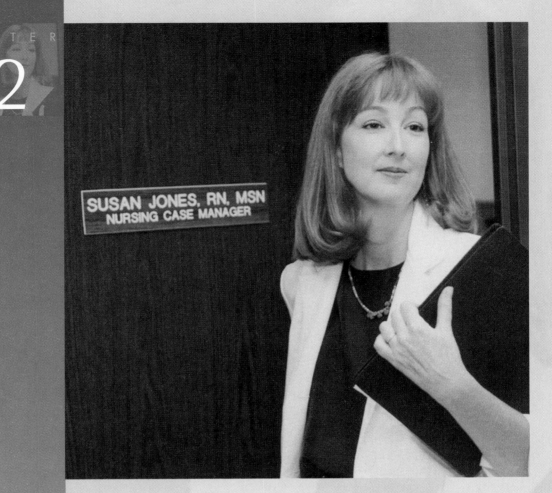

Care Delivery Strategies

Karen A. Dadich
RN, MN

This chapter introduces patient care delivery strategies that hospitals and community-based facilities currently use: the case method, functional nursing, team nursing, primary nursing, and case management. It also discusses differentiated practice. The chapter defines and discusses each strategy, summarizes its benefits and disadvantages, and discusses the nurse manager's role and the staff nurse's perspective.

Objectives

- Specify and differentiate among five patient care delivery strategies.
- Determine the nurse manager's and staff nurse's role in each strategy.
- Summarize the differentiated nursing practice model.

Questions to Consider

- What method of patient care delivery would you most enjoy working in and why?
- How does your level of nursing education affect the care you provide?
- How do you think a nurse manager influences the effectiveness of the patient care delivery system?
- How do you think the staff nurse influences the implementation of each patient care delivery strategy?

A Manager's Challenge

From a Nurse Case Manager at a Southwestern Hospital

Since the inception of nurse case management at my hospital, many changes have occurred that have affected my practice. The current director of case management services is concerned with the utilization of resources and length of stay. As the nurse case manager for oncology patients, I was affected by my manager's perspective.

I deal with complex patient care problems and challenges. These patients are critically ill with multisystem healthcare needs, including reactions to cancer, its treatments, and prolonged recovery after extensive hospitalization. I perceived that my di-

rector, who is not a nurse, is only concerned with "the bottom line" and not the care needs of the patients and families.

Compounding my dilemma is the common practice of physicians keeping patients hospitalized until the patient is ready to leave. Physicians, with whom I work very well, now perceive me as the "police" or their foe. As a nurse case manager, I am pressured to adhere to managed care principles and physician care practices.

What do you think you would do if you were this manager?

INTRODUCTION

A care delivery strategy is the method used to provide care to patients and clients (hereafter, the term *patients* refers to both patients and clients). Since nursing care is viewed as a cost, it is logical for institutions to evaluate their method of providing patient care for the purpose of saving money while still providing quality care. This chapter discusses five strategies of patient care delivery; case method (or total patient care), functional nursing, team nursing, primary nursing, or case management. The influence that differentiated practice has on care delivery is described.

Each delivery model has advantages and disadvantages and none is ideal. Some methods are conducive to large institutions while other systems may work best in community settings. Managers in any organization must examine the care delivery model and

consider the budget, staff availability, and organizational goals to determine the best system for delivery.

Exercise 22-1

You have recently accepted a position at a home health agency that provides 24-hour care to qualified patients. You are assigned a patient who has 24-hour care provided by an RN during the day, an LPN/LVN in the evening, and a nursing assistant at night. You are concerned that the patient is not progressing well and you suspect the evening and night shift personnel are not reporting changes in the patient's status. You want to change the situation. How would you justify any change in staffing? What recommendations would you make to the nurse manager and why?

CASE METHOD

The **case method**, or **total patient care** method, of nursing care delivery is the oldest method of providing care to a patient. The premise of the case method is that one nurse provides total care for one patient during the entire work period (Figure 22-1). This method was used in the 1800s when nurses cared for the sick in their homes. Nursing students have typically used this approach at some point in providing total care to a patient. Another example is a private duty nurse who cares for one person during a specific shift.

Advantages and Disadvantages

During an 8- or 12-hour shift the patient receives consistent care from one nurse. The nurse, patient, and family exchange mutual trust and can work together toward specific goals. Changes in the patient's status are apparent to the nurse during the shift, but those changes and progress to expected outcomes may not be communicated to subsequent nurses (Whitehead, 1997). **Expected outcomes** are the results of patient goals, achieved through medical and nursing interventions. When outcomes are not met, the amount of time required for care increases, leading to additional expense for the entire healthcare system.

The case method was used in the era of Florence Nightingale, when patients received total care in the home. In today's costly economy, family members participate in caring for the patient and home health visits supplement the 24-hour care that is extremely costly. Total patient care is used in critical care settings where one nurse provides total care to a small group of critically ill individuals. Total patient care by a registered nurse (RN) is very expensive. In some settings, there are not enough resources or nurses to use this model. Variations of the case method exist,

and it is possible to identify similarities after reviewing other methods of patient care delivery described later in this chapter.

Nurse Manager's Role

When using the case method of delivery, the manager must consider the expense of the system. The manager must weigh the expense of an RN versus licensed practical nurses (LPNs/LVNs) and **unlicensed assistive personnel.** Unlicensed assistive personnel are staff who are not licensed as healthcare providers. They are technicians, nurse aides, and certified nursing assistants. The patient may require 24-hour care; however, the manager must decide if the patient needs to have RN care or RN-supervised care provided by LPNs/LVNs or unlicensed personnel. To provide cost-effective care to the patients, the staff need to have adequate skills to provide total care.

The manager also needs to identify the level of education and communication skills of all staff. RNs must be educated in communicating and coordinating care as well as supervising other staff members. LPNs/LVNs and unlicensed personnel also need continuing education to provide total care according to their level of practice.

Staff Nurse's Role

The staff nurse provides holistic care to a group of patients during scheduled work time. The physical, emotional, and technical aspects of care are the responsibility of the assigned nurse. Some nurses thrive on this care delivery model, while others wish to delegate simpler, less complex aspects of care to assistive personnel. This care delivery strategy requires the total patient care nurse to complete the complex functions of care, such as assessment and teaching the patient and family, as well as the less complex functional aspects of care.

◼ FUNCTIONAL NURSING

The functional method of nursing care delivery became popular during World War II when there was a severe shortage of nurses in the United States, because many nurses went into the military to provide care to the soldiers. To provide care to patients, hospitals began to increase the number of unlicensed assistive personnel and LPNs/LVNs.

Functional nursing is a method of providing patient care where each licensed and unlicensed staff member provides a specific task for a large group of patients. For example, the RN may administer all IV

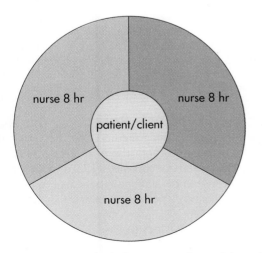

Figure 22-1   Case method of patient care for an 8-hour shift.

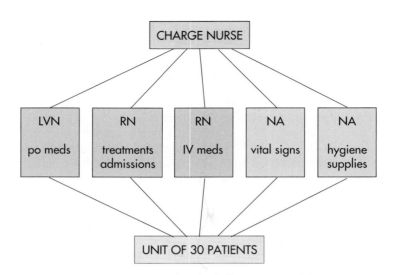

Figure 22-2   Functional method of nursing care delivery.

medications and do admissions, one LPN/LVN may provide treatments, another LPN/LVN may give all oral medication, one assistant may do all hygiene tasks, and another assistant takes all vital signs (Figure 22-2). This method is a similar to the assembly line system used by industry. A **charge nurse** coordinates care and assignments and may ultimately be the only person familiar with all needs of any patient.

Advantages and Disadvantages

There are several advantages to this method of patient care delivery. First, each person becomes very efficient at specific tasks and a great amount of work can be done in a short time. Another advantage is that unskilled workers can be trained to perform one or two specific tasks very well, such as glucometer checks or phlebotomy. The organization benefits financially from this strategy because patient care can be delivered to a large number of patients by mixing staff with a minimum number of RNs and a larger number of unlicensed assistive personnel. By decreasing the number of RNs, the hospital has fewer personnel costs.

Although financial savings may be the impetus for organizations to choose the functional system of delivering care, the disadvantages outweigh the savings (Figure 22-3). A major disadvantage is the fragmentation of care. The physical and technical aspects of care may be met, but the psychological and spiritual needs are often overlooked. Patients become confused with so many different care providers per shift. These different staff may be so busy with their assigned tasks that they do not have time to communicate with each other about the patient's progress. Since no one care provider sees patient care from beginning to the end, evaluation of the patient's response to care is difficult to assess. Fragmented care and ineffective communication can lead to patient dissatisfaction and frustration. Exercise 22-2 provides an opportunity to imagine how a patient would react to the functional method, but also to imagine how the nurse may feel.

Exercise 22-2

Imagine you are a patient at a hospital that uses the functional method of patient care delivery. You just had surgery and when you ask the nursing assistant for something for pain she says, "I'll tell the medication nurse." The medication nurse comes to your room and says that your medication is ordered IV and the IV nurse will need to administer it. The IV nurse is busy starting an IV on another patient and will not be able to give your medication to you for 10 minutes. This whole communication process has taken 40 minutes and you are still in pain. How do you feel about the functional method of patient care? How effective do you think communication between staff is when a patient has a problem?

Nurse Manager's Role

In the functional nursing method, the nurse manager must be sensitive to both the institution's budgetary constraints and the responsibility for quality patient care delivery. Since staff members are responsible only for their specific task, the role of achieving patient outcomes becomes the nurse manager's responsibility. Staff members may view this system as autocratic and become discontented with the lack of input they have into patient outcomes and departmental matters.

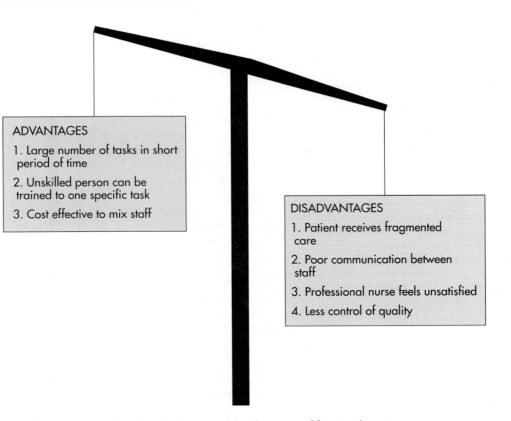

Figure 22-3   Advantages and disadvantages of functional nursing.

By using effective management and leadership skills, the nurse manager can improve the staff's perception of their lack of independence. The manager can rotate assignments among staff to alleviate boredom with repetition. Staff meetings should be conducted frequently. This would encourage staff to express concerns and empower them with the ability to communicate concerns about patient care and unit functions.

Staff Nurse's Role

The staff nurse becomes skilled at the tasks that are usually assigned. Staff follow clearly defined policies and procedures to complete the physical aspects of care in an efficient and economical manner. But the functional method leaves the professional nurse feeling frustrated because of the task-oriented role. Nurses are educated to care for the patient holistically, and providing only a fragment of care to a patient results in unmet personal and professional expectations of nursing.

The functional method of care delivery works well in emergency and disaster situations. Each care provider knows the expectations of the assigned role and completes the tasks in a quick and efficient style. Subacute care and extended care facilities use the functional method of care delivery. Severe budgetary cuts and reimbursement patterns have forced institutions to change the **staff mix** and increase the proportion of unlicensed to licensed personnel. A modification of functional nursing is team nursing.

TEAM NURSING

After World War II the nursing shortage continued. Many nurses who were in the military came home to marry and have children instead of returning to the work force. Since the functional method during the war received criticism, a new system of team nursing was devised to improve patient satisfaction.

In **team nursing** a team leader is responsible for coordinating a small group of licensed and unlicensed personnel to provide patient care to a small group of patients. The team leader assigns each member a patient or a specific responsibility. The members of the team report directly to the team leader who then reports to the charge nurse or unit manager (Figure 22-4). There are several teams per unit and patient assignments are made by each team leader.

Advantages and Disadvantages

Some advantages of the team method are improved patient satisfaction, organizational decision making occurring at lower levels, and cost-effectiveness for the agency. Many institutions and community health areas currently use the team nursing method.

Exercise 22-3

Think of a time when you worked with a group of four to six people to achieve a specific goal or accomplish a task (perhaps in school you were grouped together to complete a project). How did your group achieve the goal? Was one person the organizer or leader who assigned each member a component, or did you each determine what skills you possessed that would most benefit the group? Did you experience any conflict while working on this project? How did the concepts of group dynamics and leadership skills affect how your group achieved its goal? What similarities do you see between the team nursing system of providing patient care and your group involvement to achieve a goal?

The patient is satisfied because he receives care from a small team and when he has a specific request or concern, any team member can relay the concern directly to the team leader. The team leader can either solicit solutions from the team members or notify the charge nurse if the team is unable to solve the problem. As a result, patient concerns are addressed and the patient receives care from the most qualified team member for the job.

Each member of the team participates in the decision-making process. The team leader is responsible for facilitating a cooperative environment among team members and encouraging each member to work toward the same goals. Since decision making occurs at all levels, every member of the team feels his or her contribution is valued to have a "winning" team.

Inpatient facilities may view team nursing as a cost-effective system because it works with a high ratio of unlicensed to licensed personnel. Thus the organization saves money by hiring fewer RNs and more unlicensed assistive personnel.

The team method of patient care delivery is a good system, if implemented properly; however, one major disadvantage arises if the team leader has poor leadership skills. The team leader must have excellent communication skills, delegation abilities, conflict resolution techniques, strong clinical skills, and effective decision-making abilities to provide a working "team" environment for the members. If a team environment does not exist, team members might not assume the individual accountability necessary to provide quality patient care (Watkins, 1993). Fre-

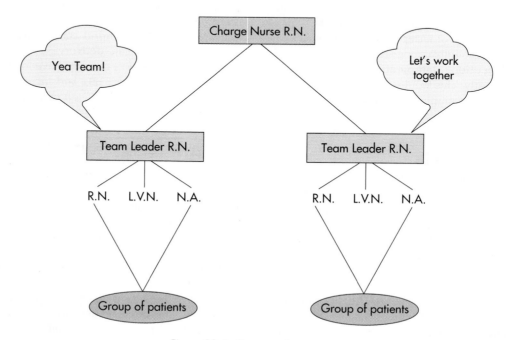

Figure 22-4   Team nursing system.

quently, the team leader is not prepared for this role and the team method becomes a miniature version of the functional method.

Nurse Manager's Role

The nurse manager, charge nurse, and team leaders must have management skills to effectively implement the team nursing method of patient care delivery. The unit manager must determine which RNs are skilled and who is interested in becoming a charge nurse or team leader. A preference should be given to the baccalaureate-prepared RNs because their basic education emphasizes critical thinking and leadership concepts. The nurse manager should also provide adequate staff mix and orient team members to the team nursing system by providing continuing education about management techniques and group interaction. By addressing these factors, the manager is aiding the teams to function optimally.

The charge nurse functions as a liaison between the team leaders and other healthcare providers. Some charge nurses have a difficult time relinquishing authority; however, the charge nurse needs to encourage each team to solve its problems independently.

The team leader plans the care, delegates the work, and follows up with members to evaluate the quality of care. In the ideal circumstance, the team leader updates the nursing care plans and facilitates patient care conferences. Time constraints during the shift may prevent scheduling daily patient care conferences.

The team leader must also face the challenge of changing team membership. Diverse work schedules may result in daily changes in the staff mix of a team and a daily assignment change for team members. The team leader assigns the professional, technical, and ancillary personnel to the type of patient care they are prepared to deliver.

Staff Nurse's Role

Team nursing uses the strengths of each caregiver. The staff nurses, as members of the team, develop strengths in care delivery. Some members become known for their expertise in the psychomotor aspects of care. If one nurse is skilled at starting IVs, she will start all IVs for her team of patients. If a nurse is especially skillful in motivating postoperative patients to use the incentive spirometer and ambulate, he should be assigned to the surgical patients. As a member of a group, each person strives to give the best care possible. Under the guidance and supervision of the team leader, the collective efforts of the team become greater than the functions of the individual caregiver.

Modular Method

A modification to team nursing is the modular method of patient care delivery. The **modular method** focuses on the geographic location of patient rooms and assignment of staff members (Magargal, 1987). The unit is divided into modules, or districts, and the same team of staff members is assigned consistently to the module. Each module has a modular, or team, leader RN who assigns the patients to module staff. Each module ideally consists of at least one RN, one LPN/LVN, and one nursing assistant. The charge nurse expects the module leaders to be accountable for patient care but assists in problem solving when necessary.

Bennett and Hylton (1990) found increased continuity of care when staff was consistently assigned to the same module and the geographic closeness of the modular system saved nursing time. The modular system could also cost money because it requires a redesign of the work environment to allow medication carts, supplies, and charts to be located in each module. Traditional long corridors are not conducive to modular nursing.

The team nursing system originated to improve staff and patient satisfaction in the 1950s. However, RNs are educated to provide holistic care to patients and they are not able to do this in the team method of patient care delivery. In the late 1960s, the nursing care delivery methods were reevaluated and the primary nursing system evolved to provide improved autonomy for nurses.

▍PRIMARY NURSING

A cultural revolution occurred in the United States during the 1960s. The revolution emphasized individual rights and independence from existing societal restrictions. This revolution also influenced the nursing profession because nurses were becoming dissatisfied with their lack of autonomy. Institutions were also aware of declining quality patient care. The search for autonomy and quality care led to the primary nursing system of patient care delivery as a method to increase RN accountability for **patient outcomes.**

Primary nursing is a method of patient care delivery where one RN functions autonomously as the patient's main nurse throughout the hospital stay. The **primary nurse** is responsible for 24-hour-a-day

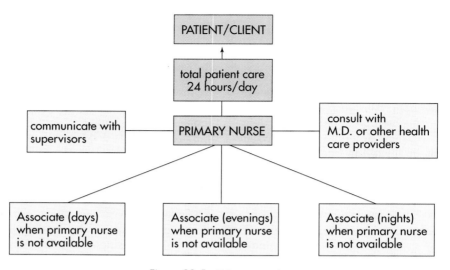

Figure 22-5   Primary nursing.

total patient care from admission through discharge. The total care involves decision making in assessing and caring for all patient needs, planning care, implementing the plan, and evaluating all goals. The primary nurse is preferably baccalaureate prepared and is held accountable for meeting **outcome criteria** and communicating with all other healthcare providers about the patient (Figure 22-5).

For example, a patient is admitted to a medical floor with pulmonary edema. His primary nurse admits him and then provides a written plan of care. When his primary nurse is not working, an associate nurse implements the plan. The **associate nurse** is an RN who provides care to the patient according to the primary nurse's specification. If the patient develops additional complications, the associate nurse notifies the primary nurse, who has 24-hour responsibility. The primary nurse makes alterations in the care plan based on the associate nurse's input.

Advantages and Disadvantages

Some advantages of the primary nursing method are professional job satisfaction, quality patient care and patient satisfaction, and a decrease in the number of nonprofessional staff (Figure 22-6).

RNs practicing primary nursing experience job satisfaction because they are able to use their education to provide holistic and autonomous care for the patient. This high level of accountability for patient outcomes encourages RNs to further their knowledge and refine skills to provide optimal patient care. If the primary nurse is not motivated or feels unqualified to provide holistic care, job satisfaction may decrease.

In primary nursing, patients are satisfied with the care they receive because they establish rapport with their primary nurse. Since the patient's primary nurse communicates the plan of care, the patient can move away from the sick role and begin to participate in his or her own recovery. The professional nurse is educated to provide holistic care. By considering the sociocultural, psychological, and physical needs of the patient, the primary nurse can plan the most appropriate care with and for the patient.

A professional advantage to the primary nursing method is a decrease in the number of unlicensed personnel. The ideal primary nursing system requires an all-RN staff. The RN can provide total care to the patient, from bed baths to patient education, even both at the same time! The unlicensed personnel are not qualified to provide this inclusive care.

A disadvantage to the primary nursing method is that the RN may not have the experience or educational background to provide total care. The agency needs to educate staff for an adequate transition from the previous role to the primary role. Additionally, the RN may not be ready for or capable of handling the 24-hour responsibility for patient care. Nursing has a large number of part-time RNs who are not available to assume the primary nurse role.

Exercise 22-4

Mr. Faulkner is admitted to the medical unit with exacerbated congestive heart failure. Mike Ross, R.N., B.S.N., is Mr. Faulkner's primary nurse who will provide total care to Mr. Faulkner. Mike notes this is Mr. Faulkner's third admission in 6 months for congestive heart failure–related symptoms.

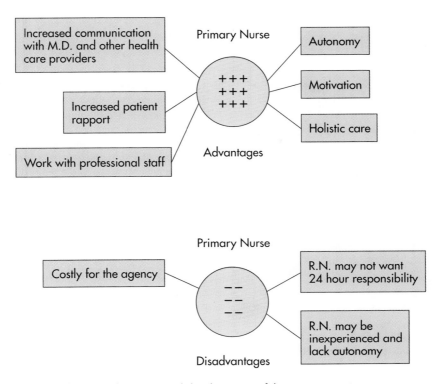

Figure 22-6 Advantages and disadvantages of the primary nursing system.

Exercise 22-4—cont'd

This is the first admission when Mr. Faulkner has had a primary nurse. What do you think will be different about this admission with Mike providing primary nursing to Mr. Faulkner? Do you think there will be any difference in continuity of care? How involved do you think Mr. Faulkner will be with his own care in the primary nursing system?

With the arrival of diagnosis-related groups (DRGs), patients' hospitalization stays are shorter than in the 1970s, when primary nursing became popular. With expedited stays, it is difficult for primary nurses to adequately provide primary nursing. If the patient is admitted on Monday and discharged on Wednesday, the primary nurse has a difficult time meeting all patient needs before discharge if she or he is not working on Tuesday. The primary nurse must rely heavily on feedback from associates, which defeats the purpose of primary nursing.

Exercise 22-5

Imagine you are a primary nurse at an inpatient psychiatric facility. The patients you are assigned to are usually suicidal. How would you feel about the added responsibility for patients even when you were not at work? How would this responsibility affect your personal life? How would you make decisions?

Nurse Manager's Role

The primary nursing system can be modified to meet patient, nursing, and budgetary demands while maintaining the positive components that spawned its conception. The nurse manager needs to determine the desire of staff to become primary nurses and then educate them accordingly. The associate nurses and all other healthcare providers need clearly defined roles. They also need to be aware of the primary nurse's role and the importance of communicating concerns directly to that nurse.

The traditional roles of delegation and decision making have been reserved for nurse managers but must be relinquished to the autonomous primary nurse. The nurse manager functions as a role model, advocate, coach, and consultant. In addition, he maintains the important roles of budget controller and unit quality manager.

Staff Nurse's Role

The primary nurse uses many facets of the professional role—caregiver, advocate, decision-maker, teacher, collaborator, and manager. With 24-hour responsibility, the primary nurse has the autonomy and authority to deliver individualized, comprehensive,

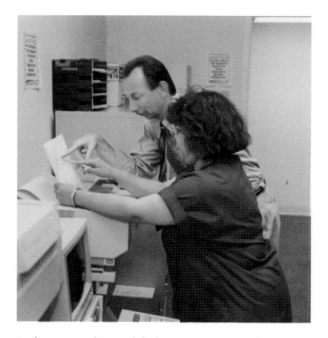

In the partnership model, the RN encourages the LPN/ LVN partner's growth and the two share patient assignments.

consistent care that is patient focused (Johnson & Tahan, 1997). The associate nurse provides care using the plan of care developed by the primary nurse. Changes in the plan of care can be made by the associate nurse in collaboration with the primary nurse. This strategy provides consistency between nurses and shifts. Since it is not usually financially possible for an agency to employ only RNs, true primary nursing rarely exists. Some institutions have modified the primary nursing concept and implemented a partnership model to use their current staff mix.

Partnership Models

In the **partnership model** (or **co-primary nursing** model) of providing patient care, an RN is paired with a technical assistant. The partner works with the RN consistently. When the partner is unlicensed, the RN allows the assistant to perform nonnursing functions. This frees the RN to provide semi-primary care to assigned patients.

A partnership between an RN and an LPN/LVN is different. The RN's role is to encourage growth in the LPN/LVN partner and the two share the patient assignments. A study by Eriksen et al. (1992) indicated that the RN-LPN/LVN partnership model, implemented in an intensive care unit, decreased the reported level of stress experienced by the RNs and improved

the quality of care provided to the patients. In some settings, the partnership is legitimized with an official contract to formalize the relationship.

Example:
You are a primary nurse in a surgical intensive care unit of a small hospital. The unit you work on uses an LPN/ LVN partnership to decrease the number of RNs required per shift. You and your partner are assigned four surgical patients. Mr. Jones had a lobectomy 5 hours ago and is on a ventilator, Mrs. Martinez had a quadruple cardiac bypass 14 hours ago, Mr. Wong had a nephrectomy 2 days ago and is receiving continuous peritoneal dialysis, and Mr. Smith has a fractured pelvis and is comatose from a motor vehicle accident 24 hours ago. How would you distribute the staff to provide primary care to these four patients? Do you think it is possible to provide primary care in this situation? What responsibilities would you assume as the primary nurse, and what could you share with the LPN/LVN?

Primary nursing can be successful in clinic settings, home health settings, and research centers. There are professional advantages for the RN; however, most agencies are unable to afford a true primary nursing system. A relatively new system that is cost-effective and allows the professional nurse to direct patient care is the case management system.

■ CASE MANAGEMENT

Case management is a strategy to coordinate care through a process of managing quality, access, and cost (Bower & Falk, 1996). Case management, as we know it today, was created because of the DRG restrictions on the length of stay patients were permitted and on the amount of care allotted during the stay.

Historically, the term *case management* first appeared in the 1970s when insurance companies, in an attempt to control extremely expensive claims, implemented *external case management*. In the 1980s, as all hospital costs began to escalate, hospitals began to develop internal mechanisms to provide quality care in a prescribed period of time with limited resources. "Within the walls," or *internal case management*, began to emerge (More & Mandell, 1997). In 1986 a Nursing Case Management system was developed at the New England Medical Center Hospital in Boston (Zander, 1988).

The case management model of patient care delivery maintains quality care while streamlining costs and seeks the active involvement of the patient, the family, and diverse healthcare professionals. Healthcare organizations have tailored the case management system to their specific needs. The elements of the case management method are the case manager and the critical pathway. This system can be used in hospitals, outpatient clinics, long-term care facilities, and community health settings.

Nurse Case Manager

The American Nurses' Association recommends the baccalaureate in nursing with 3 years of clinical experience as the minimum preparation for a nurse case manager (Bower, 1992). Many case management services prefer master's-prepared clinical nurse specialists who have advanced preparation with the specific populations being served. The case manager is client focused and outcome oriented. She or he facilitates and promotes coordination of cost-effective care, collaborates with members of the healthcare team, responds to needs of insurers, merges clinical and financial interests, and plays a role in the marketing strategies of the organization (Bower, 1992).

Depending on the facility, there may be several case managers to coordinate care for all patients, or a case manager may be assigned to a specific high-risk population (see Figures 22-7 and 22-8). The case manager may be responsible to coordinate care for 20 patients. It is essential that the case manager have frequent interaction with the patient and the healthcare provider to achieve and evaluate expected outcomes.

The case manager is assigned a patient on admission (or preadmission) to the institution based on the case manager's specialization. The case manager then coordinates patient care until discharge. The patient will have a specific care MAP, or a critical path based on a related DRG category. The case manager will implement the plan and be responsible for monitoring patient progress toward the desired outcome criteria. This progress is communicated to the physician, nurse, and other healthcare providers. All healthcare

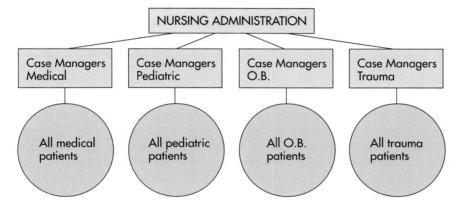

Figure 22-7 Case management system in which each patient is assigned to a case manager.

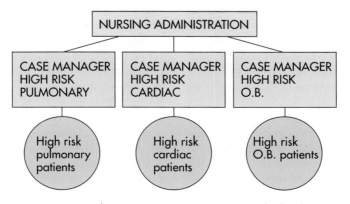

Figure 22-8 Hospital using case managers to manage high-risk patients.

providers work together to decrease the patient's length of stay while addressing patient problems.

Example:

Imagine you are the case manager responsible for pediatric patients. Margo, age 3, is admitted to the ER with severe shortness of breath and a history of asthma. You introduce yourself to Margo and her mother as the case manager responsible for coordinating Margo's case throughout her hospital stay. You implement the care MAP used at your hospital and plan her care with the ER nurse and physician. After 2 hours Margo is transferred to the pediatric ICU. The ICU nurses follow the care MAP identifying patient problems and the normal tests and treatments expected on day 1 (see Box 22-1). On day 3, Margo is transferred to the pediatric floor where you will coordinate her care with her mother, the nurse, and the physician. The nurses follow the care MAP you initiated and discuss any variations with you. When Margo is ready for discharge on day 4, you talk with her mother and arrange a follow-up phone call. You have been the pivotal person for Margo and her mother throughout this admission. Your main goal is to expedite Margo's hospitalization and prevent a readmission. If Margo is readmitted, you will be her case manager.

CRITICAL PATHWAYS AND CARE MAPS

The tool case managers use to achieve patient outcomes is a critical path. **Critical paths** are grids that outline the critical or key events expected to happen each day of a patient's hospitalization (Cohen & Cesta, 1993). The critical path component is based on the DRG services provided by all disciplines for the patient's particular DRG classification. Box 22-2 lists the various components of a critical path.

Care MAPs (multidisciplinary action plans) are a combination of the nursing care plan and the critical path. The care plan component is similar to the care plans typically used except a time is indicated for each intervention of the nursing diagnosis. (See the example in Box 22-1.) The primary reason to implement a care MAP is to provide a written system for identifying patient and family needs. All healthcare providers follow the care MAP to facilitate outcomes and reduce costs.

Development of critical paths and care MAPs can occur in various ways. Organizations can purchase paths for high-volume case types and individualize them according to the practice patterns within the organization. Retrospective chart review or concurrent chart review of patients currently receiving services for selected case types can identify patterns

that can be incorporated into the path (Cardinal, Kraushar, & Wagie, 1994). Members of the healthcare team work together to develop the paths and MAPs, which are then piloted and revised as necessary.

If a patient's progress deviates from the normal path/MAP, a variance is indicated. A **variance** is anything that occurs to alter the patient's progress through the normal critical path. Circumstances that can cause a variance include system, provider, patient, or clinical indicators (Cohen & Cesta, 1993). System causes include lost requisitions or delayed delivery of medication. Changes in the practice pattern of the healthcare provider can impact the pathway to cause a variance. Complications in the patient's condition, such as a hemorrhage into the joint after total knee replacement, may increase total hospital days. A complication can inhibit the ability of the patient to meet the clinical indicator as described in the path/MAP.

Variances can be positive or negative. A negative variance is an undesired outcome, while a positive variance is an outcome that is achieved before it is expected (Tahan & Cesta, 1995).

Advantages and Disadvantages

Case management is best used for those individuals and families who are at great risk for negative outcomes if care is not coordinated (Bower & Falk, 1996). Case management provides a well-coordinated care experience that can improve the care outcome, decrease the length of stay, and use multiple disciplines and services efficiently. Families and patients receive care across a continuum of settings (More & Mandell, 1997). Nurses receive a sense of satisfaction knowing that the patient and family received coordinated, quality care in a cost-effective manner across the spectrum of the illness or injury.

Nursing leaders across the country and in diverse health settings identified major obstacles in the implementation of case management services. Financial barriers, lack of administrative support, human resource inequities, turf battles, and the lack of information support systems have been identified as obstacles in the implementation of case management services (Rantz & Bopp, 1996). Case management is not a revenue-generating activity, but rather a "revenue-protecting" activity. It minimizes costs for those case types with the potential of high resource consumption (Rantz & Bopp, 1996). Consequently, case management is seen as an expense. Because of increased costs, nursing management may add the case management function to

Box 22-1

Pediatric Asthma Care MAP (EXAMPLE)

Critical Path

Care Category	Day 1	Day 2	Day 3	Day 4
Consults	None	None	None	None
Tests	CBC, theophylline level, SMA 6, PPD, chest x-ray, ABGs, urine dipstick, and specific gravity × 1	Theophylline level, ABGs if indicated	Theophylline level, check PPD	Theophylline level
Treatments	Pulse oximetry, postural drainage, peak exp. flow if cooperative q shift, O$_2$ therapy if indicated, IVs if indicated	Peak flow q shift, chest pt q shift	Peak flow b.i.d., chest pt q shift	Peak flow q 24 hr consider d/c if increased peak flow
Medications	(amount according to wt) Aminophylline and/or Proventil NEB/po and or steroids	Steroids may be d/ced within 48 hr or taper over 7-10 days; assess for change to p.o. meds	Assess change to p.o. meds	Consider d/c home within 24 hr of initiation of p.o. meds
Activity	As tolerated	As tolerated	As tolerated	As tolerated
Nutrition	As tolerated	As tolerated	As tolerated	As tolerated
D/C Plan	Inquire if family used home care before admission; begin initial d/c plan	Initiate social work consult as indicated	Monitor progress on discharge plan, consult with MD, SW, HH care; MD to give 24 hr notice to pt and write official d/c order	Prior to d/c confirm home plan with parents, SW, and HH care

Patient Variance (Includes variances in response to treatment or special needs on admission; for example, the patient may also have an infection.)

Patient Problems/Potential Problems

	Day 1	Day 2	Day 3	Day 4
Alteration in breathing patterns	a. Auscultate breath sounds for rales, wheezing, stridor, rhonchi b. Assess skin and mucous membrane color and nasal flaring q 4 hr	a. Auscultate breath sounds b. Assess color changes c. Assess for retractions, nasal flaring q 6 hr	a. Auscultate breath sounds, check color, retractions, nasal flaring q 8 hr and prn b. Vital signs q 8 hr	a. Auscultate breath sounds, check color, retractions, nasal flaring q 8 hr and prn b. Vital signs q 8 hr

Continued.

Box 22-1—cont'd
Pediatric Asthma Care MAP (EXAMPLE)

Patient Problems/Potential Problems—cont'd

	Day 1	Day 2	Day 3	Day 4
Alteration in breathing patterns—cont'd	c. Note agitation, anxiety d. Note changes in VS or O_2 saturation e. Monitor response to tx (notify MD of HA, agitation, tachycardia, respiratory distress) f. Chest pt q shift, position for chest expansion g. Encourage p.o. fluids, assess hydration status	d. Note changes in VS and O_2 to d/c oximeter e. Chest P/T q shift f. Monitor response to tx (report to MD changes, HA, increased respirations, distress, agitation, tachycardia) g. Peak flow q shift h. Assess pt's response to activity i. Encourage p.o. fluids	c. Assess for retractions, O_2 sat; determine d/c readiness d. Chest P/T q shift unless contraindicated e. Observe response to nebulizer treatment and check with MD f. Assess response to activity g. Assess clinical state, increased peak flow, tolerance of p.o. meds, theophylline level therapeutic	c. Assess for retractions O_2 sat. Determine d/c readiness d. Chest P/T q shift unless contraindicated e. Observe response to nebulizer treatment and check with MD f. Assess response to activity g. Assess clinical state, increased peak flow, tolerance of p.o. meds, theophylline level therapeutic
Knowledge deficit	a. Orient to environment b. Assess parent and child level of understanding c. Familiarize with hospital protocol, i.e., IV pump, meds, tx	a. Assess family and pt teaching needs for disease process and begin d/c teaching b. Assess need for visiting nurse, community referrals	a. Continue d/c teaching re meds tx and importance of follow-up b. d/c plan with parents to minimize respiratory irritants at home and in the environment	a. d/c planning b. Med review c. s/s of respiratory distress review d. Identify precipitating factors for asthma attack e. Exercise regimen f. Follow-up care g. When to call MD/come to ER
Anxiety	a. Provide calm environment b. Explore stressors and coping mechanisms c. Assess family dynamics d. Encourage parent to stay with the child	a. Encourage family to state feelings, fears, and anxieties b. Evaluate anxiety level and provide supportive measures prn	a. Continue to encourage verbalization of concerns b. Reevaluate level of anxiety	a. Reevaluate level of anxiety and provide support b. Reassure parents/child re knowledge of asthma

Adapted from Cohen & Cesta (1993).

1. Assessments
2. Consults
3. Tests
4. Treatment
5. Medications
6. Activities/safety/self-care
7. Nutrition
8. Discharge planning/teaching
9. Variants

pre-existing functions of nurses currently employed in the system.

Education and preparation of case managers are a major human resource issue. Inadequately educated staff may be assigned as case managers. The ideal case manager is a clinical nurse specialist. Performance appraisal of the case manager presents another human resource challenge. The case manager does not manage other employees; rather she manages patients and their care. How is this individual's performance evaluated? Performance appraisal criteria must be determined before implementation of the role (Rantz & Bopp, 1996).

Who should be the case manager is a hotly contested question. Physicians see themselves as the manager of care. Social workers lay claim to this role. Nursing staff see case management as utilization review. Who fills the role of case manager is determined by the population being served (Grau, 1984). Case management is a professionally autonomous role that requires clinical knowledge and clinical decision making. Publications by the American Nurses' Association have served to clarify the role, scope, and function of the nurse case manager (Bower, 1992).

Integrated healthcare information systems have to be developed to meet the needs of the case manager. Systems that include client demographics, assessment data, care plan protocols, resource data bases, and tracking delivery mechanisms must be developed to support nurse case management (Rantz & Bopp, 1996).

Nurse Manager's Role

The nurse manager has increased demands when leading the case management system. Quality improvement is constantly assessed to ensure the care MAP is DRG appropriate and the case managers are

adequately managing their case loads. Patient satisfaction is also pertinent to evaluate for quality. If the patients are not satisfied with the system, the census may decline.

Communication among all systems must be coordinated. The case manager works with all departments, so the manager needs to assist in coordinating interdepartmental communication. The communication can be facilitated by educating all departments about the case manager's role and responsibilities. The manager must also assist in educating the staff nurses.

Exercise 22-6

Imagine you are the nurse manager of a teen pregnancy clinic at the county health department. The RNs for the clients are case managers, and each RN has a specific case load. There are many agencies the case managers must communicate with to provide comprehensive care to their clients. What departments might the case managers interact with? As the nurse manager, what specific interventions could you implement to facilitate optimal communication between departments? How would you explain the case management system to nonnursing departments?

Staff Nurse's Role

The staff nurse provides patient care according to the case manager's specifications and must know the extent of the case manager's role. The case management system of patient care delivery is designed to move a patient from the illness state to optimal wellness in the quickest period of time.

It is a concern that the art of nursing may vanish with an increased emphasis on moving patients quickly through the healthcare delivery system to save money. The prospective payment system common in the managed care environment dictates that nursing must develop new systems of care delivery to maintain quality care. One way to facilitate quality care is to consider the different abilities and education of the nurses caring for the patient. According to the American Association of Colleges of Nursing (AACN), it is no longer reasonable or useful to prepare a nurse to be all things to all people (Billingsley, 1995).

DIFFERENTIATED NURSING PRACTICE

Differentiated nursing practice acknowledges the education, skill mix, and competency of each registered nurse. Nurses prepared at the associate, baccalaureate, master's, and doctorate level are integrated into the differentiated practice model. By working in a differentiated role, nurses experience career satisfaction because they are using their education, experience, and clinical expertise.

Exercise 22-7

You have been chosen to participate in a statewide committee to determine state guidelines for a plan of a differentiated practice system. Considering what you know about the preparation of nurses, what education factors will your committee recommend? How will the current nursing education systems that exist in your state influence your plan (i.e., LPN/LVN, ADN, BSN, MSN, and PhD/DNS)? What type of research would you need to do before implementing any change? What resistance do you anticipate from nurses in your state and why? What organizations or groups would your committee solicit assistance from for this project?

Skyrocketing healthcare costs, advancing technology, and an aging population mandate the re-engineering of nursing care delivery. Refinements in differentiated practice are in place in various clinical settings. Sioux Valley Hospital in Sioux Falls, South Dakota, uses a differentiated practice model in combination with a case management model. Associate, primary, and advanced practice nurses are the cornerstone of the model (Koerner & Karpiuk, 1994). Selection of role is based on competency, skill, education, and desire (Gibson, 1996).

Differentiated practice is built on the premise that the nursing roles complement each other (Drayton-Hargrove, 1995). Each role is different. For example, the associate nurse in the Sioux Valley Model is responsible for shift-to-shift patient care (Gibson, 1996). Critical paths guide the care delivered. The primary nurse coordinates care during an episode of illness for those who have complex psychosocial, educational, or discharge planning needs (Gibson, 1996). Clinical nurse specialists and nurse practitioners are advanced practice nurses who are responsible for the continuum of care that occurs beyond the walls of the hospital (Gibson, 1996).

The "right" nurse provides the most cost-effective care. Each nurse's contribution is significant in producing customer (patient and family) satisfaction. Decreased lengths of stay, declines in intensive care days, and fewer readmissions are identified outcomes of differentiated practice and nursing case management (Billingsley, 1995).

Another view of differentiated practice is the care delivered in a **patient-focused care unit.** This strategy emphasizes quality, cost, and value (Reisdorfer, 1996). During a usual hospitalization, a patient may see dozens of personnel. In an effort to reduce the number of staff and tasks performed by staff, functions become centralized on a unit (Reisdorfer, 1996). Services on a unit can include pharmacy, radiology, dietary, social services, physical therapy, and occupational therapy.

The primary nurse in this model facilitates continuity of care, enhances collaboration with the patient, the family, and the interdisciplinary team, and controls practice through autonomous decisions (Johnson & Tahan, 1997). The multidisciplinary team formulates the plan of care after the patient has been assessed by the primary nurse and the physician.

During scheduled work periods, groups of associate nurses practice with primary nurses to implement care. Patient care technicians implement basic care under the direct supervision of the primary or associate nurse. Patient care technicians are multiskilled and may have additional responsibilities, including oxygen therapy, phlebotomy, and 12-lead electrocardiography. Often patient care technicians have backgrounds as pharmacy or x-ray technicians (Reisdorfer, 1996).

In a patient-focused setting, the role and scope of the nurse manager expand. No longer is the individual a manager of nurses. Now she or he assumes the accountability and responsibility to manage nurses and staff from other traditionally centralized departments. With the care focused on the needs of the patient and not the needs of the department, the role of the manager becomes more sophisticated. The manager orchestrates all the care activities required by the patient and family.

Nurse Manager's Role

Implementation of the differentiated practice model requires a shift in managerial style. Use of participatory managerial behaviors becomes essential. The nurse manager has the responsibility as a role model and mentor to encourage the professional growth of the staff. Collaborating with the staff to expand decision-making, problem-solving, and goal-setting skills becomes essential. The manager becomes a teacher, coach, and facilitator. Leadership behaviors of the manager in a differentiated practice setting become vital to the success of the organization. Successful managers demonstrate mutual trust, respect for ideas, and consideration of feelings. This leadership and management style expands the freedom of nursing care delivered.

Staff Nurse's Role

Nursing staff practicing in the differentiated model find opportunities for more meaningful work. Increased autonomy, authority, and accountability provide opportunities to gain control over nursing practice. With greater control and responsibility comes a sense of empowerment.

Nursing competency and education can also determine advancement. Many organizations use clinical ladders for advancement. If a specific level is attainable with certain skills or education, a nurse can advance in position and salary according to the organization's structure.

The differentiated model of care delivery provides opportunities for participation in decision making and encourages initiative and responsibility (Drayton-Hargrove, 1995). See the "Research Perspective" below. Control in the work place creates more satisfied and committed employees.

Exercise 22-8

What level of education are you pursuing? Do you think the basic nursing education you have influences your perception of the differentiated nursing concept? If you were seeking ADN education, would you want to be viewed as a "technical" nurse in your RN job? What type of job do you feel qualified for? Why? Do you think that most agencies recognize a difference in nursing education? If you were in a BS program, what recognition would you want for your educa-

Exercise 22-8—cont'd

tion? Do you think there are more ADN or BSN nurses in your state? Could these numbers influence the move toward recognizing a difference in nursing practice?

COMPARISONS OF DELIVERY SYSTEMS

From the information about the different strategies of healthcare delivery, it is possible to identify strengths and weaknesses of each method. There is no perfect method of delivering nursing care to patients. A delivery strategy must be individualized per organization. With modification, each can be used by hospitals, outpatient clinics, and home health and community agencies.

Exercise 22-9

You are now familiar with five styles of patient care delivery. Which system would be the best for the following situation? You are a unit manager of a 32-bed pediatric unit in a 400-bed teaching hospital. The acuity is very high and the census averages 30 beds per day. The current staff mix is 50% RN,

Research Perspective

Koerner, J.G. (1996). Congruency between nurses' values and job requirements: A call for integrity. Holistic Nursing Practice, 10(2), 69-77.

This study is a descriptive analysis of the values of RNs working in three differentiated practice roles. The researcher sought to answer two questions: (1) Are there core values that appear across all role categories in the nursing profession as well as values unique to each role category? (2) Is there congruence between the values of the nurses in various roles and the values identified in the position description? Associate nurses, primary nurses, and advanced practice nurses completed the Hall-Tonna Inventory of Values, a paper-and-pencil test consisting of 77 forced-choice items relating to a list of 125 values.

The associate nurses' analysis did not select "rights/respect" and "adaptability" as values among the list of 10 values in their position description. This was the only group that selected obedience as a value. "Responsibility" and "adaptability" were values omitted by the primary nurses. Neither of these groups scored highly on "initiation/decision," indicating a value of responding to others' initia-

tives and decisions rather than creating them. The advanced practice nurses valued initiative, decision making, accountability, and internal locus of control behaviors. In this group there was perfect congruence between their value clusters and position description values. Consistency between the nurse's core values and the values of each role's position description was identified. Analysis of the patient care division's and organization's values identified consistency with the values of the position categories.

Implications for Practice

Matching one's values to the position assumed is often difficult. Values and skills are related. The increased complexity of nursing practice requires advanced knowledge and skills. By increasing one's knowledge and skills, more complex values are developed. Creating environments that allow a redefinition of abilities and values promotes personal and professional growth and increased self-awareness.

Exercise 22-9—cont'd

40% LPN/LVN, and 10% nursing assistants. The unit originally used the primary nursing system of delivering care;
however, as the staff mix has changed, primary nursing has
not been implemented. In analysis you find that the charge
nurse is assigning patient care according to tasks. There have
been numerous studies done by your hospital's quality management department that indicate the average length of stay
is 4 days longer than DRG requirements and 25% of the patients are readmitted. You and your staff have been receiving
complaints from the parents that "no one ever explains anything" to them and they don't know who their child's main
nurse is.

1. How would you choose a new system of patient care
   delivery?
2. What resources would you utilize?
3. How would you distribute the assignments and work
   responsibilities?
4. How would you implement the change?

A Manager's Solution

? Before my feelings of frustration escalated to a
sense of helplessness, I assessed the perspective
of other case managers within the organization.
Because the patient population I care for is sicker
with more unpredictable healthcare challenges, I
met with the director of case management services to discuss the road blocks I encounter, the
daily tasks I face, and the solutions I develop and
implement. I included the pathophysiology of
cancer, chemotherapy, and side effects, and the
details of recovery after radical surgery. Nursing
care needs of the patient and family, as well as
the time spent with each to educate for discharge
planning, were also included.

I also clarified role responsibilities. It is the
responsibility of the director of case management
to educate physicians about managed care rules
and responsibilities. Educational sessions were
conducted by the director to assist physicians in
understanding the principles of managed care.
Now I am once again their partner in the care we
provide.

Finally, my manager can be supportive because she has a comprehensive perspective of
what it means to provide quality care in a cost-
effective manner.

? *Would this be a suitable approach for you? Why?*

CHAPTER CHECKLIST

The manager and the staff nurse roles vary with
each care delivery strategy. However, regardless of the
strategy, the manager must have strong leadership/
management skills for the strategy to work. For each
strategy, the manager and staff have different issues
to consider. Without a skilled manager, none of the
patient care delivery strategies would work.

- A care delivery system is the method nurses use to
  provide care to patients.
- There are five strategies of patient care delivery,
  each with its advantages and disadvantages:
  - The case method focuses on total patient care for
    a specific time period.
    - The nurse manager must consider the expense
      of this system and identify all staff members'
      level of education and communication skills.
  - The functional method emphasizes task-oriented
    care for a large group of patients.
    - The nurse manager is responsible for achieving
      patient outcomes, whereas staff members are
      responsible only for their specific tasks.
    - The functional method is most often used in
      subacute care facilities.
  - The team method employs a small team whose
    members provide care to a small group of
    patients.
    - The nurse manager in this system needs strong
      management, critical thinking, and leadership
      skills.
    - The modular method is a modification of team
      nursing that focuses on the geographic location
      of patient rooms and assignments of staff
      members.
  - In the primary nursing method, a primary nurse
    provides total patient care and directs patient
    care from admission to discharge.
    - The nurse manager functions as role model,
      advocate, coach, consultant, budget controller,
      and unit quality manager.
    - The partnership model, or co-primary nursing
      model, pairs an RN with a technical assistant.
  - The case management system is outcome based
    and is facilitated by a case manager, who directs
    unit-based care using a critical path/care MAP.
    - The nurse manager in this care delivery system
      faces increased demands and pressure to move
      the patient through the system as quickly as
      possible.
    - Managed care is a way of organizing patient care
      delivery with cost savings as the main goal.

- The nurse manager and charge nurse are responsible for directing patient care regardless of the delivery system. Key leadership and management concepts for directing patient care include:
  - Communication
  - Delegation
  - Promotion of autonomy
  - Collaboration
- The concept of differentiated practice emphasizes two levels of nursing practice: technical and professional.
  - Each level has specific responsibilities that depend on the nurse's educational preparation, experience, and clinical expertise.
  - Nursing roles complement each other.

TERMS TO KNOW

associate nurse
care delivery system
care MAP
case management method
case manager
case method
charge nurse
co-primary nursing
critical path
differentiated nursing
  practice
expected outcomes
functional nursing
modular method

outcome criteria
partnership model
patient-focused care unit
patient outcomes
primary nurse
primary nursing
staff mix
team nursing
total patient care
unit based managed care
unlicensed assistive
  personnel
variance

TIPS FOR CARE DELIVERY STRATEGIES

- Evaluate staff mix trends to determine if there is a potential impact on your current care delivery approach.
- Remind yourself that there are only advantages and disadvantages to any strategy; there is no ideal approach.
- Know that every strategy has specific expectations for both managers and staff.

REFERENCES

Bennett, M., & Hylton, J. (1990). Modular nursing: Partners in professional practice. *Nursing Management*, 21(3), 20-24.

Billingsley, M. (1995). The differentiated nurse. *Nursing Connections*, 8(2), 12-13.

Bower, K.A. (1992). *Case management by nurses*. Washington, DC: American Nurses Publishing.

Bower, K.A., & Falk, C.D. (1996). Case management as a response to quality, cost and access imperatives. In Cohen, E.L. *Nurse Case Management in the 21st Century*. St. Louis: Mosby.

Cardinal, J., Kraushar, V.K., & Wagie, T. (1994). Implementation of episodic case management in a managed care organization. In Howe R.S., ed. *Case Management for Health Care Professionals*. Chicago: Precept Press.

Cohen, E., & Cesta, T. (1993). *Nursing Case Management: From Concept to Evaluation*. St. Louis: Mosby.

Drayton-Hargrove, S. (1995). Consider this . . . Differentiated nursing practice in all care settings. *Journal of Nursing Administration*, 25(7/8), 5-6, 11.

Eriksen, L., Quandt, B., Teinert, D., Look, D., Loosle, R., Mackey, G., & Strout, B. (1992). A registered nurse-licensed vocational nurse partnership model for critical care nursing. *Journal of Nursing Administration*, 22(12), 28-37.

Gibson, S.J. (1996). Differentiated practice within and beyond the hospital walls. In Cohen, E.L. *Nurse Case Management in the 21st Century*. St. Louis: Mosby.

Grau, L. (1984). Case management and the nurse. *Geriatric Nursing*, 5, 372-375.

Johnson, T., & Tahan, H. (1997). Care management: Outcomes-based practice for the primary nurse. *Journal of Nursing Care Quality*, 11(5), 55-68.

Koerner, J.G. (1996). Congruency between nurses' values and job requirements: A call for integrity. *Holistice Nursing Practice*, 10(2), 69-77.

Koerner, J.G. & Karpiuk, K.L. (1994). *Implementing Differential Nursing Practice: Transformation By Design*. Gaithersburg, MD: Aspen Publishers, Inc.

Magargal, P. (1987). Modular nursing: Nurses rediscover nursing. *Nursing Management*, 18(11), 98-104.

More, P.K., & Mandell, S. (1997). *Nursing Case Management: An Evolving Practice*. New York: McGraw-Hill.

Rantz, M.J., & Bopp, K.D. (1996). Issues of design and implementation from acute care, long term care and community based settings. In Cohen, E.L. *Nurse Case Management in the 21st Century*. St. Louis: Mosby.

Reisdorfer, J.T. (1996). Building a patient-focused care unit. *Nursing Management*, 27(10), 38, 40, 42, 44.

Tahan, H.A., & Cesta, T.G. (1995). Evaluating the effectiveness of case management plans. *Journal of Nursing Administration*, 25(9), 58-63.

Watkins, S. (1993). Team spirit. *Nursing Times*, 89(1), 59-60.

Whitehead, D. (1997). Leader and manager. In Kozier, B., Erb, G., & Blais, K. *Professional Nursing Practice: Concepts and Perspectives*. Menlo Park, CA: Addison Wesley.

Zander, K. (1988). Nursing case management: Strategic management of cost and quality outcomes. *Journal of Nursing Administration*, 18(5), 23-30.

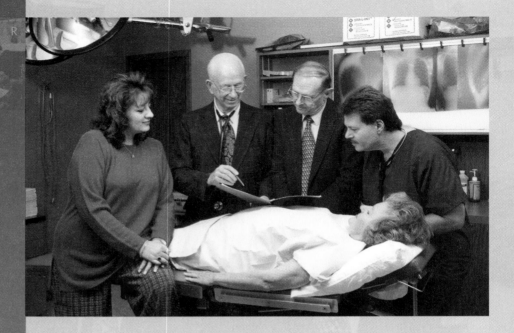

Patient Classification, Staffing, and Scheduling

**Linda Berger
  Spivack**
RN, MSN

Kerry A. Marrone
RN, MHA, CNA

This chapter explains key concepts related to patient classification, staffing, and scheduling. It defines and discusses activity reports, the staffing budget, and the staffing matrix and identifies characteristics of various patient classification systems. Many of the key points discussed are crucial to the nurse manager's ability to maintain appropriate delivery of service, ensure high-quality care in all clinical settings, and monitor resource allocation. Nurse managers' ability to use this information is crucial to leading a productive department.

Objectives

- Identify the key characteristics of a patient classification system.
- Calculate and project a staffing budget.
- Develop a staffing matrix and complete a time schedule.
- Analyze activity reports related to staffing and scheduling.

Questions to Consider

- How will a patient classification affect staffing and scheduling?
- How do I know how many full-time equivalents are needed to staff the unit?
- What activity reports can be utilized to assess unit work load levels?

 A Manager's Challenge

From the Director of Transition Planning at a Medical Center in the Northeast

Patient Care Services at my medical center applies the philosophy and values of decentralization, autonomy, collaboration, respect, caring, and teamwork among each of the departments. Given the volatility and rapid changes of patient volumes, acuity, intensity, activity, and difficult recruitment and labor relations issues, the Medical/Surgical and Critical Care Departments were challenged to max-

imize utilization of precious resources across services and departments. It was clear that to safely staff the patient care areas, relying on the centralized staffing coordinator to manage this process was not effective.

What do you think you would do if you were this manager?

INTRODUCTION

Rapid changes in the evolution of the healthcare environment have driven patient care leaders to examine the classic tools used in managing their business. These changes include addressing the expense of providing acute care, home care, and long-term care in a managed care environment that is driven by the imperative to decrease costs and improve quality.

As healthcare managers we need to be able to qualify and quantify decision-making thought processes, patient care activities, and interventions that are required to achieve desired outcomes.

Classification and acuity systems provide managers the tools to facilitate appropriate staffing and efficient scheduling to justify labor expenses.

PATIENT CLASSIFICATION

The general nature of our services makes it difficult to quantify and qualify the needs of patients. Patient classification systems give us common tools to use and a common language to share. This will become more and more important as computerization continues to grow in nursing. It has been difficult to develop

information systems and use the information for clinical data bases because we lack standardized terminology. Classification and acuity systems provide us a method to do this.

There are two basic types of patient classification systems: prototype and factor.

Prototype System

A **prototype** system is considered to be subjective. This type uses broad categories in which to place patients. These categories determine the patient care needs. The relative intensity measures (RIMs) system is a prototype system. This system classifies patient care needs based on their Diagnosis Related Group (DRG). This was first tried unsuccessfully in New Jersey in the early 1980s. Since that time, Yale New Haven Hospital, New Haven, Connecticut, has developed a RIMs system that is in use to measure work load and productivity. The data are then fed to a decision support system that integrates the clinical and financial information.

Factor System

Factor evaluation systems are considered objective. They take tasks, thought processes, and patient care activities and give each one a time or rating. These associations are then added up to determine hours of care or are weighted for each individual patient.

The Nursing Intervention Classification (NIC) system is a factor system in that it takes into consideration different interventions specific to each individual patient (McCloskey, 1997; McCloskey & Bulechek, 1996). NIC is a system that was established in 1992 by a research team at the University of Iowa. Interventions (there are now 433) are given a name and definition. They are further broken down with a list of all the associated activities. The list of interventions is comprehensive and applicable to inpatient, outpatient, home care and long-term care patients.

It is not unusual for institutions to use a combination of systems. Some patient types, i.e., outpatient hernia patients, maternal deliveries, or home care patients, would be more appropriate to a prototype system. Patients with pneumonia or a stroke whose disease courses can be very different are more appropriately evaluated using a factor system.

One of the criticisms of some factor-type classification systems has been that they are subject to inflation by those using them. Reliability and validity checks must be done to maintain the integrity of the system and credibility within the organization. This would not be an issue with the RIMs system because the patient is classified by the DRG assigned on discharge.

Selecting/Developing Systems

There are many different classification and acuity systems available: Medicus, GRASP, VanSlyk, Omaha, NIC, and RIMS (Diers et al, 1997) are just a few. Consideration of each system must include an understanding of organization-specific idiosyncrasies and unique patient care needs. The exact same system cannot be taken from one institution and carbon-copied to another. Furthermore, there is no one classification system that applies to all units. A system that may have tremendous capabilities for a medical-surgical unit may fall short on its appropriateness for a postpartum unit or a home healthcare service.

Prospective System

It is necessary to determine whether the system will be used prospectively or retrospectively. A *prospective system* is one used to predict care needs of the patients on a particular unit. This method is helpful if the system is going to be used as a method to flex or adapt staffing needs related to increases or decreases in census and/or acuity.

Retrospective Systems

Retrospective systems account for the work after it has actually been done. Areas of the hospital such as a delivery room or emergency room must use retrospective methods because there is no way to predict who will come in to deliver a baby or to be treated in the emergency department. In home care, in long-term care, or on general hospital units we can more easily predict what our work load looks like for the upcoming day or shift and are therefore able to forecast the next shift's work. In addition, the information gathered enables the flexing of staff and provides the caregiver with the ability to prioritize work. When the work load is heavy and we are not able to supplement our work force, activities can be determined as (1) critical for patient care, (2) must be done, or (3) will wait until another shift or day. In addition, the type of setting determines what the priorities of care are, based on the individual patient needs. For example, in a psychiatric setting, group therapy would be a priority, but on a rehabilitation unit, physical therapy would be a priority.

Another consideration is whether to use a prototype or a factor system. This depends on the needs of the institution and what the information will be used for. Generally speaking, a prototype system could be implemented faster and cheaper; its limitation is that it would not provide the detail possible with a factor system. Many of the systems available are computerized, and many can be combined with the documentation system, eliminating unnecessary duplicate documentation. The effective utilization of the work load measurement system in completing clinical and financial analysis is essential. This requires that the patient classification system chosen is able to interface with other components of the organization's information systems.

Significant attention must be given to analyzing the flexibility, adaptability, and applicability of patient classification systems to any patient care department. Although patient populations are different, the measuring tool must be evaluated by all departments where care is delivered.

Organizational Commitment

Organizational commitment and support are perhaps the most important considerations before purchasing or developing and implementing a patient classification system. Financial, technical, and personnel resources are required for successful development and implementation. Several decision-making options exist. One may purchase a "canned" system and, as necessary, attempt to fit it into the organization, or a patient classification system can be developed uniquely to the organization's culture and practice. Whichever decision is reached will require a major financial commitment on the part of the organization. Patient classification systems have initial costs of thousands of dollars. Additional expenses associated with the project may include consultants with experience to assist in the development and implementation of the program and software upgrades and maintenance for the system. One of the most critical requirements is to identify an in-house staff member who has the responsibility and authority commensurate to maintain upgrades, and who supports the staff in all phases of implementing and using the system.

Staff participation can result in tremendous costs to the organization, but the system/program will not be successful without a major "buy-in" by this group. Whether the system is being developed in-house or purchased as a package, staff need to participate in designing the system by representation on committees. Committee participation is important in order to develop and select tools and methodologies; define their purpose and use; identify and document expected outcomes; develop policies and procedures related to the system; and plan the implementation. The time and financial resources to train the staff must be calculated and projected. If each member using the system requires 4 hours of training and the decision has been made that all professional nurses in the department will be trained, the training hours and cost could have an impact on overall staffing, scheduling, and budget.

Exercise 23-1

Select a site that has a patient classification system. Determine the following: Is it a package purchase? Was it designed for the organization? What orientation to the system is provided for new employees?

It is the responsibility of the manager to identify these expenses and plan for the ongoing delivery of care during the process of education and the implementation of a new system.

Example
300 Nurses $\times$ 4 Hours each = 1200 Hours of training
1200 Hours $\times$ $25.00/Average hourly rate = $30,000

The next consideration for the nurse manager is deciding when the training will occur. Can these nurses be released and replaced during work hours or will they be required to attend on time off? Decisions related to who will be trained, on what shifts,

and who will provide the training may have impact on the staffing, scheduling patterns, and budget.

Patient classification systems are subject to individual judgments and biases by the reviewers. It is essential that resources be provided to support, educate, and monitor the proper application. In addition, a quality management audit must be developed to review compliance with standards and maintain accuracy of the system. This process will need to continue on an ongoing basis.

Managing Biases

Patient classification systems look at various kinds of nursing activities to determine patient care requirements. It is critical that as many categories as possible be considered. Box 23-1 presents some activities to include.

Some levels of correlation exist between severity of illness and the time it takes to provide care. In the case of an intensive care unit (ICU) patient who cannot perform activities of daily living independently, is on life support systems, and is on multiple treatment modalities, there is usually no question of the relationship between the time it takes to care for this patient and the level of illness. In the case of a newly

---

Box 23-1
Kinds of Activities to Include

- Physiological support—major body systems and the associated interventions.
- Emotional and psychosocial support—remember to include not only the patient, but also his or her significant others.
- Educational needs—learning needs relevant to the patient's condition, hospitalization, discharge, and home care needs. The patient and/or caregiver may need teaching.
- Barriers to care—language differences or impairments, for example.
- Care planning—the thought processes that go into assessing, planning, and evaluating the care we are giving.
- Indirect care—the things not directly related to a specific patient, but that are necessary, i.e., counting narcotics and answering the telephone.
- Other considerations—the physical layout of the unit we work on or, in home care, the distance we drive to reach patients.

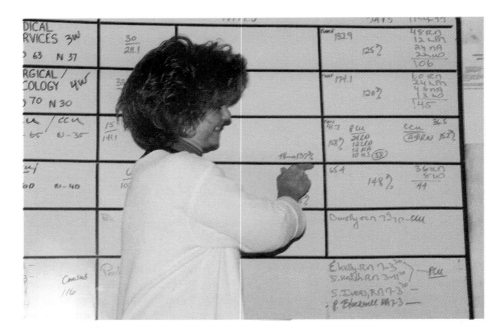

Staffing is one of the most challenging responsibilities for nurse managers.

diagnosed diabetic who is able to perform independent activities, but requires extensive teaching, the relationship may not be as clear to measure. A patient classification system, however, assists in identifying individual patient care requirements and can be instrumental in facilitating the equitable distribution of resources.

Once the system has proven to be a valid and reliable measure of the nursing work load, it can be used to predict staffing requirements and assist in the decision-making processes related to staffing. Furthermore, reports generated from the patient classification system that are indicative of variances of actual staffing needs versus predicted requirements may be used to evaluate the adequacy of staffing and unit productivity. Using the patient classification system in the board room can successfully support justification for budget requests and can be invaluable in educating top administration when trying to convert patient care needs to dollars and cents.

The mechanisms related to staffing and scheduling are complex. To facilitate knowledgeable decision making and judgment, it is essential that the nurse manager be well educated in the multiple aspects of staffing and scheduling. The integration of information from clinical and financial sources allows the nurse manager to monitor resource allocation, appropriate delivery of service, and quality of care.

STAFFING

The nurse manager's role is a complex and demanding one. Of the many responsibilities and challenges that the role entails, staffing remains one of the most arduous, but crucial, in the day-to-day operation of the unit.

It is not uncommon among new nurse managers to think of staffing as a distinct entity and process separate from the overall unit's budget. Yet the lack of proficiency in monitoring the appropriate use of personnel resources can have serious financial consequences to the organization's bottom line.

Because the fiscal resources of the entire organization go hand-in-hand with the clinical provision allocated to individual nursing divisions, nurse managers are required to assess and evaluate multiple factors when preparing their budgets and projecting staffing needs. The variables to consider are highlighted in the following sections.

Licensing Standards and Joint Commission Regulations

An important source for guidance in projecting staffing requirements is the licensing regulations of the state department of health. **Staffing regulations** or recommendations usually relate to the minimum number of professional nurses required on a unit at a given time or to the minimum staffing in an extended care facility or prison. The nurse-to-patient staffing ratios are delineated by specialty area, including, among others, adult intensive coronary care, medical-surgical, pediatric, and neonatal intensive care units. For example, in the intensive care unit the standards recommend that the overall staffing ratio be one professional registered nurse for every three patients, with the capability of decreasing this ratio depending on the acuity level and identified patient needs (New Jersey Department of Health, 1993).

Nationwide studies have researched the impact of imposing mandatory hospital nurse staffing regulations, and in 1997 the Institute of Medicine concluded that "there was insufficient quality outcome evidence to support the imposition of mandated nurse staffing" (Buerhaus, p. 66, 1997).

To comply with the 1997 Joint Commission on Accreditation of Healthcare Organizations (JCAHO) patient care standards related to staffing (H.R. 2), an institution must "provide an adequate number of staff members with the experience and training needed."

Exercise 23-2

Review an organization's policy and procedures for assigning staff. Review a specific unit's staffing plan. Note if any changes were made. Is the actual schedule reflective of the plan? Are committee meetings, educational times, and quality management activities noted on the weekly schedules? Are they noted on anyone's assignment for the day?

The Work Load of the Unit

Institution-wide reports are generated that describe the *activity level and productivity level* of each unit. Although the particular format of these reports may vary among institutions, the information that they contain is commonly used to account for:

- the number of admissions for the day
- the overall number of available patient beds
- the number of occupied beds for that period
- the number of patient days for the unit
- occupancy levels presented as both monthly and year-to-date data
- average daily census for the unit
- average acuity for the patients on the unit

Additional statistical data include average length of stay, census, transfers, and discharge information. Statistical work load reports assist the nurse manager in the decision-making process related to the allocation and use of available resources (e.g., budget, staff, supplies, and equipment).

Percentage of Occupancy

Another way of assessing a unit's activity level is by the **percentage of occupancy**, which is calculated by dividing the patient census by the number of beds actually occupied. For example, if a unit has 38 beds and 37 of those beds are occupied, the average occupancy is $37 \div 38 = 0.974$ or 97.4%. Table 23-1 is an example of a typical occupancy report.

Exercise 23-3

The next time you are in the clinical area, assume that the census is typical for the unit. Calculate the occupancy percentage.

If, on average, the 38-bed unit referred to above is occupied 97% of the time, resources, staffing, supplies, equipment, and dollars need to be budgeted to meet the requirements of the unit at that level of occupancy.

It is essential that the person responsible for staffing the unit knows the average percentage of occupancy. As in most organizations, the dollars allocated

Table 23-1	TYPICAL OCCUPANCY REPORT				
Available Beds	**Occupied Beds**	**Per Day%***	**Month-To-Date%***	**Year-To-Date%***
38	37	97.4	95.5	95.5
38	33	86.8	82.7	82.7
42	38	90.5	92.9	92.2
42	37	88.1	79.3	79.3
32	24	75.0	63.8	63.8
32	28	87.5	72.2	73.2
TOTAL: 224	197	AVERAGE: 87.55	81.25	81.96

*This percentage is derived from daily occupied beds in relation to total available for the time period to date of report.

for personnel and clinical resources are based on the average of the previous year's activity levels.

Does this figure represent occupancy rate based on the number of staffed beds or available beds? These can be two different statistics. When looking at budgeting, the manager must be sure of exactly what information is used. An important consideration that should not be forgotten is that occupancy rates are a snapshot in time. These rates reflect the midnight census or the 7 AM census, but they do not reflect the total number of patients cared for on a unit during a period of time. It is important to measure the volume of transfers in and out of a unit on a shift-by-shift basis. A unit that has the same 25 patients for a 24-hour time period is very different from a unit that has had 10 transfers in, two codes, a direct admission, six post-operative patients, and 10 transfers out. That volume of activity is not evident when you look at the average daily census, but has a great impact on how to staff the unit. In addition, the timing of these types of activities must be taken into consideration when determining shift distribution.

Average Length of Stay

Changes in the way hospitals and agencies are reimbursed by third-party payers has resulted in a focus on length of stay. Length of stay has decreased, as has the reimbursed dollar. The cost of treating the patient hasn't decreased as dramatically because the patient's acuity is greater; essentially we need to do more in less time with the same, if not better, outcomes.

Resource Use Indicator

To calculate the **average length of stay**, divide the number of patient days in a given time period by the number of discharges in that same time period. A **patient day** is considered as one patient occupying a bed for 1 day.

Example
One patient occupying one bed for 30 days of a month is equivalent to 30 patient days (1 patient × 1 bed × 30 days = 30 patient days).

Exercise 23-4

If a 40-bed unit with an 85% occupancy has an average daily census of 34 and each of those 34 beds is occupied by 1 patient for 30 days, what is the equivalent in patient days? If this same unit experiences 10 discharges a day equating to 300 discharges in 30 days, what is the average length of stay for that unit?

Staffing Budget

Full-Time Equivalent

Unit budgets are calculated by projecting how many **full-time equivalents** (FTEs) will be needed. An FTE is an employee who works 40 hours per week for 52 weeks per year, or 2080 hours. This is based on the accepted standard of an 8-hour day for 5 days per week.

$$1.0 \text{ FTE} = 8 \text{ hours per day} \times 5 \text{ days per week}$$
$$\text{for 40 hours per week}$$
$$40 \text{ hours per week} \times 52 \text{ weeks per year} = 2080 \text{ hours}$$

The 2080 hours includes all **paid time** and not just **worked time.** Hours actually worked are considered **productive time. Nonproductive time** refers to the benefit hours provided to staff, for example, vacation and sick time.

Example
- Vacation time   = to 14 days = 112 hours
- Holiday time   = to 7 days = 56 hours
- Sick time   = to 10 days = 80 hours
- Personal time   = to 3 days = 24 hours
- Education time = to 3 days = 24 hours

TOTAL	37 days	296 hours

In this example, to determine actual available time, subtract from 2080 the 296, which equals 1784 hours that the nurse is able to be scheduled. This means the benefit hours are equivalent to 14% of the full-time equivalency (296/2080 = 0.14). Generally such benefits range from 15% to 17% of the total hours. An average can be determined for a unit or a particular group of staff. The benefits percentage normally runs higher in a unit with long-term employees because many institutions base vacation time on years of service. Managers should be aware of their unit's average benefit hours.

In addition, a unit that is operational 24 hours per day, 7 days a week, must factor that into their calculations. Each 8-hour work day of a full-time employee's 5-day work week is considered to be 20%, or 0.2 FTE (5 × 0.2 = 1 FTE). To achieve 7-day coverage, an additional 0.4 FTE must be calculated into the budget.

1.0 FTE + 0.4 FTE = 1.4 FTEs required to cover 7 days/week

Departments that use different shift configurations can calculate their needs using the same method. For example, 3 × 12-hour shifts = 36 hours or 0.9 FTE.

$$3 \times 12 = 36$$
$$36/40 = 0.9$$
$$36 \text{ hours} \times 52 \text{ weeks per year} = 1872 \text{ hours per year}$$

Using the same method described earlier, we could calculate the benefit hours and replacement factor.

Exercise 23-5

Select a community health organization. Review the benefits policy. Calculate how many FTEs need to be employed to assure the presence of one registered nurse each day of operation.

VARIABLE COST

Staffing is considered a variable cost rather than a fixed cost because staffing fluctuates with census and acuity. If it were a fixed cost, we would always use the same staffing whether the unit was busy or not. Generally, as the patient census increases, so does the unit's work load, thereby requiring additional personnel. Using an acuity or classification system gives us the justification to flex up and down based on specific patient needs. Justification and its documentation are needed when the expected correlation is not observed. This could happen when we have a group of more acutely ill patients than usual for the unit or if we have an inexperienced staff or perhaps even the wrong skill mix.

Staffing Pattern/Matrix

Since staffing and census are both considered variable resource factors, a question that is usually asked by nurse managers is: How many FTEs are needed to meet the work load demands of the unit?

Since the work load and services delivered vary from unit to unit, several methods may be used to estimate the total number of FTEs needed and skill mix required.

One of the easiest ways of accomplishing this task is to develop a **staffing matrix/pattern.** A staffing matrix is a plan that outlines the number of individuals and job classifications needed by unit, per shift, per day. This is accomplished by assessing the current daily staffing patterns and asking the question: Does the current staffing meet the patient care needs of the unit?

Daily staffing patterns are developed based on historical data that relate to the patient population being served. If there is a shift or change in that patient population on a particular unit, the staffing pattern or matrix may require adjustments.

The staffing matrix may change by day and by shift, depending on the services provided. For example, if a hospital performs cardiac surgery Monday through Friday, and those patients are cared for on a one-to-one basis, the required staffing will be reflected in the staffing pattern Monday through Saturday until 3:00 PM. However, it will not be reflected from 3:00 PM Saturday to 7:00 AM on Monday. If the demand for cardiac surgery on Saturday and Sunday increases, the staffing pattern will change to meet the identified change in patient care requirements.

Another method that may be used to arrive at the FTEs is to calculate the number of hours to be staffed. For example: An outpatient endoscopy unit that operates from 7:00 AM to 3:00 PM, Monday through Friday, 52 weeks per year will require staffing for 2080 hours. If the unit is closed on the holidays observed by the organization, those hours may be deducted from the total.

Example
7 Holidays/Year × 8 Hours/Day = 56 Hours that the unit is closed for holidays. 2080 Total Hours/Year − 56 Holiday Hours = 2024 Hours that the unit is in operation and requires staff.

If the available productive hours for each employee working in this unit are 1680 hours, the actual number of staff to be hired to cover the 2024 hours per year is approximately 1.2 FTEs.

Example
2024 Hours of Operation ÷ 1680 Hours/FTE = 1.204

$$\frac{Desired}{Available} = \frac{2024}{1680} = 1.204$$

The nurse manager then determines the categories of staff needed to cover these hours of operation. If there are two endoscopy rooms that are used simultaneously, and one nurse is required to be in each room during a procedure, the nurse manager's staffing would be:

2 RN FTEs × 1.2 = 2.4 RN FTEs to cover both rooms during the hours of operation

This same method is completed for each category of staff required to adequately meet the needs of the unit, as follows:

Endoscopy Unit Staffing
2 RNs × 1.2 = 2.4 FTE RNs
1 Secretary × 1.2 = 1.2 FTE Secretaries
1 Endo Tech × 1.2 = 1.2 FTE Endo Techs
TOTAL **4.8 FTEs + Nurse Manager**

This endoscopy unit required a total of 4.8 FTEs plus the nurse manager to cover the two rooms and meet the standards of patient care and staffing requirements.

Projected patient days and the **patient care standard** or hours of patient care per patient day may also be used to calculate FTEs. A medical-surgical unit that has 12,000 patient days per year providing 5 hours of patient care per patient day will require 60,000 productive hours for patient care.

Example

12,000 Patient Days × 5 Hours per Patient Day = 60,000 Productive Hours

If on the average, each FTE is available to work 1680 productive hours, this unit will require 35.7 FTEs.

Example

60,000 Hours ÷ 1680 = 35.7 FTEs

Once the total number of FTEs has been calculated, this total is divided among all shifts. This *division of resources* is usually calculated in percentages and is related to work load and activity. Historically, the majority of staff was placed on the day shift and the remaining numbers were divided between the remaining two shifts.

A shift in this trend is occurring and is related to shorter stays, sicker patients, and extension of hours and services, particularly in the outpatient setting, to accommodate customers' needs. It is imperative to identify the specific time of day activity occurs in the unit(s) to determine appropriate shift distribution and allocation of resources.

Example

50% allocated to 7:00 AM-3:00 PM
30% allocated to 3:00 PM-11:00 PM
20% allocated to 11:00 PM-7:00 AM

If the activity and work load have shifted to later in the day, the staffing resources would be divided in a different manner:

45% allocated to 7:00 AM-3:00 PM
35% allocated to 3:00 PM-11:00 PM
20% allocated to 11:00 PM-7:00 AM

If the work load is evenly distributed throughout the 24-hour period, as in a *critical care unit*, the division may be:

33 ⅓% allocated to 7:00 AM-3:00 PM
33 ⅓% allocated to 3:00 PM-11:00 PM
33 ⅓% allocated to 11:00 PM-7:00 AM

For a medical-surgical unit with a total budget of 35 FTEs, the staffing allocation for each shift, assuming the historical approach is used, would be:

50% allocated to 7:00 AM-3:00 PM	17.50 FTEs
30% allocated to 3:00 PM-11:00 PM	10.50 FTEs
20% allocated to 11:00 PM-7:00 AM	7.00 FTEs

After deciding the *percentage of allocation* of the total staff, the nurse manager then projects what the *staffing mix* will be for the unit on each shift. The nurse manager, using historical, current, and projected data of the unit, determines the number of RNs, LPNs/LVNs, unlicensed assistive personnel, and unit secretaries to be placed on each shift. Using the example of the medical-surgical unit, the nurse manager would create the following staffing pattern:

Total FTEs = 17.50 **7:00 AM-3:00 PM (Day Shift)**
8.00 RN
1.58 LPN/LVN
4.65 UAP
1.55 US
15.78 TOTAL

Total FTEs = 10.50 **3:00 PM-11:00 PM (Evening Shift)**
4.77 RN
1.58 LPN/LVN
3.10 UAP
1.55 US
11.00 TOTAL

Total FTEs = 7.00 **11:00 PM-7:00 AM (Night Shift)**
3.49 RN
1.58 LPN/LVN
1.55 UAP
6.62 TOTAL

Total FTEs = 35.0   **Total FTEs = 33.40**

The total staffing pattern initially established accounts for 35.0 FTEs. There is still 1.60 FTE (35.0 FTEs – 33.40 FTEs) available for the nurse manager to use on whatever shift requires the additional resources. Although the proposed staffing pattern does not exactly equal the original number of personnel, it is still considered within the total FTE allocation and provides reasonable coverage for the unit.

If the nurse manager decides to have five RNs on the 7:00 AM to 3:00 PM shift each day, she or he must calculate the total coverage required for 7 days/week as well as the coverage required for the paid nonproductive time. As referred to in a previous example (Staffing Budget section), the paid nonproductive time factor equates to 1.6 FTE (1.54 rounded to the nearest whole number). (As noted in this example, 1.0 FTE + 0.4 (days off) + 0.14 (paid nonproductive time) = 1.54 FTEs × 5 RNs = 7.7 RN FTEs). The nurse manager then takes the 1.6 FTE and multiplies it by the chosen number of FTEs in that category/skill mix. After these calculations have been completed, the nurse manager needs to allocate 8.0 FTE RN positions to the 7:00 AM-3:00 PM shift to provide five RNs on duty each day. This step is then completed for each category of staff to meet the projected staffing patterns.

SCHEDULING

Time Schedule

The next issue facing the manager is to take the FTEs that were allocated to each shift and prepare the time schedule. At this point, the manager is faced with variables that need serious consideration when preparing the actual staffing schedule.

The nurse manager also needs to be aware of any rules or regulations that dictate minimum staffing requirements or recommended nurse-patient ratios. Labor contracts that stipulate the terms and conditions of employment also require careful consideration when preparing the schedule. A variable that is difficult to project is illness, either short- or long-term, and a leave of absence. The nurse manager must be aware of labor laws and personnel policies regarding these issues. For instance, a personnel policy may require that the positions of employees on sick leave remain open for a minimum period of time before they can be filled.

Variables That Affect Staffing Schedules

- Each FTE or portion of an FTE position carries certain obligations. For example, in one institution, all FTE nurses work every other weekend, but a 0.6 FTE nurse is required to work only one weekend per month.
- Either there is no shift rotation or there is a plan for which staff rotate to another shift.
- There will be requests from staff members for specific days off, which may include holidays, personal days, vacation, and days to attend school and educational programs.
- The nurse manager may need to consider staff participation in committees, when the personnel may be off the unit for long periods of time.

Taking all these issues under consideration, the nurse manager sets out on the quest of preparing the staffing schedule, always keeping in mind the goal of delivering safe, effective, quality patient care. Using as an example a medical unit, a completed time sched-

ule is presented in Figure 23-1. Since nurse managers are responsible for achieving appropriate staffing levels, they may need to negotiate with RNs to ensure that daily staffing is balanced.

Exercise 23-6

Replicate Figure 23-1. Assume the following policies are present, and complete the staffing schedule for the month.

Weekends:	Every other weekend off
Holiday:	(The second Monday of the schedule is a holiday)
	Time and one-half for working a holiday
	Equivalent must be taken in same schedule period
Committees:	Two 1-hour meetings scheduled for all RNs in weeks 2 and 3
Education:	Two RNs to attend conference last Friday of month

Flexible Staffing

Numerous flexible staffing/scheduling options have been developed. The weekend incentive program allows employees to work only weekends, receiving monetary incentives with minimal weekends off and fulfilling a holiday work commitment only if the holiday falls on a weekend. A popular innovation is the 12-hour shift plan. Some 12-hour shift programs offer a "work 36 hours, pay for 36 hours," while others provide the added incentive of work 36 hours and pay for 40 hours. A 10-hour shift plan allows nurses to work 40 hours in 4 days with 3 days off each week. Night shift programs also abound, attracting staff with a "work four shifts, pay for five" option. These programs may appear to offer the best of all worlds. While in and of themselves, these staffing arrangements appear harmless, they may contain caveats not apparent at first.

Primarily, these incentive/flexible staffing programs attract employees to the organization, which in turn is able to fulfill staffing needs on shifts that are considered less desirable to work (that is, nights, weekends) or more difficult to attract staff. But do these programs really meet the needs of the unit, and what is the cost to the organization? Nurse managers need to assess their units and their hours of operation and patient populations to be confident about a particular staffing/scheduling option. For example, a 12-hour shift alternative may be requested by the staff. If the unit currently uses 8-hour shifts, what impact will a 12-hour staffing plan have on the staff and the unit? Are all staff on the unit going to be required to work 12 hours or will some be allowed to

```
                         VETERANS MEMORIAL MEDICAL CENTER
RS22        GRASP MIStro:Schedule for Period:      03/03/96 03/30/96
                                                          Run:08/21/97
Dept: MED     MEDICAL SERVICES
```

Name	Hr	Title	CL	Sun 03/03	Mon 03/04	Tue 03/05	Wed 03/06	Thu 03/07	Fri 03/08	Sat 03/09	Total	Sun 03/10	Mon 03/11	Tue 03/12	Wed 03/13	Thu 03/14	Fri 03/15	Sat 03/16	Total
RN																			
	40	DIR			D	D	D	D	D		40.00		D	D	D	D	D		40.00
	40	AAD			D	D	D	D	D		40.00		D	D	D	D	D		40.00
	40	AD			A	A				A	36.00*	A			A	A			36.00*
	40	AD		A				A	A		36.00*		A	A				A	36.00*
	36	RN		A			A	A			36.00			A	A			A	36.00
	36	RN				A	AV			AG8	28.00*	AGC			A	A			24.00*
	36	RN				A	A			A	36.00	A			AGC	A			24.00*
	36	RN			A			A	A		36.00		A	A			A		36.00
	36	RN			A	A				A	36.00	A				A	A		36.00
	36	RN			A		A		A		36.00				A		A	A	36.00
LPN																			
	36	LPN		A	A		A	A			48.00*	A	A		A				36.00
	24	LPN					A	A			24.00						AS	AG8	16.00*
	24	LPN			A	D	v		uG6	u	32.00*	A				A			24.00
		LPN	P								0.00								0.00
NURSE AIDES																			
	36	NA		A		A	A				36.00		A	A		A			36.00
	36	NA		AV	AV	AV					36.00	AV	AV	AV					36.00
	36	NA			A		A		A		36.00		A	A		AA			24.00*
	36	NA				AS		A	A		36.00				A	A	A		36.00
	36	NA				A	u	A		v	36.00		A	A	A				36.00
	36	NA	Z	A			H		A		32.00*		P	H		A		A	44.00*
	36	NA	Z	H							8.00*								0.00*
	24	NA		A			A		A		36.00*			A	A			A	36.00*
	24	NA									0.00*								0.00*
	24	NA							A	A	24.00					A	A		24.00
U.SECRETARIES																			
	40	US			D	D	D	D	DV		40.00		DS	D	D	D		D	40.00
	40	US		D	D		D	D	D	D	48.00*		D	D	D	D	D		40.00
	25	US		j		a	j		j		24.50*			j	j		a	j	24.50*
	25	US			d	G		d		E	22.50*	E	d			d	G		22.50*
	8	US								D	8.00	D							8.00
		US	P								0.00		xF8						8.00*

Name	Hr	Title	CL	Sun 03/17	Mon 03/18	Tue 03/19	Wed 03/20	Thu 03/21	Fri 03/22	Sat 03/23	Total	Sun 03/24	Mon 03/25	Tue 03/26	Wed 03/27	Thu 03/28	Fri 03/29	Sat 03/30	Total
RN																			
	40	DIR			D	DE	DE	D	D		40.00		D	D	D	D	D		40.0
	40	AAD			D	DE	DE	D	D		40.00		D	D	D	D	D		40.0
	40	AD			A		A			A	36.00*	A			A		AM		36.0
	40	AD		A		DE			AV		32.00*			A		A		A	36.0
	36	RN				Dn	A	A			32.00*			A	AG8			A	28.0
	36	RN			A	A			A		36.00		A			A	A		36.0
	36	RN			A	A		DQ		A	44.00*	A			A	A			36.0
	36	RN				A		AGC		A	24.00*	A		A					24.0
	36	RN				A	A			A	36.00	A		A	A				36.0
	36	RN			A			A	A		36.00		A		A			A	36.0
LPN																			
	36	LPN				DP		A		A	32.00*		AGC			A		A	24.0
	24	LPN						A	A		24.00			A	A				24.0
	24	LPN			A	u	A				30.00*	A	A						24.0
		LPN	P			Af					12.00*								0.0
NURSE AIDES																			
	36	NA		A		A	A				36.00		A	A				A	36.0
	36	NA		AV	DP	Dg					28.00*				A	A	A		36.0
	36	NA					A	A		A	36.00	A			A	AV			36.0
	36	NA			A	A			AS		36.00		A			A	AV		36.0
	36	NA		A		A	A				36.00					A	A	A	36.0
	36	NA	Z	A	A		HG8		A		36.00		A	A			A		36.0
	36	NA	Z				rG4				0.00*								0.0
	24	NA		A		s			A		28.00*			A	A		A		36.0
	24	NA				DG8					0.00*								0.0
	24	NA			AS8			AS			24.00			A		A			24.0
U.SECRETARIES																			
	40	US		Z		D	D	D	D		32.00*		DV	DV	D	D	D		40.0
	40	US			D	D	D	D			32.00*		D	D	D	DS		D	40.0
	25	US		q			j	j	a		25.00		a	j	j			js	24.5
	25	US			d	G			G	E	25.00	E	G			G	G		27.5
	8	US								D	8.00	D							8.0
		US	P		xF4						4.00*								0.0

Figure 23-1 Example of a completed time schedule using a computer base scheduling package (MISTRO) based on the GRASP Patient Classification System. (Used with permission of GRASP Systems, Inc.)

Legends of Codes:

Time Codes	Shift Begins	Shift Ends
A	0700	1900
C	0600	1630
D	0700	1530
E	1500	2330
H	2300	0700
a	0900	1730
d	1700	2100
j	1100	1900
r	1500	1900
u	0700	1300
v	1300	0700

Leave Codes	
F	Float In
G	Float Out
Q	Committee
S	Sick
V	Vacation
s	selfcancel

remain at 8 hours? If all staff on the unit are required to switch to 12 hours, are positions available on another unit or area for staff who cannot make the change? With a 12-hour shift schedule, will the FTE weekend, holiday, and personal day commitment and hours alter? How will the nurse manager schedule with a combination of 8- and 12-hour shifts? Look closely at the weekend commitment. An example might be an FTE working 8 hours per day, 5 days per week, who is required to work every other weekend, usually two weekends per month. When this same FTE employee changes to a 12 hours per day, 3 days per week schedule, the weekend commitment is altered to every third weekend or usually one weekend per month. This unit has now reduced its available coverage by nine weekends per year and, unless these days do not require coverage, an increase in personnel resources will be needed to staff the hours required by the nine weekends.

The financial impact of special incentive programs on the department's staffing budget can be staggering. A weekend incentive program of "work 24 hours, pay for 36 hours" equates to 24 hours of paid productive time and 12 hours of paid nonproductive time for each weekend.

Example
24 Hours at $25.00/Hour = $600
12 Hours at $25.00/Hour = $300
TOTAL: **36 Hours**   **= $900 per Staff Nurse**

Furthermore, the additional 12 hours of paid nonproductive time may need to be covered as well. In this instance the organization may need to double the projection for nonproductive time.

Overtime related to special staffing incentive programs may harbor additional hidden costs. The impact on FTEs and dollars is of utmost importance to the nurse manager and thus requires analysis and evaluation before implementation. For example, the 12-hour shift employee who works 36 hours but is paid for 40 hours may receive overtime after 40 hours if all time paid is considered time worked. Overtime for this employee really occurs beginning with the thirty-seventh hour that the employee works. This occurs because the 4 hours of paid nonproductive time each week is considered as time worked. This same scenario may be true for other incentive programs. The impact on FTEs and dollars is of utmost importance to the nurse manager and requires analysis and evaluation before implementation.

Different patient classification systems provide managers with various reports that can guide them in determining the implications of proposed options or the retrospective review of utilization patterns and overall productivity.

A nurse manager may be adequately budgeting FTEs related to activity, acuity, and history, but a change in composition protocols may indicate that rather than paying for 35 FTEs, the unit is now actually allocating dollars for 40 FTEs (even though the staffing has not changed). Although the nurse manager may not have additional resources to use for providing patient care or to increase the productivity of the unit, the financial report indicates that the costs equivalent to five more FTEs than were originally budgeted are now being paid by that unit. It is the responsibility of the nurse manager to be aware of the contrast in the FTE allocation and to be able to justify all staffing variances.

The Schedule

Schedules are usually prepared in blocks of time. That provides management and staff with enough time to plan proactively. Typically there are mechanisms in place within the organization for staff to use in requesting days off and to know when the final schedule will be posted. Staffing schedules may be prepared by a centralized staffing coordinator or by the manager of an individual unit. There are pros and cons related to each method.

One benefit to centralized staffing is that the coordinator is usually aware of the abilities, qualifications, and availability of supplemental personnel. In many organizations the centralized staffing coordinator is also aware of the budget and number of shifts allocated to supplemental staffing agencies. On the other hand, a disadvantage to centralized staffing is the limited knowledge related to specific patient care needs, activities, and resource allocation for individual units. A combination of both mechanisms usually meets the needs of the majority of staff involved.

The staffing schedule for a 4- to 6-week period is prepared by the nurse manager of each unit and submitted to a centralized staffing coordinator for review. The centralized staffing coordinator cross-references the established approved staffing pattern with the one submitted. To ensure a coordinated effort in achieving the established staffing pattern, any variance in the pattern is brought to the attention of the appropriate nurse manager.

The centralized staffing coordinator either has control of the supplemental staffing, whether it is float, per diem, or agency personnel, or facilitates shared decision making among departments to determine allocations of supplemental staff available. These personnel are used on an as-needed basis throughout the department and are best allocated by the centralized staffing coordinator, who takes the bigger picture into consideration when facilitating the overall staffing of the department.

The process used in an organization depends on a large number of variables, including the size of the organization and the complexity of staffing schedules.

Self-Scheduling

A self-scheduling process has the opportunity to promote autonomy and accountability and to improve communication, problem-solving, and negotiation skills. Successful self-scheduling is achieved when each nurse and the whole department can balance patient care needs with the staff's personal needs. The literature reports that there are several factors that can influence the successful implementation of self-scheduling (Hoffart & Wildermood, 1997):

- Committee structure
- Staff education
- Negotiation skills
- Managerial support

Self-scheduling has become more complicated in the wake of care delivery changes and the decentralization of many activities to patient care departments. The professional nursing staff cannot work in isolation from other care team members when creating a schedule. Assessing the readiness of support staff to participate in this type of initiative is critical, as resource utilization and cost containment continue to be major focal points of our attention.

Float staff are personnel prepared to work in various patient care settings throughout the hospital. The per diem staff also work on an as-needed basis or a few days per month and may or may not be assigned to a regular unit. Float and per diem staff are employed by the hospital and may be paid at a higher hourly rate than a full-time or part-time employee. This rate is usually less than overtime because these employees do not accrue benefits or paid time off (paid nonproductive time). Float and per diem staff are used to supplement regular staffing before overtime costs are incurred. Agency personnel are contracted through an outside staffing service and are used in various areas to fill temporary staffing needs.

The JCAHO standards require that all nursing staff, regardless of their employment criteria or status, are competent to fulfill the duties and responsibilities of their position. Competency levels may be ascertained through the implementation and use of generic and unit-specific performance skills lists. Generic skills are those that can be carried out by the majority of personnel who deliver care and perform skills in various clinical settings. Unit-specific skills are activities that relate to a more defined patient population.

Another important consideration when the nurse manager is preparing the schedule is given not only to the staffing pattern and availability of staff, but also to the qualifications needed for each day. A patient care unit requires and demands various duties and responsibilities of each individual staff member. One may be responsible to take charge. This nurse usually has seniority, education, and experience in caring for the patient population on the unit, is current in technical skills, and has experience in the charge nurse role. This unit may also be required to care for patients on cardiac monitors. Ideally, the nurse manager would want all nurses on duty to have that ability; however, a nurse orientee has been assigned to the unit and has not had the opportunity to attend staff development education to acquire this skill. The nurse manager must then determine how best to achieve the desired staffing. The decision may be that as long as the charge nurse and the other three nurses on the unit can interpret readings from the monitor, there may be sufficient coverage and resources available to the staff nurse who is unable to use the equipment. Another approach may be not to assign cardiac monitored patients to this nurse. Another consideration for the nurse manager is that although everyone may have received education and training in an area, for example, the charge nurse role, certain nurses perform the duties and responsibilities of that role more

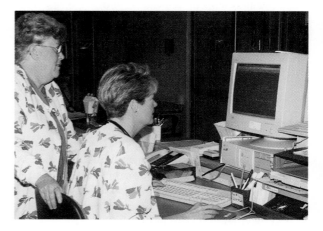

Computerized programming has dramatically reduced the amount of time spent preparing staffing schedules.

expertly than others. On a busy day or a day when the nurse manager may be out of the building, the appropriate decision may be to schedule and assign the most experienced charge nurse on duty.

On a daily basis, staffing sheets are used to make shift-to-shift revisions that may occur related to census, acuity, sick calls, and emergencies. These daily staffing sheets are reviewed by the nurse manager to assess attendance of staff and unplanned variances. Once the schedule is posted and the staff arrives on duty, the daily assignment is completed. The actual assignment of the staff may be accomplished by the nurse manager or delegated to the charge nurse. When completing this task, two major factors are considered: the needs of the patients and the qualifications of the staff. Determining the skills and qualifications of the staff has historically been the responsibility of the organization. These standards for practice are evaluated annually or semiannually and are reflected in the staff's performance evaluations.

A large amount of time spent preparing the staffing schedule has been alleviated by computerized programming. Currently there are several computerized staffing and scheduling packages on the market. These systems, though expensive, have the ability to save countless hours for the nurse manager and centralized staffing coordinator, streamline record keeping, and generate staffing justification and utilization reports.

These computerized staffing systems have the ability to retain multiple variables about each employee in every category entered and develop a schedule. Once a pattern by an employee has been developed and programmed into the computer, the system can generate a schedule in a matter of minutes. This is far more expedient and productive than the most experienced nurse manager can be.

CHAPTER CHECKLIST

Multiple patient classification systems are available on the market and are supported by information systems technology (computers).

- Working with a classification system currently in place or assisting the department in the decision-making process of selecting and/or developing a patient classification, the nurse manager should remember several important points:
  - Does the system designate levels of care using critical indicators?

A Manager's Solution

A project team was formed that included representatives from all levels of management and staff from each patient care department. In addition, the nursing coordinator who is the administrative representative on evening, nights, weekends, and holidays was included. The project team was led by the systems coordinator, who is accountable for the patient classification system and supports the decentralized management teams by ensuring staffing needs are met and providing information and data to manage efficiently. The project team used the organization's continuous quality improvement process to identify opportunities for improvement of the shift-to-shift resource allocation process.

The staff was very committed to using the results of the patient classification system they designed as the framework for distributing available resources. The result of this empowering process was that staff agreed to meet two times a day in the centralized nursing office and collaborate on the staffing for the next shift. A large white board was placed on the wall; where each patient care department, the census, and the total patient care hours required is recorded. The shift distribution for each department is multiplied by the total patient care hours required to determine the needed nursing care hours in each unit. The board also displays the available nursing care hours. As a team, the percentage utilization numbers are analyzed, activity is discussed, skill mix is evaluated, and the available nursing care hours are assigned.

Staff nurses who participate are then confident that available staff have been distributed appropriately. This process has improved the relationship between patient care departments. The staff have come to acknowledge and support each other's staffing needs and the limited availability of additional staff to augment their resources. This process has been invaluable in response to the changes that occur hour to hour within the acute care environment. The solution and process have promoted and supported effective teamwork across the organization.

Would this be a suitable approach for you? Why?

- Can staffing requirements be projected related to the patient's level of illness?
- Do the critical indicators consider multiple aspects of care?
- Can the data generated by the system be used to trend and determine resource allocation for the department/hospital, and can they support a manager in justifying staffing requirements?
- How will care providers be involved in monitoring the system to ensure validity and reliability?
- Can the patient classification system integrate to other systems within the organization? (Ledwitch, 1988)

■ Nurse managers must be familiar with licensing regulations such as those affecting the organization and the nursing populations, and with accreditation standards.

■ Careful consideration must be given to the multiple impacts flexible scheduling can have.

TIPS FOR PATIENT CLASSIFICATION SYSTEMS

■ Determine the intended use of the system—will it be used to support day-to-day operations?

■ Will the patient classification system be retrospective and/or prospective?

■ Will the system be automated and able to integrate with the organization's other information systems?

■ Involve staff in the design and implementation process.

■ Obtain senior leadership support.

TERMS TO KNOW

average length of stay	percentage of occupancy
factor evaluation	productive time
full-time equivalent (FTE)	prototype
nonproductive time	staffing matrix/pattern
paid time	staffing regulations
patient day	worked time

REFERENCES

Buerhaus, P. (1997). What is the harm in imposing mandatory nurse staffing regulations? *Nursing Economics*, 15(2), 66.

Diers, D., Bozzo, J., & RIMS/Nursing Acuity Project Group. (1997). Nursing resource definition in DRGs, *Nursing Economics*, 15(3), 124-130.

Hoffart, N. & Wildermood, S. (1997). Self scheduling in five Med-Surg units: A comparison. *Nursing Management*, 28(4), 42-45.

Joint Commission. (1997). *Accreditation Manual for Hospitals Volume I: Standards*. Oakbrook Terrace, IL: Joint Commission.

Ledwitch, L. (1988). Expanded utilization of the patient classification system. In Scherubel, J.C., & Schaffer, F.A., eds. *Patient and Purse Strings* II. New York: National League for Nursing.

McCloskey, J. (1997). Nursing Interventions Classification Program facilitates data gathering, study of nursing, *Clinical Data Management*, 3(12), 3-5.

McCloskey, J.C., & Bulechek, G.M. (1996). *Nursing Interventions Classification* (NIC). St. Louis: Mosby.

New Jersey Department of Health. (1993). *Licensing Standards for Hospitals*. Trenton, NJ: New Jersey Department of Health Division of Health Facilities Educational Licensing, CN 367.

SUGGESTED READINGS

Bradley, V. (1995). Innovative informatics. NIC: What is it? *Journal of Emergency Nursing*, 21(4), 338-340.

Bulechek, G.G., & McCloskey, J.C. (1989). Nursing interventions: Treatments for potential diagnoses. In Carroll-Johnson R.M., ed. *Proceedings of the Eighth Conference*, NANDA, Philadelphia: J.B. Lippincott.

Daly, J.M., Button, P., Prophet, C., Clarke, M., & Androwich, I. (1997). Nursing interventions classification implementation issues in five test sites, *Computers in Nursing*, 15(1), 23-29.

Finkler, S. (1992). *Budgeting Concepts for Nurse Managers*. Philadelphia: W.B. Saunders.

Massaro, T., Munroe, D., Schisler, L., White, R., Stone, A., Gambill, A., Shirkman, N., Tittle, M. A professional practice model: two key components, *Nursing Management*, 27(9), 43-47.

Moorehead, S.A., McCloskey, J.C., Bulechek, G.M. (1993). Nursing Interventions Classification: A comparison with the Omaha System and the Home Healthcare Classification, *JONA*, 23(10), 23-29.

O'Brien-Pallas, L., Irvine, D., Peereboom, E., & Murray, M. (1997). Measuring nursing workload: Understanding the variability, *Nursing Economics*, 15(4), 171-182.

Prescott, P.A. (1986). DRG prospective reimbursement: The nursing intensity factor, *Nursing Management*, 17(1), 43-48.

Saba, V.K. (1997). Why the home health care classification is a recognized nursing nomenclature, *Computers in Nursing* (Supplement), 15(2), s69-s74.

Stevens, B., & Mallard, C. (1989). *Essentials of Nursing Management: Concepts and Context of Practice*. Rockville, MD: Aspen.

Van Slyck, A. (1991). A system approach to the management of nursing services, Part I-Part VII. *Nursing Management*, 22(3,4,5,6,7,9).

Weidmann, J., & North, H. (1987). Implementing the Omaha Classification System in a public health agency. *Nursing Clinics of North America*, 22, 971-979.

Managing Personal Resources

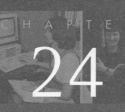
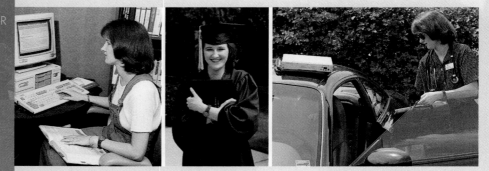

Role Transition

Jennifer Jackson
Gray
RN, PhD

This chapter provides information about role transition, the process of moving from a clinically focused position to a supervisory position with increased responsibility. A basic overview of management roles illustrates the complexity of managing work done by others and provides a foundation for understanding role transition. The exercises offer opportunities to recognize one's own expectations, resources, and management potential.

Objectives

- Construct a nonnursing role using *responsibilities, opportunities, lines of communication, expectations, and support* (ROLES).
- Analyze specific examples of role transitions as a leader, manager, and follower.
- Hypothesize the phases of role transition using comparisons to the phases in developing an intimate relationship.
- Compare the phases of an unexpected role transition to the grieving process.
- Compare the strategies used during a previous transition: strengthening internal resources, negotiating a role, growing with mentors, or learning necessary skills.

Questions to Consider

- What do I need to know about a management position before accepting it?
- How can I quickly make the transition from clinical nurse to nurse manager?
- Am I currently in a role transition?

A Manager's Challenge
From the Area Nurse Manager of a Physician Network in The Southwest

I was working such long hours doing infusion therapy for a home health agency that it seemed that I did not have a life away from work. A nurse that I knew through the Oncology Nurses Society offered me a brand new position in a company that was rapidly expanding. The company provided management services to oncologists in clinics and offices. I had helped several physicians establish practices so I knew insurance, Medicare, and pay-ment issues inside and out. Nurses in the clinics and offices had little support, so they wanted me to be an area nurse manager over several locations. I did not realize the enormity of the job. I floundered some. There wasn't even a position description for an area nurse manager.

What do you think you would do if you were this manager?

INTRODUCTION

Role transition involves transforming one's professional identity. Consider the staff nurse who becomes a nurse manager. The staff nurse performs tasks related to the care of patients. As a team member, the staff nurse has accountability and responsibility for the work that is accomplished. A staff nurse who becomes a nurse manager must transition into the new role as a generalist, orchestrating diverse tasks and getting work done through others.

A staff nurse who moves from an acute care setting to a home health agency must also undergo a role transition (ANA, 1996). In fact, Porter-O'Grady (1996) asserts that all nursing roles are being radically altered, forcing nurses into role transition. Whether it is moving to a management position or from one setting to another, a new professional identity must be forged. Without forging a new professional identity through the process of role transition, the nurse may be uncomfortable and ineffective in the new role (Robinson, Murrells, & Marsland, 1997).

A new graduate makes a transition from the student role to the nurse role. Expectations of students are clearly specified in course and clinical objectives. Expectations for a new nurse as an employee may not be as clear. The new graduate nurse faces the first of several professional transitions.

Knowing what to expect during the transformation can reduce the stress of accepting and transitioning into a new role. Following an overview of the roles of leader, manager, and follower, this chapter describes the process of role transition with an emphasis on strategies that can be used to ease the transition.

TYPES OF ROLES

Accepting a management position dictates accepting three roles that involve complex processes. The processes comprising the roles of leader, manager, and follower are complex because they involve working through and with unique individuals in a rapidly changing environment. Examples of the people with whom you interact and the processes involved in each role are shown in Box 24-1. In nursing, each of these roles relates to patients and clients.

The *leader* role involves creating an interface between providers and supporting innovation (Porter-O'Grady, 1997). The nurse leader brings employees together to discuss concerns, solve problems, and dream about possibilities. The nurse leader listens to employees and cares about them as people. Providing feedback on their performance, the nurse leader encourages the employees to set individual goals that will contribute to team and organizational outcomes. The nurse leader provides team members with opportunities to access the information and develop the skills needed to reach these goals. New ideas are encouraged by the leader providing an

environment in which it is safe to take reasonable risks (Prather & Gundry, 1995).

Changes in the processes of delivering patient care and organizing healthcare agencies have led to the roles and responsibilities of managers being reviewed and revised (Hammer & Stanton, 1995). The role of *manager* involves linking the team or nursing unit to the larger organization. The nurse manager translates information into a usable format and makes it available to those making patient care decisions (Porter-O'Grady, 1997). Organizational outcomes are communicated to the group, and team outcomes are developed. The nurse manager links the unit or team to the resources necessary to achieve the outcomes and rewards success.

The role of *follower* involves respecting the authority of others and working within the system to contribute to the organizational outcomes. Managers as followers recognize their accountability to the persons above them on the organizational chart. Within a team, the manager recognizes the leadership being provided by others and supports decisions made by the group.

In the evolving healthcare environment, the nurse providing direct patient care also must function as a leader, manager, and follower. As leader, the nurse recognizes the uniqueness of each patient and provides feedback on clinical progress. As manager, the nurse links the patient to the resources to achieve clinical outcomes. Medical information is translated into a format that the patient can use to make informed decisions about treatment and self-care. Through referrals, the nurse facilitates continuity of care within the larger system. As a follower, the nurse is accountable to the team and the supervisor by completing the work that is assigned. The nurse as a follower practices within the policies and procedures of the organization and the standards of the profession.

Learning the leader, manager, and follower aspects of any new role can be overwhelming! Another approach to the complexity of role transition is the acronym "ROLES," in which each letter represents a component common to all roles.

"ROLES": THE ABCs OF UNDERSTANDING ROLES (Box 24-2)

Acronyms help us retain and organize information. "**ROLES**" (see Box 24-2) is an acronym useful in role transition.

Box 24-1

Leader, Manager, and Follower Roles: People With Whom You Interact and Processes Involved in Each Role

PEOPLE WITH WHOM INTERACTIONS OCCUR	PROCESSES INVOLVED IN THE ROLE
Leader	
Persons being led	Listening
Peers	Encouraging
	Motivating
	Organizing
	Problem solving
	Developing
	Supporting
Manager	
Persons being supervised	Organizing
Administrators	Budgeting
Supervisors	Hiring
Regulating agencies	Evaluating
	Reporting
	Disseminating
Follower	
Supervisors	Conforming
Peers	Implementing
	Contributing
	Completing assignments

"**R**" stands for *responsibilities*. What are the specified duties in the position description for the management position? What tasks are to be completed? What decisions are made by the person in this position? The answers to these questions may vary depending on the respondent. Each position has specific tasks for which the position holder is responsible.

"**O**" stands for *opportunities*, which are untapped aspects of the position. In the employment interview the nurse executive may have said that the previous manager did not encourage the staff nurses to participate in continuing education. Or while touring the unit, a manager observes that the report room is lacking in amenities. Maybe there is a new method of delivering patient care appropriate for the unit. These possibilities represent opportunities for a manager to have impact on organizational and unit goals.

"**L**" represents *lines of communication*. All roles involve relationships with other people. Some of these people are above the manager on the organizational chart; others are below. Still others are peers. Roles incorporate patterns of structured interactions between the manager and people in these groups. The nurse manager receives and sends messages. Being a skillful listener can be more important than being skillful in sending messages. Skill is required to effectively communicate both the content and the intent of the message; skill can only be developed through practice. Chapter 15 describes techniques of effective communication that are extremely important to a new manager.

"**E**" stands for *expectations*. Staff nurses have specific expectations of their manager and particularly want the manager to be a facilitator and a leader. The nursing executive or administrator will likely have expectations about how managers spend their time on the job—even about how much time they spend at work. Nurse executives' expectations evolve from their perspective of the manager's accountability and duties.

Box 24-2
"ROLES" Acronym

Responsibilities
Opportunities
Lines of communication
Expectations
Support

Exercise 24-1

Observe communication on a clinical unit. Choose one registered nurse. Diagram lines to represent what you see as that person's involvement in communication.

Finding out in advance what the expectations are of the people involved can facilitate a smoother role transition (Wells, Erickson, & Spinella, 1996) by decreasing role ambiguity (Hardy, 1978). Hardy's work with role theory suggests a strong relationship between role ambiguity (one type of role stress) and role strain. The major concepts of role theory are presented in the theory box.

There are also personal expectations related to performance as a manager. New managers may have imagined what it would be like to be a manager and be in control. Stereotypes about the work and people involved may have developed (Michelozzi, 1996). The process of role transition unfolds as a new manager identifies expectations from without and within, recognizes the similarities and differences, and develops the roles of leader, manager, and follower.

"**S**" stands for *support*, which is closely tied to expectations about performance. All roles are shaped to some degree by the support and services others provide. The acute care nurse has peers readily available when a second opinion is needed about an assessment finding. The same nurse may feel lost when confronted with questionable findings during a home visit. The nurse manager who must develop the unit's budget in a skilled care facility may have no accounting department to provide services such as a detailed analysis of the facility's expenditures. Each role has some support available. When considering a new position, it is important to evaluate whether support is available in areas where a manager may lack knowledge or skill. When implementing changes in roles, the organization needs to develop support services to facilitate role transition. The "Research Perspective" on p. 404 describes the support needed to facilitate role changes when unlicensed assistive personnel are added to the care delivery team.

Exercise 24-2

Assume you are seeking a management position. When considering this position, write down the information related to each of the letters in ROLES. Writing the information down may help you organize your thoughts so that you can make the best decision. Complete the "Roles Assessment" exercise found in Box 24-3 for your potential management position.

Text continued on p. 407

Role Theory

THEORY/KEY CONTRIBUTOR	KEY IDEAS	APPLICATION TO PRACTICE
Hardy (1978) is credited with applying role theory with healthcare professionals.	**Role** is the expected and actual behaviors associated with a position. **Role expectations** are the attitudes and behaviors others anticipate a person in the role will possess or demonstrate. **Role stress** is a social condition in which role demands are conflicting, irritating, difficult, or impossible to fulfill. **Role strain** is the subjective feeling of discomfort experienced as the result of role stress. Role stress is a precursor to role strain. Role stress is associated with low productivity and performance. Role stress and role strain can lead to the person psychologically withdrawing from the role.	Clear, realistic role expectations can decrease the role stress for a new nurse manager. Clear, realistic role expectations can increase productivity.

Research Perspective

Barter, M., McLaughlin, F.E., & Thomas, S. (1997). Registered nurse role changes and satisfaction with unlicensed assistive personnel. Journal of Nursing Administration, 27, 29-38.

The investigative method used was a descriptive, cross-sectional study of the perceptions of registered nurses (RNs) whose roles had changed with the hiring of unlicensed assistive personnel (UAP). The researchers also reported the degree to which the nurses were satisfied with the performance of the UAP. The convenience sample consisted of 171 nurses employed in three acute care community hospitals with UAP.

The RNs reported moderate to profound changes in six aspects of their role: delegation of patient care responsibilities, allocation of personnel, assignment of tasks, performance as a team leader, managing patient care, and evaluating team performance. The role as a team leader had become increasingly complex with difficult and conflicting demands resulting in role overload. Increased stress due to the role change was reported by a number of respondents.

Implications for Practice

Ideally, the nurses should be involved in the process of selecting and training the UAP. Data bases need to be developed that allow the RN to access information about the specific competencies of individual UAPs. A process for communicating vital patient information must be implemented. Nurse managers and staff nurses must recognize that the addition of UAPs may increase the stress on a unit until role changes can occur. The organization must provide support for the nurses in the form of inservice education about the role of any UAP and delegating.

Box 24-3
ROLES Assessment

Answer these questions for a position in management that you are considering.

Responsibilities

1. From the position description, what are the responsibilities?

2. For what decisions are you responsible?

3. Consider information about the management position that you learned during the interview (this may be role played). Also consider the responsibilities of managers you have observed. Are there other responsibilities to add to your list?

Opportunities

4. What would you like to do differently from the previous manager?

5. How could your strengths or expertise benefit the people or nursing unit you would manage?

6. Dream a little (or a lot). If a person who had been a patient on the unit was describing the nursing care to another potential patient, what would you want the first patient to say? Describe the unit as you want it to be known.

Continued.

Box 24-3
ROLES Assessment—cont'd

Lines of Communication

7. Draw yourself in the middle of the space provided. Now fill in the people above you and below you with whom you would communicate. Draw lines from you to each person or group. On the line, identify the form of communication. For example, if you communicate with the director of nursing through a weekly report, write on the line, "Written report."

Expectations

8. This may be the most difficult part to assess. List in short sentences or phrases the expectations each person or group may have for you in relation to your management position.

SELF   FAMILY

ADMINISTRATION   IMMEDIATE SUPERVISOR

PEOPLE YOU WILL MANAGE

Now compare the lists. Place a star next to those expectations that are held by more than one person or group. For example, you want to handle the budget of the unit efficiently, an expectation shared with nursing administration. Circle those items that could cause conflicts. Read the strategies section in the chapter for ideas on how to resolve these conflicts.

Support

9. What people do you know in the organization who could provide information that you will need to do your job?

10. What departments provide services that you could access for assistance?

Save your responses to these questions to review in 3 months. You may be surprised how your own perception of your ROLES may change over time.

ROLE TRANSITION

Unlearning old roles while learning new roles requires an identity adjustment over time. The persons involved must invest themselves in the process. In this way, **role transition** can be compared to relationships. The process of developing an intimate relationship with another person provides a familiar framework for considering role transition. Relationships typically move through the phases of dating, commitment, honeymoon, disillusionment, resolution, and maturity.

During the dating phase, the interested persons spend structured time together. Both parties present their best characteristics and dedicate a lot of energy to developing the relationship. While both parties present their best characteristics, both are also alert to clues that the other party cannot meet their expectations.

When you are interviewing for a management position, it is like dating. An interview involves touring the unit, visiting with people, and attempting to make a good impression. The potential employer is also attempting to make a favorable impression. Questions are asked about the role of the manager, and the potential manager mentally evaluates whether the described role matches personal expectations about management. Both of these examples represent the phase "role preview."

Through the dating process, two people decide that they want to spend the rest of their lives together and commit to the relationship. Sometimes one or both of the people decide that they do *not* want to establish a long-term relationship. In a similar way, following the role preview of the interview process, both parties may agree to establish a relationship as employee and employer. Or one or more of the parties may decide not to establish the relationship. In dating, the public decision to leave other similar relationships and establish this new relationship represents a formal commitment. In role transition, the formal commitment of the employment contract implies acceptance of the management role, or "role acceptance."

In new relationships, a time of dating and commitment is usually followed by a honeymoon. More than a trip to a vacation spot, the honeymoon has become synonymous with excitement, happiness, and confidence. In a new position in management, people also experience a honeymoon phase. The employer is excited that the new manager is available. The staff is happy to have a leader, especially if staff members had input into the hiring decision. The new manager is happy, excited, and, most of all, confident in exploring the new roles involved in the management position.

Maybe it is a gradual process or maybe there is a particular event as the turning point. Either way, the honeymoon is over and disillusionment about the relationship occurs. For example, one person makes an expensive purchase without consulting the partner. An argument is followed by a period of painful silence. Similarly, the honeymoon phase in a new position can be followed by a period of disillusionment.

Role discrepancy, a gap between role expectations and role performance, causes discomfort and frustration. Role discrepancy can be resolved by either dissolving the relationship or by changing expectations and performance. The importance of the relationship and the perceived differences between performance and expectations, the basis of role discrepancy, must be considered in light of personal values. When the relationship is valued and the differences are seen as correctable, the decision is made to stay in the relationship. This decision requires the couple or the manager to develop the role.

Choosing to change either role expectations or role performance or both is the process of **role development.** In an intimate relationship, open communication can clarify expectations. Negotiation may result in reasonable expectations. Certain behaviors may be changed to improve role performance. For example, one person in the relationship learns to call home to let the other know about the possibility of being late.

To reduce role discrepancy in a new management position, the same open communication and negotiation must occur. Expectations need to be clarified and stipulated by both parties. New managers evaluate management styles and techniques to determine which ones best fit them and the situation. The personal management style evolves as the individuals develop the management roles in their own unique ways. If role discrepancy can be reduced and the role developed to be satisfactory to both parties, the new manager can focus on developing the roles of the position and proceed to the phase of **role internalization.**

Exercise 24-3

Think about a difficult time you have experienced while developing a relationship. Maybe you chose a best friend who had different goals for the relationship. Maybe you had to work through a conflict about roles in the relationship. What did you learn from the difficult time? How could what you learned apply to the process of role transition?

Role internalization occurs in relationships as they mature. No longer do the persons in the relationship consciously consider their roles. They have learned the behaviors that maintain and nurture the relationship. The behaviors become second nature. The energy spent on establishing and developing the relationship can be redirected toward achieving mutual goals. In the same way, managers who have been in management positions for several years have internalized their roles. Most of the time they do not consciously consider their roles. Managers know they have reached the stage of role internalization when they focus on accomplishing mutual goals instead of contemplating whether their role performance matches their role expectations. Managers who have internalized their roles have developed their own unique personal style of management. Table 24-1 summarizes the comparison between the phases of developing an intimate relationship and the phases of role transition to a nurse manager.

UNEXPECTED ROLE TRANSITION

Not every relationship is successful. Some relationships end in an argument, divorce, or death. When a relationship ends unexpectedly, a person goes through a grieving process. In a similar way, when a person is fired, a position is eliminated, or a job description changes dramatically, the person may have to grieve before being able to engage in role transition. Restructuring demands that those affected embrace a tremendous amount of change in a short period of time (Hammer & Stanton, 1995). To be successful, restructuring must be undertaken with the same sensitivity afforded a person who has lost a relationship through death or divorce. Any role change will have an impact on the lives of the nurse, not just their work (Glynn, Ardnt, Beal, & Bennett, 1996). Role transition takes time, even in reverse.

The initial response to a change in role can be shock and disbelief. The person may feel numb and unable to function. As the numbness wears off, the person may become angry. The anger fuels resistance to the change and may be directed toward those who initiated the role change. The anger may be directed internally, leading to depression. If the person is unable to acknowledge and talk about the loss, the period of grief may be extended or emotional baggage may be created that is carried into the next role. Grieving can eventually resolve in acceptance. Lessons learned from the experience are identified and

Table 24-1	COMPARISON OF PHASES IN DEVELOPING AN INTIMATE RELATIONSHIP AND IN UNDERGOING ROLE TRANSITION AS A NURSE MANAGER	
Phase in Developing an Intimate Relationship	**Phase in Role Transition as a Nurse Manager**	**Characteristics of Phase**
Dating	Role preview	Presentation of best characteristics to make favorable impression; both parties evaluate each other to determine likelihood of the other being able to fulfill one's expectations
Commitment to relationship	Role acceptance	Public announcement of mutual decision to initiate contract
Honeymoon	Role exploration	Experience of excitement, confidence, and mutual appreciation
Disillusionment	Role discrepancy	Awareness of difference between role expectations and role performance; reconsideration of whether to continue with contract
Resolution	Role development	Negotiation of role expectations; adjustment of role performance to approximate expectations and to find own unique style
Maturation of relationship	Role internalization	Performance of role congruent with own beliefs and individual style; achievement of mutual goals

internalized. A new role is sought, and the "dating" begins again.

When a relationship is dissolved in the case of death or divorce, a legal document is prepared to formally dissolve the financial and social obligations between the persons involved. The loss of a position as a result of restructuring or a buy-out should involve a similar process. The employer may offer the nurse a severance package that includes reasonable financial compensation and outplacement services. If a written agreement is not offered by the employer, the nurse should formally request and negotiate reasonable compensation and assistance. Similar to signing a prenuptial agreement, a nurse may have signed a contract with the employer when hired. The terms of that agreement may require the employer to buy out (pay the salary and benefits) for the time remaining on the contract.

■ STRATEGIES TO PROMOTE ROLE TRANSITION

Becoming a manager requires a transformation—a profound change in identity. Such a transformation invokes stress as the manager unlearns old roles and learns the management role. Several strategies can be helpful in easing the strain and quickening the process of role transition (see Box 24-4).

Exercise 24-4

List reasons for being a nurse manager. What goals can be reached as a manager that cannot be reached as a staff nurse? How strong is your need to manage?

Internal Resources

A key strategy in promoting role transition is to recognize, utilize, and strengthen the internal resources of commitment, character, and self-respect. Work commitment is a function of the fit between the role and the person's professional goals and commitments in other areas of life, such as family or church. Being a manager is not for everyone. Consider whether personal goals and professional fulfillment

---

Box 24-4

Strategies to Promote Role Transition

- Strengthen internal resources
- Negotiate the role
- Grow with a mentor
- Develop management knowledge and skills

---

can best be achieved through management. One's commitment to the challenges of managing can provide the desire to persevere during the process of role transition.

Another internal resource is character. Character is the essence of the person—the values, beliefs, and habits of a person. Centering one's character on correct principles creates power to realize dreams (Covey, 1990). Persons whose characters are based on principles continue to be educated by their experiences and are service oriented. Principle-centered people believe in others, creating a climate that promotes growth and opportunity. A manager with a principle-centered character can be trusted.

People with principle-centered character lead balanced lives, taking time for self-renewal. Living a life congruent with ethical principles guides the individual and sets an example for others (Covey, 1990). The nurse manager can rely on tested life principles during the transition to management, especially when those principles are embedded in the values of the profession (see the following "Research Perspective").

Closely related to character is another internal resource—self-respect. Self-respect allows managers to weather the difficult times when there may be little external recognition. Always remember that a person's value does not depend on the quality or quickness of the adjustment to the management role. Knowing what you believe in is especially important during a transition period. Writing down short statements of belief or self-affirmations and posting this information may be helpful as a visual reminder.

Role Negotiation

A strategy that is helpful during conflicting role expectations is role negotiation. The ROLES assessment (Box 24-3) may have identified areas of significant conflict. Writing the expectations down provides the first step in resolving areas of conflict. It is important to review the expectations listed to determine if they are realistic. Unrealistic expectations strongly held by others may require diplomatic reeducation so their expectations can become more realistic.

The priority of different role expectations may also require role negotiation with the nursing administrator. Ask for input as to which expectations have the highest priorities. Explain personal and family expectations and clearly state the priority that meeting those expectations has. The process may have to be repeated several times before agreement on the expectations related to roles and the priority of each expectation is found. Rewriting the unrealistic expectations to be

📖 Research Perspective

Fagermoen, M.S. (1997). Professional identity: Values embedded in meaningful nursing practice. Journal of Advanced Nursing, 25, 434-441.

The values underlying the professional identity of nurses were the focus of a two-phase descriptive study. A survey was completed by 767 randomly selected nurses in Norway with different levels of work experience. The second phase involved in-depth interviews with six nurses as to the meaning of work. Instead of questioning the nurses directly about the values that guided their work, the researcher asked these six subjects to tell stories about meaningful patient care situations.

The moral orientation to care was identified as altruism. Ten patient-oriented values were identified that were expressed in the role of the nurse, with the core value being human dignity. The transcultural core of the professional identity of nurses was described as being the "actualization of the values of dignity, personhood, being a fellow human, and reciprocal trust" (p. 439).

Implications for Practice

Patient-oriented values are the core of one's professional identity. These values must not be ignored or violated when the nurse is transitioning to a new role or creating a new role. All nursing roles should be consistent with these values. Ignoring or violating these values may lead to a role that lacks meaning, a threat to both the professional and personal identity of the nurse. Positive work environments and supportive relationships are created when management decisions are based on the values of dignity, personhood, being a fellow human, and reciprocal trust.

---

achievable can reduce three common sources of role stress—ambiguity, overload, and conflict.

Exercise 24-5

Identify one area of conflict between your personal expectations and your immediate supervisor's (clinical instructor) expectations. Decide how you would like your supervisor to respond to you when you discuss this area of conflict. Write out the desired response. Now consider how you can present your viewpoint to elicit this response.

Mentors

In Greek mythology, Mentor was the name of a character who advised and counseled (Parsloe, 1992). The word **mentor** refers to an older, more experienced adult who helps a younger adult navigate the world. The mentor serves as a role model and supports, guides, and counsels the young adult (Kram, 1985).

Mentors can be a tremendous source of guidance and support for staff nurses and managers, serving both career functions and psychosocial functions (see Box 24-5). Career functions are possible because the mentor has sufficient professional experience and organizational authority to facilitate the career of the "mentee." Psychosocial functions are possible because of an interpersonal relationship based on mutual trust (Kram, 1985).

Sponsorship involves volunteering or nominating the mentee for additional responsibilities. A mentor can be a sponsor by creating opportunities for individual achievement. The mentor may suggest the mentee be appointed to a key nursing committee or volunteered for a special assignment. Sponsorship leads to exposure or opportunities for the mentee to build a reputation of competence. With exposure, the mentor provides protection by absorbing negative feedback, sharing responsibility for controversial decisions, and teaching the unwritten rules. These unwritten rules about "how things are done around here" may be more important to job success than the written rules.

Box 24-5

Functions of a Mentor

Career functions
Sponsorship
Exposure/protection
Coaching
Challenging assignments

Psychosocial functions
Role modeling
Mutual positive regard
Counseling
Social interaction

Adapted from Kram (1985).

Coaches provide information about how to improve performance, including feedback on current performance. Coaching requires frequent contact and willingness on the part of the mentee to accept feedback. Challenging assignments are given to the mentee that will stretch the limits of knowledge and skill. The mentor helps the mentee learn the technical and management skills necessary to accomplish the task, such as which numbers on the budget printout are added to get the total expenditures.

The interpersonal relationship between the mentor and the mentee involves mutual positive regard. Because the mentee respects the career accomplishments of the mentor, the mentee identifies with the mentor's example. This role modeling is both conscious and unconscious. The mentee with character and self-respect will evaluate the behaviors of the mentor and select those behaviors worthy of being emulated.

Counseling, as another psychosocial function of the mentor, allows the mentee to explore personal concerns. Confidentiality is a prerequisite to this sharing of personal information. Since the opinion of the mentor is respected, the mentor may provide guidance to the mentee. The best mentors can provide guidance, while recognizing that the mentee may choose to disregard the advice.

Being mentored is a learning process. A mentee may have to develop an openness to receiving support and guidance. A mentee can identify potential mentors by noting whose names are frequently mentioned in favorable terms and developing a broad network of contacts (Kaponya, 1990). Invest time and energy in getting to know more about the potential mentors. Admiration for a mentor and a recognition of the mentor's commitment to self-success can provide an environment of trust in which a mentor-mentee relationship begins. Both persons develop positive expectations of the relationship and both take the initiative to nurture the new relationship. As more of the mentor functions are experienced, the bond between the mentor and mentee grows stronger.

Relationships between mentors and mentees vary due to individual characteristics and to the career phase of each. During early phases of a career, a nurse manager is concerned about competence and a mentor can provide valuable coaching. As the nurse manager develops, sponsorship by a mentor can prepare the manager for a promotion. A mentor nearing the end of the work career can find fulfillment in sharing knowledge with new managers and at the same time benefit from the counsel of a recently retired colleague.

Management Education

Management performance can be hindered by a specific knowledge deficit. For example, the manager may lack business skills or knowledge about legal aspects of supervision. Most healthcare organizations have little or no management orientation. Instead of depending on others for management development, a manager should identify areas where competence will require new information and actively pursue acquiring this information through educational programs, workshops, books, professional journals, and electronic sources (see end of chapter for URL addresses). Graduate education in nursing administration or business is a valuable professional investment. Membership in the American Organization of Nurse Executives is another avenue for networking with more experienced managers and learning through continuing education programs.

Experience and education provide a firm basis for seeking additional credentials. A nursing administrator with a baccalaureate degree and 24 months of experience at a middle management level can take an examination to become a Certified Nursing Administrator. Nursing administrators with master's degrees and experience at the executive level can take an examination to become a Certified Nursing Administrator, Advanced. The website of the American Nurses Credentialing Center has more detailed information about certification examinations (http://www.nursingworld.org/ancc).

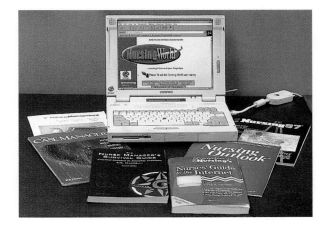

Reading professional books and journals and attending conferences are effective management education strategies.

FROM ROLE TRANSITION TO ROLE TRIUMPH

Developing an intimate relationship can be a difficult process but the majority of people still value relationships enough to make the effort. Making the transition and transformation into a management role is also worth the effort. Leading lives of integrity and commitment, nurse managers set examples, bringing out the best in staff nurses and thereby multiplying their influence on quality patient care. The self-assessment in Box 24-6 is designed to determine readiness for management.

CHAPTER CHECKLIST

Role transition is a process that takes time and energy—two scarce resources for nurse managers. Knowing what to expect and how to facilitate the process can speed role transition and minimize the expenditure of energy as the nurse manager negotiates new roles.

- Responsibilities, opportunities, lines of communication, expectations, and support are aspects common to all roles. When considering a management role, gather information about each of these aspects.
- Managerial roles vary.
  - Figurehead, leader, and liaison rely heavily on interpersonal skills.
  - Monitor, disseminator, and spokesperson are the roles that emphasize on collecting and sharing information.
- Role transition is a process of unlearning old roles and learning new roles.
  - The phases of role transition are as follows:
    - role preview
    - role acceptance
    - role exploration
    - role discrepancy
    - role development
    - role internalization
- Unexpected role transitions involve a grieving process. Financial and social obligations of the manager and the employer may need to be formally dissolved with appropriate compensation and outplacement services.
  - The phase of role preview is similar to dating in that both parties present their best characteristics in order to make a favorable impression.
  - Commitment to a relationship is analogous to role acceptance, a public announcement of a mutual decision to initiate a contract.

Box 24-6
Self-Assessment

Respond to each item using the scale. Add up your score.
1 = strongly disagree
2 = disagree
3 = unsure
4 = agree
5 = strongly agree

1. I am responsible for my own professional development.
2. I feel confident about my ability to learn the skills I need to be an effective manager.
3. I am able to balance multiple priorities and activities.
4. I have a strong psychological desire to influence others.
5. I can develop a personal network of support.

There is no magical score that indicates your readiness for management. A person who is unsure in every category will score 15. A score of 20 or above indicates that you are confident that you could master the management role. If you currently have a mentor, ask that person to respond to each item to analyze your abilities. Compare those responses with your own. Do you have a realistic view of yourself?

- Role exploration compares to the honeymoon phase of an intimate relationship.
- Role discrepancy has its roots in the disillusionment experienced when role expectations do not match role performance.
- Role development is a time of resolution, when role expectations are negotiated and performance is adjusted to approximate expectations.
- A maturing relationship is similar to role internalization; during role internalization, the performance of the role is congruent with one's own beliefs.
- Commitment, character, and self-respect are internal resources that can facilitate the process of role transition.
- Role negotiation involves communicating with your supervisor to come to an agreement as to role expectations.
- Mentors can provide career and psychosocial functions enhancing the career development of the manager.

A Manager's Solution

? Personal characteristics made my transition to the role of nurse manager successful. I had a lot of self-confidence and I had the people skills I needed. I enjoy meeting new people. I had learned a lot from the nurses I worked with in the Oncology Nurses Society. They validated me by valuing my input. I was willing to take the risk.

As a manager I learned that when I visit a site about a problem, I have to pay more attention to the personalities involved. I used to be much more resolution focused. Now, I take time to collect more data—there are times when it is best to do nothing. I use honest, open, and direct communication, something I believe in strongly.

As the company continued to grow rapidly, expanding from 20 to 108 sites in less than a year and a half, my role changed. My role was seen as valuable, so the company created five more area nurse manager positions, except now our role has changed from nurse manager to that resembling consultants. I spend most of my time focused on educating, developing, and mentoring new managers. I developed an orientation program that provides managers with the knowledge, skills, corporate contacts, and resources in the field that they need to make a successful role transition.

? *Would this be a suitable approach for you? Why?*

■ Educational programs provide information needed by nurses to fulfill management roles.

TIPS IN ROLE TRANSITIONING

■ Role transition is a normal process. Anticipate and prepare for role changes.
■ Identify the responsibilities, opportunities, lines of communication, expectations, and support for the role.
■ Use your internal resources to negotiate a role consistent with your values and life commitments.

TERMS TO KNOW

mentor	role internalization
ROLES	role negotiation
role development	role strain
role discrepancy	role stress
role expectations	role transition

REFERENCES

American Nurses Association. (1996). *The Acute Care Nurse in Transition*. Washington, D.C.: American Nurses Publishing.

Barter, M., McLaughlin, F.E., & Thomas, S. (1997). Registered nurse role changes and satisfaction with unlicensed assistive personnel. *Journal of Nursing Administration*, 27(1), 29-38.

Covey, S.R. (1990). *Principle-centered leadership*. New York: Simon & Schuster.

Fagermoen, M.S. (1997). Professional identity: Values embedded in meaningful nursing practice. *Journal of Advanced Nursing*, 25, 434-441.

Glynn, P., Arndt, J., Beal, J., & Bennett, N. (1996). The interconnectedness of nurses' lives: Implications for nursing management. *Journal of Nursing Administration*, 26(5), 36-42.

Hammer, M. & Stanton, S.A. (1995). *Reengineering revolution*. New York: Harper Collins Publishers.

Hardy, M.E. (1978). Role stress and role strain. In Hardy, M.E., & Conway, M.E., eds. *Role Theory: Perspectives for Health Professionals*. New York: Appleton-Century-Crofts.

Kaponya, P. (1990). *How to Survive the First 90 Days at a New Company*. Hawthorne, NJ: Career Press.

Kram, K.E. (1985). *Mentoring at Work*. Glenview, IL: Scott, Foresman & Co.

Michelozzi, B.N. (1996). *Coming Alive from Nine to Five: A Career Search Handbook* (5th ed.). Mountain View, CA: Mayfield Publishing.

Parsloe, E. (1992). *Coaching, mentoring, and assessing*. London, EN: Kogan Page Limited.

Porter-O'Grady, T. (1996) Nurses as advanced practitioners and primary care providers. In Cohen, E.L., ed. *Nurse Case Management in the 21st Century*. St. Louis: Mosby.

Porter-O'Grady, T. (1997). Quantum mechanics and the future of healthcare leadership. *Journal of Nursing Administration*, 27(1), 15-20.

Prather, C.W. & Gundry, L.K. (1995). *Blueprints for Innovation: How Creative Process Can Make You and Your Company More Competitive*. New York: American Management Association.

Robinson, S., Murrells, T., & Marsland, L. (1997). Constructing career pathways in nursing: Some issues for research and policy. *Journal of Advanced Nursing*, 25, 602-614.

Wells, N., Erickson, S., & Spinella, J. (1996). Role transition: From clinical nurse specialist to clinical nurse specialist/case manager. *Journal of Nursing Administration*, 26(11), 23-28.

ELECTRONIC RESOURCES

http://www.mgma.com

Site for the Medical Group Management Association that links to discussion groups, on-line resources, and a virtual exhibit hall.

http://www.albany.edu/hcm/

Home page of The Institute for the Advancement of Health Care Management; resource for videoconferences related to healthcare management.

http://www.aboutwork.com

Networking and career planning resources.

http://www.hsj.macmillan.com/

Weekly journal entitled Health Services Journal published in the United Kingdom; links to 500 other sites.

http://www.aupha.com/

Association of University Programs in Health Administration; national calendar of conferences related to management.

http://nursequest.com/board.htm

Bulletin board to which concerns about role transitions can be submitted or even clinical questions.

http://www.nursingworld.org

Access to the American Nurses Association and Credentialling Center.

http://www.lib.umich.edu/hw/nursing.html

Link to career information and numerous nursing-related sites.

SUGGESTED READINGS

Dieneqann, J., & Shaffer, C. (1993). Nurse manager characteristics and skills: Curriculum implications. *Nursing Connections, 6*(2), 15-23.

Everett, M. (1995). *Making a Living While Making a Difference.* New York: Bantam Books.

Graen, G.B. (1989). *Unwritten Rules for Your Career: The 15 Secrets for Fast-Track Success.* New York: John Wiley & Sons.

Hill, L.A. (1992). *Becoming a Manager: Mastering a New Identity.* New York: Penguin Books.

Holton, B., & Holton, C. (1992). *The Manager's Short Course.* New York: John Wiley & Sons.

Kaponya, P. (1990). *How to Survive the First 90 Days at a New Company.* Hawthorne, NJ: Career Press.

Kriegel, R.J., & Patler, L. (1991). *If it ain't broke . . . Break it!* New York: Warner Books.

McCormack, M.H. (1984). *What They Don't Teach You in Harvard Business School.* New York: Bantam Books.

Westmoreland, D. (1993). Nurse managers' perspectives of their work: Connection and relationship. *Journal of Nursing Administration, 23*(1), 60-64.

Wheatley, M.J. (1994). *Leadership and the New Science: Learning about Organization from an Orderly Universe.* San Francisco, CA: Berrett-Koehler Publishers.

Power, Politics, and Influence

Karen Kelly
RN, EdD, CNAA

This chapter describes how power and politics influence the roles of leaders and managers. It focuses on contemporary concepts of power, empowerment, types of power exercised by nurses, key factors in developing a powerful image, and personal and organizational strategies for exercising power. Having the opportunity to relate to politics in the work place is critical for effective leadership and management.

Objectives

- Apply the concept of power to leadership and management in nursing.
- Employ different types of power in the exercise of nursing leadership.
- Develop a power image for effective nursing leadership.
- Choose appropriate strategies for exercising power to influence the politics of the work setting, professional organizations, and legislatures.

Questions to Consider

- What kind of image does the phrase "a powerful nurse" conjure up in your mind?
- Do you ever think of yourself as a powerful nurse?
- What factors, persons, and events have influenced your development as a nurse?
- What kinds of behaviors do you observe in people that tell you whether they are powerful? Which of these behaviors do you consider socially desirable? Which are undesirable?
- What are your own powerful behaviors?
- What are your beliefs and values about power and politics in organizations?

A Manager's Challenge

From a Nurse Manager of a Mental Health Unit in the Midwest

A nurse on the mental health unit I manage experienced recurrent episodes of schizophrenia. At times she was as sick as some of her patients on the mental health unit. She was being treated by a psychiatrist on the hospital's staff who hospitalized her on the very unit where she would return to work. Counseling had only limited impact on her; she asked the psychiatrist to admit her at another hospital when she became acutely ill again. With each acute episode of her illness, she was less and less able to cope with the demands of her work. Yet, her psychiatrist kept giving her a full release to return to work in the mental health setting.

Disciplinary action was difficult to institute; when I sought guidance from human resources personnel, they were concerned about the implications of the Americans with Disability Act if we took action that was too strong. I was concerned about her ability to separate her own problems from those of her patients. Her colleagues increasingly had to work to compensate for her deteriorating performance. At first, the deterioration was almost nebulous; it was very difficult to describe her deficiencies in the kind of concrete terms that were required for the hospital's disciplinary process. She was not open to seeking a less stressful nursing job outside of mental health. She could not be influenced to seek another position.

What would you do if you were this manager?

INTRODUCTION

The profession of nursing was born in the United States at a time when women had limited legal rights (for example, most were prohibited from voting and many could not own property). Women were viewed as neither powerful nor political; in the late nineteenth century, *feminine* and *powerful* were practically contradictory terms. In the twentieth century, as the status and role of women have changed in contemporary American society, so have the status and role of nurses. As the economic and social power of women has evolved, so has the power of nurses.

As the healthcare environment changes rapidly and, in many cases, drastically, the need for nurses to exercise power becomes essential if nursing is to have a strong voice in shaping these changes. In an era of rapid and often unplanned change, nurses must exercise their power and flex their political muscles in order to serve as healthcare advocates for the public.

HISTORY

Power was once considered almost a taboo in nursing. In the profession's earliest years, the exercise of power was considered inappropriate, unladylike, and unprofessional. Many decisions about nursing education and practice were often made by persons outside of nursing (Ashley, 1976). Nurses began to exercise their collective power with the rise of nursing leaders like Lillian Wald, Isabel Stewart, Annie Goodrich, Lavinia Dock, M. Adelaide Nutting, and Isabel Hampton Robb, and the development of organizations that evolved into the American Nurses' Association and the National League for Nursing.

Many social, technological, scientific, and economic trends have shaped nursing, nurses, and our ability to exercise power over the last century. As we move toward the next century, nurses must be skilled and confident in exercising power to ensure the continuing development of the profession and that nursing's voice will be heard in shaping the future of the healthcare system.

The media, politicians, organized medicine, and some healthcare executives have traditionally viewed nurses and nursing as powerless. That view began to change radically in the 1990s as nurses began to appear frequently on local and national news and talk shows as experts on the changes occurring in the healthcare system and the impact of these changes on the public. As nurses have become increasingly visible in political campaigns on the local, state, and national levels, both as candidates and as political influentials, nurses and nursing have gained new respect in the political arena.

However, even in the contemporary profession of nursing, there are a few nurses who see themselves as powerless and oppressed, who demonstrate aspects of oppressed group behavior. Like many politically and economically oppressed people, some nurses still persist in engaging in intragroup conflicts (e.g., "infighting") and they distance themselves from other nurses (e.g., the failure of many nurses to join professional organizations) (Roberts, 1983). Hence, nurses have a continued need to expand their understanding of the concept of power and to develop their skills in exercising power. Avoiding involvement in the politics of nursing, either in the work place or in the profession at large, limits the power of the individual nurse and the profession as a collective whole.

Some nurses are still uncomfortable about politics, treating "politics" as if it is a "dirty" word. Politics can be defined in many ways (e.g., the science of government, the process of allocation of scarce resources, or a process of formal human interactions). **Politics** is simply a process of human interaction within organizations. Politics permeates all organizations, including work places, legislatures, professions, and even families. Young children often learn that one parent is more likely than the other to give permission for special activities and more likely to buy toys and other desired items. They quickly learn to ask permission or ask for a desired item from that parent before asking the other. This is an unwritten political rule in many families.

Cohen et al. (1996) have identified four stages of political development for the profession of nursing:

1. *Buy-in*: recognition of the importance of activism
2. *Self-interest*: developing and using political expertise to further the profession's self-interests
3. *Political sophistication*: moving beyond self-interests, recognizing the need for activism on behalf of the public
4. *Leading the way*: providing true leadership on broad healthcare interests

Cohen et al. contend that the fourth stage represents nursing's current level of political evolution, with the possibility of further stage development.

This model can also be applied to the political development and activism of individual nurses related to both professional and legislative political arenas, with the addition of an initial stage:

1. *Apathy*: no membership in professional organizations; little or no interest in legislative politics as they relate to nursing and healthcare
2. *Buy-in*: recognition of the importance of activism within professional organizations (without active participation) and legislative politics related to critical nursing issues
3. *Self-interest*: involvement in professional organizations to further one's own career; developing and using political expertise to further the profession's self-interests
4. *Political sophistication*: high level of professional organization activism (e.g., holding office at the local and state level) moving beyond self-interests, recognizing the need for activism on behalf of the public
5. *Leading the way*: serving in elected or appointed positions in professional organizations at the state and national level; providing true leadership on broad healthcare interests within legislative politics

Political activism is a powerful form of professional involvement. Kalisch and Kalisch (1982) describe four levels of political participation or activism:

- *apathetics*, who engage in little or no political activity, may not even be registered to vote, and, if registered, they are unlikely to vote;
- *spectators*, who vote, may wear a political button or display a political bumper sticker, and engage in political discussions with family and friends;
- *transitionals*, who attend meetings and rallies and other political events, lobby their legislators, and contribute to political campaigns and political actions committees (PACs); and
- *gladiators*, who work in political campaigns of candidates, solicit campaign funds, become active within a political party, or run for political office (pp. 315-316).

These same levels of political activism can be applied to professional involvement in nursing:

- *apathetics*, who belong to no professional organizations, serve on no committees in the work place; if assigned to such a committee, they fail to do the work of the committee
- *spectators*, who pay dues to one or more professional organizations, but rarely, if ever, attend meetings or serve on committees; or they serve on committees in the work place occasionally and, perhaps, reluctantly; they read an occasional article on national issues and trends in nursing and discuss these with colleagues
- *transitionals*, who are actively involved in local professional organizations and may attend state and national conventions of these organizations; they read extensively about trends and issues in nursing and knowledgeably discuss these with colleagues; they assume leadership roles on committees and task forces in the work place and in professional organizations
- *gladiators*, who serve in leadership roles in professional organizations on the state and national level

Not surprisingly, nurses who are active participants in the politics of the profession of nursing tend also to be involved in legislative politics because of the close interaction of the two forms of political activism.

FOCUS ON POWER

Power comes from the Latin word *potere*, to be able. Simply defined, **power** is the ability to influence others in the effort to achieve goals. Nurses have sometimes viewed power as if it were something immoral, corrupting, and totally contradictory to the caring nature of nursing. However, the above definition demonstrates the essential nature of power to nursing. When providing health teaching to patients and their families, the nurse's goal is to provide needed information and to change behavior to promote optimum health. That is the exercise of power in nursing practice. Nurses regularly influence patients in an effort to improve their health status as an essential element of nursing practice. Changing a colleague's behavior by instructing her about a new policy being implemented on the nursing unit is another example of how a nurse can exercise power. Coaching a nurse to improve his or her performance is the exercise of power.

Exercise 25-1

Recall a recent opportunity you had to observe the work of an expert nurse. Think about that nurse's interactions with patients, family members, nursing colleagues, and other professionals. What kinds of power did you observe this nurse exercise? What did the nurse do that suggested to you, "This is a powerful person?"

Social scientists have studied the use and abuse of power in human organizations. They have analyzed and categorized the sources and applications of power in human experience. Hersey, Blanchard, and Natemeyer (1979) offer one formulation on the bases of social power. They identified seven bases of power, which are most easily understood as sources or types of social power (see theory box on page 419). These types of power are not mutually exclusive. They are frequently used in concert to exert influence on individuals or groups.

Nurses use all of these types of power frequently in both clinical practice and management. Nurses who teach parents about the care of their newborn use *expert* and *information* power by virtue of the information they share with parents; they also exercise *legitimate* power because they are registered nurses and, thus, are accorded a certain status by society. New graduates are employed on probationary status until they successfully meet and demonstrate the initial clinical competencies of a position. They may view the nurse manager as exercising both *coercive* and *reward* power related to their evaluation for continued

Theory of Types or Bases of Social Power

THEORY/KEY CONTRIBUTOR	KEY IDEAS	APPLICATION TO PRACTICE
Types or bases of social power were formulated by Hersey, Blanchard, and Natemeyer (1979) to explain the use of power within the human experience.	**Coercive power:** based on fear, coercion, and the ability to punish. *Parents are viewed as powerful by children because of their ability to punish inappropriate behavior.* **Reward power:** based on the ability to grant rewards and favors. *Parents are also viewed as powerful by children because of their ability to reward appropriate behavior.* **Expert power:** results from the knowledge and skills one possesses that are needed by others. *A professor is viewed as the expert within the classroom and as a relatively powerful person.* **Legitimate power:** possessed by virtue of one's position with an organization or status within a group. *The president of the United States is viewed around the world as a powerful person as a result of election to this office.* **Referent power:** results from followers' desire to identify with a powerful person. *Teenagers may dress like their favorite rock stars in order to copy an aspect of the performers' behavior.* **Information power:** stems from one's possession of selected information that is needed by others. *A student who seems to grasp the day's math assignment easily may be sought out by classmates for assistance with their homework.* **Connection power:** gained by association with people who are perceived as powerful. *Some people go to political conventions and meetings just to be seen with people they perceive as politically powerful.*	These categories help explain how we use power to influence others. The categories are not mutually exclusive and usually are used in concert with one another.

employment. Nursing faculty and skilled clinicians often serve as role models to nursing students. The faculty and clinicians exercise *referent* power as students emulate their behavior. Examples of *connection* power are evident at any kind of social gathering in the work place. People of high status (e.g., vice presidents or directors) within an organization may be sought out for conversation by managers who want to move up the organizational hierarchy. Consistent with this concept of connection power, Ferguson (1993) notes that, early in her administrative career, a senior nurse executive advised her: "Find out where the power lies. Be there" (p. 119).

These types of power describe the potential for power. Having a high-status position in an organization immediately provides stature, but power depends on the ability to accomplish goals within that position. While we frequently hear that "knowledge is power," power is derived from what we do with that knowledge (Curtin, 1989). Sharing knowledge expands one's power and, in turn, empowers our colleagues by giving them information or skills that they need to take action in a situation.

Nursing's early history in this country was marked by powerlessness (Ashley, 1976). Nurses were absent from the decision-making processes about their education, practice, and employment. As the social, political, and economic status of women and nurses changed, so did nursing's exercise of power. We recognize today that powerlessness results in apathy, anger, and indifference (Ferguson, 1993). This can result in a work place culture that is marked by conflict, anger, and other dysfunctional behaviors (see "Research Perspectives"; Seago, 1996). Sharing power and facilitating the empowerment of colleagues are strong forces in creating revitalized work place cultures.

Influence is the process of using power. Influence can range from the punitive power of coercion to the interactive power of collaboration. Teaching a patient the skills necessary to empower him or her to give self-care at home uses the expert, information, and legitimate power to influence the behavior of the patient. Coaching a new graduate nurse in orientation to complete a complicated nursing procedure successfully vividly demonstrates the ability of the experienced nurse to influence that orientee. That coaching uses reward, expert, legitimate, referent, and information power to influence the orientee not only at that moment, but also perhaps over the span of a career. *Power* is a set of behavioral and cognitive skills that are used through the process of *influence* to create change in others and in ourselves.

EMPOWERMENT

Empowerment is a term that has come into common usage in nursing in recent years. It has been used extensively in the nursing literature related to administration and management; it is also highly relevant to the domain of clinical practice. **Empowerment** is the process by which we facilitate the participation of others in decision making and taking action within an environment where there is an equitable distribution of power. Empowerment is power sharing and a form of feminine-feminist leadership (Mason, Backer, & Georges, 1991). This concept of empowerment is consistent with the contemporary view of leadership, a paradigm that is exemplified by behaviors characteristic of nurses: facilitator, coach, teacher, and collaborator. These leadership skills are an essential component of professional nursing practice, whether a nurse is a clinician, an educator, a researcher, or an administrator/manager. Nursing leaders, whether in the employment setting or in professional organizations, exercise power in making professional judgments as they do their daily work.

These leadership skills are essential to effective followers, too. Powerful nurse managers empower their staffs, influencing them to grow professionally. Powerful nurses empower their patients and the families in their care. Hence these leadership skills can be viewed as an essential component of professional nursing practice whether one is a clinician, an educator, a researcher, or an executive/manager. Nursing leaders, whether in their employment settings or within their work in professional organizations, exercise power in making a range of professional judgments as they do their work.

Empowerment is the process by which power is shared with colleagues and patients as part of the nurse's exercise of power. This is in sharp contrast to traditional conceptualizations of power, a patriarchal model of power, which relies on coercion, hierarchy, authority, control, and force. Empowerment, by embracing a feminist conceptualization of power, emphasizes cooperation as a vital element for the exercise of power (Wheeler & Chinn, 1989). Nurses have too often viewed power as a finite quantity: "If I give you some of my power, I will have less." Empowerment emphasizes the notion that power grows when shared. Nurses who view power as finite will avoid cooperation with their colleagues and refuse to share their expertise. Nurses who conceptualize power as infinite are strong collaborators who gain satisfaction by helping their colleagues expand their expertise and their power base.

Research Perspective

Seago, J.A. (1996). Culture of troubled work groups. Journal of Nursing Administration, *26(9), 41-46.*

Troubled or conflicted work groups can make tremendous demands on a manager and may result in or from manager turnover. As many nurse managers have had their span of responsibility expanded to include two or more patient care units, dealing with troubled work groups can become overwhelming. This descriptive study served to identify characteristics of troubled work groups and to identify strategies used by successful managers in dealing with such groups.

Troubled work groups may be conceptualized as demonstrating collective anger, high absenteeism, lack of collaboration with high levels of internal competition, signs of isolation and absence of peer support, verbal hostility toward the manager, extreme criticism of care given by peers, and the formation of subgroups (cliques). Individuals in such a unit may tend to scapegoat others, seek undue attention, demonstrate high levels of defensiveness, engage in power struggles and covert activities, and unrealistically expect the manager to attend to their needs and demands.

One hundred fifteen nurse managers or executives, in a voluntary sample, were surveyed at the 1995 American Organization of Nurse Executives and Organization of Nurse Executives–California meetings. They responded to a 25-item survey describing troubled units they had managed and successful strategies they had employed in managing such units and a demographic questionnaire.

Most commonly identified as troubled units were medical-surgical units, intensive care units, and emergency departments. Eighty percent of the respondents had managed a troubled unit, with almost 70% knowing about the unit's negative reputation before accepting the position.

Troubled units were characterized as having two or three "significant employees with poor attitudes" (p. 43), high levels of staff anger, difficulties in dealing with change, high levels of stress, a reputation for "eating their young," and a difficult work load.

Among the successful strategies for managing such units were appropriate confrontation; strengthening the positive skills of staff; reducing stressors; increasing and improving communication with the manager; increasing visibility of the manager on the unit; setting clear expectations for performances; regular meetings with problem employees; addressing issues consistently; dealing with the manager's own feelings of anger and avoidance; and counseling employees regarding transfer out of the unit.

Implications for Practice

Employees on troubled units display the signs of both powerlessness (e.g., poor attitudes, anger) and the misuse of power (e.g., "eating their young"). Successful strategies reflect the effective exercise of power by the manager (e.g., appropriate confrontation, dealing with own feelings) and efforts to empower the staff (e.g., strengthening positive staff skills, counseling employees).

The empowerment of nurses makes truly professional practice possible, the kind of professional practice that is satisfying to both managers and clinicians. Empowered clinicians are essential for effective nursing management, just as empowered managers set the stage for excellence in clinical practice. Encouraging a reticent colleague to be an active participant in committee meetings serves to empower that nurse. Guiding a novice nurse in exercising professional judgment empowers both the senior nurse and the novice clinician. Coaching a patient on how to be more assertive with a physician who is reluctant to answer the patient's questions is another form of empowerment. Teaching a newly diagnosed diabetic patient and the family about diabetic care is an exercise both of the nurse's expert and legitimate power and of the empowerment of the patient and family.

Exercise 25-2

Think about a recent clinical experience when you empowered a patient. What did you do for and/or with the patient (and family) that was empowering? How did you feel about your own actions in this situation? How did the patient respond?

STRATEGIES FOR DEVELOPING A POWERFUL IMAGE

As Margaret Thatcher, former prime minister of Great Britain, said, "Being powerful is like being a lady. If you have to tell people you are, you aren't."

The most basic power strategy is the development of a powerful image. Lady Thatcher's statement emphasizes the importance of this powerful image. If nurses think they are powerful, others will view them as powerful; if they view themselves as powerless, so will others. A sense of self-confidence is a strong foundation in developing one's "power image," and it is essential for successful political efforts in the work place or within the profession. Such self-confidence is simply the belief that one has the power to make things happen (Grainger, 1990). Several key factors contribute to one's power image:

- Self-image: thinking of one's self as powerful and effective
- Grooming and dress: well-groomed hair and appropriate make-up; clothing and appearance that are neat, clean, and appropriate to the situation
- Good manners: treating people with courtesy and respect
- Body language: good posture, gestures that avoid too much drama, good eye contact, and confident movement
- Speech: a firm, confident voice, good grammar and diction, an appropriate vocabulary, and good communication skills

Exercise 25-3

Think about a powerful public figure whom you admire. What key factors contribute to this person's powerful image? Think about a powerful nurse you have met. Identify this person's key image factors.

Concern about a powerful image may seem superficial. However, the impressions we make on people influence the way they view us now and in the future and how they value what we do and say. First impressions are important. Given similar educational and experiential backgrounds, who is more likely to be hired for a nursing position: the candidate who comes dressed in a suit or the candidate who arrives in jeans and sandals? Who will be seen as the more competent professional by a patient: the nurse in wrinkled scrubs or the nurse in neat street clothes and a freshly laundered lab coat? A powerful image signals to others that you are professionally competent and capable of exercising appropriate judgments, influential, and powerful.

Attitudes and beliefs are another important aspect of a powerful image; they reflect one's values. Believing that power is a positive force in nursing is essential to one's powerful image. It is also important to believe firmly in nursing's value to society and the centrality of nursing's contribution to the healthcare delivery system. Powerful nurses do not allow the phrase "I'm just a nurse" in their vocabulary. Behavior reflects one's pride in the profession of nursing. This not only increases a nurse's own power, but also helps to empower nursing colleagues.

Make a commitment to nursing as a career. Nursing is a profession; professions offer careers, not just a series of positions. For a long time, nursing marketed itself to recruits as the perfect preparation for marriage and family. Even some contemporary job advertisements hint at romance as an outcome of employment at the agency featured. Some people still view nurses only as members of an occupation who drop in and out of employment, not as members of a profession with a long-term career commitment. Having a career commitment does not preclude leaving employment temporarily for family, education, or other demands. Having a career commitment implies that a nurse views himself or herself first and foremost as a member of the discipline of nursing with an obligation to make a contribution to the profession. Status as an employee of a particular hospital, home health agency, long-term-care facility, or other healthcare agency is secondary to the person's status as a member of the profession of nursing. This is a prevalent view of how careers will be focused in the future.

Value continuing education in nursing. Valuing education is one of the hallmarks of a profession. The continuing development of one's professional skills and knowledge is an empowering experience, preparing the nurse to make decisions with the support of an expanding body of knowledge. Seminars, workshops, and conferences offer opportunities for continued professional growth and empowerment. Returning to school for advanced degrees is also a powerful growth experience and reflects commitment to the profession of nursing. Change will continue in the healthcare system, necessitating continuing education to empower nurses to be proactive, not just reactive. A well-educated nursing work force is essential if nursing is to have a strong voice in shaping the changes in healthcare. An additional advantage of participating in educational experiences is that it creates opportunities for networking, a strategy that will be discussed later in this chapter.

PERSONAL POWER STRATEGIES

Developing a collection of power strategies, or power tools, is an important aspect of personal empowerment. These strategies should be used in situations that demand the exercise of leadership. Such strategies are techniques for building a professional power base and for developing political skills within an organization (see Boxes 25-1 and 25-2). They also indicate to others that one is a powerful nurse and a leader. These boxes identify personal power strategies beyond those discussed in this section.

Communication Skills

The most basic tool is effective verbal communication skills, which help define a power image. These are the same communication skills nurses learn to ensure effective interaction with patients and families. Listening skills are essential leadership skills. Just as the clinician listens to the patient to collect assessment data, the manager uses listening skills to assess and evaluate. Managers who are good listeners develop reputations for being fair and consistent. Listening to recurring themes related to minor issues of staff dissatisfaction in informal conversations may enable the manager to take action before a staff crisis occurs.

Verbal and nonverbal skills are important personal power strategies; the ability to assess these messages is a critical power strategy. Experts in communication estimate that 90% of the messages we communicate to others are nonverbal. When nonverbal and verbal messages conflict, the nonverbal message is more powerful. The basic lessons on the power of nonverbal communication most nurses learn in an introductory psychiatric course are relevant in all nursing arenas!

Networking

Networking is an important power strategy and political skill. A **network** is a system of contacts that are developed, nurtured, and maintained as sources of information, advice, and moral support (Schutzenhofer, 1992). Networking supports the empowerment of participants through interaction and the refinement of their interpersonal skills. Most nurses have relatively limited networks within the organizations where

---

Box 25-1

Strategies for Developing a Powerful Image

- Self-image
- Grooming and dress
- Speech
- Body language
- Belief in power as a positive force
- Belief in value of nursing to society
- Career commitment
- Continuing professional education

Box 25-2

Additional Personal Power Strategies

- Be honest.
- Always be courteous; it makes other people feel good!
- Smile whenever appropriate; it puts people at ease.
- Accept responsibility for your own mistakes and learn from them.
- Be a risk taker.
- Win and lose gracefully.
- Learn to be comfortable with conflict and ambiguity; they are both normal states of the human condition.
- Give credit to others where credit is due.
- Develop the ability to take constructive criticism gracefully; learn to let destructive criticism "roll off your back."
- Use business cards when introducing yourself to new contacts and collect the business cards of those you meet when networking.
- Always follow through on promises.

---

they are employed. They tend to have lunch or coffee with those people with whom they work most closely. One strategy to expand a work place network is to have lunch or coffee with someone from another department, including managers from nonnursing departments, at least two or three times a month.

Active participation in nursing organizations is the most effective method of establishing a professional network outside one's place of employment. Participation in professional organizations can propel a nurse into the politics of nursing. State and district

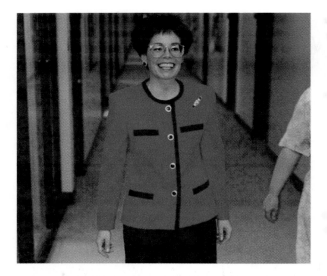

Professional grooming and dress are basic strategies for developing a powerful image.

nurses' associations offer an excellent opportunity to develop a network that includes nurses from various clinical and functional areas. Membership in specialty organizations, especially organizations for nurse managers and executives, provides the opportunity to network with nurses with similar expertise and interests. Additionally, membership in civic, volunteer, and special interest groups and participation in educational programs (for example, formal academic programs and conferences) also provide networking opportunities.

The successful networker identifies a core of networking partners who are particularly skilled, insightful, and eager to support the development of colleagues. These partners need to be nurtured. For example:

- Send them articles on topics of interest to them.
- Call them to keep in touch if face-to-face contact is sporadic or infrequent.
- Never argue the merit of advice given by a networking partner; consider its value later.
- Be reasonable in making requests for help or information; ask for only one thing at a time and be specific about what is wanted.
- Most importantly, be prepared to reciprocate with networking partners (Schutzenhofer, 1995).

Mentoring

In recent years mentoring has become a driving force in nursing. Mentors are competent, experienced pro-

fessionals who develop a relationship with a novice for the purpose of providing advice, support, information, and feedback in order to encourage the development of the individual. Mentoring has been an important element in the career development of men in business, academia, and selected professions. Mentoring has become a significant power strategy for women in general and for nurses in particular during the last 20 years. Mentoring provides novices with expanded access to information, power, and career opportunities. Mentors have historically been a critical asset to novices trying to negotiate work place and professional politics. Effective mentoring in nursing can be characterized by certain attributes (Stewart & Kruger, 1996):

1. Mentoring is a teaching-learning process for both the mentor and the mentee.
2. It is a reciprocal relationship for the mentor and mentee, a give-and-take situation for both parties.
3. There is a knowledge or competence differential between participants.
4. The focus of the relationship is on career development.
5. The relationship will endure over several years.
6. Mentees will in turn become mentors to others.

Mentoring is an empowering experience for both mentors and novices. The process of seeking out mentors is an exercise in growth for novices or proteges. Mentors frequently come from one's professional networks. Some mentors select their proteges; sometimes the reverse is true. Novices may attract mentors by implementing these strategies:

- Demonstrate a developing expertise.
- Develop a sensitivity to the attention of powerful people within the organization.
- Volunteer to serve on committees and do good work.
- Openly discuss professional goals and personal desire to grow.
- Ask experienced and talented people within the network for advice and help (Black, 1989).

Novices learn new skills from influential mentors and gain self-confidence. Mentors gain stature within their peer groups, extend their scope of influence through relationships with novices, refine their professional skills, and gain self-confidence through the satisfaction experienced in observing the development of novices.

Exercise 25-4

You encounter an old friend in a restaurant. You greet one another warmly, each stating how good it is to see the other. Yet your friend visibly backs away when you extend your arms to embrace. What is your immediate reaction? Despite the warm words of greeting, do you question your old friend's sincerity because of the strong nonverbal message regarding physical contact? Consider other situations you have experienced recently when words and actions contradict one another. Which message, the verbal or the nonverbal, did you accept as the person's "real" communication to you? Practice with a friend: pretend you are greeting a visitor to your home, a colleague, or a patient. In the first trial, state your greeting warmly, extend your hand to shake the other person's hand, smile, and make eye contact. In the second trial, use the same words of greeting, but use an angry tone of voice, avoid eye contact, and fold your arms across your chest while moving one step back from the other person. Observe the physical actions and listen carefully, especially to the tone of voice. Repeat the exercise, switching roles. Discuss your response to these interactions.

Goal Setting

Goal setting is another power strategy. Every nurse knows about setting goals. Students learn to devise patient care goals or patient outcomes as part of the care planning process. Nurses may be expected to write annual goals for performance reviews at work. Even a project at home, for example, painting rooms, may necessitate setting goals, like painting a room each day of one's vacation. Goals help one to know if what was planned was actually accomplished. Likewise, a successful nursing career needs goals to define what one wants to achieve as a nurse. Without such goals, one can wander endlessly through a series of jobs without a real sense of satisfaction. As the Cheshire Cat told Alice during her trip through Wonderland: Any road will take you there if you don't know where you are going.

Well-defined, long-term goals may be hard to formulate early in a career. For example, few new graduates know specifically that they want to be chief nurse executives, deans, managers, or researchers. Yet, eventually some will choose those career paths. However, developing such a vision early in a career is an important personal power strategy. Once this career vision is developed, one must create opportunities to move toward that vision. Such planning is empowering; it puts the nurse in charge, rather than letting a career unfold by chance. Having this sense of vision is consistent with the commitment to a career in nursing that is part of developing a power image. This vision is always subject to change as new opportuni-

ties are experienced, and new interests, knowledge, and skills are gained. Education and work experiences are tools for achieving the vision of one's career.

Developing Expertise

As noted earlier in this chapter, expertise is one of the bases of power. Developing expertise in nursing is an important power strategy. Expertise must not be limited to clinical knowledge. Leadership and communication skills, for example, are essential to the effective exercise of power in a range of nursing roles. Education and practice provide the means for developing such expertise in any of the domains of nursing: clinical practice, education, research, and management. Developing expertise expands one's power among nursing colleagues, other professional colleagues, and patients. A high level of expertise can make one nearly indispensable within an organization. This is a very powerful position to have within any organization, whether it is the work place or a professional association. A high level of expertise can also lead to a high level of visibility within an organization.

High Visibility

This strategy of high visibility within an organization also requires volunteering to serve as a member or the chairperson of committees and task forces. High visibility can be nurtured by attending the open meetings of committees and other groups of which one is not a member in the work place, professional associations, or the community. Review the agendas of such meetings if they are circulated ahead of the meeting. Use opportunities both before and after meetings to share one's expertise, providing valuable information and ideas to members and leaders of such groups. Share this expertise at open meetings when appropriate. Speak up confidently, but have something relevant to say. Be concise and precise; members of the committee will ask for more information if they need it.

Exercise 25-5

Almost everyone has attended a class, meeting, or workshop with a "know-it-all." These group members are capable of commenting on everything at great length without saying anything of substance. These self-appointed experts tend to create great tension within a group: members begin to shift in their seats, give one another frustrated looks, and may eventually lose interest in the topic at hand. In a highly effective group with strong leadership, someone may intervene to end the speaker's soliloquy. No matter how this situation is resolved, the unfortunate speaker at least suffers a loss of respect from members of the group. Compare this unfortunate
Continued.

Exercise 25-5—cont'd

scenario to another kind of experience you may have had. A member of the group, or perhaps a nonmember who is simply sitting in on the meeting, offers a comment or piece of information that energizes the group and propels them toward more effective action. This individual gains the respect of those in attendance by virtue of this valued contribution. Compare your reactions to these two types of experiences. How do you feel? Are you embarrassed by or for the first kind of speaker? Why? Compare your interactions with both kinds of speakers after these kinds of events. Do you handle these situations differently? Why?

EXERCISING POWER AND INFLUENCE IN THE WORK PLACE AND OTHER ORGANIZATIONS

To use influence effectively in any organization, understanding how the system works and developing organizational strategies are critical. Developing *organizational savvy* includes identifying the real decision makers and those persons who have a high level of influence with the decision makers. Recognize the informal leaders within any organization. In the work place, an influential senior staff nurse may have more decision-making power than the nurse manager on significant aspects of the nursing unit's operations. The senior staff nurse may have more clinical expertise and a greater wealth of knowledge about the history of the unit and its personnel than a nurse manager with excellent management and leadership skills who is new to the unit.

Secretaries of chief nurse executives (CNE), for example, are usually very powerful people, although they are not always recognized as such. The CNE's secretary has a great deal of control over information, making decisions about who gets to meet with the nurse executive and when, screening incoming and outgoing mail, letting the CNE know when a letter or memo needs immediate attention, or placing another memo on the bottom of the stack of mail for review at a later time.

Collegiality and Collaboration

Nursing does not exist in a vacuum, nor do nurses work in isolation from one another, other professionals, and support personnel. Nurses function within a wide range of organizations, such as schools, hospitals, community health organizations, government agencies, professional associations, and universities. Nursing's historic lack of unity on important issues, such as

basic educational preparation for entry into professional practice, has weakened our power base and political clout in the healthcare and educational systems (Huston & Marquis, 1988). Developing a sense of unity requires each nurse to act collaboratively and collegially in the work place and in other organizations (e.g., professional associations). Collegiality demands that nurses value the accomplishments of nursing colleagues and express a sincere interest in the efforts of colleagues. Turning to nursing colleagues for advice and support empowers them and expands one's own power base at the same time. Unity of purpose does not contradict diversity of thought. It is important for colleagues to agree that disagreement based on differences of ideas, not on the basis of personalities, is healthy for professional growth (Vance, 1985). One does not have to be a friend to everyone who is a colleague. Collegiality demands mutual respect, not friendship.

Collaboration and collegiality require that nurses work collectively to ensure that the voice of nursing is heard in the work place. Volunteer to serve on committees and task forces in the work place, not only within the nursing department but also on organization-wide committees. Get involved in the politics of the organization. If the organization uses shared governance or continuous quality improvement models, get involved in these councils, committees, task forces, and work groups to share your energy, ideas, and expertise. Many organizations have instituted joint practice committees that bring together nurses and physicians to improve the quality of interdisciplinary collaboration and, in turn, the quality of patient care. Become an active, productive member of such groups within the work place, as well as community groups dealing with healthcare issues and problems.

An Empowering Attitude

Demonstrate a positive and professional attitude about being a nurse to nursing colleagues, patients, and their families and other colleagues in the work place. This attitude is very contagious and can empower colleagues. A power image is an important aspect of demonstrating this positive professional attitude. The current practice of nurses to identify themselves by first name only may decrease their power image in the eyes of physicians, patients, and others. When physicians are always addressed as "Dr." but are free to address others by their first names, a notable difference in social status is apparent, thus limiting the collegial relationship between physician and nurse (Campbell-Heider & Hart, 1993). The use of first names among colleagues is not inappropriate, so long as everyone is playing by the same rules. Managers may want to enhance the empowerment of their staffs by encouraging them to introduce themselves as "Dr.," "Ms.," or "Mr." Arriving at work, appointments, or meetings on time; looking neat and appropriately attired for the work setting or other professional situation; and speaking positively about one's work are examples of how easy it is to demonstrate a positive professional attitude.

Developing Coalitions

The exercise of power is often directed at creating change. While an individual can often be effective at exercising power and creating change, in many situations creating change within most organizations requires collective action. Coalition building is a very effective political strategy for collective action. **Coalitions** are groups of individuals or organizations that join together temporarily around a common goal. This goal often focuses on an effort to effect change. The networking between organizations that results in coalition building requires members of one group to reach out to members of other groups. This often occurs at the leadership level and may come through formal mechanisms, such as letters that identify an issue or problem, a shared interest, around which a coalition could be built. For example, a state nurses' association may invite the leaders of organizations interested in child health (for example, organizations of pediatric nurses, public health nurses and physicians, elementary school teachers, and day-care providers) to discuss collaborative support for a legislative initiative to improve access to immunization programs in urban and rural areas. Informal mechanisms may also lead to coalition building. For example, members of a practice council at a small hospital are developing a parent education program to increase awareness about immunizations in the community served by the hospital. Public health nurses in the community are developing a similar program. A nurse who serves on the practice council mentions this effort to a friend who is a public health nurse. They both go back to their own work groups, informing their colleagues about the other group's work. A coalition of the two groups of nurses creates a very effective community education program by working collaboratively and collectively. The coalition of over 60 nursing and healthcare organizations that joined together to support "Nursing's Agenda for HealthCare Reform" offers one example of such collective action (American Nurses' Association, 1991). The efforts of nurses in Illinois to pass a nurse-friendly, patient-friendly practice act offers another example of coalition building (see Box 25-3).

Exercise 25-6

How do you routinely introduce yourself to patients, families, physicians, and other colleagues? A powerful and positive approach involves making eye contact with each individual, shaking hands, and introducing yourself by saying, "I'm Ann Jones (Dan Jones), a registered nurse (or nursing student)." If you do not currently use this technique, try it out. Note any difference in the responses of people whom you meet using this technique in comparison with your usual approach.

Box 25-3

New Illinois Nurse Practice Act Goes to Governor

A coalition of over 30 nursing organizations, including the Illinois Nurses' Association and the Illinois Organization of Nurse Leaders, was successful in getting unanimous support in both the House and the Senate for a new nurse practice act. The old act "sunseted" (i.e., expired) at the end of 1997. The coalition, known as the Nursing Act Planning Group, began their work almost 2 years before the expiration of the current practice act.

The new act provides a comprehensive and contemporary definition of professional nursing that includes recognition of the nursing process as a framework for practice, recognition of the role of the nurse as patient advocate, and provisions for an impaired nurse assistance program.

Opposition to statutory recognition of advanced practice registered nurses (APRNs) by the Illinois State Medical Society necessitated withdrawing an amendment on advanced practice at the eleventh hour in order to ensure passage of the basic practice act language in the spring legislative session. The Nursing Act Planning Group will continue negotiations with the medical society over advanced practice and will continue to build a coalition with other healthcare and consumer organizations who support the role of APRNs in order to introduce an APRN amendment in the next legislative session. The chief legislative sponsors in both the House and the Senate support this strategy to finally gain recognition for APRNs in Illinois (Clark, 1997).

Enlisting the support of others who share the same goal or interest often results in greater success in effecting change and exercising power in the work place and within other organizations. Expanding networks in the work place, as suggested earlier in this chapter, facilitates creating a coalition by developing a pool of candidates for coalition building before they are needed. Invite people with common goals to lunch or coffee. Discuss this shared interest and gain the commitment of the individual. Meet over lunch or coffee with members of the committee or task force that is working on this issue. Share ideas on how to create the desired change most effectively.

Coalition building is an important skill for involvement in legislative politics. Nursing organizations frequently use coalition building when dealing with state legislatures and Congress. Changes in nurse practice acts to expand opportunities for advanced nursing practice have been accomplished in many states through coalition building. Such changes are often opposed by state medical societies or the state agencies that license physicians. Efforts by a single nursing organization (for example, a state nurses' association or a nurse practitioners' organization), representing a limited nursing constituency, often lack the clout to overcome opposition by the unified voice of the official voice of the state's physicians. However, the unified effort of a coalition of nursing organizations, other healthcare organizations, and consumer groups can be very powerful in effecting change through legislation.

Negotiating

Kritek (1994) points out nursing's vulnerability in the title of her book, N*egotiating* A*t an* U*neven* T*able*. **Negotiating,** or bargaining, is a critically important skill for organizational and political power. It is a process of making trade-offs. Children are natural negotiators. Often they will initially ask their parents for more than what they are willing to accept in the way of privileges, toys, or activities. The logic is simple to children: ask for more than is reasonable and negotiate down to what you really want! Negotiating often works the same way within organizations. People will sometimes ask for more than what they want and be willing to accept less. In other situations, both sides will enter a negotiation asking for radically different things, but each may be willing to settle for a position that differs significantly from their original positions. In the simplest forms of bargaining, each participant has something that the other party values, for example, goods, services, or information. At the "bargaining table," each party presents an opening position

and the process moves on until they reach a mutually agreeable result or until one or both parties walk away from the unsuccessful process.

Bargaining in the work place may take many forms. Individuals may negotiate with a supervisor for a more desirable work schedule or with a peer to effect a schedule change so the nurse can attend an out-of-town conference. A nurse manager may sit at the bargaining table with the department director during budget planning to expand training hours for the nursing unit in the next year's budget. A group of nurses may bargain with nursing and hospital administration over wages, staffing levels, other working conditions, and the conditions and policies that govern clinical practice. This is called "collective bargaining," a specific type of negotiating that is regulated by both state and federal labor laws and that usually involves representation by a state nurses' association or a nursing or nonnursing labor union (see Chapter 10).

Successful negotiators are well informed about not only their own positions, but also those of the opposing side. Successful negotiators must be able to discuss the pros and cons of both positions. They are able to assist the other party in recognizing the costs versus the benefits of each position. These same skills are also essential to exercising power effectively with the arenas of professional and legislative politics.

Exercise 25-7

Consider a situation in which you engaged in bargaining or negotiating. Have you ever bought a car? Negotiating the price of the car is a great American tradition. Few people enter into the purchase of a car intending to pay the sticker price. Most sticker prices are set by the manufacturer at a level that gives the dealer room to negotiate the price down. Have you ever negotiated a schedule change at work/school? What was the trade-off you made in the process? How far did the other person move from his or her original position? What factors led to your success or failure in this negotiation?

CHAPTER CHECKLIST

Power was once a taboo issue in nursing. The exercise of power in nursing conflicted sharply with the historic feminine stereotypes that surrounded nursing. The evolving social and political status of women has also opened nursing to the exercise of power. Power is essential to the effective implementation of both the clinical and the managerial roles of nurses.

- Contemporary concepts of power focus on power as influence and a force for collaboration rather than coercion, an infinite quality rather than a finite quantity.

A Manager's Solution

❓ After her most recent hospitalization, several of this nurse's colleagues began to complain about her performance. A review of some of her recent charting demonstrated poor assessment skills, but, more significantly, she began to experience serious trouble with administering medications. The most serious problem was her inability to calculate drug dosages. She seemed to have lost basic math skills. She was counseled regarding the problem, and an action plan was initiated when she was unable to pass the drug administration test required of all newly employed nurses. The nurse was suspended until she could meet the basic job responsibility of administering medications safely and accurately. I informed her that she would be terminated if she could not demonstrate her ability to safely and accurately administer medications. My director and I provided her with pharmacology books, independent learning materials, and practice opportunities. Our clinical specialist worked with her, trying to teach and coach her. I gave her repeated opportunities to complete the simulated drug administration exercises with the clinical specialist, as well as the written test, within a defined time frame. She failed both the demonstrations and the written test repeatedly; her performance grew worse instead of better. After reviewing the outcomes with my director and the director of human resources, I made an appointment with her; she would be terminated. She tendered her resignation to me instead.

❓ *Would this be a suitable approach to you? Why?*

- Empowerment is a feminine-feminist process of power sharing and leadership.
- Contemporary views of leadership in social systems are consistent with the concept of empowerment.
- Seven types of power exercised by nurses include:
  - coercive
  - reward
  - expert
  - legitimate
  - referent
  - information
  - connection
- Key factors in developing a powerful image include:
  - self-confidence
  - body language
  - self-image
  - career commitment
  - grooming and dress
  - speech
  - attitudes, beliefs, and values
  - continuing professional education
- Key personal and organizational strategies for exercising power include:
  - communication skills
  - career goal setting
  - high visibility
  - a sense of unity
  - coalition building
  - networking
  - expertise
  - organizational savvy
  - collaboration and collegiality
  - negotiation skills
  - mentoring
  - an empowering attitude

TIPS ON POWER AND POLITICS

- Remember that power is not a "dirty word" nor an undesirable professional characteristic for nurses; it is the ability to influence others effectively.
- By exercising power in the work place and other professional activities, you empower patients, families, and colleagues to accomplish their goals.
- Believing in one's own ability to create change (i.e., exercise power), valuing the exercise of power, and projecting a powerful image (e.g., grooming, manners, body language, and verbal communication skills) are essential to functioning as an influential professional nurse.
- Participating in networking and mentoring, setting clear career goals, and developing one's expertise are key power strategies.

TERMS TO KNOW

coalitions	network
empowerment	politics
influence	power
negotiating	

REFERENCES

American Nurses' Association. (1991). *Nursing's Agenda for Health Care Reform* (PR-3 25M, revised). Kansas City, MO: American Nurses' Association.

Ashley, J.A. (1976). *Hospitals, Paternalism, and the Role of the Nurse*. New York: Teachers' College Press.

Black, K.S. (1989, September). Why it pays to have a mentor. *Working Mother*, pp. 33-34, 36.

Campbell-Heider, N., & Hart, C.A. (1993). Updating the nurses's bedside manner. *Image: Journal of Nursing Scholarship*, 25, 133-139.

Clark, S. (1997, June). Nursing act goes to the governor's desk. *Chart*, 1,3.

Cohen, S.S., Mason, D.J., Kovner, C., Leavitt, J.K., Pulcini, J., & Sochalski, J. (1996). Stages of nursing political development: Where we've been and where we ought to go. *Nursing Outlook*, 44, 259-266.

Curtin, L.L. (1989). Powers: The traps of trappings. *Nursing Management*, 20(6), 7-8.

Ferguson, V. (1993). Perspectives on power. In Mason, D.J., Talbott, S.W., Leavitt, J.K., eds. *Policy and Politics for Nurses*, 2nd ed. Philadelphia: W.B. Saunders.

Grainger, R.D. (1990). Self-confidence: A feeling you can create. *American Journal of Nursing*, 90(10), 12.

Hersey, P., Blanchard, K., & Natemeyer, W. (1979). Situational leadership, perception and impact of power. *Group and Organizational Studies*, 4, 418-428.

Huston, C.J., & Marquis, B. (1988). Ten attitudes and behaviors to overcome powerlessness. *Nursing Connections*, 1(2), 39-47.

Kalisch, B.J., & Kalisch, P.A. (1982). *Politics of Nursing*. Philadelphia: J.B. Lippincott.

Kritek, P.B. (1994). *Negotiating At an Uneven Table: Developing Courage in Resolving Our Conflicts*. San Francisco: Jossey-Bass.

Mason, D.J., Backer, B.A., & Georges, C.A. (1991). Toward a feminist model for the political empowerment of nurses. *Image: Journal of Nursing Scholarship*, 23, 72-77.

Roberts, S.J. (1983). Oppressed group behavior: Implications for nursing. *Advances in Nursing Sciences*, 5, 21-30.

Schutzenhofer, K.K. (1992). Essential for the year 2000. *Nursing Connections*, 5(1), 15-26.

Schutzenhofer, K.K. (1995). Networking and professionalism. In Strader, M., Decker, P.J., eds. *Role Transition to Patient Care Management*. Norwalk, CT: Appleton & Lange.

Seago, J.A. (1996). Culture of troubled work groups. *Journal of Nursing Administration*, 26(9), 41-46.

Stewart, B.M., & Kruger, L.E. (1996). An evolutionary concept of mentoring in nursing. *Journal of Professional Nursing*, 12, 311-321.

Vance, C.N. (1985). Political influence: Building effective interpersonal skills. In Mason, D.J., & Talbott, S.W., eds. *Political Action Handbook for Nurses: Changing the Workplace, Government, and Organizations, and Community*. Menlo Park, CA: Addison-Wesley.

Wheeler, C.E., & Chinn, P.L. (1989). *Peace and Power: A Handbook of Feminist Process*, 2nd ed. New York: National League for Nursing.

SUGGESTED READINGS

Ashley, J.A. (1980). Power in structured misogyny: Implications for the politics of care. *Advances in Nursing Science*, 2, 3-22.

Borman, J., & Biordi, D. (1992). Female nurse executive: Finally, at an advantage? *Journal of Nursing Administration*, 22(9), 37-41.

Costello-Nikitas, D.M., & Mason, D.J. (1992). Power and politics in health care organizations. In Decker, P.J., & Sullivan, E.J., eds. *Nursing Administration: A Micro/Macro Approach for Effective Nurse Executives*. Norwalk, CT: Appleton & Lange.

del Bueno, D. (1986). Power and policy in organizations. *Nursing Outlook*, 34, 124-128.

Dobos, C. (1997). Understanding personal risk taking among staff nurses: Critical information for nurse administrators. *Journal of Nursing Administration*, 27(1), 12-13.

Fisher, R., Ury, W., & Patton, B. (1991). *Getting to Yes: Negotiating Agreement Without Giving In*, 2nd ed. New York: Penguin.

Flaherty, M.J. (1991). Global empowerment in nursing: Personal, professional, and environmental. *AORN Journal*, 54, 1200-1210.

Goldwater, M., & Zusy, M.J.L. (1990). *Prescription for Nurses: Effective Political Action*. St. Louis: Mosby.

Gorman, S., & Clark, N. (1986). Power and effective nursing practice. *Nursing Outlook*, 34, 129-134.

Heim, P., & Goliant, S.K. (1993). *Hardball for Women: Winning at the Game of Business*. Los Angeles: Plume Books.

Hoelzel, C.B. (1989). Using structural power sources to increase influence. *Journal of Nursing Administration*, 9(11), 10-15.

Holloran, S.D. (1993). Mentoring: The experience of nursing service executives. *Journal of Nursing Administration*, 23(2), 49-54.

Kippenbrock, T.A. (1992). Power at meetings: Strategies to move people. *Nursing Economics*, 10, 282-286.

Klakovich, M.D. (1996). Registered nurse empowerment: Model testing and implications for nurse administrators. *Journal of Nursing Administration*, 26(5), 29-35.

Laschinger, H.K.S., & Havens, D.S. (1996). Staff nurse work empowerment and perceived control over nursing practice: Conditions for work effectiveness. *Journal of Nursing Administration*, 26(9), 27-35.

Laschinger, H.K.S., & Shamian, J. (1994). Staff nurses' and nurse managers' perceptions of job-related empowerment and managerial self-efficacy. *Journal of Nursing Administration*, 24(10), 38-47.

Manthey, M. (1992). Leadership: A shifting paradigm. *Nurse Educator*, 17(5), 5, 14.

Manthey, M. (1992). Power: Grace under pressure. *Nursing Management*, 23(4), 22-26.

Mason, D.J., Talbott, S.W., Leavitt, J.K., eds. *Policy and Politics for Nurses* 2nd ed. Philadelphia: W.B. Saunders.

Newton, M., & Chaney, J. (1996). Professional image: Enhanced or inhibited by attire. *Journal of Professional Nursing*, 12, 240-244.

Pike, A.W. (1991). Moral outrage and moral discourse in nurse-physician collaboration. *Journal of Professional Nursing*, 7, 351-363.

Schorr, T., & Zimmerman, A., eds. (1988). *Making Choices, Taking Chances: Nurse Leaders Tell Their Stories*. St. Louis: Mosby.

Schutzenhofer, K.K., Shelley, S.R., & Pontious, S.L. (1992). Communication systems. In Decker, P.J., & Sullivan, E.J., eds. *Nursing Administration: A Micro/Macro Approach for Effective Nurse Executives*. Norwalk, CT: Appleton & Lange.

Tannen, D. (1994). *Talking from 9 to 5*. New York: William Morrow.

Wolf, G.A. (1989). The effective use of influence. *Journal of Nursing Administration*, 19(11), 8-9.

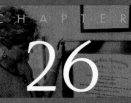

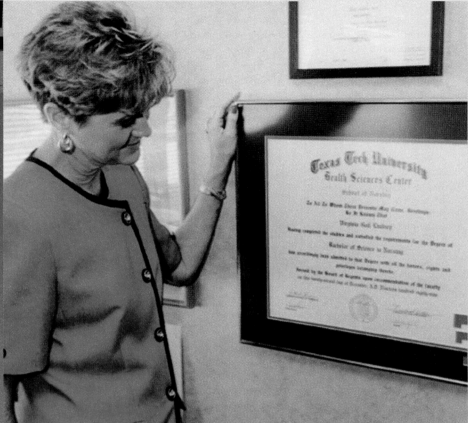

Career Management: Putting Yourself in Charge

Patricia S. Yoder-Wise
RN, C, EdD, CNAA, FAAN

This chapter focuses on career development, identifying career styles and describing the importance of continuing learning and certification to professional development. Linking career goals with specific strategies provides a way to enhance career success. Attending to professional expectations before beginning a career can further develop successful outcomes. The appendix to this chapter contains tools to use in preparing a curriculum vitae, résumé, and cover letter, as well as a checklist for interviewing, in essence, the tools that create the opportunities for you to manage your career.

Objectives

- Differentiate career styles and how they influence career options.
- Analyze person/position fit.
- Evaluate the relevance of curriculum vitae and résumés as entrees to interviews.
- Use critical elements of curriculum vitae and résumés to develop each.
- Analyze critical elements in an interview.
- Compare and contrast different types of professional learning opportunities.
- Value professional expectations.

Questions to Consider

- What clinical nursing experience thus far was most stimulating and challenging? Why?
- What excites you about nursing? What excites you about leadership and management options?
- What do you want to be doing in three years? (Describe as much as possible about your desirable future.)
- What are your strengths in teamwork? How do you function as a leader? What about as a follower?

A Manager's Challenge

From the Vice President for Patient Care Services at a Hospital in the Southwest

As I've moved along in my career, I thought it was important to gain academic and continuing education and to be certified in nursing administration. I had done all the "right things" to assure what I thought would be a solid career at the new hospital where I had just been named as the chief nursing executive.

Within weeks, a new CEO arrived and informed us we could all vie for the positions we held, but they were all open for reconsideration. I also knew some of the external competition and knew I would not retain my current position. As best I could tell, my choices would be to stay in a position I didn't necessarily want or to find another comparable position in town.

What would you do if you were this manager?

INTRODUCTION

Although it is important to take advantage of opportunities as they develop during a career, it is also important to make decisions about what you want to do in nursing and how you can go about doing it. Because nursing extends across the life span and is not institutionally based (that is, not defined by the institution but rather by law), the options for careers in nursing are vast. Some options build primarily on experience, others build primarily on educational background, and still others require a mix of education and experience. In general, you can assume that you must continue to learn and to develop your expertise. How you reach a career goal, however, depends on what goals you set and how you manage your own development.

CAREER MANAGEMENT

A **career** can be defined as progress throughout a person's professional life. If life, in general, is seen as

a series of changes, that is, positive, growth-producing experiences (Jeska & Rounds, 1996), career management holds great potential. Some people, including professional nurses, have a series of positions with no connection among them. Others can have divergent positions that are connected in some way. Irrespective of how careers develop, the real focus is continued competence.

Example

Nurse A moves between hospitals each time one of the hospitals offers a major new benefit or opens a new service. Nurse A also has worked in a few community settings and served on a cruise ship one summer. When asked about career patterns, Nurse A says, "I've capitalized on any opportunity that has come along. I really want to work in long-term care; but there don't seem to be openings to fit my needs." Nurse B also moves between hospitals and community organizations providing the positions always relate to care of newborns. This nurse has worked in entry positions and nurse manager positions. The clinical areas have ranged from labor and delivery to pediatrics and neonatal intensive care units. Nurse B belongs to the state nurses' association and the Association of Women's Health, Obstetrics, and Neonatal Nurses (AWOHNN). In addition to volunteering as a professional resource person at a local day-care center, nurse B has attended many professional conferences about newborns and recently applied to a graduate program to become a pediatric nurse practitioner. When asked about career patterns, nurse B states, "Well, I've sort of been all over the map; but I know that each time I've changed positions, I've had opportunities to work in a different phase of pediatric nursing."

There are several ways to develop a career. Basing career decisions on goals is a useful beginning. Some of the most notable work about careers has been conducted by Friss (1989), who identifies four career styles. Box 26-1 summarizes the key points related to each style. One career pathway is not better than another; rather, each is different. For example, the types of positions sought differ. Steady state and linear are the traditional career styles. The first remains at a plateau positionally and becomes increasingly competent; the second moves up the hierarchy of the organization and becomes more diversified. The entrepreneurial and transient style is one that has fostered many nurses' creative bent. For a great deal of flexibility and, in a time of rapid changes in healthcare, this style can permit creative solutions to traditional problems. Finally, the spiral style is one seen in situations where nurses move in and out of active practice and in situations where nurses move in and out of subcareer foci, such as general pediatrics and neonatal nursing.

The motivations and resultant leadership and management implications vary among the styles. Providing the same structure, feedback, and guidance for all would not capitalize on varying career styles. Similarly, nurses who choose a less traditional path (one that is not steady state or linear) may need to describe to others how they see their careers and how they have managed them. Sometimes because of a personal need or geographic location, a particular approach to a career in nursing may need to be modified.

To achieve a good person/position fit, there are several strategies that can be employed to elicit appropriate information before selecting a position. A good fit is built on strong similar goals and tolerable or growth-producing differences. Figure 26-1 suggests that the whole of any work situation is composed of two elements interacting in an environment with other elements. That whole is symbolized by blending a person's talents with the position's expectations to create a productive whole.

In today's rapidly changing society, it is possible that a position that was a fit no longer works for the person. The position is as likely to change as is the person. Some "promotions" occur without the traditional view of a-position-above-mine-opened-up event (Breen, 1996). In other words, some promotions result from a person expanding beyond his or her designated position. As a result, a new title/position description is created. Another nontraditional approach to promotions occurs when a major reorganization occurs and creates different positions to meet the redefined demands. While neither of these promotion approaches may have been a part of an individual's career plan, both are likely to happen as healthcare continuously reshapes itself.

▎MARKETING STRATEGIES

Irrespective of career style, core career development strategies are important. Selecting professional peers and mentors to share your development is important. Even the steady-state nurse who is not typically seeking a new position needs to develop a curriculum vitae or résumé that can document continued development of expertise. Interviewing, a two-way process, is also an important strategy to develop.

Few nurses have achieved a significant nursing career without assistance from peers and mentors. Heeding the "naysayers" can dampen career prospects. It is important to have a few well-chosen peers and mentors who can respond openly with various perspectives to help with career decisions. For example, a nurse who seeks a career as a direct-care provider in an acute care setting should seek support from a mentor (see this chapter's "Research Perspective"). Such a person could also provide honest appraisals of an individual's career development, suggest specific strategies to enhance development, and help with meeting the leaders in an organization.

Exercise 26-1

Turn to part I of the appendix to this chapter, "The Curriculum Vitae and the Résumé: Writing to Sell Yourself." Even if you have limited time right now, stop and draft a data set or two so you know how to prepare them. If you have sufficient time, draft a CV and résumé now. The appendix contains an example of each. As a checkpoint for yourself, make a list of four to five professional facts/qualities that you want others to know about. You can use this list in checking your CV or résumé and in interviewing. Keep in mind that a CV or résumé serves one primary purpose—letting others know enough about you that they want to meet you, advance your career, or gain more information.

Box 26-1
Career Styles

STEADY STATE
Example: staff nurses
Description: constancy in position with increasing professional skill
Motivation and characteristics:
- Increasing expertise
- High professional identity
- Obligation to serve
- Maintenance of standards
- Autonomy in performance of care
- Preference for action
- Personal accountability
- The work itself
- Stability

Managerial implications:
- Hold work in high esteem
- Decentralize
- Utilize and recognize abilities
- Provide feedback about client outcomes
- Reward competence and tenure
- Provide continuing education
- Provide permanent assignment

LINEAR
Example: nursing service administrator
Description: hierarchical orientation with steady climb
Motivation and characteristics:
- Requisite authority and power
- Had a challenging first job
- Guided by internalized norms
- Money
- Recognition
- Opportunities for self-development

Management implications:
- Provide management development
- Reward and value both education and competence
- Modify management selection and development systems
- Provide decreasing supervision

ENTREPRENEURIAL AND TRANSIENT
Example: nurses in private practice; temporary assignments
Description: desire to create new service; meeting own priorities
Motivation and characteristics:
- Limited organizational commitment
- Opportunists
- Novelty/creativity
- Other people
- Achievement

Managerial implications:
- Use flexibility to organization's benefit
- Avoid burdening them with organizational and practice decisions
- Provide immediate feedback

SPIRAL
Example: nurse who returns after raising a family
Description: rational, independent responsibility for shaping career
Motivation and characteristics:
- Novelty
- Prestige
- Intense period of employment followed by nonemployment or a different employment
- Care for others
- Opportunities for self-development
- Typically well paid, service oriented recognition

Managerial implications:
- Configure specific job that needs doing
- Be flexible about terms and length of commitment
- Find challenging initial assignment
- Negotiate
- Encourage creativity

Adapted from Friss (1989).

The current popular literature is replete with information about forming relationships. Although not all career development occurs through the influence of a mentor, being in a relationship with a strong role model is valuable. Although Yoder's study (1995) fo-

cused only on staff nurses in the Army, she found that coaching relationships were most valued by staff nurses. Both managers and advanced practice nurses (APNs) can provide such development. In fact, Yoder says, "it may be appropriate to use career development of the staff as one criterion in the annual evaluation of nurse managers and APNs" (p. 296). If the profession of nursing is to continue to develop its greatest strengths, all of us must determine how we contribute to each other's growth, especially as the business field, a driving force for healthcare, moves to a future of self-coaching (Kane, 1996).

A **curriculum vitae** (CV) is a listing of professional life activities. It is designed to be all-inclusive, but not detailed. The reverse is true of a résumé. A **résumé** is a summary of professional abilities and facts. It is designed for specific opportunities to illustrate a fit of a person with a position. For the steady-state nurse, a résumé could be used to reflect increasing skills and abilities; for others, a résumé can create specific messages about an individual's unique experiences, education, and abilities in relation to a new opportunity. In other words, a CV or résumé opens doors.

The exercise "Writing to Sell Yourself" (found in the appendix to this chapter) is designed to help create a system for developing and maintaining professional data and create both a CV and a résumé in a print format. Electronic résumés, while emerging rapidly in some fields (Fryer, 1995), are currently undeveloped in nursing.

A cover letter conveys the quality of experience when paired with a CV. Because a CV is merely a set of facts, it conveys little quality. A cover letter serves to describe specific assets or qualities you have. When seeking a position, you can make several key points about yourself and how you fit the position. When providing your CV or résumé for career advancement purposes, you can highlight specific qualities that enhance your potential to be seen as the right choice.

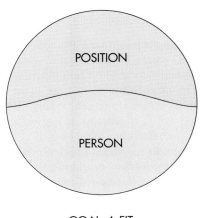

GOAL: A FIT

Figure 26-1 Person/position fit.

Research Perspective

Angelini, D.J. (1995). Mentoring in the career development of hospital staff nurses: Models and strategies. Journal of Professional Nursing, 11(2), 89-97.

An exploratory, descriptive, qualitative study of 37 white female staff and eight managerial nurses was conducted to determine what mentoring for staff nurses exists in hospitals, where the majority of nurses remain employed. Triangulation of audiotaped interviews (one with staff, the other with managers), biographies/career histories, and such documents as position descriptions and philosophies was performed. Each of the nurses worked 32 hours or more per week and had at least 5 years' experience, although the average number of years the staff nurses had worked in their current settings was 12.2 years.

Mentoring of hospital staff nurses was viewed from two models: structural and process. The structural model was influenced by people (especially peers and the nurse manager), events (such as patient situations and political circumstances), and environments (such as values, advancement, and work conditions). The process model used four phases that conclude in one of three outcomes: positive interaction within the organizational climate, development of career building relationships, and facilitation of career transition points.

Implications for Practice
Peers and managers alike can be influential on a staff nurse's career development, and that influence is especially important in patient care situations. Because mentoring can be a large influence on a staff nurse's career development, gaining insight about how staff and managers perceive their role in mentoring others is critical in an interview.

Exercise 26-2

Using part II of the appendix to this chapter, "The Cover Letter," write a letter that highlights information from at least two of your data sets.

Assuming you are using these strategies to secure a new position, the next logical step is seeking an interview. Interviewing is a two-way proposition; the interviewee should be gathering as much information as the interviewer is. Both should be making judgments throughout the process so that if a position is offered, the interviewee will be prepared to accept, decline, or explore further. Interviews may take place with one or more individuals and may include a range of activities. To be at ease, the interviewee should wear comfortable, but professional, clothing. Rehearsing specific questions to ask and points to make can create comfort for these somewhat challenging situations. Be prepared to cite challenges and dilemmas you faced and what you did and why, because these types of questions may be posed to you.

Resources, such as Tye's *Personal Best* (1997), provide a variety of general career tips from thinking positively about yourself to determining various career strategies. Other resources, such as Allen's *Complete Q and A Job Interview Book* (1997), need to be used care-fully. Although it is helpful to have targeted answers in mind, answers that sound "canned" are as limiting as are "canned" résumés. It is critical to listen to what is being asked and respond genuinely. Skills can be developed; honesty and attitude must come with the employee.

Exercise 26-3

Select a partner and role play an interview. The potential employer role should include questions and scenarios about common conflicts and challenges seen in clinical settings. The interviewee role should include responses from experiences and concerns.

If you have prepared well, you will know what the organization's stated beliefs are and whether they are compatible with yours. The challenge in an interview is to determine if those beliefs are lived or merely printed words. If numerous people can relate how the mission actually is translated in a specific role, it is likely that the beliefs are lived ones.

The appendix to this chapter includes three tools designed to be used in preparing for an interview: "Checklist for Interviewing," "Questions to Ask/to be Asked," and "Interview Topics and Questions of Concern." One other tool, "The Successful Thank You," is included to illustrate an additional opportunity to market yourself.

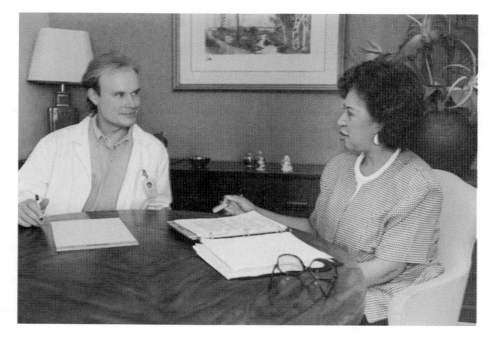

Interviewing is a two-way proposition in which both participants gather as much information as possible.

The interrelationship of these strategies allows people to emphasize specialization or diversity. Each strategy leads to the next so that the potential for attaining a preferred position is enhanced. As careers progress, factors other than the specific nursing school or in-school activities take precedence in influencing career development and how an individual is seen by others. Thus, updating a CV or résumé is important. Keeping a passion alive must be evident. The "Career Tips" (page 442) will help to keep your career vibrant.

CONTINUING LEARNING

One of the keys to maintaining competence is continued learning. Learning occurs in various ways. It can occur in a conversation with colleagues, by reading an article in the general literature, or sometimes in an "ah hah" experience that provides sudden enlightenment. Although nurses could share these experiences with others, the continued learning that the profession, healthcare employers, boards of nursing, and professional associations are most concerned with is formal study—graduate education and continuing education.

A graduate degree opens numerous career opportunities and leads to new levels or areas of expertise. A graduate education may focus on a clinical area, a functional area, or a combination of both. Admission to graduate programs typically requires taking a test (frequently the Graduate Record Examination [GRE]), having an above-average grade point average (GPA), and graduating from a professionally accredited school of nursing.

Graduate education consists of both master's- and doctorate-level study. In some employment situations or career specialties, graduate education is required. For example, expectations for nurse practitioner preparation are centered on graduate-level preparation as opposed to the earlier certificate programs. As healthcare becomes more complex, it would be fairly easy to argue that persons licensed as individual practitioners, such as nurses, would need more education to continue to meet the healthcare system's demands.

Deciding to pursue graduation education may be very simple. Some applicants to baccalaureate programs already have a specific career focus in mind and the required graduate preparation is a given. New graduates are sometimes encouraged (or even required) to gain experience before seeking a master's degree or doctorate. While experience enriches previous learning, it may not be relevant to specific graduate programs such as those entailing a major career redirection. Working while attending a graduate program may be difficult; but it is common among graduate students in nursing. Box 26-2 lists some factors to consider in selecting a graduate program.

Exercise 26-4

Analyze your preparation in your current program. Do you feel confident in your knowledge basis and clinical skills? Can you effectively juggle multiple roles? Based on these answers, determine if you should pursue graduate education immediately or wait. Then determine how you would pursue it. Would you pursue it full-time or juggle multiple roles?

If you are geographically bound, your fields of study may be limited. If you are not and you know what general area you want to pursue, consider the following illustration:

Example
You know you want to work with the elderly. Your library subscribes to *The Journal of Gerontological Nursing* and *Geriatric Nursing*. Pull the most recent year's issues of both. Scan the masthead (the page with the editors, board members, etc.). Where are these individuals affiliated? Now scan the articles. Are there some that are particularly intriguing? Where are the authors affiliated? Finally, look back over your lists. Are there any places emerging as where the leaders in the field may be? You now have a good starting place.

Exercise 26-5

Assume you are interested in graduate education. Talk with your local financial aid official to determine how you can learn about financial assistance for graduate education. Go to the library and locate some reference about graduate education in nursing. What specialties exist at the master's level? What programs are near you? What programs stimulate clinical interest? What about doctoral programs? What do they provide?

Continuing education also contributes to professional growth. **Continuing education** is defined as "those learning activities intended to build upon the educational and experiential bases of the professional nurse for the enhancement of practice, education, administration, research, or theory development to the end of improving the health of the public" (American Nurses Credentialing Center, 1991, p. 76).

Numerous opportunities for continuing education exist at local, state, regional, and national levels. Selecting which opportunities to pursue may be a difficult choice. Box 26-3 lists several factors to consider in selecting any offering, but, depending on your particular goal, certain factors may be more influential than others. For example, if cost is a major factor, length and speaker may be less influential factors.

Box 26-2
Factors to Consider in Selecting a Graduate Program

Accreditation	• Does the program have national nursing accreditation? (master's level)
	• Is the institution regionally accredited? (for example, North Central Association of Colleges and Schools)
Clinical/functional role	• How closely do the descriptions of clinical/functional courses of study meet career goals?
Credits	• How many graduate credits are minimally required to complete the degree?
	• How many are devoted to gaining experience?
	• How many relate to classroom experiences?
Thesis/research	• Is a thesis required?
	• If not, what opportunities exist for research development?
	• What support is available for graduate students?
Faculty	• What credentials do faculty hold?
	• Are they in leadership positions in the state/nation?
	• Are they competent in your field of interest?
	• What is their reputation?
Current research	• What are the current research strengths of the institution?
Flexibility	• Do these strengths fit with your interests or is there flexibility to create your own direction?
	• Is flexibility present in scheduling, progress through the program?
Admission	• What is required?
	• Is the GRE used?
	• What is the minimum undergraduate GPA expected?
	• Is experience required? What kind? How much?
Costs	• What are the total projected costs?
	• What financial aid is available?

In addition to increasing your knowledge base, continuing education opportunities provide professional networking opportunities, contribute to meeting certification and licensure requirements, and document additional pursuits in maintaining or developing clinical expertise. Sponsors of continuing education include employers, professional associations, schools of nursing, and private entrepreneurial groups.

Both types of formal continued learning, graduate education and continuing education, are valuable to your professional development, and both can contribute to a specific area of career development—certification.

Exercise 26-6

Even though you are not an organization, you still develop strategic plans for yourself. Imagine you have decided to earn a master's degree in nursing. This decision can be enhanced by a strategic plan. What values do you have that influence your plan? Are your interests in primary care, administration, or education? What is your target date for completion of the master's program? What are other factors that

Exercise 26-6—cont'd

would interfere with your strategic plan? Do you have specific short-term goals, or operational plans, that must be attained first? Even though you are not an organization you do use the same type of planning method. Do you see the similarities?

CERTIFICATION

In 1989 Styles identified at least 45 different types of certification. These include clinical areas such as cancer as well as functional areas such as administration. Many of these include an expectation for participation in continuing education, as reported annually in the January-February issue of T*he Journal of Continuing Education in Nursing* (Yoder-Wise, 1997). **Certification** is the designation of special knowledge beyond basic **licensure.** It is an expectation in some employment settings for career advancement; in the field of advanced practice nursing, it is viewed as an expectation of practice. Furthermore, in some states certification

---

Box 26-3

Factors to Consider in Selecting a Continuing Education Course

Accreditation/approval	• Is the course accredited/approved? If so, by whom?
	• Is that recognition accepted by a certification entity, by the board of nursing (if continuing education is required for reregistration of licensure)?
Credit	• Is the amount of credit appropriate in terms of the expected outcomes?
Course title	• Does it suggest the type of learner to be involved? (e.g., advanced)
	• Does it reflect the expected outcomes?
Speaker(s)	• Is the instructor known as an expert in the field?
	• Is the instructor experienced in the field?
Objectives	• Are the objectives logical and attainable?
	• Do they reflect knowledge, skills, or attitudes, or a combination of these?
	• Do they fit a learner's needs?
Content	• Is the content reflective of the objectives?
	• Is the content at an appropriate level?
Audience	• Is the audience designed as a general or target one? (e.g., all RNs or experienced nurses in state health positions)
Cost	• Is it equitable with what similar nursing conferences cost?
	• Is travel required?
	• What is the actual direct expense for an individual to attend? Is it affordable?
Length	• Is the total time frame logical in terms of objectives, personal needs, and time away from work?
	• Does the time frame permit breaks from intense learning?
Provider	• Does the provider have an established reputation?

---

in advanced practice is the avenue to designation by the state as an advanced practitioner and to reibursement and practice privileges of advanced practice. Obtaining certification may range from testing and continuing education to documented time in practice in the specialty area plus testing and continuing education. Recertification is a process of continued recognition of competence within a defined practice area. As an example, the American Nurses Credentialing Center (ANCC) provides for recertification every 5 years. The ANCC provides two certification examinations in nursing administration: one is basic (CNA), the other is advanced (CNAA). Nurses certified through this process initially provide a variety of information and sit for a licensure examination. Effective in 1998, all generalist examinations will require a baccalaureate in nursing for initial certification. During each subsequent 5-year period, nurses complete a stipulated practice requirement and choose either to retake the examination or to document participation in appropriate continuing education activities.

The American Nurses' Credentialing Center in 1998 began work to credential baccalaureate gradu-ates to distinguish the knowledge and abilities that are different than those tested in the licensure examination. The intent of this strategy is to help employers of nurses know that an individual prepared at the baccalaureate level has documentable differences at the point of entering the profession. This certification does not replace those related to defined clinical practice areas.

Certification plays an important part in the advancement of a career. In some fields, more than one examination exists; in some, there is an examination in the broad field and numerous options for very defined subspecialties; and in other fields, no examination exists. If certification does exist, however, the current trend is to expect commensurate recognition in the work place if career advancement is anticipated.

PROFESSIONAL EXPECTATIONS

In addition to the expectations of being a professional that have already been cited, other strategies have been proposed. For example, Archibald and

Bainbridge, risk consultants for a health insurer, suggest that nurses move to a process of privileging, whereby nurses could be authorized to perform procedures or to work with specific diagnoses or patient care problems (1994). Once privileged, nurses then would collect and document their specific practice experiences. This approach is, in a sense, a form of proactive (and positive) peer review, a concept adopted by the Texas Legislature in 1997. Because both of these strategies depend heavily on peer groups, the challenge for leaders—and followers—to be proactive is evident. In addition to advancing nursing's accountability as a profession, these strategies emphasize the individual as a professional and allow for recognition of individual quality. Although more and more work is accomplished through teams, a savvy nurse manager knows which staff have which abilities so that individual resources are most fully utilized.

Being a professional holds both privileges and obligations. The legal privileges and expectations are codified in the state nursing practice acts, rules, and regulations. Because licensure is designed to provide the baseline, that is, the minimum expectation, it does not identify or obligate any practitioner to function in a professional manner as defined by the profession itself. For example, no practice act identifies membership in a professional association as an expectation. Nor is there an expectation for community service or scholarship. Yet the profession, through various professional organizations, holds the expectation that nurses will belong to professional associations and provide leadership in improving communities. How to incorporate these activities in a busy, committed life can at times seem difficult. The key is to use a concept known as **reintegration** (Langford, 1990), which refers to the process of returning to a whole of nursing. It designates an incorporation of four role aspects into the role of professional nursing: education, scholarship, practice, and service. For example, the nurse who is expert in geriatrics nursing might provide guest lectures at a nearby university in problems related to aging (*education*). This same nurse might help explain the latest research related to dementia, a common concern of institutionalized elderly, to the staff of a nursing facility (*scholarship*). This individual might also be certified as a gerontological nurse through the American Nurses Credentialing Center as an example of expertise in a specialized area of practice (*practice*). Additionally, this nurse might provide community blood pressure screenings at a senior citizens center and belong to the Gerontological Nurses' Association (*service*). Thus, each of the four elements of reintegration capitalizes on all other

areas to contribute to this nurse's expertise in caring for the elderly. Figure 26-2 reflects the reintegration model. Each element could stand alone as a major role; instead the synthesis of these functional elements in an area of expertise contributes to the totality of professional competence.

Belonging to a **professional association** not only demonstrates professional leadership but also provides numerous opportunities to meet other leaders, participate in policy formation, continue specialized education, and shape the future of the profession. To learn more about an association, it is probably useful to write to the national association and ask for information. Each April in the *American Journal of Nursing* all state boards of nursing and professional associations are listed, including addresses and telephone numbers. Requesting information should provide insight into both direct and indirect benefits of organizational membership. For example, a direct benefit may be receiving a publication or attending a meeting at reduced, or no, cost. An indirect benefit is knowing that your association actively lobbies on behalf of professional nurses. It is also possible to contact numerous organizations through the American Nurses' Association's web page, www.nursingworld.org.

Depending on the type of career you want to have, it might be very important to belong to a specific association because it is synonymous with leadership in the field. In nursing, in general, the American Academy of Nursing and Sigma Theta Tau are such non-clinical, specific focus entities. Determining a logical level of involvement in an association at the local, state, regional, or national level is important. When a bright, articulate, committed member is discovered, that individual is frequently asked to meet other expectations of the association's work. Once again, knowing what is important in professional goals can help you decide what level of involvement is desirable and acceptable.

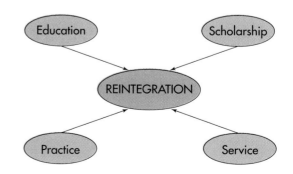

Figure 26-2 Reintegrated nursing.

Because the public places its trust in any licensed profession, there are numerous other obligations and privileges to being a professional. Some are exciting, for instance providing testimony related to healthcare concerns. Others are troublesome, for instance reporting a colleague to the state nursing board for incompetent practice. These are opportunities to improve the profession and the resultant care the general public can expect.

CAREER POTENTIAL

Traditionally, nursing has been seen by the public as hospital based; but that has changed dramatically recently. There are numerous other nursing careers, such as teacher, administrator, manager, clinical specialist, researcher, organizational executive, entrepreneur, and practitioner. Additionally, the number of clinical specialties continues to increase. Some have been a part of nursing for a long time and are experiencing major growth and recognition because of the financial impact on healthcare. These include such foci as occupational health, school health, and public health. Concomitantly, the traditional hospital careers are simultaneously focusing and expanding. Nurses with these focused, expert skills need to be able to function with more than one clinical population. This ability to increase expertise and flexibility will continue to be in demand. Positioning within the profession to achieve this flexibility and expertise requires career commitment, continuous self-development, a passion for nursing, and a strong foundation as a leader.

A Manager's Solution

❓ Because there was a "buy-out" (or outplacement) package available, I decided to totally rethink my nursing career. I really focused on what I valued in *life*, not just nursing. As a result, I left my native state, a major decision for me, and moved to New Mexico to be in charge of a division of nursing services. I live on a ranch, own five llamas, and am now the chief nursing executive. I'd say that being willing to take risks dramatically enhanced my life and my career in nursing. I wish everyone courage!

❓ *Would this be a suitable approach for you? Why?*

CHAPTER CHECKLIST

It is important for nurses to make decisions about career goals and career development. Managing a career requires a set of planned strategies designed to lead systematically toward the desired goal. The use of each strategy should be geared toward finding a good person/position fit. Career management is focused on continual competence. Continued learning, whether via graduate education or via continuing education, is a crucial component of success as a nurse.

■ Career styles contribute to the diversity of the nursing profession and reflect different ways of achieving success.
  • The four career styles are:
    – Steady state: characterized by constancy with increasing professional skill.
    – Linear: a hierarchical orientation with a steady climb.
    – Entrepreneurial/transient: focused on new services and personal priorities.
    – Spiral: rational, independent responsibility for shaping the career.

■ Certain career control strategies are effective with every career style:
  • Selecting professional peers and mentors helps shape professional development.
  • Interviewing at its best is a two-way interaction that enables both people to determine whether there is a good person/position fit.
  • Designing personal/professional documents that open doors for further action includes
    – The curriculum vitae (a listing of facts) (quantitative)
    – The résumé (a sampling of the most relevant facts, with details) (qualitative)

■ Both graduate education and continuing education contribute to a nurse's ability to provide competent care.
  • Graduate education (master's- or doctorate-level study) may focus on:
    – A clinical area
    – A functional area
    – A combination of both
  • Factors to consider in selecting a graduate program include:
    – Accreditation
    – Clinical/functional role
    – Credits
    – Thesis/research requirements
    – Faculty
    – Current research

- Flexibility
- Admission policy
- Cost
- Continuing education opportunities exist at local, state, regional, and national levels.
- Certification is the designation of special knowledge beyond the basic licensure and is a requirement in some employment settings. Being a professional carries additional obligations and privileges to ensure that the nurse remains competent, advances the profession, and improves healthcare.

CAREER TIPS

- Use an expanding file to organize your accomplishments such as continuing education certificates by year so you can report accurate data for licensure or certification.
- Update your curriculum vitae at least once a year (6 months is better and 3 months is ideal) so you always have an accurate, current set of data to share with someone should a special opportunity appear.
- Keep connected with people.
- Find a mentor; be a mentor; self-mentor.
- Review the most difficult events of the day immediately and determine how to improve yourself (Kane, 1996).
- Improve your abilities, especially those you use all of the time—get better at being better (Kane, 1996).
- Think about the future and what you need to be employable.
- Join two professional organizations—such as the American Nurses' Association (broad professional) and American Association of Critical Care Nurses (a specialty).
- Read professional journals and, on a regular basis, at least one other journal external to nursing to keep current with the world.
- Attend at least one professional meeting each year, especially outside of your geographic area, to network.
- Volunteer in your profession and your community.

TERMS TO KNOW

career	licensure
certification	professional association
continuing education	reintegration
curriculum vitae	résumé

REFERENCES

Allen, J.G. (1997). *The Complete Q and A Job Interview Book*. 2nd ed. New York: John Wiley & Sons.

American Nurses Credentialing Center. (1991). *Manual for Accreditation as a Provider of Continuing Education in Nursing*. Kansas City, MO: ANCC.

Angelini, D.J. (1995). Mentoring in the career development of hospital staff nurses: Models and strategies. *Journal of Professional Nursing*, 11(2), 89-97.

Archibald, P.J., & Bainbridge, D.D. (1994). Capacity and competence: Nurse credentialing and privileging. *Nursing Management*, 25(4), 49-51, 54-56.

Breen, B. (June-July, 1996). Getting promoted without promoting yourself. *Fast Company*, 130-132.

Bronstein, E. & Hisrich, R.D. (1983). *The MBA Career: Moving on the Fast Track to Success*. Woodbury, NY: Barrons Educational Series.

Friss, L. (1989). *Strategic Management of Nurses: A Policy Oriented Approach*. Owings Mills, MD: AUPHA Press.

Fryer, B. (March, 1995). Job hunting the electronic way. *Working Woman*, 59-60, 78.

Jeska, S., & Rounds, R. (1996). Addressing the human side of change: Career development and renewal. *Nursing Economics*, 14, 339-345.

Kane, K.A. (June-July, 1996). Do-it-yourself mentoring. *Fast Company*, 133.

Langford, T.L. (1990). *Managing and Being Managed: Preparation for Reintegrated Professional Nursing Practice*. Lubbock, TX: Landover Publishing.

Styles, M.M. (1989). *On Specialization in Nursing: Toward a New Endowment*. Kansas City, MO: American Nurses Foundation.

Tye, J. (1997). *Personal Best: 1001 Great Ideas for Achieving Success in Your Career*. New York: John Wiley & Sons.

Yoder, L.H. (1995). Staff nurses' career development relationships and self-reports of professionalism, job satisfaction, and intent to stay. *Nursing Research*, 44, 290-297.

Yoder-Wise, P.S. (1997). Annual CE survey: State and association/certifying boards CE requirements. *The Journal of Continuing Education in Nursing*, 28, 5-9.

SUGGESTED READINGS

Bolles, R.N. (1997). *What Color is Your Parachute?: A Practical Manual for Job Hunters and Career-Changers*. Berkeley: Ten Speed Press.

Case, B. (1997). *Career Planning for Nurses*. Albany: Delmar.

Fast Company. http://www.fastcompany.com

Glaxo Wellcome. (1995). *Pathway Evaluation Program for Nursing Professionals: Specialty Profiles*. Research Triangle Park, NC: Glaxo Wellcome.

RN. (1996). *Nursing Opportunities: Getting the Job You Want*. Montvale, NJ: Medical Economics.

CHAPTER 26 APPENDIX

MARKETING YOURSELF AS A COMPETENT PROFESSIONAL*

THE CURRICULUM VITAE AND THE RÉSUMÉ: WRITING TO SELL YOURSELF

Objectives
Using this material, you will be able to:

- compile a curriculum vitae (CV)
- write a professional résumé
- access professional data in an organized manner

Things you will need: computer, printer (laser-preferred), and disk; or index cards, file box, pencil, scratch paper, typing paper, and access to a professional typing service.

Time to allocate: Depending on your unique background, this assignment varies considerably. It is not necessary to set aside a block of time in the data collection stage, but it may be useful to do so in the data assembly stage for the résumé.

Although there are numerous ways to record professional data, the fact remains that most nurses do not do so in a systematic manner. Therefore, when asked a question, it is often difficult to recall the information needed. The goal of this exercise is to develop a systematic plan that you can use throughout your professional career so that developing a CV or a résumé will be relatively easy.

Curriculum vitae (note there is no singular form of the word *vitae*) means one's life story. It need not include personal facts, but it should include *all* professional facts. A résumé (the word is French, meaning summary) is a summary of one's professional abilities and facts. It is designed to match a certain position or type of work. A third approach, the biosketch, is a listing of *key* facts. It is used infrequently in nursing.

Data Collection
The first step is to collect all previous professional information about yourself. If you are fairly new in the profession, it would help to analyze anything special you did in school, e.g., electives, offices held, or special assignments or awards. If you have an employment history, you can start with your nursing positions. Keep in mind, also, that you should include other relevant information. For example, serving as a volunteer in a day-care center may augment a brief professional history; serving on voluntary health association committees or boards may be useful to secure a position related to a particular position; and both convey a professional commitment to community life.

It may be most useful to start where you are and think back. If you have limited "thinking back" to do, you are in great shape for starting a systematic plan. If, however, you have been practicing nursing for a long time, you may have some difficulty. In fact, some information may be irretrievable—do not dwell on that aspect, just record as much as you can.

At the end of this first step, you will have a series of entries with one data element in each data set. The areas in Box 26-4, however, should be considered, even if you currently have nothing to record under these topics. Create topic listings (file headings) and place each data set for each with experience, committee, article, activity, etc. behind the appropriate topic. This collection is for your use only. In other words, this serves as your professional career memory.

Data Assembly
The "checklist" in Box 26-5 will help you keep track of your data and assemble the facts attractively.

Curriculum Vitae
The hard part is over. To develop a CV, simply select a logical flow of information and assemble the CV. Information should be in a chronological order. Most recent first (reverse chronological) draws attention to your latest contributions and is a better presentation of your information than a historic chronological sequence. You need to include your name, credentials, degrees, address, phone number, and fax and e-mail data. This set of information should be distinct so you are easy to contact. Using the information facts by category, assemble a CV that reflects all professional involvement. A sample CV appears in Box 26-6. A CV must be typed and appear organized. Therefore, since you are providing facts only, it is helpful to have subheadings, such as:

---
*Copyright Patricia S. Yoder-Wise, R.N., Ed.D.

Box 26-4
Data Collection

Topics	Facts Needed
1. Education	Years of attendance, year of graduation, name of school, location, name of degree (diploma) received, special recognition—e.g., two concurrent degrees, minor or with honors.
2. Continuing education	Dates attended, places, topics and any special outcomes, type and amount of credit earned during the last few years.
3. Experience	Dates of employment, title of position, name of employing agency, location and phone number, name of chief executive officer, chief nursing officer, immediate supervisor, salary range, typical duties (role description).
4. Community/institutional service	Dates of service, name of committee/task force and the parent organization (e.g., name of hospital or district nurses' association), your role on the committee (e.g., chairperson or member), general description of the committee's functions, any unique accomplishments.
5. Publications	Articles: author(s) name(s), year of publication, title, journal, volume, issue, pages.
	Books: author(s) name(s), year of publication, title, city, publisher.
	If appropriate, description of item (e.g., internal policy manual, first article on quality assurance in a rural hospital, or letter to the editor). Be sure to note your contribution if the project was a group effort. Keeping the sequence of authorship straight is important.
6. Honors	Date, description of award, special factors related to the award (e.g., competitive, community-wide, national.)
7. Speeches/presentations (made)	Date, place, title of speech made, name of sponsoring group and nature of the presentation (e.g., keynote), your honorarium.
8. Workshops/conferences (made)	Date, place, title of conference conducted, name of sponsoring group, nature of the presentation, brief description of the effort, your honorarium.
9. Certification	Date, certifying body, area/type of certification.

Education

Name of Institution/

Location	Dates Attended	Degree	Year
•			
•			
•			

Experience

Name of Institution/

Location	Dates of Service	Title of Position
•		
•		
•		

Develop a CV (typed). Be sure to have the CV error-free and on quality bond paper.

Résumé

To "sell" yourself to someone, you need to provide more than the facts, and the information needs to be brief and to the point. Thus the résumé is the best choice for selling your abilities to a potential employer. A résumé focuses on a particular position's expectations or an individual's special abilities. A sample résumé appears in Box 26-7.

Box 26-5
Checklist for Constructing a Curriculum Vitae/Résumé/Qualifications Brief

Data Collection

_____ 1. Data sets for information development.

_____ 2. Information assembled in categorical manner.

Data Assembly

_____ 1. Discrete categories are used.

_____ 2. Assembly addresses *specific* position (or cover letter for CV).

_____ 3. Current name, address, telephone number, voice mail, and e-mail are prominent (use as many as are appropriate for you).

_____ 4. Career summary (if used) (or cover letter for CV) is prominent.

_____ 5. Key points about positions/experiences are evident.

_____ 6. A logical flow is evident.

_____ 7. Grammar, spelling, and syntax are correct.

_____ 8. Writing style is positive and direct, but not terse.

_____ 9. Action verbs are evident.

_____10. If writing in full sentences, third person and passive voice are avoided, i.e., write in the active voice.

_____11. "Canned" résumé language is avoided—e.g., "distinguished" and "all phases of . . ."

_____12. Emphasis is on competence, not years (cover letter for CV).

_____13. Specific examples of key competencies are cited (cover letter for CV).

_____14. The format is consistent throughout.

_____15. Personal information (e.g., health, marital status) is absent.

Appearance and Format

_____ 1. There are no typographical errors.

_____ 2. The product is "clean"—e.g., no smudges, no discrepant margins.

_____ 3. It is readable—e.g., layout design is pleasing: white space, capitalization, etc.

_____ 4. The paper is *high*-quality bond (24-pound paper), white or cream.

_____ 5. The type is businesslike (no script); text is at least 9 to 10 points and fonts are limited to one or two.

_____ 6. Emphasis is evident—e.g., centering and bold print or underlining.

_____ 7. It is only one or two pages in length (not applicable for a CV).

Overview

_____ 1. It is attractive, interesting, quick-reading, and competency-based.

_____ 2. The package *sells you*.

_____ 3. You are pleased to have it precede you.

_____ 4. Additional items are enclosed or they are assembled for personal handling at an interview.

_____ 5. If you were receiving this CV or résumé, would *you* want to interview this person?

There are basically two ways to develop a résumé—conventional and functional.

- The *conventional* approach provides:
  NAME
  ADDRESS
  PHONE NUMBER/FAX/E-MAIL

  CAREER SUMMARY (optional)

TITLE OF POSITION

Name or type of employer (compression of experiences may be necessary to keep the résumé brief)

Inclusive dates

Responsibilities and achievements

OTHER CATEGORIES OF SPECIAL MEANING FROM FACT CARDS

Box 26-6

Sample Curriculum Vitae (Excerpts)

SALLY JONES, R.N., B.S.N.
4370 South Sunset Drive
Columbus, Ohio 43213
(614) 555-2736 (home)
(614) 555-2937 (fax)
sjones@aol.com

EXPERIENCE

Institution	Position	Dates
Childrens' Hospital Columbus, Ohio	Staff Nurse, Adolescents	February 1997-present
Health Services Hospital Troy, Texas	3-11 Charge Nurse Maternal Child Division	July 1994-December 1996
Llano Estacado Hospital Troy, Texas	Staff Nurse Maternal Child Division	June 1993-June 1994

EDUCATION

Institution	Degree	Year
The Ohio State University Columbus. Ohio	6 Graduate Credits	1997
Texas Tech University Health Sciences Center	Bachelor of Science in Nursing	1993

HONORS

Sigma Theta Tau, Inc., inducted into Iota Mu Chapter, 1991.

MEMBERSHIPS/OFFICES/COMMITTEES

Member	District 18 Program Committee	1993-94
Member	American Nurses' Association-Texas Nurses' Association	1993-94
	Ohio Nurses' Association	1994-Present
Secretary	Evening Shift Staff Council, Llano Estacado Hospital	1993
Member	Sigma Theta Tau, Inc.	1991-present

PRESENTATIONS/PUBLICATIONS

Testimony to the legislature of the State of Texas on diabetes education	January 13, 1993
Certification ACLS	current

MISCELLANEOUS

Member of YWCA Community Advisory Board Bilingual (oral Spanish)	1995-96
Delivered Meals on Wheels	1992-1996

- The *functional* approach provides:
  NAME
  ADDRESS
  PHONE NUMBER/FAX/E-MAIL

  CAREER SUMMARY

  FUNCTION (e.g., neonatal nursing)
  Paragraph description of activities and for whom

NEW FUNCTION (e.g., management)
  Same

NEW FUNCTION
  Same

EDUCATION

OTHER CATEGORIES OF SPECIAL MEANING

Box 26-7
Sample Résumé (Conventional)

SALLY JONES, R.N., B.S.N.
4370 South Sunset Drive
Columbus, Ohio 43213
(614) 555-2736 (home)
(614) 555-2737 (fax)
sjones@aol.com

CAREER SUMMARY: Maternal child health is the general focus of my career with a specialty in adolescent care. In addition to taking elective credit in this area in my undergraduate program and completing 6 credits as a special student at the graduate level, I have worked in general maternal child service areas since graduating with my Bachelor of Science in Nursing.

EXPERIENCE:

STAFF NURSE Children's Hospital Columbus, Ohio February, 1997-present	While pursuing graduate education, I am working part-time on an adolescent unit that includes acutely ill and unstable chronically ill patients.

CHARGE NURSE
Health Services
  Hospital
Troy, Texas
July, 1994–
  December, 1996
	As 3-11 charge nurse in a 50-bed postpartum unit, I assigned staff nurses and managed the unit. I had responsibility for orientation to the unit on evenings. During this time, I designed a reporting format for change-of-shift report and unit standards for care of adolescent patients.

STAFF NURSE
Llano Estacado
  Hospital
Troy, Texas
June, 1993–
  June, 1994
	As primary nurse typically caring for six normal newborns or two critically ill newborns, I refined skills in this specialty. Additionally, I helped institute standardized care plans with individual modifications and designed a plan for overflow to the normal newborn area.

HONORS:	Member of Sigma Theta Tau, Inc., 1991-present. Recipient of C.W. Smith Scholarship, 1992-93

Both of these honors were based on the fact that I carried a 3.9 GPA while working 20 hours a week as a nursing assistant.

SPECIAL SKILLS: I speak Spanish, am computer literate, and hold ACLS certification.

PROFESSIONAL COMMITMENTS: As a student, I joined the Texas Nursing Students' Association and served as president of my local chapter for a year. Upon graduation, I joined the Texas Nurses' Association and served on the program committee of the local district. As a result of serving as secretary of the evening shift staff council at Llano Estacado, I also joined AWOHNN, the Association of Women's Health, Obstetrics, and Neonatal Nurses.

EDUCATION: After completing my B.S.N. at Texas Tech University Health Sciences Center in 1993, I enrolled in six graduate credits at The Ohio State University. These courses focus on management and computer science. I have earned approximately 20 contact hours of continuing education credits per year since graduation.

Keep in mind that a résumé should be brief—a one- or two-page summary is best. The "other categories of *special* meaning" should relate to the specific career goal you have or position you seek. Sometimes a career goal is included on the résumé; other times it is described in a cover letter. A functional approach is best if you are planning a sharp departure from present positions. The focus is on what you've done, not when or what you can/will do.

Develop a résumé (typed). Be sure to have the résumé error-free and on quality bond paper.

THE COVER LETTER

Using the information in this section, you will be able to write a cover letter that is brief and that contains the essential information.

Things you will need:
- Your curriculum vitae or résumé, computer, printer, and disk (or scratch paper, pencil, and access to a professional service)

Time to allocate:
- Approximately 20 minutes

The cover letter can be a vital source of information and the opportunity to assure yourself of an interview. It is a brief (generally no more than one page) statement that says why you are writing, why you "fit" the organization and a specific position (or type[s] of position[s]), and how you will follow up (e.g., write or call).

Numerous positions may be advertised by a major organization simultaneously. Thus it is crucial to state immediately why you are writing. If a particular advertisement or referral does not include the name of the key nursing contact, you could obtain this information and send your letter to that person (even if you are writing directly to the personnel office). (NOTE: This assumes the position you are seeking is in the purview of the nursing division.)

Once you have stated your reason for writing, i.e., referencing a particular position or type(s) of position(s), you should address the issue of "why you." That is, why should someone take time to read your attached résumé or curriculum vitae? This statement should reflect what you know about the organization and how you will fit in. This point may take the form of comparable experience, or diverse experiences that will blend in a unique way, or how your educational program prepared you to work in such a place. Reference to the enclosed résumé or curriculum vitae is appropriate. Examples of competencies can be included to clarify your strengths.

> **Box 26-8**
> **Checklist for Interviewing**
>
> 1. Check interviewing guides, such as *What Color Is Your Parachute?*
> 2. Check out the new organization
>   a. Read, call, network, visit
>   b. Obtain statistics, facts, etc.
>   c. Learn the buzz words
>   d. Ask about new directions
> 3. Recheck your résumé or curriculum vitae for
>   a. emphasis
>   b. new information
> 4. Practice using "action" words
> 5. Decide about
>   a. appearance
>   b. key points
>   (1) to make
>   (2) to learn
>   c. format for quick check (for example, a file card with key points)
> 6. Arrive on time and alone
> 7. Make a memorable entrance:
>   a. make eye contact
>   b. shake hands
>   c. smile
>   d. say "Hello, I'm (name)"
> 8. Position yourself with the interviewer
> 9. Keep in mind your key points
> 10. Appear interested—project confidence, energy, and ability
> 11. Accentuate the positive!
> 12. Answer questions directly, or know when not to
> 13. Ask for more information
> 14. Say only positive things about your present employer
> 15. Thank interviewer, at the time and later
> 16. Write thank you
> 17. Let interviewer know your decision
> 18. Put commitments in writing

The closing comment should convey optimism—that is, you anticipate being interviewed. If you want to *assure* yourself of having an additional opportunity to sell yourself, you should indicate when you will follow up with a phone call.

The letter should include your name as it appears on your résumé or curriculum vitae, and your address and telephone number(s). It is especially helpful to designate both daytime and evening telephone numbers. Quality bond paper reflects the image you wish

---

Box 26-9

Questions to Ask/To be Asked

1. What kinds of experiences did you have in your _____ program? [new graduates]
2. Why did you select that type of program? [new graduate]
3. Tell me what your strengths are.
4. What can you contribute to *this* position? *This* organization?
5. Tell me what you believe to be a major ethical dilemma. What would you do in such a situation?
6. Why should I hire you?
7. What do you expect to get from this position?
8. What do you expect to be doing in 3 years?
9. What do you do best?
10. What would people who report to you say was your best ability? Your worst?
11. If I met your current manager at a special function and mentioned your name, what would he or she say in 10 seconds or less?
12. What do you like best about your present (last) job? Least?
13. How do you reach decisions in relation to your job?
14. What have you done for your professional development?
15. What do you like to do to relax?
16. How did you prepare for this interview?
17. How does this position fit with your goals?
18. What criteria are you using to evaluate and choose a position?
19. What are some adjectives that describe you?
20. How do you handle criticism?
21. What is your philosophy of nursing care?
22. Describe how you interact with physicians. Nurses. Assistive personnel.
23. Have you ever reported anyone for improper care? How did you feel about it?
24. How would your peers describe you—as a leader?
    as a member of the profession?
    as a manager?
    as a nurse?
    as a follower?
25. Picture this situation: (a typical one). How would you respond?
26. What percentage of registered nurses belong to the state nurses' association? To the specialty association in your clinical field?
27. Who chairs your peer review committee? Quality committee?

*From Bronstein & Hisrich (1983).

---

to portray. A printed letterhead can be used, but it is not necessary. If you have a business card, you can enclose it, paper-clipped to the letter and résumé or curriculum vitae. Only blue or black ink or ballpoint pens should be used for signature.

If you already know the person, it may be easy to use first names in conversation. Using the appropriate title and last name is generally more acceptable for written communication, however. A personal note, using the person's first name, can be handwritten on an enclosed note or at the bottom of the letter.

■ THE INTERVIEW

Box 26-8 provides key activities to help you prepare for an interview. Box 26-9 presents questions you may want to ask (e.g., questions 26 and 27), questions that will be asked of you (e.g., questions 4 and 20), and questions that can serve either the interviewer or interviewee when modified. For example, question 6 can be reworded to ask, "Why should I work for you?"; question 9 can be something each of you wants to know about the other.

> ## Box 26-10
> ### Sample of Inappropriate Questions
>
> 1. How old are you?
> 2. What does your husband (wife) do?
> 3. Who takes care of your children?
> 4. Are you working "just to help out"?
> 5. Do you have any handicaps?
> 6. Where were you born?
> 7. What are the names of all organizations to which you belong?
> 8. What is your religious preference?

Interview Topics and Questions of Concern

During interviews, employers should ask all applicants for a given position the same questions. In addition to providing comparable information as the basis for a decision, the applicant's expectation for equal treatment is upheld. Only questions related to the position and its description are legitimate. Employers should not ask other questions (see Box 26-10), and applicants should express appropriate concern if asked such inappropriate questions.

If the interviewer asked an inappropriate question, the applicant can choose not to answer the direct question by addressing the content area. For example, if asked about your spouse's employment, you might say, "I believe what you are asking is how long I will be able to be in this position. Let me assure you that I intend to be here for at least 2 years."

Each of the content areas in Box 26-10 may be acceptable, but the question as phrased is inappropriate. The following examples are ways to verify/secure the information as an employer, in a manner that is both appropriate and legal.

1. Do you know that this position requires someone at least 21 years old?
2. This position requires that no one in your immediate family be in the healthcare field or own interest/shares in any healthcare facility. Does this pose a problem for you?
3. Attendance is important. Are you able to meet this expectation?

4. What are your short-term and long-term goals?
5. Is there anything that would prevent you from performing this work as described?
6. This position requires U.S. citizenship. May I assume you meet this criterion?
7. What professional organizations do you belong to?
8. As you have read in our philosophy, we subscribe to a Christian philosophy. Do you understand that all employees are expected to promote that philosophy?

The key to assuring a fair interviewing process is being prepared ahead of time and knowing what can be asked legitimately and what a reasonable answer is.

The Successful Thank You

This may be the last chance you have to sell yourself. As a result, careful thought should be given to what you need to say in your "thank-you" letter.

Use the full inside address (name, title, division/department, organization's name and address). This action conveys accuracy and detail. The greeting should use the title the interviewer prefers (ask the personnel office/secretary). It should read: "Dear Mr./Ms./Dr./Miss/Mrs./Ms. (last name):". The lead sentence should recall the interview date and purpose so the reader can place you. If you discussed more than one position, list your preference first or follow it with "as well as other positions."

To help the interviewer remember you, the body of the letter should focus on some key point the interviewer defined as crucial and your abilities to focus on that point. Use "action" words in describing your "fit" in this organization.

Your closing should reference specific time frames if necessary, for example, when you are available. Be sure to sign your full name above a typed name with credentials including degrees.

Proof the letter for layout, typographical errors, spelling, and content. Mail it promptly. The interviewer should receive it within a week of the interview if it is to be most effective. You may also want to add a handwritten note to someone who was exceptionally helpful.

Epilogue:
Thriving in the Future

Leading and managing in nursing constitute a consistent challenge. Nurses who choose to be followers find that the new demands call for sporadic leadership and increased self-management skills. More importantly, the work of the future is being accomplished in teams, and a strong team does not emerge from weak members. You may have heard President Harry S. Truman's often quoted phrase, "The buck stops here." But Michael Hammer, author of *Beyond Reengineering*, in a videotape, "The Secrets of Shared Leadership," says "The buck stops everywhere!" Nurses who seek leadership opportunities will find that there are many available . . . in the employment setting, in professional organizations, and in voluntary, community organizations. Balancing the multiple demands in an era of rapid changes and the resultant new expectations becomes an even greater challenge. To be valued in the future, it is important to know what predictions about the future might encompass. As Rosabeth Moss Kanter (1997) says, "Security no longer comes from being employed. It comes from being employable."

VISIONING

Whether you are a leader, a follower, or a manager, being able to visualize in your mind what the ideal future is becomes a critical strategy. Sigma Theta Tau used a "think tank" approach to creating its vision (Sigma Theta Tau, 1997). The report, commonly called the *Arista* II *Report*, sets expectations for the organization and for the profession in relation to creating nursing's contribution toward healthy communities. A vision can range from that of an individual to that of a group or to a whole organization. But, as Tyrrell (1994) says, "we must engage in open dialogues about them" (p. 93). Peter Senge, author of *The Fifth Discipline: The Art and Practice of the Learning Organization* (1990), says that all leadership is really about is people working at their best to create the future.

This epilogue is designed to share some views about the future so that you can think about them in relation to what it means to lead and manage. This "thinking about" the future, like visions, is further enriched through sharing in open dialogues.

Although no one knows the future for certain, there are many entities that engage in formal discussions and predictions. These range from structured groups, such as the World Future Society, to regular reports such as CNN's Sunday afternoon program, "Future Watch." But not everyone is a futurist. What is important to us all, however, is that we are aware of

trends. As Mintzberg (1994) says, strategy-making is an ongoing process that cannot be structured. Thinking about the future should be mind expanding; it is the most nonstereotypical thinking you can do. The leader of tomorrow, as Porter-O'Grady (1997) says, will be "a gatherer of people and a facilitator of the processes that they might use to come to agreement or to find common ground with regard to an issue or direction" (p. 18).

If the future is about teams and group work (which it is), there are many implications for nursing. For example, what will evaluations and compensation be like in the future? Will you receive favorable reviews because the group you work with is productive? Will a group of us receive a bonus or merit salary increase? If you are not a team player, will you be useful to the organization at all? This is one example of how to rethink the future.

SHARED VISIONS

The concept of shared visions suggests that several of us buy into a particular view. If we think of a familiar concept, *stress*, and what Selye (1976) described as *eustress* and *distress*, we have a continuum (see figure below).

Eustress   Distress

←——————————————————→

Stress

Again, if you think about stress, you recall that each of us views an event differently and that having no stress results in death. Comparably, we can think about how society is evolving currently. Stability and total chaos are the ends of a continuum. Moving in some way between those two ends suggests we live in a constant state of disequilibrium in which we strive toward stability but recognize we experience chaos. The figure below suggests that in times of great stability, society makes little progress (but life probably seems serene). In times of great chaos, in contrast, society may transform itself (and life may seem uncontrollable). Today we are closer to chaos than we are to stability. Thus, it is even more important to think about the projections for the future.

Stability   Chaos

←——————————————————→

Society

PROJECTIONS FOR THE FUTURE

If you watch CNN's "Future Watch," or read Tom Peter's *Fast Forward*, *Trend Letter*, *The Futurist* (The World Society publication), or Popcorn's *Clicking* (1996), you will find comparable themes about the future. The following are some forecasts for the future that could affect nursing:

- Knowledge will change dramatically, requiring that we all be dedicated learners.
- Technology will continue to revolutionize healthcare.
- Increasing diversity will result in:
  - More people who are older.
  - More people moving to different parts of the country or the world.
  - More need for speaking two or three languages.
- People no longer are satisfied with service—they want an experience.
- There will be increased violence and simultaneously an increased expectation for civility.
- Stores will be either very small or huge.
- Macromarketing (targeting masses) is out; micromarketing (targeting specific populations) is in.
- Job security is out; career options are in.
- Competition is out; cooperation is in.
- Work will be sporadic.
- More people will be living with chronic diseases.
- Emphasis on prevention will redirect care efforts.
- Work will be accomplished by teams.
- Everyone must be a leader.

IMPLICATIONS

So should we be concerned with these forecasts? Are they likely to come true? Cornish (1997) analyzed the predictions from the February 1967 issue of *The Futurist*. Of the 34 forecasts that could be judged, 23 were accurate, and 11 were not. However, some of the 11 were accurate trends that did not meet the targeted date, frequently due to shifting national priorities such as funding. If this is true historically, we might assume that forecasting, which becomes better refined each year, will continue to be a valuable tool for the future. For those who want to thrive, the future forecasts are like the gold ring on the merry-go-round. If you risk and reach far enough, you can! Lead on . . . Adelánte!

REFERENCES

Cornish, E. (January-February, 1997). The Futurist forecasts 30 years later. *The Futurist*, 45-48.

Kanter, R.M. (1997). In *Changing Workplace Alert*, Sample Issue, p. 7.

Mintzberg, H. (1994). The fall and rise of strategic planning. *Harvard Business Review*, 72, 107-114.

Popcorn, F. (1996). *Clicking: 16 Trends to Future Fit Your Life, Work and Business*. New York: Harper Collins.

Porter-O'Grady, T. (1997). Quantum mechanics and the future of healthcare leadership. JONA, 27(15-20).

Selye, H. (1976). *The Stress of Life*. New York: McGraw-Hill.

Senge, P. (1990). *The Fifth Discipline: The Art and Practice of the Learning Organization*. New York: Doubleday Currency.

Sigma Theta Tau International. (1997). *Nursing Leadership in the 21st Century: A Report of Arista II*. Indianapolis: Sigma Theta Tau.

Tyrrell, R.A. (1994). Visioning: An important management tool. *Nursing Economics*, 12, 93-96.

SUGGESTED READING

Begun, J.W. & White, K.R. (1995). Altering nursing's dominant logic: guidelines from complex adaptive systems theory. *Complexity and Chaos in Nursing*, 2(1), 5-15.

Glossary

Absenteeism The rate at which an individual misses work on an unplanned basis. (Ch. 20)

Acceptance The second phase of the change process when change is willingly used.

Accommodation An unassertive, cooperative approach to conflict in which the individual neglects personal needs, goals, and concerns in favor of satisfying those of others. (Ch. 19)

Accountability The expectation of explaining actions and results. (Ch. 18)

Acknowledgement Recognition that an employee is valued and respected for what he or she has to offer to the work place, team, or group; acknowledgements may be verbal or written, public or private. (Ch. 17)

Active listening Focusing completely on the speaker and listening without judgment to the essence of the conversation; an active listener should be able to repeat accurately at least 95% of the speaker's intended meaning. (Ch. 17)

Advocacy Multidimensional concept that refers to acting on or in behalf of another who is unable to act for himself or herself.

Agenda A written list of items to be covered in a meeting and the related materials that meeting participants should read beforehand or bring along. Types of agendas include structured agendas, timed agendas, and action agendas. (Ch. 12)

Apparent agency Doctrine whereby a principal becomes accountable for the actions of his or her agent; created when a person holds himself or herself out as acting in behalf of the principal; also known *as apparent authority.* (Ch. 3)

Assertions Statements about the truth of a matter; often these are only assumptions, postulations, or individual points of view that have little or no basis in fact or relevant evidence. (Ch. 15)

Associate nurse A licensed nurse in the primary nursing system who provides care to the patient according to the primary nurse's specification while the primary nurse is not working. (Ch. 22)

Autonomy Personal freedom and the right to choose what will happen to one's own person. (Ch. 3)

Average length of stay The number of patient days in a specific time period divided by the number of discharges in that same time period. (Ch. 23)

Avoiding An unassertive, uncooperative approach to conflict in which the avoider neither pursues his or her own needs, goals, and concerns nor helps others to do so. (Ch. 19)

Awareness The first phase of the change process when the need for change or innovation emerges.

Barrier A factor, internal or external to the change situation, that interferes with movement toward a desirable outcome. (Ch. 5)

Beneficence Principle that states that the actions one takes should promote good. (Ch. 3)

Biomedical technology The use of machines and implantable devices to provide physiologic monitoring, diagnostic testing, drug administration, and therapeutic treatments in patient care. (Ch. 13)

Budget A detailed financial plan, stated in dollars, for carrying out the activities an organization wants to accomplish in a specific period of time. (Ch. 14)

Budgeting process An ongoing activity of planning and managing revenues and expenses in order to meet the goals of the organization. (Ch. 14)

Bureaucratic organization Characterized by formality, low autonomy, a hierarchy of authority, an environment of rules, division of labor, specialization, centralization, and control. (Ch. 9)

Burnout Disengagement from work characterized by emotional exhaustion, depersonalization, and decreased effectiveness. (Ch. 12)

Capital expenditure budget A plan for purchasing major capital items, such as equipment or a physical plant, with a useful life greater than 1 year and exceeding a minimum cost set by the organization. (Ch. 14)

Capitation A reimbursement method where healthcare providers are paid a per person per year (or per month) fee for providing specified services over a period of time. (Ch. 14)

Care delivery strategy A method nurses use to provide care to patients and clients. (Ch. 22)

CareMAP An abbreviation for a care multidisciplinary action plan, which combines a nursing care plan with a critical path. The purpose is to expedite patient care by improving the expected outcome during a designated day. (Ch. 22)

Career Progressive achievement throughout a person's professional life. (Ch. 26)

Caring Behaviors and attitudes that denote special concern, interest, and/or feeling.

Case management A person-oriented service that reflects multidisciplinary cooperation and coordination. (Ch. 2)

Case management method A method of delivering patient care based on patient outcomes and cost containment. Components of case management are a case manager, critical paths, and unit-based managed care. (Ch. 22)

Case manager A baccalaureate or master's degree prepared clinical nurse who coordinates patient care from preadmission to and through discharge. (Ch. 22)

Case method A method of care delivery in which one nurse provides total care for one patient during an entire work period. (Ch. 22)

Case mix The volume and type of patients served by a healthcare provider. (Ch. 14)

Cash budget A plan for an organization's cash receipts and disbursements. (Ch. 14)

Centers for Disease Control and Prevention The federal agency. (Ch. 10)

Certification Designation of special knowledge beyond basic licensure. (Ch. 26)

Change Any condition or circumstance that is new or different from what existed previously. (Ch. 5)

Change agent Synonymous with change leader. (Ch. 5)

Change complexity continuum A progression of levels of change ranging from low to high complexity determined by the rapidity and quantity of factors present and interacting in a change situation. (Ch. 5)

Change leader An individual with formal or informal legitimate power whose purpose is to initiate, champion, and direct or guide change. (Ch. 5)

Change management The overall processes and strategies used to moderate and manage the preparation for, impact of, responses to, and outcomes of any condition or circumstance that is new or different from what existed previously. (Ch. 5)

Change models Structured approaches selected to guide change management. (Ch. 5)

Change outcome The end product of a change process. (Ch. 5)

Change principles Generally accepted truths predicting that applying a particular action will result in a specific outcome.

Change process The series of ongoing efforts applied to managing a change. (Ch. 5)

Change situation The field composed of various factors and dynamics within which change is occurring. (Ch. 5)

Chaos theory Theoretical construct defining the random-appearing, yet deterministic characteristics of complex organizations (see *Nonlinear change*). (Ch. 5)

Charge nurse A registered nurse responsible for delegating and coordinating patient care and staff on a specific unit. A resource person for all staff, there is usually one charge nurse each shift. (Ch. 22)

Charges The cost of providing a service plus a markup for profit. (Ch. 14)

Chemically dependent A psychophysiological state in which an individual requires a substance such as drugs or alcohol to prevent the onset of symptoms of abstinence. (Ch. 20)

Coaching The strategy a manager uses to help others learn, think critically, and grow through communications about performance. (Ch. 16)

Coalitions Groups of individuals or organizations that join together temporarily around a common goal. This goal often focuses on an effort to effect change. (Ch. 25)

Collaboration Conjoint, interdisciplinary problem solving from an equal power base on the client's behalf; also, an assertive, cooperative approach to conflict in which the individual is able to work creatively and openly with others to find the solution that best achieves all important goals. (Ch. 19)

Collective action A mechanism for achieving professional practice through group decision making. (Ch. 10)

Collective bargaining Mechanism for settling labor disputes by negotiation between the employer and representatives of the employees. (Ch. 10) (Ch. 3)

Commitment A state of being emotionally impelled; feeling passionate about and dedicated to a project or event. (Ch. 17)

Common law System of jurisprudence that is derived from principles rather than rules and regulations and that consists of comprehensive principles based on justice, reason, and common sense. (Ch. 3)

Community health information networks An electronic highway that provides access to data that have been collected and stored in a central data repository. (Ch. 13)

Competing An assertive, uncooperative approach to conflict in which the individual pursues his or her own needs at the expense of others. (Ch. 19)

Complaints Statements in which one asserts that a prior promise has been broken and requests that a new promise be made to complete the prior promise. (Ch. 15)

Compliments Statements that show appreciation or gratitude to a person who has accomplished goals and/or achieved results in accordance with a prior agreement. (Ch. 15)

Compromising A moderately assertive, cooperative approach to conflict in which the individual's ability to negotiate and willingness to "give and take" results in conflict resolution and fulfillment of important priorities for all involved.

Computerized patient record Technology allowing for immediate and complete access to patient information for clinical decision making, outcome evaluation, and coordination of patient care resources and patient flow through the healthcare delivery system. (Ch. 13)

Confidentiality Right of privacy to the medical record of a patient or client; also, a respect for the privacy of information and the ethical use of information for its original purpose. (Ch. 13) (Ch. 3)

Conflict A perceived difference among people and a four-stage process including frustration, conceptualization, action, and outcomes. (Ch. 19)

Consent A voluntary action by which one agrees to allow someone else to do something; may be oral, written, or implied based on the circumstances.

Consolidated systems A group of healthcare organizations that are united based on common characteristics of ownership, regional location, or mutual performance objectives for the purpose of optimizing utilization of their resources in achieving their missions. (Ch. 7)

Constructive confrontation A means by which group or team members can deal with issues by openly expressing their ideas and feelings, thereby using interactive skills to accomplish tasks and improve outcomes. (Ch. 17)

Consumer focus Centering of action or attention on the participant or user as a whole. (Ch. 21)

Continuing education Those learning activities intended to build upon the educational and experiential bases of the professional nurse for the enhancement of practice, education, administration, research, or theory development to the end of improving the health of the public (ANCC, 1991, p. 76).

Continuous quality improvement (CQI) A program designed to improve the quality of care. Also, an ongoing process that involves a multidisciplinary team for planning or problem solving. Similar to quality improvement but emphasizes the continuous nature of the process. (Ch. 11)

Contractual allowance A discount from full charges. (Ch. 14)

Controversy A situation in which opinions, ideas, information, theories, and conclusions are perceived as incompatible with those of another person or group (Johnson & Johnson, 1997). (Ch. 19)

Coping The immediate response of a person to a threatening situation. (Ch. 12)

Co-primary nursing See *partnership model.* (Ch. 22)

Cost The amount spent on something; the national healthcare costs are a function of the price and utilization of healthcare services; a healthcare provider's costs are the expenses involved in providing goods or services. (Ch. 14)

Cost-based reimbursement A retrospective payment method where all allowable costs are used as the basis for payment. (Ch. 14)

Cost center An organizational unit for which costs can be identified and managed. (Ch. 14)

Creativity Conceptualizing new and innovative approaches to solving problems or making decisions. (Ch. 6)

Critical path A component of a care MAP that is specific to diagnosis-related group reimbursement. The purpose is to ensure patients are discharged before insurance reimbursement is eliminated. (Ch. 22)

Critical thinking A composite of knowledge, attitudes, and skills; an intellectually disciplined process. Also, the ability to assess a situation by asking open-ended questions about the facts and assumptions that underlie it and to use personal judgment and problem-solving ability in deciding how to deal with it. (Ch. 6)

Cross-culturalism Involving or mediating between two cultures, one's own and that of another (Simons et al, 1993). (Ch. 8)

Cultural diversity A vast range of cultural differences related to institutional, ethnic, gender, religious, or other variables that convey a set of beliefs or values that have become factors needing attention in living and working together. Often applied to an organization that seeks to deal with the interface of people who are different from each other (Simons et al, 1993). (Ch. 8)

Cultural sensitivity The capacity to feel, convey, or react to ideas, habits, attitudes, customs, or traditions that help to create standards for a group of people to coexist. (Ch. 8)

Culture A way of life. It is developed and communicated by a group of people, consciously or unconsciously, to subsequent generations. It consists of ideas, habits, attitudes, customs, and traditions that help to create standards for a group of people to coexist. It makes a group of people unique (Simons et al, 1993). (Ch. 10) (Ch. 8)

Culture broker One who interprets, mediates, and/or negotiates cultural or racial differences between people. (Ch. 21)

Curriculum vitae A listing of professional life activities. (Ch. 26)

Cybernetics Regulation of systems by managing communication and feedback mechanisms. (Ch. 5)

Data Discrete entities that describe or measure something without interpretation. (Ch. 13)

Data processing Structuring, organizing, and interpreting of data into information. (Ch. 13)

Database A collection of data elements organized and stored together. (Ch. 13)

Decision making Purposeful and goal-directed effort using a systematic process to choose among options. (Ch. 6)

Declarations Statements that create and describe a new set of available possibilities. (Ch. 15)

Defendant The party against whom a suit is brought; in a criminal action, the person accused of committing a crime.

Delegatee The individual who becomes accountable for performing delegated activities. (Ch. 18)

Delegation Achieving performance of care outcomes for which an individual is accountable and responsible by sharing activities with other individuals who have the appropriate authority to accomplish the work. (Ch. 18) (Ch. 12)

Delegator The individual with authority to share activities with another. (Ch. 18)

Deontologic theory From the Greek for "duty," derived norms and rules from the duties that human beings owe one another by virtue of commitments made and roles assumed; has sometimes been subdivided into situational ethical theory. (Ch. 3)

Depersonalization Inability to become involved in human relationships and interactions. (Ch. 12)

Descriptive/behavioral model A problem-solving/decision-making approach used when not all options or consequences are known; as uncertainty exists, options that are acceptable are chosen. (Ch. 6)

Diagnostic testing Systems that provide ongoing information for the establishment of diagnoses from data such as blood gases, pulmonary functions, intracranial pressure, and drug levels.

Differentiated Nursing Practice Recognizing a difference in the level of education and competency of each registered nurse. The differentiation is based on education, position, and clinical expertise. (Ch. 22)

Drug Administration Systems Equipment that can be programmed to deliver medication at a preestablished rate for a defined period. (Ch. 13)

Dualism An "either/or" way of conceptualizing reality in terms of two opposing sides or parts (right or wrong, yes or no), limiting the broad spectrum of possibilities that exists between. (Ch. 17)

Emancipated minor Persons under the age of adulthood who are no longer under the control and regulation of their parents and who may give valid consent for medical procedures; examples include married teens, under-aged parents, and teens in the armed services. (Ch. 3)

Employee Assistance Programs Programs designed to provide counseling and other services for employees through either in-house staff or a contracted mental health agency. (Ch. 12)

Empowerment A sharing of power and control with the expectation that people are responsible for themselves; also, the process by which we facilitate the participation of others in decision making and taking within an environment where there is an equitable distribution of power. (Ch. 25) (Ch. 16) (Ch. 10)

Environmental influences Factors, internal or external to an organization, that positively or negatively influence the movement of the change process toward a desired outcome. (Ch. 5)

Ethics Science relating to moral actions and moral values; rules of conduct recognized in respect to a particular class of human actions. (Ch. 13) (Ch. 3)

Ethics committees Groups of persons who provide structure and guidelines for potential healthcare problems, serve as an open forum for discussion, and function as patient advocates. (Ch. 3)

Ethnocentrism Using the culture of one's own groups as a standard for the judgment of others, or thinking of it as superior to other cultures that are merely different (Simons et al, 1993). (Ch. 8)

Expected outcomes The result of patient goals that are achieved through a combination of medical and nursing interventions with patient participation. (Ch. 22)

Expert system A program that mimics the inductive and deductive reasoning of a human expert. (Ch. 13)

Expert witness Person testifying who has special knowledge about a given subject or occupation; knowledge of an expert witness must generally be such that it is not normally possessed by the average person; contrasts with a lay witness. (Ch. 3)

Facilitator A factor, internal or external to the change situation, that promotes movement toward a desired outcome. (Ch. 5)

Factor evaluation A patient classification system that incorporates specific elements or critical indicators and rates patients on each of these elements. Each indicator is assigned a weight or numerical value. (Ch. 23)

Failure to warn Newer area of potential liability for nurse managers that involves the responsibility to warn subsequent or potential employers of nurses' incompetence or impairment. (Ch. 3)

Fee-for-service See Fee-for-service system. (Ch. 7)

Fee-for-service system A system in which patients have the option of consulting any healthcare provider, subject to reasonable requirements that may include utilization review and prior approval for certain services, but does not include a requirement to seek approval through a gatekeeper. (Ch. 7)

Fidelity Keeping one's promises or commitments. (Ch. 3)

Fit The possession of characteristics that are suitable to the work that is to be carried out and the technologies by which the work is to be accomplished. (Ch. 9)

Five-why technique Asking the question "Why?" at least five times to attempt to get to the root of a problem. (Ch. 11)

Fixed costs Costs that do no change in total as the volume of patients changes. (Ch. 14)

Flat organization Characterized by decentralization of decision making to the level of personnel carrying out the work. (Ch. 9)

Follower A person who contributes to a group's outcomes by implementing activities and providing appropriate feedback. (Ch. 2)

Followership Those with whom a leader interacts; involves the assertive use of personal behaviors in contributing toward organizational outcomes, while still acquiescing certain tasks to the leader or other team members. (Ch. 10) (Ch. 1)

Foreseeability Concept that certain events may reasonably be expected to cause specific consequences; third element of negligence/malpractice. (Ch. 3)

For-profit Term used when financial gains are distributed to stockholders.

Full-time equivalent (FTE) An employee who works full-time, 40 hours per week, 2,080 hours per year. (Ch. 14) (Ch. 23)

Functional leadership A theory of leadership based on task and maintenance behaviors, in which every member of a group contributes verbally and/or nonverbally to the group at a particular time. (Ch. 15)

Functional nursing Care provided by each member providing a specific task for a large group of patients. (Ch. 22)

Gatekeeper Liaison between the consumer and the healthcare market. (Ch. 21)

General Adaptation Syndrome A pattern of response to stress (Selye, 1956). (Ch. 12)

Group A number of individuals assembled together or having a unifying relationship. (Ch. 17)

Governance System by which an organization controls and directs formulation and administration of policy. (Ch. 10)

Halo or Recency Effect Only positive (halo) or recent (recency) performances are acknowledged. (Ch. 16)

Healthcare consumer Client/patient/customer that uses healthcare provider resources. (Ch. 21)

Healthcare provider Agencies, insurers, physicians, nurses, allied health people providing health-related business to consumers. (Ch. 21)

Hierarchy Chain of command that connotes authority and responsibility. (Ch 9)

High-complexity change A complicated change situation characterized by the interactions of multiple variables of people, technology, and systems. (Ch. 5)

High tech Mechanistic perspective that relates to the use of technology in the diagnosis and treatment of disease. (Ch. 21)

High touch Caring, humanistic perspective that relates to the use of human skills in the care and treatment of patients. (Ch. 21)

Hospital information system A large integrated computer system that focuses on hospital processes. (Ch. 13)

Hybrid organization Possessing characteristics from several types of organizational structures. (Ch. 9)

Hygiene factors Factors that motivate workers by meeting safety and security needs and helping prevent job dissatisfaction. These include working conditions, salary, status, and security. (Ch. 1)

Indemnification Obligation resting on one person to make good any loss or damages another has incurred because of the person's actions or non-actions; refers to the total shifting of the economic loss to the party chiefly responsible for that loss. (Ch. 3)

Independent contractor One who makes an agreement with another to perform a service or piece of work and retains in himself/herself control of the means, method, and manner of producing the result to be accomplished; sometimes called an independent practitioner. (Ch. 3)

Influence The process of using power; may range from the punitive power of coercion to the interactive power of collaboration. (Ch. 25)

Informatics The use of knowledge technology. (Ch. 13)

Information Communication of reception of knowledge, consisting of interpreted, organized, or structured data. (Ch. 13)

Information overload A state of stress brought about by a lack of information processing skills. (Ch. 12)

Information technology The use of computer hardware and software to process data into information to solve problems. (Ch. 13)

Informed consent Authorization by patient or patient's legal representative to do something to the patient. (Ch. 3)

Innovation See *Change*. (Ch. 5)

Innovator One who leads a change. (Ch. 5)

Integrated systems Computer systems that link one mainframe containing a central data base with terminals or personal computers in all departments of the organization. (Ch. 13)

Interpersonal conflict Conflict that occurs between or among people. (Ch. 19)

Intrapersonal conflict Conflict that occurs within the individual. (Ch. 19)

Justice Principle that person should be treated equally and fairly. (Ch. 3)

Knowledge Information that is combined or synthesized so that interrelationships are identified. (Ch. 13)

Knowledge base Produces decisions in standard manner for administrative and clinical decisions. (Ch. 13)

Knowledge technology The use of expert and decision support systems to assist in making decisions about patient care delivery. (Ch. 13)

Labor Acts Examples of these federal mandates include the 1935 Wagner Act, which established election procedures for collective bargaining representatives, and the 1947 Taft-Hartley Act, which placed curbs on some union activity and excluded employees of not-for-profit hospitals from coverage. (Ch. 10)

Labor union Association of workers that exists for the purpose of bargaining, either in whole or in part, on behalf of the workers with management about the terms of employment. (Ch. 3)

Law Sum total of rules and regulations by which a society is governed; rules and regulations established and enforced by authority or custom within a given community, state, or nation. (Ch. 3)

Leader A person who demonstrates and exercises influence and power over others. (Ch. 2)

Leadership the use of personal traits to constructively and ethically influence patients, families, and staff through a *process* where clinical and organizational outcomes are achieved through collective efforts. (Ch. 1)

Learning organization The designation of a type of organization where continual learning as an expectation permeates all levels to promote adequate responses required by dynamic, accelerated change. (Ch. 5)

Liable Refers to one's responsibility for his or her actions or inactions. (Ch. 3)

Licensure A right granted that gives the licensee permission to do something that he or she could not legally do absent such permission. Also, the minimum form of credentialing, providing baseline expectations for those in a particular field without identifying or obligating the practitioner to function in a professional manner as defined by the profession itself. (Ch. 26)

Low complexity change An uncomplicated change situation characterized by the interactions of the limited influences of people, technology, and systems. (Ch. 5)

Mainframe computer The largest, fastest computer that can collect, store, and process large amounts of data. (Ch. 13)

Malpractice Failure of a professional person to act in accordance with the prevalent professional standards or failure to foresee potential consequences that a professional person, having the necessary skills and expertise to act in a professional manner, should foresee. (Ch. 3)

Managed care Care purchased through a public or private healthcare organization whose goal is to promote quality healthcare outcomes for its clients at the lowest cost possible through planning, directing, and coordinating care delivered by healthcare organizations that it may own, have contractual agreements with, or have authority over by virtue of the fact that it reimburses the organization for services provided its clients. This model rewards healthcare providers for low utilization of care that is relatively low in cost; also, a system of care in which a designated person determines the services the patient uses. (Ch. 14) (Ch. 7) (Ch. 2)

Management The activities needed to plan, organize, motivate, and control the human and material resources needed to achieve outcomes consistent with the organization's mission and purpose.

Management theory The theory related to the activities described in management. (See above) (Ch. 1)

Manager A person who directs a team of workers. (Ch. 2)

Marketing Analysis, planning, implementation, and control of programs for the purpose of meeting organizational objectives. (Ch. 4)

Matrix organization An organizational structure influenced by dual authority such as product line and discipline. (Ch. 9)

Mentor An experienced adult who helps someone younger navigate into expertise. (Ch. 10, 24)

Mission Statement of an organization's reason for being. (Ch 9, 17)

Modular method A modified team nursing approach focused on geographic location of patient rooms and assignment of staff members. (Ch. 22)

MORAL Mode An ethical decision-making model consisting of five distinct steps. (Ch. 3)

Motivator factors Factors that promote job enrichment by creating job satisfaction. These include achievement, recognition, and the satisfaction of the work itself. (Ch. 1)

Multiculturalism Maintaining several different cultures. (Ch. 8)

Negligence Failure to exercise the degree of care that a person of ordinary prudence, based upon the reasonable person standard, would exercise under the same or similar circumstances; also known as ordinary negligence. (Ch. 3)

Negotiating Conferring with others to bring about a settlement of differences. (Ch 9, 25)

Network A resource of colleagues upon whom you can draw for advice, a formal system to provide services. (Ch. 7) (Ch. 25)

Networked systems Several computers that are supported by another computer that acts as a file server. (Ch. 13)

Nonlinear change Change occurring from self-organizing patterns, not human-induced ones, in complex, open system organizations.

Nonmaleficence Principle that states that one should do no harm. (Ch. 3)

Nonproductive hours See *Nonproductive time*. (Ch. 14)

Nonproductive time Benefit time such as vacation or sick time. (Ch. 23)

Nonpunitive discipline A disciplinary measure, usually verbal, describing existing standards and goals to which the parties agreed; pay is not withheld; employee either agrees to adhere to the standards in the future or to be terminated. (Ch. 20)

Norms Authoritative standard that guides behavior. (Ch. 15)

Normative/prescription model An anlytical approach to finding the ideal option or solution, used when options and consequences are known. (Ch. 6)

Not for profit Organization that has funds redirected to maintenance and growth rather than as dividends to stockholders. (Ch. 7)

Nurse practice act Legal scope of practice allowed by state legislation and authority. (Ch. 3)

Nursing administration systems Administrative data, such as census, personnel and forecasting data that have been automated. (Ch. 13)

Nursing governance The methodology or system by which an organized department of nursing controls and directs the formulation and administration of policy.

Nursing information system (NIS) A system that uses computers to process nursing data. (Ch. 13)

Nursing minimum data set Uniform standard for collecting comparable essential patient data. (Ch. 13)

On-line interactive systems Organizational level patient information systems. (Ch. 13)

Operating budget A financial plan for day-to-day activities of an organization. (Ch. 14)

Optimizing decision Selecting the most ideal solution or option to achieve goals. (Ch. 6)

Organizational conflict Conflict that occurs when a person confronts an organization's policies and procedures for patient care and personnel and its accepted norms of behavior and communication. (Ch. 19)

Organizational structure A framework that divides work within an organization and delineates points of authority, responsibility, accountability, and non-decision-making support. (Ch. 9)

Organized delivery system Networks of healthcare organizations, providers, and payers who provide a comprehensive package of healthcare services at a competitive price. (Ch. 14)

Organizational chart A graphic representation of the chain of command. (Ch. 9)

Orientation The initial development of new employees to make them "job-ready."

Outcome criteria See *Expected outcomes*. (Ch. 22)

Overwork A situation in which employees are expected to become more productive without additional resources. (Ch. 12)

Paid time A combination of productive and nonproductive hours. (Ch. 23)

Paraphrase An oral rephrasing of the original communication in one's own word. (Ch. 15)

Partnership Interaction built on common goals, concerns, intentions, aspirations, and/or problems. (Ch. 15)

Partnership model A system of providing patient care when an RN is paired with an LPN or an unlicensed assistive person to provide total care to a number of patients. (Ch. 22)

Paternalism Principle that allows one to make decisions for another; often called *parentalism*. (Ch. 3)

Patient care standard The hours of patient care per patient day. Also, the criteria statements related to quality of patient care.

Patient classification system A method of quantitatively estimating and assessing patient needs in relation to nursing care.

Patient day One patient occupying a bed for 1 day. (Ch. 23)

Patient focused care unit A system in which staff functions become centralized on a unit in order to reduce the number of staff required; emphasizes quality, cost, and value. (Ch. 22)

Patient outcomes See *Expected outcomes*. (Ch. 22)

Patterns of behavior Varying attitudinal and behavioral responses to change. (Ch. 5)

Payer mix The volume and type of reimbursement sources for a healthcare provider. (Ch. 14)

Payers Sources of healthcare financing or payment for health services; includes government, private insurance, and individuals (self-pay). (Ch. 14)

Percentage of occupancy The patient census divided by the number of beds actually occupied. (Ch. 23)

Perfectionism The tendency to never finish anything because it isn't quite perfect. (Ch. 12)

Performance appraisal Individual evaluation of work performance. (Ch. 16)

Personal liability Serves to make each person responsible at law for his/her own actions. (Ch. 3)

Personal motives Driving factors that are influenced by values or beliefs. (Ch. 1)

Philosophy Values and beliefs regarding nature of work derived from a mission and the rights/responsibilities of people involved. (Ch. 9)

Physiological monitoring Equipment that monitors patients' physiological functions, such as heart rate and blood pressure. (Ch. 13)

Plaintiff Party bringing a civil lawsuit seeking damages or other relief; usually synonymous with the injured patient or his/her representative. (Ch. 3)

Planned change Change expected and deliberately prepared beforehand by using systematic directional processes to develop and carry out activities to accomplish a desired outcome. (Ch. 5)

Point of Service An interconnected or free-standing unit that provides specific healthcare services. (Ch. 8).

Polarities Situations involving two interdependent opposites between which a shifting of emphasis naturally occurs. (Ch. 19)

Politics A process of human interaction within organizations. (Ch. 25)

Position description A general overall description of the duties and responsibilities of the employee. (Ch. 16)

Possibility A new future beyond the predictable extension of what already exists. (Ch. 15)

Power The ability to influence others in the effort to achieve goals. (Ch. 25)

Preceptor An experienced staff member who is paired with a less experienced preceptee in order to share expertise and serve as a role model.

Price See charges. (Ch. 14)

Primary care First access to care. (Ch. 7)

Primary nurse One who is the deliverer of autonomous care. (Ch. 22)

Primary nursing A method of patient care delivery where one registered nurse functions autonomously as the patient's main nurse throughout the entire hospital stay. (Ch. 22)

Principlism Emerging theory of ethics that incorporates existing ethical principles and attempts to resolve conflicts by applying one or more of the ethical principles. (Ch. 3)

Prioritization Placing activities in the order of their importance. (Ch. 12)

Privacy The right to protection against unreasonable and unwarranted interference with one's solitude; the right of an individual to be left alone. (Ch. 3)

Private Owned and operated by an individual citizen or group of citizens. (Ch. 7)

Problem solving Using a systematic process to solve a problem. (Ch. 6)

Procrastination Doing one thing when you should be doing something else. (Ch. 12)

Productive hours Paid time that is worked. (Ch. 14)

Productive time Time an employee actually works. (Ch.23)

Productivity The ratio of outputs to inputs or, in nursing terms, of services to resources used to provide services. (Ch. 14)

Professional association An alliance of practitioners within a profession that provides opportunities for its members to meet leaders in the field, hone their own leadership skills, participate in policy formation, continue specialized education, and shape the future of the profession. (Ch. 26)

Profit An excess of revenues over expenses. (Ch. 14)

Progressive discipline A step-by-step process of increasing disciplinary measures, usually beginning with an oral warning, followed by a written warning, suspension, and termination, if necessary. (Ch. 20)

Promises Pledges to do something, reflecting a commitment to action and a stake in getting it done. (Ch. 15)

Prospective reimbursement A method of payment where the third-party payer decides in advance the flat rate that will be paid for a service or episode of care. (Ch. 14)

Prototype system System of classifying in broad categories. (Ch. 23)

Providers See Healthcare Providers. (Ch. 14)

Public organization Organization providing health services under the support and direction of local, state, or federal government. (Ch. 7)

Quality assurance A process that focuses on the clinical aspects of a provider's care, frequently in response to an identified problem. (Ch. 11)

Quality care The end product of a process that demonstrates excellence. (Ch. 2)

Quality control On-going process of monitoring completed products and services to detect and correct deviations. Processes and products are compared to previously established norms and specifications.

Quality improvement An ongoing process of innovation, error prevention, and staff development used by an organization who has adopted quality management philosophy. (Ch. 11)

Reengineering A complete overhaul of an organizational structure. (Hammer & Champy, 1993) (Ch. 9)

Reintegration A concept that focuses on a return to the whole of nursing, incorporating all aspects of the professional nurse's role: education, scholarship, practice, and service. (Ch. 26)

Relatedness Logic that binds people together in their interactions. (Ch. 15)

Reporting statutes Laws that mandate healthcare providers or their employees to give certain information to the proper state or federal agencies.

Requests Asking others to take action for themselves and/or become active in the things the speaker asks. (Ch. 15)

Respect for others The highest ethical principle, respect for others acknowledges the right of individuals to make decisions and to live by those decisions. (Ch. 3)

Respondeat superior A doctrine by which the employer is given accountability and responsibility for an employee's negligent actions incurred during the course and scope of employment. (Ch. 3)

Responses to change The varied reactions of people, technology, systems, and organizations to change. (Ch. 5)

Responsibility The condition of being reliable and dependable and being obligated to accomplish work. (Ch. 18)

Résumé A summary of professional abilities and facts designed for specific opportunities. (Ch. 26)

Revenue Money earned by an organization for providing goods or services. (Ch. 14)

Risk management Process of developing and implementing strategies that will minimize the adverse effects of accidental losses on an organization. This includes preventing client injury, minimizing financial loss after a problem/error occurs, and preserving agency reputation. (Ch. 11)

Role Expected or actual behavior, determined by a person's position or status in a group. (Ch. 24) (Ch. 2)

Role ambiguity A condition in which individuals do not have a clear understanding about performance and evaluation. (Ch. 16)

Role conflict A condition in which individuals understand the role but are unwilling or unable to meet the requirements. (Ch. 16) (Ch. 2)

Role development Choosing to change role expectations and/or role performance. (Ch. 24)

Role discrepancy A gap between role expectations and role performance. (Ch. 24)

Role expectations The attitudes and behaviors another anticipates a person in the role will possess or demonstrate. (Ch. 24)

Role internalization The stage at which a person has learned the behaviors that maintain the role so thoroughly that the person performs them without consciously considering them; energy once spent on establishing these behaviors can now be redirected toward other goals. (Ch. 24)

Role model A person who enacts a role, typically in a positive way, so that others can follow the example. (Ch. 10)

Role negotiation Resolving conflicting expectations about personal management performance through communication. (Ch. 24)

Role strain The subjective feeling of discomfort experienced as a result of role stress; may manifest through increased frustration, heightened emotional awareness, or emotional fragility to situations. (Ch. 24) (Ch. 20)

Role stress A social condition in which role demands are conflicting, irritating, or impossible to fulfill. (Ch. 24) (Ch. 20)

Role theory A framework used to understand how individuals perform within organizations. (Ch. 16)

Role transition The process of unlearning an old role and learning a new role. Transforming one's identity from being an individual contributor as a staff nurse to being a leader as a nurse manager. (Ch. 24)

Satisficing decision Selecting an option that is acceptable, but not necessarily the best option. (Satisfy + suffice = satisfice) (Ch. 6)

Scope of practice Refers to legally permissible boundaries of practice for a health professional; the allowable boundaries are defined by statute, rule, or a combination or statute and rule. (Ch. 3)

Secondary care Disease restorative care. (Ch. 7)

Self-management The ability of individuals to actively gain control of their lives; components include stress management, time management, meeting management, and the ability to delegate. (Ch. 12)

Service In healthcare context, the interaction between a consumer and the system to the extent needs were addressed. (Ch. 21)

Service lines A functional unit of management where all related concepts of medical care are grouped. (Ch. 21)

Shared governance A term used to describe a flat type of organizational structure with decision making decentralized. (Ch. 9, 10)

Smart card Credit-card like devices that store data. (Ch. 13)

Staff mix Proportion of licensed to unlicensed personnel in a specific setting. (Ch. 22)

Staffing Matrix/Pattern A plan that outlines a number of individuals by classification needed by a unit per shift, per day. (Ch. 23)

Staffing regulations Licensing regulations required by the state department of health, usually related to the minimum number of professional nurses on a unit at a given time. (Ch. 23)

Stand-alone systems Systems internal to a department to automate processes. (Ch. 13)

Standard of care Level or degree of quality considered adequate by a given profession; skills and learning commonly possessed by members of a profession; also written at minimum level. (Ch. 3)

Statute Rule/regulation created by elected legislative bodies; also known as statutory law. (Ch. 3)

Strategic planning A process designed to achieve goals through allocation of resources. (Ch. 4)

Strategy Approaches designed to achieve a specific purpose. (Ch. 5)

Stress Perceived adversity, pressure, and/or strain related to events or anticipated events.

Synergy A phenomenon in which teamwork produces extraordinary results that could not have been achieved by any one individual. (Ch. 17)

Systems perspective Ability to detect sources of immediate problems. (Ch. 12)

Teaching institution Academic health centers and affiliated hospitals. (Ch. 7)

Team A number of people associated together in specific work or activities. (Ch. 17)

Team nursing A small group of licensed and unlicensed personnel, with a team leader, responsible for providing patient care to a group of patients. (Ch. 22)

Technology A method, process, or system for providing services. Also, a scientific method of achieving a practical purpose. (Ch. 13) (Ch. 9)

Telehealth The use of modern telecommunications and information technologies for the provision of healthcare to individuals at a distance and the transmission of information to provide that care; involves the use of two-way interactive video-conferencing, high-speed phone lines, fiber/optic cable, and satellite transmissions. (Ch. 13)

Teleological theory From the Greek for "end," derived norms and rules for conduct from the consequences of actions. (Ch. 3)

Tertiary care Rehabilitative or long-term care. (Ch. 7)

Therapeutic systems Equipment that can be programmed to calculate and regulate specific conditions/factors such as IV drip rate, arterial pressure, drug therapy, fluid resuscitation, and serum glucose levels. (Ch. 13)

Third party payers See p. 564 of ed 1. (Ch. 7)

Time management The use of tools, techniques, strategies, and follow-up systems to control wasted time and to assure that the time invested in activities leads toward achieving a desired, high-priority goal. (Ch. 12)

Total patient care See *Case method*. (Ch. 22)

Total quality management A combination of quality improvement ideas. (Ch. 11)

Transculturalism Bridging significant differences in cultural practices. (Ch. 8)

Transformational leadership An act of encouraging followers to follow your style and change their interests into a group interest with concern for a broader goal. (Ch. 2)

Triangulation A technique used by risk managers using multiple data sources and data collection to gather information about unusual occurrences. (Ch. 11)

Unit based managed care Control of costs and quality at the unit level. (Ch. 22)

Unit of service A measure of the work being produced by the organization, such as patient days, patient or home visits, or procedures. (Ch. 14)

Unlicensed assistive personnel Healthcare workers who are not licensed and who are prepared to provide certain elements of care under the supervision of a registered nurse (for example, technicians, nurse aides, or certified nursing assistants). (Ch. 22)

Utilization The quantity or volume of services provided. (Ch. 14)

Values Inner force that influence decision making and priority setting. Ch. 1, 3)

Variable costs Costs that vary in direct proportion to patient volume or acuity. (Ch. 14)

Variance Anything that occurs to alter a patient's progress through a normal care path. (Ch. 14, 22)

Variance analysis Budget control process to determine differences between income and expense, projected and actual costs. (Ch. 14)

Veracity Principle that compels the truth be told completely. (Ch. 3)

Vicarious liability Imputation of accountability upon one person or entity for the actions of another person; substituted liability or imputed liability. (Ch 3)

Vision Assess current reality, determine the desired state, and then manage the distance between them. (Ch. 1)

Voice technology Control of computer by vocal input. (Ch. 13)

Wireless messaging An extension of an existing wired network that uses radio-based systems to transmit data signals through the air without any physical connections. (Ch. 13)

Worked time See *Productive time*. (Ch. 23)

Workbook Activities

Managing and Leading

■ INTRODUCTION

Effective *managers* focus efficiently on objectives, tasks, procedures, and policies. But recently, the emphasis has been on *leaders* who provide vision, inspiration, and empowerment. Exactly what does each of these terms mean? Who should lead, manage, or follow, and when? The activities in this section are designed to help you recognize the differences between leading, managing, and following and to recognize how and why these behaviors are essential for organizations to move forward.

■ ACTIVITY 1-1

1. What are words that come to mind when you think of the word, "leader"?

2. What are words that come to mind when you think of the word, "follower"?

3. Analyze the differences between the two lists. Do you think of leaders in different ways than you think of followers?

4. Recall pairs of leaders-followers from politics, science, education, the media, or personal experience. As you recall these pairs of individuals, what made one the "leader" and the other the "follower"? How did the "leader" contribute to the "follower's" success? How did the "follower" contribute to the "leader's" success? Were there times when the leader functioned more as the follower? Were there times when the follower functioned more as the leader? What does this analysis tell you about the nature of leader-follower relationships?

ACTIVITY 1-2

Write a short analysis of the similarities and differences between managers and leaders on a unit of a hospital with which you are familiar. Discuss these similarities and differences with others (staff nurses, nurse managers, and other students).

ACTIVITY 1-3

1. In the spaces below, write a list of the positive consequences (beneficial outcomes) that occur when one manages well, when one leads well, and when one follows well.

Beneficial Outcomes or Consequences

Managing well	**Leading well**	**Following well**
a) Orderly, organized unit	a) Progressive, creative unit	a) Balanced teamwork
b)	b)	b)
c)	c)	c)
d)	d)	d)
e)	e)	e)
f)	f)	f)

2. Write any observations, questions, and/or conclusions you have about the above lists.

3. Write a list of the negative consequences/outcomes of (or difficulties caused by) overemphasizing managing to the exclusion of leading, and then overemphasizing leading to the exclusion of managing.

Negative Outcomes or Consequences

Overemphasizing managing	**Overemphasizing leading**
a) Limited freedom for staff	a) Out of touch with reality
b)	b)
c)	c)
d)	d)
e)	e)

List negative outcomes of ineffective or passive followership.
a) Waits for others to assume responsibilities
b)
c)
d)
e)

4. Write any questions, observations, and/or conclusions you have about the above three lists.

5. Discuss with at least one other person the benefits and negative results (all lists) of leading and managing. List specific ways you could (or have seen others) shift emphasis between leading and managing.
   a) What behaviors, policies, procedures, etc. facilitate a shift of emphasis from managing to leading and back again **in the institution(s) you have chosen?**

   b) What behaviors, policies, procedures, etc. block this shifting emphasis **in the institution(s) you have chosen?**

   c) What new behaviors, policies, procedures, etc. would produce an effective shifting in the future **in the institution(s) you have chosen?**

ACTIVITY 1-4

Read at least three articles concerning managing and leading. Notice the degree to which the articles focus on the benefits of either leading or managing and the consequences of the other. When this occurs the article tends to be a "crusade" for one side of this dilemma as though the author's favored approach is the solution to a particular problem. By overemphasizing the favored side, you could eventually experience its negative consequences, just as walking on top of a seesaw will at some point make it tip downward (see your negative consequences listed above). Do any of your articles call for both leading and managing together, or mix them into a "superperson" profile? This may lead to clouding the distinctions and ignoring the need to emphasize leading or managing when appropriate.

1. What do the articles recommend about shifting focus?

2. With what level of certainty do the authors speak about the most needed behaviors?

3. What recommendations could you use in your clinical or work setting?

4. Why?

ACTIVITY 1-5

1. Team up with another student in your class. Separately, compile a list of what you each believe are leadership behaviors. Try to list at least 10.

1.	6.
2.	7.
3.	8.
4.	9.
5.	10.

2. Review your lists, and mark your initials beside each behavior that you believe can be used to describe some of your own behaviors. Do this without input from anyone else. Using the same lists, indicate by marking your partner's initials which behaviors you have observed in the other student. Do this activity without any input from the other student. When finished, compare lists.

3. What do you both notice about the differences in how you view yourselves and how you view one another?

4. What did you learn about yourselves?

5. Do others see you as having more, or fewer, leadership traits than you believe you have? Why?

Role Development

INTRODUCTION

Does the role of nurse manager intrigue you? Do you think you would like to be nurse manager? To use a cliche . . . It is the best of times for nursing because this era of healthcare calls for creativity, flexibility, and tenacity—three attributes that students often possess. The exercises you are about to complete should heighten and soar these attributes to higher peaks of excellence. Try them with your peers, share them with your peers, and, most importantly, learn from them with your peers.

ACTIVITY 2-1

Role play the following scenario in a group of 9-12 peers. Use your experience in clinical settings as the basis for your knowledge.

Roles: Nurse manager of a home health agency
Staff nurses—3 to 4
Home health aides—5 to 8

Scenario: The agency needs to develop a new care delivery model based on the influence of managed care. Work as a group to develop different roles for this new model—do not limit yourselves to what you currently see in practice. For each new role (see below) identify assets and liabilities, such as costs, inherent in each role (recruitment, education, benefits).

HOME HEALTH AGENCY PROBABLE PERSONNEL NEEDS

Position	Assets	Liabilities
Case manager	Can coordinate care	Requires extraordinary "people skills"
1.		
2.		
3.		
4.		
Home health aide	Delivers many aspects of basic care	Not prepared for delivering complex nursing care
1.		
2.		
3.		
4.		
Medication aide/pharmacy aide	Can be very proficient in delivery of care with a defined scope of practice	May not be cost effective due to lack of role versatility
1.		
2.		
3.		
4.		

◼ ACTIVITY 2-2

In what ways can technology be used by a home health agency in a home setting? For example, list client data that might be computer-based for entry or retrieval at home site. What teaching aspects for health promotion/disease prevention can be done with your client using computer technology?

◼ ACTIVITY 2-3

You are about to downsize your hospital unit. You have been told that your role as nurse manager will expand to cover more patient care areas and that the staff for each shift on your present unit will be reassigned. How can you prepare yourself and your staff for this change? Consider small staff meetings to let people talk about the new changes; also consider your own and your staff's adaptability traits. Write down a tentative plan for addressing the downsizing and staff relocation.

◼ ACTIVITY 2-4

You have been repeatedly asked to change the quality care program so that it reflects evaluation of outcomes. You have changed the program at least twice, yet your supervisor is not satisfied with the quality outcomes, especially in relation to cost containment. What other strategies can you use to meet management and customer expectations? Write a paragraph that reflects your plan and your ability to maintain objectivity and sustain the demands of the job. Consider research strategies, collaboration with others (in and out of the institution) and patient care standards.

Legal and Ethical Issues

▌ INTRODUCTION

The increasing demands in healthcare for cost containment and quality in patient care services, combined with increasing technology, pose escalating ethical and legal questions. As the healthcare scene changes, so do the questions that are posed to staff nurses and managers. This section presents dilemmas that can assist in heightening your awareness of legal and ethical issues prominent today. These exercises are designed to offer an opportunity to experience some of the dilemmas that are posed to managers and staff. The exercises were selected as representative of current examples of common dilemmas that nurses may encounter.

▌ ACTIVITY 3-1

Required Request has been made into law in a majority of states. This law requires that after all deaths all families must be made aware of the possibility of donation of organs and tissues. The nurse manager at the time of death, or just before, may be expected to request the organs.

1. Identify the ethical principles underlying the Required Request law by giving specific examples of how these principles are used by nurses when requesting organs after death.

2. Review the three ethical theories presented in the text. Which theory most guides your position regarding the Required Request law? State three reasons to support your position.

Position:

a)

b)

c)

ACTIVITY 3-2

You are the nurse manager on a busy intermediate coronary care unit. You have just received a request from the admitting department for a bed on your unit, but there are no beds available. You inform the admitting department and request more information on the patient. The information you receive is that the patient is a 73-year-old woman with severe congestive heart failure who needs to receive IV medications. The physician has requested that she be on a monitored bed while receiving the medication. There are no telemetry beds available.

After reviewing all of the patients on the unit, the director decides to transfer a 48-year-old man who had a myocardial infarction 2 days earlier. The patient is transferred and you receive the woman with congestive heart failure. The next day you find out that during the night the patient who was transferred was found in complete arrest when the nurse on the other unit made rounds at 2:00 AM. The man was resuscitated but is now in intensive care with brain damage resulting from the anoxia that occurred before he was resuscitated.

1. Was the decision to transfer the patient out of the intermediate care unit appropriate? Provide a rationale for your answer.

2. Use the MORAL model discussed in the text to review this ethical dilemma.
M Massage the dilemma; identify and define the issues in the dilemma.

O Outline the options.

R Resolve the dilemma.

A Act by applying the chosen option.

L Look back and evaluate the entire process.

ACTIVITY 3-3

As a nurse manager, you are responsible for review of all incidents that occur on your unit to determine if they were reported according to protocol and if appropriate follow-up has been completed.

On the previous day, one patient received injuries to her hand while ambulating when an IV controller slipped on the IV pole and pinned her hand between the controller and a platform designed to be used as a flat surface to hold equipment while working with the IV.

The incident report states: "Patient was ambulating to bathroom at 10:30 PM and used the IV pole to stabilize herself while walking. The controller fell down the pole and pinned her right hand to the small table beneath it. Injury evident to right hand. Hand immediately began to swell and patient had acute pain. X-ray revealed a fracture of the third and fourth metacarpal of the right hand. Physician notified, responded, and orthopedic consult ordered."

The nurse's note in the chart states: "Patient ambulating to bathroom using IV pole to stabilize herself. IV controller fell, pinning hand, resulting in injury. This would not have happened if I had been present to help her. She stated that she turned on her light but no one answered because the unit was very busy at the time. Physician notified and responded. Incident report filed."

1. Identify and examine potential liability from this incident.

2. How does the note made in the chart affect the potential liability for (a) the nurse involved, (b) the nurse manager, and (c) the institution?
   a) nurse

   b) nurse manager

   c) institution

3. Rewrite the nurse's note so that you could advise someone in a similar situation.

Strategic Planning, Goal Setting, and Marketing: Planning for the Future is the Key

▌ INTRODUCTION

In Chapter 4, you have been learning the importance of planning strategically, developing clear goals and objectives, implementing in a disciplined manner, and marketing concepts in the field of healthcare. You have also considered the critical importance of integrating the planning, targeting, implementing, and marketing functions. This section provides processes to enable you to develop skills in performing these functions.

▌ ACTIVITY 4-1

1. To identify the marketing strategies of a healthcare organization, obtain a copy of at least one marketing brochure or plan for your own organization or one with which you are familiar.
2. Analyze the completeness and effectiveness of your brochure or plan according to the following criteria:
   a) Is the market for each product or service clearly defined?

   b) Are organization resources (capacity to deliver the product or service) quantified for each product or service?

   c) What are the marketing objectives? Are they realistic, specific, measurable, and mutually consistent?

   d) Are specific market segments identified for increased penetration?

   e) Is the planned mix of products and services clearly defined or will the mix be reactive to market requirements?

ACTIVITY 4-2

Select a healthcare organization and assess its current state with regard to the planning, targeting, implementing, and marketing functions. You can conduct this type of assessment by reviewing such relevant documents in the organization as mission statements, strategic plans, tentative budgets, etc. In reviewing documents to assess the current state, what would you use as review criteria? List those criteria below.

Reviewing the Strategic Plan

Review criteria	Not met	Partly met	Fully met
1.			
2.			
3.			

Reviewing Goals and Objectives

Review criteria	Not met	Partly met	Fully met
1.			
2.			
3.			

Reviewing the Marketing Plan

Review criteria	Not met	Partly met	Fully met
1.			
2.			
3.			

ACTIVITY 4-3

1. Participate in independent activity or small group discussion with students outside of class.

2. The case study in the Chapter 4 Appendix lists four forthcoming changes and develops a strategic planning document that responds to those changes. With your group members, discuss (or reflect by yourself on) how the plan would have to be altered if the changes included the following, rather than those mentioned in the case:

   a) The advisory committee was comprised mainly of health care professionals.

   b) The marketing plan was targeted to lower socioeconomic groups only.

   c) The health promotion expectations were divided among existing agencies.

   d) Costs and outcomes were the only basis for evaluation.

3. What are the main principles inherent in the concepts of budget reductions and increased regulation?

ACTIVITY 4-4

Planning is a critically important function. Without plans, we cannot sustain long-term initiatives. But planning must exist within a context of spontaneity, just as spontaneity must exist within a context of planning. To value one and eliminate the other will lead to system dysfunction!

1. List the benefits of planning.

2. List the problems associated with planning. Think about the problems that would occur if everything were planned and people were prohibited from taking any spontaneous action.

3. List the benefits associated with spontaneous action.

4. List the problems associated with spontaneous action. Think about the problems that would occur if no one in the organization did any planning.

ACTIVITY 4-5

Planning requires effective vision, goals, and objectives. The text discusses guidelines for effective goals. Using these guidelines and examples, write some specific short-term, medium-range, and long-term goals for a department or team. Discuss them with another student and revise them as needed.

Leading Change

INTRODUCTION

This section contains two application activities. The ultimate outcome is the development of effective change management skills by further enhancing students' conceptual foundations about roles and approaches in leading change.

The first activity asks students to analyze an actual change situation initially using their basic knowledge of change management gleaned from Chapter 5, Leading Change, and subsequently applying a set of structured questions to the situation. The second activity requests that students propose a plan for the actual or hypothetical change. Guidelines and a sample provide a descriptive blueprint for the development of the plan. The best outcome for this activity is for the students to implement their plans in actual healthcare organizations.

ACTIVITY 5-1

Using planned change models for relatively uncomplicated change where the quantity and interactive influences of people, technology, and systems is limited can be effective. Most organizational change, however, takes place in groups, units, and departments responsive to influences outside and inside (open system). Thus, managing the influencing factors of a change situation in conjunction with a plan's elements for the change can lead to creative results. Using the change planning worksheet, guidelines for planning a change, and the sample of a plan for a hypothetical change, develop a plan for a change. Select a change situation, either an actual or a hypothetical one, follow the problem-solving format of the planning worksheet to assess the change situation, develop an activity plan supported by sound change theories and principles, and decide on methods to evaluate the change process and outcomes. The activity plan should reflect several potentially feasible outcome scenarios to work toward and specifically identified resources, time lines, responsible parties, and strategies to achieve each outcome. Discuss your proposed plan with your peers, instructors, and individuals in the change situation.

This following worksheet provides a general framework for planning low-complexity change. The worksheet headings and sections outline essential points to consider. The guidelines explain the completion of the worksheet section by section. A completed sample worksheet is included as a model to follow.

▌GUIDELINES

Section I: Situational Assessment and Analysis

Developing an appropriate plan requires an accurate understanding of the situation before the implementation. Effective assessment results in accurate identification of the need, not to be confused with symptoms of the need. The need may be a problem needing resolution, a need requiring innovative action, or a measure improving quality.

Part A

Describe the actual situation needing change, addressing the who, what, when, where, why, and how elements.

Part B

Using your initial assessment data in question A, identify current and anticipated facilitators and barriers operating in the change situation. Using a numerical weighting system, rate each factor's strength or potential to either promote or hinder the change process (1 is low and 5 is high). Choose strategies that have the most potential to increase the influences of facilitating factors and reduce or eliminate the effects of interfering factors.

Part C

Analyze all factors assessed. State whether you will proceed with the plan.

Section II: Implementation Plan

Clearly write acceptable change outcomes and corresponding objectives and evaluation methods. State predictable unexpected occurrences.

Part A

Describe several desired outcomes using specific, concrete terms. Though broad in nature, the outcomes contain the criteria against which progress is measured throughout and at the end of the change.

Part B

Objectives are specific descriptions of the processes needed to achieve change outcomes. State objectives in terms of needed resources (materials, space, finances, staff) and desired time lines for each scenario. List objectives in the approximate order in which they will occur.

Part C

It is probable that unexpected occurrences and circumstances will have impact on the change process. Predict these and designate potential actions to respond to them if they do happen.

Part D

Various methods exist for collecting information throughout and at the end of the change process. Choose appropriate methods as needed to measure attitude, behavior, or knowledge during the change and after the change, the influences or concerns hampering the implementation process, or the degree to which objectives are met and the outcomes achieved.

Section III: Evaluation and Revision

It is important to judge the effectiveness of the plan for change and its implementation. Both the processes and outcomes of the change should be evaluated for effectiveness to project what could be improved in future endeavors.

Worksheet for Planning a Change

Section I: Situational Assessment and Analysis

A. Describe actual situation in terms of who, what, when, where, how, and why.

B. Complete a force field analysis by identifying the facilitators and barriers in the change situation, numerically rate their potential strength (1=low; 5=high), then indicate strategies appropriate to managing the influences of the factors. Focus on information, relationships, and possible alterations in the pool of outcome scenarios.

Facilitators (+/pro)	Strength	Strategies	Barriers (−/anti-)	Strength	Strategies
1.			1.		
2.			2.		
3.			3.		
4.			4.		
etc.			etc.		

C. State how influences of the facilitators and barriers are equal to or different from each other based on your assessment of their strength. State whether you will proceed with plan.

Section II: Implementation Plan

A. State several desirable outcomes for proposed change in specific, measurable terms:

1.

2.

3.

Worksheet for Planning a Change—cont'd

B. State and sequence objectives in terms of specific resources, time lines, strategies, and responsible parties for each outcome scenario (some may overlap).

1. Outcome 1:   2. Outcome 2:   3. Outcome 3:

a.   a.   a.

b.   b.   b.

c.   c.   c.

d.   d.   d.

e.   e.   e.

etc.   etc.   etc.

C. Identify unexpected occurrences and potential actions to handle.
  1.

  2.

D. State methods for measuring the progress and outcome of the change process.

Ongoing/Process   Outcome/Summative
  1.   1.

  2.   2.

  3.   3.

Section III: Evaluation and Revision
A. State to what degree outcome(s) was met.

B. Indicate ways to improve the change process or outcome quality.

Sample Worksheet

Section I: Situational Assessment and Analysis

A. Describe actual situation in terms of who, what, when, where, how, and why.

RNs/LPNs/LVNs hear patient information only on assigned patients at shift change due to unit's 15-month-old policy of nurse-to-nurse shift reports. Frequent complaints exist due to nursing staff's inability to knowledgeably assist other patients, families, and healthcare providers. Miscommunications increase the risk for errors.

B. Identify facilitating and interfering (barrier) factors in the change situation, numerically rate their potential strength, and then indicate strategies appropriate to managing the influences of the factors.

Facilitators (+/pro)	Strength	Strategies	Barriers (−/anti-)	Strength	Strategies
1. *Nurse manager supportive*	*+4*	*Communication Facilitation*	1. *Two nurse rejectors*	*−4*	*Coercion Co-optation*
2. *Staff's desire for patient information*	*+3*	*Communication Support*	2. *Perceived late start to provide care*	*−2*	*Communication Facilitation*
3. *Effectiveness of S.O.P. committee*	*+3*	*Involvement Support*	3. *Increased accountability for all patients*	*−2*	*Negotiation Support*
4. *Staff's desire to reduce frustration*	*+2*	*Participation Encouragement*	4. *Possible change in reporting with new information system*	*−2*	*Education Support Participation*
Total Wt. = *+12*				*Total Wt.* = *−10*	

C. State how influences of the facilitators and barriers are equal to or different from each other based on your assessment of their strength. State whether you will proceed with the plan.

Will proceed with plan as facilitators outweigh barriers by +2. Will carefully monitor during implementation.

Section II: Implementation Plan

A. State acceptable outcomes for proposed change in specific, measurable terms

1. *By June 25, all RNs/LPNs/LVNs will be knowledgeable about all patients on unit due to comprehensive shift report using the patient care Kardex as tool for standardization of information reported.*

2. *By September 1, all RNs/LPNs/LVNs will be knowledgeable about all unit patients due to computer printout of key information on each patient and brief status reports at shift change.*

Sample Worksheet—cont'd

B. State and sequence objectives in terms of specific resources, time lines, strategies, and responsible parties.

1. *By May 1, S.O.P. committee representatives meet with all nursing staff (on all three shifts) to define problem, identify solutions, and seek staff involvement.*

2. *By May 15, staff will complete short survey to determine overall willingness to adopt specific options for change in report method.*

3. *By June 1, S.O.P. committee will communicate most acceptable options with rationale and then field staff comments (survey results).*

4. *By June 7, S.O.P. committee and nurse manager will conduct sessions at staff meetings to update progress on two possible solutions.*

5. *On June 20 or September 1, begin new shift report method for the transition between each shift change.*

C. Identify unexpected occurrences and potential actions to handle.

1. *Lack of general agreement on new shift report method: Reassess problems, solution(s), and associated legal-ethical issues with staff.*

2. *Reluctance/harmful resistance of staff members: Identify at beginning and during change process and use appropriate strategies to prevent sabotage of change process (communication → manipulation → coercion).*

D. State methods for measuring the progress and outcome of the change process.

Ongoing/Process	Outcome/Summative
1. *Survey of six to 10 questions to poll attitudes and abilities to support one or more options for new shift report method.*	1. *Conduct discussions with individual RNs/LPNs/LVNs on all three shifts at random to assess knowledge of all patients on unit after change has been implemented for one to five weeks.*
2. *Informal interviews of RNs/LPNs/LVNs during change process that include random attendance/ discussion.*	

Section III: Evaluation and Revision

A. State to what degree outcome(s) was met.

After 6 weeks of full implementation, evaluation measures with staff and attendance at all three shift report times show almost all staff knowledgeable about all unit patients. Patient, family, and provider information needs met more quickly and accurately.

B. Indicate ways to improve the change process or outcome quality after outcome evaluated.

Conduct quality study at monthly intervals to attain threshold of 95% consistently for 6 months at minimum. Build in more frequent points of seeking input from and giving feedback to staff (each shift initially, then weekly) related to movement toward outcome, with recognition provided for achievement and effort. Provide redirection for inability and unwillingness.

Problem Solving and Decision Making

INTRODUCTION

As proper problem identification is key to effective problem solving and decision making, the exercises in this section provide an opportunity to enhance your skills in this area. Activity 6-1 involves utilization of a "gap analysis" technique to differentiate a problematic state from the ideal state. Activity 6-2 provides an opportunity to collaborate with a colleague to reflect on the possible causes to a problem (select an actual problem currently affecting you) and possible remedies to solve it.

ACTIVITY 6-1

Gap Analysis

A gap analysis is another way of envisioning problem solving. Pick a personal or professional problem and describe the elements of the problem under the heading "description of present undesired state and conditions." Then, identify the desired future state/conditions that would ideally solve the problem, and list the elements under the heading in the right column.

Description of Present Undesired State and Conditions

Description of Desired Future State/Conditions

ACTIVITY 6-2

Problem Definition

There are many different ways to define a problem, starting with the way that you and I see it. One way is ask and answer the four questions below. Select a problem, select a partner, and follow through with the questions below.

1. Who and what are affected in what "problematic ways"?

   Who (as I see it):

   Who (as you see it):

   What (as I see it):

   What (as you see it):

2. Who and/or what is causing it?

   Who (as I see it):

   Who (as you see it):

   What (as I see it):

   What (as you see it):

3. What type of a problem is being confronted?

   The problem (as I see it):

   The problem (as you see it):

4. What are the intended goals/specific results to remedy the situation?

   Specific goal, results (as I see it):

   Specific goal, results (as you see it):

   Using these four guidelines requires other considerations related to each element of the problem definition. As you formulate and write problem definitions, you can reflect about the following:

1. Who and/or what is affected in what problematic ways? Consider these possibilities: How many people, and who specifically, are negatively affected? What other things are affected and how?

2. Who and/or what is causing this problem? What people are causing this problem, especially in the ways they are interpreting the circumstances and what is happening?

3. What type of problem is being confronted? What is this problem really about: Is it missing resources; a lack of training/skills; power struggles; inaccurate, inadequate, or superfluous communication; a lack of clarity of mission, priorities, roles, and/or norms; poor performance and/or results; misunderstandings; unethical actions; poor public relations, etc.?

Is this really a conflict over information, goals, means, or values/standards rather than a problem to solve? Is it a dilemma that has been mismanaged, or treated like a solvable problem?

4. What are the specific goal(s) and intended result(s) to remedy this situation?
Goals:

Intended results:

How would the situation look if this problem was completely solved? What will be the same and what will be different?

Adapted from Jung, Pino, & Emory (1973).

Healthcare Organizations

▮ INTRODUCTION

Changes in the healthcare system, its organizations, and its financing are bringing about rapid developments in the modes and sites of care delivery. As acute care facilities become more focused on the acutely ill, community facilities that focus on people who are less acutely ill are being developed. No longer are people who are ill or who need surgery cared for in acute hospitals. They are in intermediate-care agencies, clinics, and at home. This chapter focuses on how the community is changing its healthcare facilities, changes in healthcare delivery that have occurred in the past 5 years, and the emerging trends.

▮ ACTIVITY 7-1

Community Scavenger Hunt

Form a group with three to five of your classmates who identify themselves as highly committed and productive. Assume that you have been charged with the responsibility to provide the local health planning community with definitive information that they can use for future planning.

1. Scan community publications (e.g., newspapers, magazines, brochures, etc.) to develop a scenario of what the healthcare scene in your community was like 3 years ago and how it has changed in yearly increments. Write your description of the agencies and services available in the space below.

   What healthcare was like 3 years ago:

   2 years ago:

   1 year ago:

   Today:

2. Answer the following questions.

How many new agencies have been established? What are they?

How have existing ones been modified by adding programs, redesigning facilities for different services, combining with others, etc.?

Describe the patients (clientele) served then and now, using the following questions as guidelines:

How has acuity changed?

How have census and access changed?

How has professional nursing staffing changed?

How have their healthcare demands changed?

How have reimbursement systems (insurance, HMOs, etc.) changed, expanded, declined?

3. Using your answers to the questions in item 2 above, develop a visual representation (such as a form, grid, mindmap, graph, chart, table, etc.) to depict the changes in the agencies.

4. Based on the information you have gathered, what are your conclusions? What trends can you identify?

5. Using the information you have gathered, and keeping in mind the trends you just described, write a scenario that predicts the future. You already have all the data you need to do so. You know as much as anyone! Keep in mind that nurse-owned and nurse-managed organizations may be essential components of networks in the evaluation.

ACTIVITY 7-2

Build a Collage

1. Collect news articles, magazine articles, photos, advertisements, brochures, etc. regarding local healthcare services, or services in some identifiable region. List your article titles below.

2. Organize them into time frames or developmental stages. Highlight new agencies and services within the time period(s) you select.

3. Identify geographic areas with the newest developments and expansions, perhaps with a creative visual or map.

4. On a poster board, create a visual collage that displays the historical trends in healthcare delivery in the area(s) you have selected.

5. Present your collage to the class.

Cultural Diversity

▋ INTRODUCTION

The purposes of the exercises in this section are, first, to help you examine your own cultural attitudes to determine how they influence your behavior, and second, to compare and contrast your cultural beliefs and practices with those of others who come from a different cultural background.

▋ ACTIVITY 8-1

Cultural Diversity Exercise: Cultural Awareness

1. Describe the differences among the terms *culture*, *race*, and *ethnicity*.

2. List at least six common characteristics usually associated with the middle-class American culture.
   a)
   b)
   c)
   d)
   e)
   f)

3. Describe common characteristics found in the culture of Western scientific medical practice (e.g., belief in medical model, germ theory).

4. Identify the four most prominent cultural groups in your area.
   a)
   b)
   c)
   d)

   Choose two groups for an in-depth study. Identify the groups in relation to their health beliefs/customs in the areas of birth and death, and their use of folk healers or folk medicines.

5. Determine four similarities and four differences between the "folk medicine" and "Western, scientific medicine" systems. (You may need to think broadly.)

Similarities	**Differences**
a)	a)
b)	b)
c)	c)
d)	d)

■ ACTIVITY 8-2

Cultural Values Checklist

The following is a short checklist regarding culturally determined values, attitudes, and beliefs, especially as they pertain to healthcare. You must choose to strongly agree, agree, disagree, or strongly disagree with each statement as it is written. This requires that you be as introspective as possible to determine where you stand on each of the issues presented. Please remember that there is no right or wrong answer, just individual attitudes and beliefs. By answering as honestly as possible, this exercise will help you be more conscious of your own culturally determined beliefs.

Read each statement carefully, then circle the answer that most closely reflects your beliefs regarding each statement.

    SA=Strongly Agree   A=Agree   D=Disagree   SD=Strongly Disagree

1. Only a small percentage of Americans use alternate forms of healing other than traditional medical science.

   SA   A   D   SD

2. People can change the outcome of serious medical conditions with prayer.

   SA   A   D   SD

3. True grief is expressed with loud sobbing and copious crying.

   SA   A   D   SD

4. Life support should be removed from a person who is brain-dead with no possible hope for recovery.

   SA   A   D   SD

5. Patients should be allowed to have family members at their bedside 24 hours a day.

   SA   A   D   SD

6. Family members should donate a deceased person's organs (as appropriate) so others may be helped.

   SA   A   D   SD

7. Good health is largely determined by a person's diet, exercise, and other similar activities.

   SA   A   D   SD

8. It is important for nurses to question a physician if the nurse is unsure of the rationale behind the physician's orders.

   SA   A   D   SD

9. To get a good patient history, it is important for the nurse to write down the information as the patient is speaking to make sure that none of the information is missed.

   SA   A   D   SD

10. Family members should not be allowed to perform support tasks such as bathing the patient while the patient is hospitalized.

    SA   A   D   SD

11. To be an effective communicator, it is important to maintain good eye contact with people.

    SA   A   D   SD

12. If an employee is not performing satisfactorily, it is important for the manager to speak directly to that person, even if it involves giving straightforward criticism.

    SA   A   D   SD

13. Patting an employee on the back is a friendly gesture to say thanks for a job well done.

    SA   A   D   SD

14. Providing psychosocial care is an important part of being a nurse and nurse manager.

    SA   A   D   SD

For each of the 14 statements in the previous checklist, identify one cultural group that would agree and one that would not:

1. AGREE _____   DISAGREE _____

2. AGREE _____   DISAGREE _____

3. AGREE _____   DISAGREE _____

4. AGREE _____   DISAGREE _____

5. AGREE _____   DISAGREE _____

6. AGREE _____   DISAGREE _____

7. AGREE _____   DISAGREE _____

8. AGREE _____   DISAGREE _____

9. AGREE _____   DISAGREE _____

10. AGREE _____   DISAGREE _____

11. AGREE _____   DISAGREE _____

12. AGREE _____   DISAGREE _____

13. AGREE _____   DISAGREE _____

14. AGREE _____   DISAGREE _____

Meet in groups of three or four students to discuss your responses to this exercise. Determine three areas of commonality and three areas of difference among members of your group.

Commonality:
1.
2.
3.

Difference:
1.
2.
3.

■ ACTIVITY 8-3

One responsibility of a family is to provide healthcare for its members by helping them stay well and taking care of members who are ill. Health promotion activities and care given during illness vary greatly among families. Each function is very much influenced by the family's cultural orientation. Friedman (1992) describes six stages of family health/illness interaction that greatly influence each individual's response to healthcare. These stages are health promotion, illness recognition, care seeking, healthcare system, acute response, and adaptation to illness/recovery.

It is important to note that the family will not make contact with the healthcare delivery system until at least the fourth stage of this interaction continuum. Therefore the family may have engaged in various health activities before they ever have contact with anyone in a professional setting.

The Family Health/Illness Practices Inventory is designed to increase awareness of family and cultural values that shape health and illness practices. It is a tool that can increase self-awareness of the cultural factors that shape your current approach to healthcare. When used as an interview tool, it can increase awareness of other cultural perspectives regarding healthcare.

Complete your own Family Health/Illness Practices Inventory. Try to remember what it was like for you as a child growing up and answer the questions based on what your family did before you became a nurse.

Family Health/Illness Practices Inventory

Questions to ask:
1. Health promotion:
   Cite three health promotion/disease prevention activities done by your family.
   a)
   b)
   c)
   Did you consider your parents to be healthy, frail, sickly? What about your siblings?
   How did your family define *health*?

2. Illness recognition:
   Who was the primary person in the family responsible for determining if a family member was ill?
   Who was primarily responsible for determining what should be done about the illness?
   Who in the family was seen as the "health expert"?

3. Care seeking:
   Who did the family turn to for information regarding the illness if the family was unable to resolve the problem on its own?
   Did the family discuss the problems with extended family members, neighbors, or friends, or go straight to a health professional?

4. Healthcare system:
   Did the family use folk practitioner/healers?
   Where was the initial contact with the healthcare delivery system made (e.g., healer, private physician, clinic, hospital)?
   Who in the family was responsible for deciding where to seek help?

5. Acute response:
   What did it mean to be "sick" in your family?
   What behaviors were expected of the sick person and of other family members in relation to the sick member?
   If it was a serious illness or crisis, how did the family cope with a crisis?
   Who was seen as the leader in times of crisis?
   What happened if the traditional leader was sick?

6. Adaptation to illness/recovery:
   Did anyone in the family have a chronic illness?
   How did that affect the other family members?
   Who did the family depend on for support (physical, emotional)?

After completing your own Family Health/Illness Practices Inventory, interview someone from a different cultural background. Explain that you are trying to learn more about how different cultures and families view health and illness. Assure the person that the information will be kept confidential. Or seek out a classmate whose cultural background is different from yours, and mutually compare and discuss your responses.

REFERENCE

Friedman, M. (1992). *Family Nursing: Theory and Practice*, 3rd ed, Norwalk, CT: Appleton & Lange.

Understanding and Designing Organizational Structures

INTRODUCTION

Technology, which is defined as all the work required to carry out the nursing care of clients, has a major impact on the design of the organizational structure. The technology is determined by the type of setting, e.g., critical care, long-term care, rehabilitation, home care, hospice, etc. A primary factor to be considered is the amount of autonomy required in decision making. In settings where clients' conditions are unstable and unpredictable, structures are needed that provide for a great deal of independence in decision making. In community settings where access to higher levels for decision making is not available, a structure providing independence in decision making is also required. A good fit is required between organizational structure and technology.

Making decisions at the level where client care is occurring provides many advantages to clients and their nurses. When decision making is delegated to this level, there has to be some means of assuring that clients are treated equally and that one client is not provided with advantages that are not granted to another. Agency guidelines for care established by nurses providing the care are one method of ensuring that all clients are treated equally.

ACTIVITY 9-1

Describe and illustrate with concrete examples the relationship between technology and structure, e.g., how does one influence the other; how does organizational structure vary in different types of institutions and what are resultant technology demands?

ACTIVITY 9-2

Describe a decentralized organization and list the positive factors of working in such an organization. Describe chaos that might occur in a completely decentralized organization and methods that could be used to avoid such chaos.

ACTIVITY 9-3

Obtain at least 2 organizational charts. Compare them in terms of their missions. Describe the placement, authority, and reporting for nursing.

ACTIVITY 9-4

The new chief nursing officer for the Cady Institute is reviewing several theories and philosophies in preparation for implementing one that can carry the organization into the next century. In perusing the literature, it became apparent that the concept of shared governance was most appealing for it seemed consistent with the mission of the institution as well as that of the nursing division. You have been appointed to the new committee that has been formed to review the requirements to be considered prior to this change. As a responsible member of this committee deliberating the proposed change, you have been requested to review the literature and cite at least three advantages and three disadvantages for this proposal.

Advantages of shared governance:

1.

2.

3.

Disadvantages of shared governance:

1.

2.

3.

Having completed this assignment, you report your findings to the committee at large. The committee then requests you to compare shared governance to participatory management and formulate a response supporting either management style.

You respond, "I have listed the pros and cons of each type of governance for your consideration prior to recommending adoption of one or the other."

Participatory management has the following advantages:

1.

2.

3.

Participatory management has the following disadvantages:

1.

2.

3.

The reasons you give reflect that you have also compared the advantages and disadvantages of participatory management.

YOUR RECOMMENDATION:

I recommend that (select one) be adopted for the following reasons:

Your recommendation was based on the following considerations (please describe each in one or two sentences):

1. How does the educational level of staff affect the decision?

2. What style(s) of managerial leadership are preferred?

3. How are nursing staff members demonstrating autonomy?

CHAPTER 10 WORKBOOK

Collective Action

INTRODUCTION

These activities ask you to reflect on your skills that will contribute to your success in collective action within the practice of nursing. Activity 10-1 begins with the personal you and will influence your performance within the professional context. The remaining activities give you an opportunity to consider your role within nursing practice.

ACTIVITY 10-1

1. You have developed many interpersonal skills within your life. List four interpersonal skills that are essential for nurses within a shared governance model.
   a.
   b.
   c.
   d.

2. In the space below, describe activities that will help you refine these skills.
   a.
   b.
   c.
   d.

3. Identify other skills that you think will assist you in collective action within your nursing practice.
   a.
   b.
   c.
   d.

ACTIVITY 10-2

Eden Valley is a community hospital. That is, it is an institution that operates solely within the community in which it is located. It is experiencing financial pressures. The options it is considering include selling to a national company, joining a multi-hospital group in the surrounding area, or trying to preserve its identity. Employees, including nurses, are experiencing stress related to the uncertainty. Employees in other job categories are unionized. Several nurses believe that it is a good time to consider organizing a staff union. They contact the state nurses' association (SNA) and other unions to discuss their concerns.
   1. What factors will influence the establishment of a union?

2. What factors will be a barrier to the establishment of a union?

3. Identify goals for establishing a union.

4. What criteria are important in the selection of a union?

ACTIVITY 10-3

Obtain a copy of a collective bargaining contract between nurses and their employer. (If there are no contracts for nurses in your area, obtain a copy of a collective bargaining contract used by another group.) Identify three features of the contract that are important to you. Identify any features of the contract that are objectionable to you.

Contract Features

Features Important to You	Objectionable Features

ACTIVITY 10-4

Nurses can no longer ignore or be uninformed about the business side of healthcare delivery. Knowledge of the facilities in which you practice and trends in the industry is necessary to make informed decisions. Imagine you have been informed that the hospital must decrease the number of registered nurses within the new business practices designed to reduce costs. From your perspective and those of your nurse colleagues, the hospital is doing fine. Identify three sources of public information related to an organization's financial health. Who would you contact to assist you in obtaining the information?

ACTIVITY 10-5

Read two articles related to the 1994 Supreme Court decision that struck down the nursing exception used by the National Labor Relations Board (NLRB) to determine supervisory status and the February 1996 ruling by the NLRB that upheld the nonsupervisory status of nurses in Anchorage. These decisions reflect two versions of the same ruling. Identify the implications for nurses within each decision.

Managing Quality and Risk

INTRODUCTION

Planning is necessary to improve quality and decrease risk. Total quality management (TQM) and continuous quality improvement (CQI) programs will help to improve the quality of care that is provided in an institution. Planning is an essential part of these programs, and the planning time is well spent. The occurrence of incidents may be costly for the institution. Decreasing those risks will decrease costs, improve the quality of care you provide, and improve client satisfaction.

ACTIVITY 11-1

1. Form groups of four in which each group member will conduct his or her own interview with a healthcare professional regarding quality improvement. Select interviewees from the institutions in which you work or have clinical experience. Ask the interviewees to address quality improvement in their institution. You will want to interview people at different levels of the organization to gain a broad perspective of everyone's understanding of the process. Suggested people to interview include the head nurse, staff nurse, unit secretary, physician, director of quality improvement, people from other departments, etc.

2. After interviewing these people, reflect on and answer the following questions:
   a) Did each person give you a similar picture of the quality improvement process? Why or why not?

   b) If there were differences, were they significant? Why or why not? (If the differences are significant, they can have an impact on how well the quality improvement process works.)

   c) Discuss the interviews in your groups and determine what similarities and differences you found.

ACTIVITY 11-2

Use the following steps to apply quality improvement principles to your own practice.
 1. Identify a process or procedure that you perform routinely and wish to improve.
 2. Using a flowchart, delineate each step of the procedure.
 3. Collect data that show your present ability to do this process or procedure.
 4. Set a measurable standard of excellence for this procedure. Use established standards if available, but remember to also determine what your customers value and expect.
 5. Develop a plan to improve your practice to meet this standard. This could include further reading, education, or consultation with peers.
 6. Collect data to document your improvement in this procedure.
 7. When you successfully meet your performance standard, reward yourself.

ACTIVITY 11-3

Obtaining information from your customers is very important when assessing quality of care. Interview five clients regarding quality of care. The following are some suggested questions to use in your interview:

1. What was most satisfying about the care you have received?

2. What was least satisfying about the care you have received?

3. Have there been any delays in the care that was provided (pain medication delayed, meal tray served late, call light not answered)?

4. Who was most attentive to your specific needs (physician, nurse, nursing assistant, housekeeper)?

5. What would you like to see changed?

6. What would you like to see stay the same?

7. Would you recommend this institution to others?

8. Is there anything else you would like to share regarding the quality of care you have received?

ACTIVITY 11-4

Obtain a copy of the form used in an institution to report incidents or occurrences. Review the related policy and procedure. Interview a nurse manager or staff nurse regarding the following if the policy and procedure do not provide the information.

1. What happens to the occurrence report after it is filled out?

2. What types of incidents are to be reported?

3. What is the most frequently occurring incident?

4. How is corrective action taken after an occurrence has taken place?

Self-Management: Stress and Time

▌ INTRODUCTION

The following activities afford the reader opportunities to put the principles described in this chapter into action. The first activity invites you to analyze how stress and time management are related. Identifying your own coping skills and seeking more positive ways of managing stress are the focus of the second activity. The third exercise invites you to use your time management skills to plan a successful meeting.

▌ ACTIVITY 12-1

Self-Management

1. Have a classmate describe his or her most stressful clinical day. What did your classmate do to deal with the stress during the day and after leaving the clinical area?

2. Analyze the description in terms of the time management skills of goal setting, prioritization, organization, use of time tools, and dealing with information.

3. Review the principles of time management in Chapter 12 and identify how the day might have been made to be less stressful.

4. Analyze the appropriateness of your classmate's stress management strategies.

ACTIVITY 12-2

Stress
Use the following questions as a guide to understanding how you perceive stress, respond to it, and attempt to gain mastery.

1. Think about a recent situation in which you experienced a high level of distress. Indicate how you responded:

   Emotionally

   Behaviorally

   Physically

   Review what you have written and identify whether your coping strategy was negative or positive.

   Consider an alternative approach for those coping strategies you have identified as negative.

2. Describe a situation in which you were in conflict with another person. How was that situation influenced by your expectations and behavior? Could the conflict have been avoided or resolved differently?

ACTIVITY 12-3

Meeting Management
Examine the Tips box on how to manage a meeting at the end of Chapter 12. Given the list of agenda items below, organize a 2-hour meeting to address them all. List them in an agenda with specific time limits for each item. Be able to give the rationale for the specific order you choose. When would you hold this meeting? What site might you choose for this meeting?

Agenda Items
a. 10 minutes to discuss how to make team meetings more effective
b. 30 minutes to decide on a new schedule format
c. 10 minutes to share the news
d. 20 minutes to discuss new possibilities for continuous improvement on the unit
e. 5 minutes to decide when to hold a shift party
f. 10 minutes to review last meeting's minutes
g. 10 minutes to revise a report form
h. 5 minutes to discuss agenda items for the next meeting
i. 10 minutes to give out assignments
j. 10 minutes to answer questions

Managing Information and Technology: Caring and Communicating with Computers

▌ INTRODUCTION

These exercises will help you use the information presented in the chapter. The Managing Information and Technology Self-Assessment Tool can be used to assess the current state of information technology for a patient care area, and to help you determine what data are gathered and how they are used for patient care. This exercise should help you determine how computer technology might help to improve the process.

The second activity helps you to subscribe to the student nurse listserv. Other list addresses are also provided for you. Try a few of them; they all provide valuable information for students and nurses in practice.

The third activity will help you find information on the Internet World Wide Web. A list of search engines and instructions for accessing them is provided. Be sure to use the help function to learn more about using these engines.

▌ ACTIVITY 13-1

Managing Information and Technology Self-Assessment Tool

Instructions: The purpose of this tool is to lead you through the process of assessing the current state of information technology for the patient care area in which you work or learn, as well as identifying problems or areas for improvement, planning for the improvement, implementing it, and evaluating it. It's an application of the nursing process to the process for using technology for the improvement of patient care.

1. List the biomedical technologies available to you for patient care and the data that you gather from these devices:

_____

_____

_____

_____

_____

2. For each type of technology that you listed, explain what you do with the data gathered:

_____

_____

_____

_____

_____

3. Describe how you aggregate and process these data to gain information:

_____

_____

_____

_____

_____

4. Explain how you use this information to make patient care decisions:

_____

_____

_____

_____

_____

5. Think of ways to improve the manual system for gathering data and aggregating and processing it. List every idea you have—brainstorm!

_____

_____

_____

_____

_____

6. List the ways that a computerized system might eliminate steps in the manual system.

_____

_____

_____

_____

_____

7. If you do not have any of the automated technologies for patient care (biomedical, information, knowledge), what steps might you as an individual take to get the process started?

_____

_____

_____

_____

_____

8. Think about your fellow staff members. Are they accepting of change? Would they resist computerization of the patient care process? How would you handle this?

_____

_____

_____

_____

_____

9. Name some ethical issues you might want to consider when computerizing patient care data:

_____
_____
_____
_____
_____

10. After you have installed and implemented patient care systems, how would you evaluate whether or not they have helped nurses provide patient care?

_____
_____
_____
_____
_____

11. Describe what you see as the "big picture" for healthcare computerization:

_____
_____
_____
_____
_____

12. List as many new roles for nursing in the field of nursing informatics and technology as you can think of:

_____
_____
_____
_____
_____

ACTIVITY 13-2

Using a Listserv

Using the instructions in the box below subscribe to the SNURSE-L listserv. Be sure to save the instructions returned to you by e-mail. They explain how to unsubscribe to the listserv when you are finished using it. Read the messages for a few days to see what other students are saying. This is called "lurking." You will notice that there are many responses and additions to a topic of interest. These messages become a "thread." When you are comfortable and have something to contribute, you may send a message to the list by clicking the reply button. Do NOT use all capital letters in your reply; this is considered to be shouting (rude); keep your messages short and to the point.

1. Did you have problems subscribing to the listserv? Were you able to find help?

2. Once you were subscribed, what information did you find useful for you? What information did you provide that was interesting and informative for others?

3. Did the listserv members respond to you?

4. Click on the print button to make a copy of your latest message.

How to Subscribe to a Listserv

1. Log on to your e-mail server at home or at school.
2. To subscribe to a listserv, type the server address (listserv section of the mail screen).
3. Tab to the message section (leave the subject blank) and type the information following subscribe under listserv addresses (remember to type the word *subscribe*).
4. Click the send button.
5. You will receive confirmation of your subscription and instructions for using the listserv in your e-mail.
6. If your message bounces, read it carefully. Make sure that you typed the server address exactly.

NOTE: Some schools do not allow access to listservs because they greatly increase the amount of mail processed by the servers.

Listserv Addresses

5. Remember to send subscribe and unsubscribe commands to the server address. Send the command message to the message address. Be sure to type the commands subscribe or unsubscribe (see the example screen) in your message.

Student Nurse (snurse-1)		General Nursing (nursenet)	
Server	listserv@listserv.acsu.buffalo.edu	listserv@listserv.utoronto.ca	
Subscribe	snurse-1 firstname lastname	nursenet firstname lastname	
Unsubscribe	snurse-1	nursenet firstname lastname	
Message	snurse-1@ubvm.cc.buffalo.edu	nursenet@listserv.utoronto.ca	

Nursing Education (nrsinged)		Nursing Research (nurseres)	
Server	listserv@ulkyvm.louisville.edu	listserv@listserv.kent.edu	
Subscribe	nrsinged firstname lastname	nurseres firstname lastname	
Unsubscribe	nrsinged	nurseres	
Message	nrsinged@ulkyvm.louisville.edu	nurseres@listserv.kent.edu	

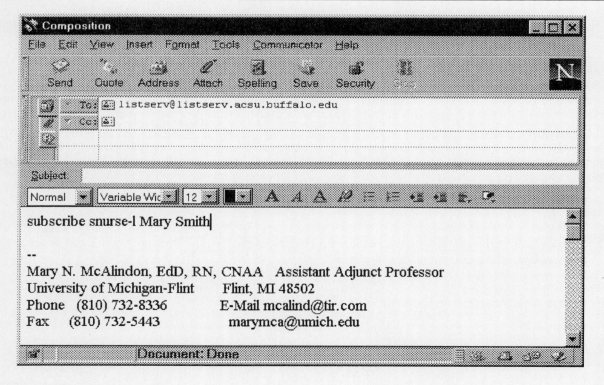

■ ACTIVITY 13-3

The Internet and the World Wide Web contain so much information that sometimes you can't find what you are looking for. Search engines were developed to search through millions of web pages to find exactly what you need. Below is a list of the common search engines and their functions.

Search Engine	Address (called the URL)	Description
Alta Vista	http://www.altvista.digital.com	Fast searches, indexes every word on millions of pages. If the information is on the web, you'll find it here.
Lycos	http://www.lycos.com	Unique options will work around misspellings. Is an older useful site.
Webcrawler	http://www.webcrawler.com	Handles searches in an orderly and logical manner. Reviews and recommends the best web sites. Not as fast as the others.
Yahoo	http://www.yahoo.com	Well-organized categories, easy to find useful information, finds only keywords. A good place to start.

Go to your school computer lab and ask the personnel to show you how to access the Internet (if you don't already know) and the browser needed to access the World Wide Web. These examples illustrate the use of the browser Netscape; if you are using Microsoft Explorer, your screen may look different.

1. Access your browser and enter the address (called the Uniform Resource Locator or URL) of one of the search engines listed above. Search for information that you need for patient education or for a paper that you are writing. What did you find? Was there too much information? Try searching for the keyword *diabetes* or *cystic fibrosis*. What did you find? Click the print icon on the tool bar to print and keep your findings.

2. Use the World Wide Web to access the Centers for Disease Control and Prevention (CDC).

   Type the Uniform Resource Locator (URL) for the CDC in the location or Netsite:

   http://www.cdc.gov/

   When the CDC home page opens, click on an icon (picture) or underlined topic with your mouse and follow the links. Use the Back and Forward buttons on the toolbar to move between the pages.

3. Check some of the statistics. Find information that might be useful in writing a paper about HIV or diabetes. Find health information for travelers.

4. Do you know how to write a reference for information that you find on the Internet? Check with your library for the latest APA format for citing electronic information, as this is now an accepted form of reference. You can also access the web site containing this information. The URL is

   http://www.nyct.net/~beads/weapas/

Managing Costs and Budgets

▌ INTRODUCTION

This section provides additional opportunities to consider how to manage both costs and budgets.

▌ ACTIVITY 14-1

1. You are a staff nurse in an ambulatory care clinic that is making a transition from fee-for-service reimbursement to capitation. Review the incentives for cost control in both methods of reimbursement. How are they different? How will this change affect the nursing practices in the clinic? What will be the important considerations when caring for patients under capitation?

2. Torrell Medical Center grants all full-time employees 10 paid holidays and 12 paid vacation days annually. In addition, the Nursing Department experiences 6.4 average annual sick days and 1.6 other paid and non-paid days off (bereavement, jury duty, education, etc.) per employee.
   a. How many productive hours are worked per full-time employee?

   b. One of TMC's medical-surgical units is expanding its capacity from 38 to 45 beds. It is anticipated that the average daily census will be increased by 4 patients. The unit's average patient care standard is 5.4 hours of nursing care per patient day. How many *additional* FTEs will be needed due to the proposed expansion?

3. How is productivity measured on the unit or at the agency where you practice? What is the process for monitoring productivity? What is the role of staff nurses in monitoring and improving productivity?

4. For the past 3 months nursing salaries have exceeded the budgeted amount by 10%. Is this a positive or negative variance? How would you begin to investigate this variance? What factors might contribute to it? Which factors are controllable by the nurse manager? Are unfavorable or negative variances always a problem? Why or why not?

ACTIVITY 14-2

Do this exercise with a partner. Develop charts or other graphic ways to illustrate the following activities.

SCENARIO: EXPANSION!

You have been informed that because of your statistical justification efforts, administration has recognized the need for more monitored beds. This means that your department will expand from its current eleven beds to twenty monitored beds. As a nurse manager, you are initially very pleased about this expansion, but then you feel dismay because you will have a lot of work to do and only a little time in which to accomplish it. You also have an additional 12 FTE's to add to your current 20.5 FTE's. The current staffing mix is as follows:

> RN FTE's = 12 (10 full-time and 4 part-time)
> LPN FTE's = 3.5 (2 full-time and 3 part-time)
> Nursing Assistant FTE's = 1.5 (6 work every other weekend and one works the Friday along with her weekend)
> Nursing Aide FTE's = 1.0 (full-time, works only Monday to Friday)
> Unit Clerk FTE's = 2.5 (2 full-time, work 9 to 5:30 during the week and every other weekend, and 1 part-time, works 6 P.M. to 10 P.M. Monday through Friday)

The additional 12 FTE's include all support personnel (unit clerks, nursing assistants, and aides as well as RNs and LPNs).

Establish the following:

1. List three goals for the new expanded unit. Include patient outcomes such as discharge criteria, acuity level, and patient teaching.

   a)

   b)

   c)

2. Make a list that differentiates the allocation of FTE's of caregivers and support personnel. Some of the support personnel may also be listed as caregivers, such as nursing assistants and/or unit clerks that are cross-trained as nursing aides. Consider the following when doing the allocation.
   a) There are nine more patients who require care.
   b) There are times when there is no unit clerk available and the daytime clerks have to work overtime to cover the period from 5:30 to 6:00 P.M.
   c) Who will be observing nine additional monitors? Would you want to consider a monitor tech or cross-training some of the other available personnel?
   d) Consider patient outcomes—will your patients be on the monitor during their entire stay in the unit and when the monitor is discontinued they are transferred, or will they remain on the unit until discharge and require a lower level of care?
   e) Currently the acuity level is higher than the original staffing plan was designed for, which is resulting in the nursing staff working overtime on a daily basis.

3. Decide how many part-time versus full-time positions you will need to accomplish the goals set forth in #1 above.

   Remember that when a part-time person works overtime it is not usually paid at time and a half and they frequently are asked to contribute more to receive benefits.

4. Determine the minimum number of staff necessary for all three shifts. Keep in mind that the staffing ratio on your unit is currently one RN or LPN to four patients. Take into account that full-time staff on your unit currently work twelve-hour shifts and every third weekend.

5. Discuss with your partner and develop a clear rationale to demonstrate your understanding of overbudgeted hours and overtime.

Communication and Partnership

▌ INTRODUCTION

Partnership and communication are the building blocks of leadership, team effectiveness, and management. Nurse managers have to be able to promote conversations for relatedness, possibility, structure, action, and functional leadership while partnering with others to deal with common concerns. The following activities are aimed at your identifying (1) your own present strengths and practical uses for them, and (2) new ways to be more effective in the future.

▌ ACTIVITY 15-1

Go back to the self-examination activity in Chapter 15 where you completed the questionnaire. Using another color of pen or pencil, answer the questions again, considering what would be more ideal ways of acting based on what you have read. Then compare your actual behaviors with these ideal ones. List the following:

1. What natural strengths do you have in communication for results?

2. What new behaviors will you work on that would increase your effectiveness in the future?

▌ ACTIVITY 15-2

Study the observation sheets for task, maintenance, and individualistic behaviors on pp. 55-56. Use them to observe a real group. Do the following:

1. What are the strengths of the group in the task and maintenance areas?

2. What individualistic behaviors did you see?

3. What recommendations would you make to the leader and/or the team?

4. What natural strengths do you have?

5. What will you do to increase your effectiveness in the future?

Observing Task Behaviors

Observer Name _____
Observation Date _____

Group Member Numbers

	1	2	3	4	5	6
Task starting						
Initiators						
Information seekers						
Information givers						
Opinion seekers						
Opinion givers						
Procedural facilitators						
Doers						
Recorders						

	1	2	3	4	5	6
Task accomplishment						
Orienters						
Elaborators						
Coordinators						
Evaluators						
Energizers						

Observing Maintenance Behaviors

Observer Name _____
Observation Date _____

Group Member Numbers

	1	2	3	4	5	6
Maintenance						
Encouragers						
Gatekeepers						
Harmonizers						
Conflict managers						
Standard setters						
Welcomers						
Levelers						
Followers						
Observers						

Observing Individualistic Behaviors

Observer Name _____
Observation Date _____

	1	2	3	4	5	6
Individualistic behaviors						
Blockers						
Aggressors						
Recognition seekers						
Dominators						
Avoiders						
Special interest pleaders						

Selecting, Developing, and Evaluating Staff

▌ INTRODUCTION

The following exercises provide an opportunity for you to identify personal preferences for various types of appraisals as well as the strengths and weaknesses for methods commonly used. You may wish to critique an appraisal from a system in which you are currently employed or where you have had clinical experience. Finally, you may develop and critique typical dialogs among professionals. Behaviors that foster empowerment and disempowerment, whether verbal or nonverbal, should be identified.

▌ ACTIVITY 16-1

Design a performance appraisal process that you believe would help you to grow professionally.

Which of the performance appraisal types listed below would be a part of your preferred process? In the spaces below, identify the strengths and limitations of each. State a rationale for each regarding how the process could help you professionally.

a) *Graphic rating scales* provide feedback that can:

Strengths:
Limitations:
b) *Forced distribution* provides feedback that can:

Strengths:
Limitations:
c) *Peer review* provides feedback that can:

Strengths:
Limitations:
d) *Management by objectives* provides feedback that can:

Strengths:
Limitations:

e) *Behaviorally Anchored Rating Scales* provide feedback that can:

Strengths:
Limitations:

State three performance criteria that should be included in your process.
a)
b)
c)

Meet with one to three students to construct a performance appraisal form incorporating each of the performance criteria that you have identified.

Share the group process that has been developed with a person responsible for appraising you, or someone who would. Will that person agree to use your process to assist you to grow professionally? Remember, because your organization uses a particular system does not preclude the use of an *additional* system!

ACTIVITY 16-2

Assess the state of performance appraisal in a clinical organization (setting) by using the checklist below.

_____ 1. Does your organization have a formal performance appraisal system? (If "no," see last item on this list.)
_____ 2. Does it use graphic rating scales?
_____ 3. Does it use forced distribution?
_____ 4. Does it include peer review?
_____ 5. Is it based on management by objectives?
_____ 6. Are the objectives based on a strategic plan?
_____ 7. Does it include a behaviorally anchored rating scale?
_____ 8. Does it influence compensation?
_____ 9. Does it serve as the basis for discipline?
_____ 10. Is it used to determine training needs?
_____ 11. Does it increase role clarity?
_____ 12. Do appraisal meetings occur at least quarterly?
_____ 13. Is the system based on up-to-date position descriptions/criteria?
_____ 14. Is there a clearly defined training process for appraisers?
_____ 15. Every organization has an appraisal process! If your organization has no formal process, you can be sure that an informal process exists. Your performance is assessed!

Cite three examples of criteria used in the informal system in the organization.
1.
2.
3.

What is your opinion regarding the workings of the informal system of appraisal in your organization?

How does the informal system of performance appraisal reflect the values, climate, or cultural of the setting? Cite two ways.

1.

2.

■ ACTIVITY 16-3

Examine and analyze typical dialogues among nurses, managers, and other health professionals. Cite three instances of both empowering and disempowering behaviors.

Empowering behaviors

1.

2.

3.

Disempowering behaviors

1.

2.

3.

Team Building

▌ INTRODUCTION

Teamwork is the name of the game these days. In almost every type of institution there is an emphasis on building and maintaining effective teams. Despite this focus on teamwork, many of us still have old habits and beliefs about being effective individuals. Remember all those times you decided, and others encouraged you, to "do it yourself." "Be strong and handle it alone!" Now the games has been changed to cooperating and collaborating. This chapter aims to increase your understanding of what produces high-performing teams. You will learn the power of focusing your attention on commitment to a particular task. You will also discover how to maintain the cohesiveness of a group and how individualist behaviors affect groups.

▌ ACTIVITY 17-1

1. List at least five criteria for effective teamwork.
   a)
   b)
   c)
   d)
   e)

2. Identify what was missing from the team's performance. Apply criteria to your observations and experience in the group.

3. Based on your reading of Chapter 17 and various articles, list three specific ways to enrich team performance.
   a)
   b)
   c)

4. Identify and commit to at least two new actions you could take to improve your role as a team member. Write them down and set deadline dates.
   a) I will   by

   b) I will   by

ACTIVITY 17-2

Examine a work group that you are familiar with, either currently or from the past. Select two people you have worked with: one person with whom you enjoyed working, and one with whom you were very reluctant to work. For each person, list two behaviors that are characteristic of that person's interactions with others.

PERSON I USUALLY ENJOYED WORKING WITH	PERSON I WAS USUALLY RELUCTANT TO WORK WITH
1.	1.
2.	2.

Next, respond to the following:

Do you demonstrate behaviors from either list   YES   NO

Would you fall exclusively in one list or the other?   YES   NO

Cite two examples of your behavior to support your answer.
1.

2.

In considering the person you were reluctant to work with, cite two positive behaviors for him/her:
1.

2.

In what ways could you encourage growth and expansion of those behaviors?
1.

2.

What could this person contribute to a team?
1.

2.

ACTIVITY 17-3

Make a list of your strengths and limitations as a team member and as a team leader.

Team Member	**Team Leader**
Strengths	
1. _____	1. _____
2. _____	2. _____
3. _____	3. _____
Limitations	
1. _____	1. _____
2. _____	2. _____
3. _____	3. _____

Now examine each of the above and determine how each enhances or interferes with the team process.

Delegation: An Art of Professional Practice

INTRODUCTION

Delegation is a critical strategy for nurses to accomplish their work. It has legal and ethical implications and it is a complex decision. Delegation requires that the nurse know many facts, both about patients or clients and about other workers. This chapter provided some of the key information for making appropriate delegation decisions. The following activities are designed to strengthen your skills in determining assignments from two perspectives: one requires knowing about specific patients in terms of the criteria set by a national organization; the other requires hypothesizing what to anticipate in an unknown patient population.

ACTIVITY 18-1

Arrive for your next clinical assignment 1 to 2 hours early. Using the actual patients on your unit or in your population actively served and the projected staffing, apply the factors for delegation for the anticipated tasks. Complete this assignment for at least five patients with five tasks each.

Factors	Patient 1 Tasks 1 2 3 4 5	Patient 2 Tasks 1 2 3 4 5	Patient 3 Tasks 1 2 3 4 5	Patient 4 Tasks 1 2 3 4 5	Patient 5 Tasks 1 2 3 4 5
Potential for harm					
Complexity of task					
Need for problem solving/innovation					
Unpredictability of outcomes					
Level of interaction (patient)					
TOTALS					

Scale: 0 = best outcome
|
|
|
3 = least desirable outcome

Which factors were most difficult to assess? Why? When assignments were actually made, did delegation occur as you anticipated? If not, were the actual choices better than yours? Why? Why not?

ACTIVITY 18-2

Select a partner. Each of you choose an uncommon (and preferably previously unstudied) chronic disease condition. In the space below, identify the condition and your literature source. Then list what tasks you would delegate to a new nursing assistant. Provide rationale and method of evaluating your decision.

Condition:

Source:

Delegated Tasks	**Rationale**	**Method of Evaluation**

Conflict: The Cutting Edge of Change

INTRODUCTION

The following activity assumes you have completed and scored the Conflict Self-Assessment (p. 323) and responded to the questions in Boxes 19-5, 19-7, 19-9, 19-11, and 19-13. Effective conflict resolution and polarity management lead to effective leadership for change.

ACTIVITY 19-1

After you have read Chapter 19 in the textbook, complete and score the Conflict Self-Assessment on page 323 in the text. Next, write out your responses to the self-assessment questions for each of the five approaches to conflict on pages 324, 325, 326, 327, and 328 of the textbook (avoiding, accommodating, competing, compromising, and collaborating), focusing only on conflicts in your professional life. (If you are not yet in a professional position, you might instead focus on conflicts during your "career" as a student.) Use the Conflict Reflection Form below to focus your thinking. What new behaviors have you committed to for the future?

Conflict Reflection Form

Look at your scores on the Conflict Self-Assessment and responses to the five sets of self-assessment questions in the textbook. Reflect on how you act during conflict (professional and/or personal). Be honest with yourself without being critical.

1. How do you tend to balance the following polarities related to conflict?
   a) Unassertiveness and assertiveness?
   b) Uncooperativeness and cooperativeness?
   c) Avoidance and involvement?
   d) Escalating and minimizing any conflict?
   e) Rigid control and loose improvisation?
   f) Revealing and concealing information?
   g) Intellectual and emotional reactions?

2. Which two approaches to conflict resolution do you tend to underemphasize? Why?

   a)

   b)

3. Which two do you tend to use most frequently? Why?

   a)

   b)

4. How might you be overemphasizing some approaches? Are they situation specific, or are they just the ones you rely on? Why?

5. When and how might you be matching approaches effectively to the particular nature of conflicts in which you are involved?

6. When and how might you be matching approaches ineffectively with the particular nature of conflicts in which you are involved?

ACTIVITY 19-2

Playing Twenty Questions: Conflict Analysis

Reflect on past and present conflicts in which you have been directly involved. Choose one conflict to focus on, particularly if it seems to be reappearing with the same or with other people. Check the textbook to determine whether it is a polarity. If it is, choose another conflict that is not a polarity. Then write out your responses to each of the 20 questions below.

Defining the Conflict

1. Who was the conflict between? How were they affected?
   Who:
   How:
   Who:
   How:

2. Who else was affected and how?
   Who:
   How:

3. What was the actual conflict? What were the perceived incompatibilities?

Conflict Process Analysis

Frustration Stage

4. What did you feel at the start and in the early stages of the conflict?

5. Why did you feel this way?

6. How did you act as a result of these feelings?

7. What do you think the other people felt at the start and in the early stages of the conflict?

8. Why do you think they felt this way?

9. How did they act as a result of these emotions?

10. After the conflict moved into the conceptualization stage (see below), what other emotions, or changes in your initial emotions, occurred? Why?

Conceptualization Stage

11. What did you think the real conflict, or issue, fight, disagreement, etc., was? Why?

12. What do you think now that the other people believed the conflict, or issue, fight, disagreement, etc., was? Why?

13. Where did you and others have serious differences: facts and information, goals and objectives, means and methods of action, and/or standards and values?

14. Describe why you had the following differences:

   a) Exposure to different data?

   b) Different interpretations of the information?

   c) Differences in your roles and position?

   d) Different values and beliefs?

   e) Cultural differences?

   f) Different directions from someone else?

15. After the conflict moved into the action stage, what new views of the conflict (conceptualizations) were created by anyone involved? Why?

Action

16. How did you act specifically (and which of the five approaches to conflict were tried)? Why?

17. How did the other people act? Why?

18. After the conflict clearly was in the outcome stage, were there any new actions by anyone that were aimed at resolving this conflict or in changing any of the outcomes below?

Outcomes

19. What happened to the quality of task accomplishment and efficiency of action as a result of the actions taken? Why?

20. What happened to the quality of the relationships among those involved?

ACTIVITY 19-3

Imagine that you will be in a conflict in the future similar to the one you just analyzed in Activity 19-2. Knowing what you do about this past conflict, your tendencies to approach conflict (review the self-assessments in Chapter 19), and the five different approaches to conflict, write out a short scenario below (including all four stages of the process) describing how you could act to resolve the conflict.

Managing Personal/ Personnel Problems

◼ INTRODUCTION

Successfully managing personal/personnel problems is a crucial element of the role of a nurse manager. To master this role function requires that the manager be able to accurately identify personnel problems, develop intervention strategies, implement those strategies, and then evaluate the effectiveness of the interventions. The exercises in this section will help you develop the assessment and intervention skills necessary to successfully manage personnel problems.

◼ ACTIVITY 20-1

Personal/Personnel Problems: Chemical Dependency

1. Review the following documents:
   a) Your state board of nursing's policy and procedure regarding chemically impaired nurses.
   b) The American Nurses' Association *Code for Nurses* and the policy statement regarding chemical dependency.
   c) A healthcare agency's policy and procedures regarding chemically dependent employees.
   d) A healthcare agency's policy regarding employee drug screening.

2. Define the differences between substance dependence and substance abuse.

   Substance dependence is:

   Substance abuse is:

3. List three factors leading to substance abuse in employees.
   a)
   b)
   c)

4. List five of the most common types of abused substances.
   a)
   b)
   c)
   d)
   e)

5. Describe four signs and symptoms of dependence/abuse that may be evident in a chemically impaired employee.

a)

b)

c)

d)

6. Write a short paragraph either supporting or contesting the following statements regarding chemically impaired healthcare employees.

a) Substance dependence/abuse is a disease and therefore not fully under the control of the affected person. Substance abusers should be treated, not punished.

b) Nurses and other health professionals, with their knowledge about drugs as well as their social contract with patients, should be held to higher standards than the general population.

7. Obtain a copy of personnel policies from an agency in which you have clinical experience. Analyze the policy in relation to the following factors, recording your answers in the space provided.

a) Is the *Diagnostic and Statistical Manual* (DSM-IV) definition used to define substance dependence/abuse in the agency policy?

b) Is there a policy for reporting suspected or known impaired employees? If so, what is the role of the nurse manager? Staff nurse?

c) Does the policy include plans for intervention and treatment? Is an employee assistance program (EAP) provided for employees? What is the manager's role in intervention?

d) Does the policy include a notification procedure? If so, who within the agency administration is to be notified? What is the policy for notifying the state board of nursing if the impaired worker is a nurse?

e) List three key elements that you think should be included in an "ideal" agency policy.

f) Does the return-to-work section of the policy identify how the recovering nurse will be monitored?

g) Are there conditions within the policy to address how a relapse will be handled?

ACTIVITY 20-2

Personal/Personnel Problems: Mandatory Drug Testing for Healthcare Professionals

1. Review a copy of the following documents:
   - An agency's policy and procedure regarding chemically dependent employees.
   - An agency's policy regarding employee preemployment and on-the-job drug screening.
   - Your state board of nursing's policy and procedure on reporting suspected chemically dependent nurses.
   - The American Nurses' Association *Code for Nurses.* Determine their policy statement regarding substance abuse.
   - An agency's policies on nondiscrimination in employment under the Americans with Disabilities Act.

2. Prepare to debate the issue of mandatory drug testing for healthcare employees. Read the following debating statement. Prepare five key points to argue for each side (pro and con) of the issue, drawing support for your arguments from the list of readings in item 1 above: *Whereas approximately 70 percent of all cases handled by state boards of nursing are related to chemically impaired nurses, and whereas nurses have entered into a social contract with their clients to provide safe care, Therefore, mandatory, random drug testing should be done on all practicing nurses.*

	Pro	Con
a)		
b)		
c)		
d)		
e)		

■ ACTIVITY 20-3

1. Read about the legal, regulatory, and ethical issues related to termination of an employee. Refer to the following reading as a guide.

   Curtin, L. (1996). *Ethics, discipline, and discharge. Nursing Management*, 27(3), 51-52.

2. Review an agency's policies and procedures for terminating employees.
3. Read the scenario below. Carefully weigh the pros and cons of each termination decision, considering the legal, ethical, and personal factors that enter into your decision.

Downsizing Scenario

You are a nurse manager in an agency that is experiencing financial difficulties. This problem affects more than just your agency. You are located in a county that is economically depressed and unemployment is high. You have just received the budget for the next financial year and note that you have lost one full-time position, meaning you must lay off one of your full-time nurses. Due to the poor economic situation, it is not possible to transfer within the agency and the layoff will most likely be a permanent one. Also, no other agencies in the area are hiring, although some jobs may be available through a staffing pool or on a contingency basis. You must decide which of the following three employees to lay off. This is a nonunion agency, each of the nurses has the same number of years of service with the hospital, and all have had very similar performance evaluations for the last 3 years.

Nurse A: Nancy is 50 years old and entered nursing later in life after raising a family of four. She is married to the hospital's chief of staff, and some of the younger nurses on the unit resent her "country club" attitude. They think she is not really serious about nursing and only works to escape being bored. Nancy does a good job, but does have some difficulty working with other staff nurses. You personally like Nancy a great deal. She is closer to you in age and life experience than the other staff nurses, and you find yourself turning to her for advice and support. Nancy has confided in you that she really enjoys her newfound career. She says that for the first time in her life she has an identity of her own instead of always being somebody's daughter, spouse, or mother. Nancy has missed 4 days of work in the last 6 months, two times to take her mother to the doctor for evaluation of Alzheimer's disease, one because her husband unexpectedly told her that she had to accompany him to an important hospital social event, and one time she called in sick.

Nurse B: John is 35 years old and the only male nurse on your unit. He has suffered a great deal of personal crises and losses in the past 2 years. His 2-year-old son has Down syndrome, and his 10-year-old son was killed in an automobile accident last year. Six months ago his father died unexpectedly from a heart attack. John had confided in you that he is really struggling with these personal losses. He is especially having difficulty with losing his son because he says he will never be able to do all the "father/son" things with his 2-year-old son that would have been possible with the older son. John says he just doesn't feel the same kind of bond with either his 2-year-old son or his 6-year-old daughter. John also states that he's having difficulty with his wife. Their relationship is very strained and stressful. He's not sure if the marriage will survive. He says that he has been very depressed over all of these crises and has sought professional counseling. He also tells you in confidence that the psychiatrist has him on antidepressants to help him cope. John has missed 4 days of work in the last 6 months. All of them have been on Mondays. He says that the depression has at times made it difficult for him to start another week.

Nurse C: Carrie is 33 years old and very well liked by her peers. She is an informal leader in the group. You personally don't like Carrie very much. She was working on the unit before you became manager and she has constantly challenged you since you arrived. She is argumentative and resistant to change, but she always ends up doing what you have asked her to do. You worry about the effect that she has on unit morale. Yet you note that none of the staff nurses has ever reported having difficulties working with her. Nine months ago Carrie seriously injured her back when a patient she was ambulating started to fall. Carrie saved the patient from injury, but was on medical leave for 6 weeks because of the incident. Her recovery may have been hindered by the fact that she is 40 pounds overweight. Due to her back injuries, she often requests that she be assigned to Charge (desk) duty. Other staff nurses have offered to give her their Charge duty or volunteered to help her with patient care if she needs any assistance. Carrie has missed 4 days in the past 6 months, 2 days on two separate instances, both for complaints of back pain.

Which nurse will you lay off?

List two reasons to terminate or retain each of the nurses.

Nancy: 1.
       2.

John: 1.
       2.

Carrie: 1.
       2.

Indicate one personal, ethical, and legal issue that may be raised in terminating each of the three nurses.

Nancy: Personal:
       Ethical:
       Legal:

John: Personal:
       Ethical:
       Legal:

Carrie: Personal:
       Ethical:
       Legal:

Consumer Relationships

▊ INTRODUCTION

It is essential to be aware of how consumer relations affect the provision of nursing care. Consumers are faced with many changes in the healthcare delivery system. When patients enter the healthcare system they lose a significant amount of control. The following exercises are to help you identify how nurses can promote positive experiences with healthcare.

▊ ACTIVITY 21-1

Mr. Irons is transferred to your unit after having a myocardial infarction (MI). He is the C.E.O. at Interplast, an internationally known plastics manufacturer, specializing in healthcare supplies. One report stated he has been very unhappy because of the limitations that have been placed on him in the ICU and is happy to go to the telemetry unit so that he can "carry on with his life." Mr. Irons has made arrangements for a laptop computer to be brought in and his secretary to be present for four hours a day. The staff has expressed concern regarding how wise it is for him to work while recovering from an MI and have witnessed many "type A" behaviors.

You are the nurse manager of the unit and when you return from a meeting you have a message to call the vice president for nursing regarding a patient complaint. When you call her, you are told that Mr. Irons has called the hospital administrator and demanded that a nurse on the unit be fired. His physician wants the "usual" procedures used. You have been asked to investigate the situation.

Upon investigation you find that Mr. Irons is very upset because the nurse has been attempting to do some patient education regarding reducing stress and providing time for relaxation. He feels that he rests adequately at night and if he does not take care of business there will be serious consequences at his company. The staff nurse is upset and fearful of being fired. The physician has ordered Valium for the patient.

Review the textbook pages promoting successful consumer relationships: service, advocacy, teaching, and leadership. Then answer the following questions.

1. How can your staff effectively provide services for Mr. Irons? List four ways.
   a)
   b)
   c)
   d)

2. If Mr. Irons refuses to collaborate with the staff in the plan of care, cite three effective ways to support staff regarding Mr. Irons' demands.
   a)
   b)
   c)

3. How are you going to respond to the vice president for nursing and to the hospital administration? Cite three critical areas to include in your response.
   a)
   b)
   c)

4. How will you handle Mr. Irons' demand for the staff nurse to be fired? Cite your approach and give supportive rationale for your selection.
   Approach

   Rationale

5. How will you be an advocate for Mr. Irons?
   Approach

   Rationale

ACTIVITY 21-2

In some institutions there are designated patient representatives who act as ombudsmen (advocates) for the hospital and the patient. (These persons may also be designated as "risk managers.") They are frequently first in line and highly skilled in handling patient complaints. Consider how a person in such a position may effectively respond to Mr. Irons' concern? Make a list of at least three possible actions the patient representative could take.

   1.

   2.

   3.

   Compare your responses with at least two other classmates. Were your responses the same? Different? What would *you* do?

   1.

2.

3.

Give rationale for each of these actions.

1.

2.

3.

■ ACTIVITY 21-3

(Refer to Activity 21-1.)

Role Play

Time limit: three to five minutes.

1. Divide into small groups of five to seven students. Two students will role play while the others observe.
   Role players for Mr. Irons and the staff nurse: Don't be afraid to express feelings of anger, fear, disappointment, etc. Think about how you would respond (both in words and in feelings) as if you were the person.
   Observers make notes about:
   a) what is said.
   b) what may be said differently.
   c) report on body language of the role players.
2. Discuss what was observed. (Note: Be open to make and receive recommendations regarding the nurse role play from your peers. This is your chance to receive nonthreatening feedback from your peers prior to confronting this possible situation clinically.)
3. *Role play repeat*: After completing one role play, two other members of the group rotate roles and complete the same process. Everyone should have the opportunity to have played at least one role, either nurse or patient.
   Other possible role combinations: Mr. Irons and hospital administrator; nurse manager and vice president for nursing; Mr. Irons and nurse manager; nurse manager and staff nurse (the one Mr. Irons wants fired); nurse manager and Mr. Irons' physician; you, the ombudsman, and any one of the above.
4. Identify how it would feel to be in the role you are assigned. For example, as the patient, you want to make your own decisions; as the staff nurse you feel concerned because you know his behavior may be detrimental to his health.
   I felt:

5. Discuss the feelings that were identified as a group. For example, as the nurse manager, while you were discussing the situation with the vice president for nursing you felt defensive.
List five suggestions generated by the group to avoid defensiveness.
a)
b)
c)
d)
e)

6. Consider what responses would have made you feel better. For example, you become angry while talking to Mr. Irons and tell him you are going to have his doctor talk to him. With the assistance of the group, list five ways that this might have been said differently.
a)
b)
c)
d)
e)

ACTIVITY 21-4

It is the practice of some institutions to have patient care conferences. It is the goal of these conferences to handle problems that may occur and design a plan to provide quality care for the patient. It is also a good time to support your peers who may be having difficulties in providing care when there are problems.

You are responsible for leading a patient care conference and outlining a plan of care for Mr. Irons. Outline your plans for the conference. The patient should be involved in decisions made regarding the provision of care. Will you invite Mr. Irons to attend your patient care conference? Why? (Provide rationale.)

How will you involve Mr. Irons in his plan of care in the future? Identify five ways.

1.

2.

3.

4.

5.

ACTIVITY 21-5

(Refer to Activity 21-4)

Form a group of five to seven and compare and discuss your individual responses. Develop group responses and provide rationale, using the space below to write out your rationale and plan in detail.

Care Delivery Systems

▌ INTRODUCTION

Healthcare delivery has been significantly impacted by many factors. Managed care and financing reforms will continue this rapid transformation in care delivery strategies. Identifying characteristics, strengths, and liabilities of each system will enable the nurse to match the care delivery strategy with the agency's philosophy, goals, organizational and financial structure.

▌ ACTIVITY 22-1

You are the charge nurse on a 10-patient subacute care unit. There are two RNs, one LPN/LVN, and one nursing assistant working today. Each care delivery strategy has different functions for care providers, e.g., in primary care, RNs have different functions than in the functional method. Describe the role of each care provider in each of the care delivery strategies below.

Case Method
RN #1 role:

RN #2 role:

LPN/LVN role:

Nursing assistant role:

Functional
RN #1 role:

RN #2 role:

LPN/LVN role:

Nursing assistant role:

Team
RN #1 role:

RN #2 role:

LPN/LVN role:

Nursing assistant role:

Primary
RN #1 role:

RN #2 role:

LPN/LVN role:

Nursing assistant role:

Case Management
RN #1 role:

RN #2 role:

LPN/LVN role:

Nursing assistant role:

Additional considerations for the above activity:

1. Cite one advantage and one disadvantage of each care delivery strategy.

2. Cite two care delivery strategies that would require a different staff mix to make them work.

3. As a baccalaureate prepared nurse, which care delivery method would you be satisfied to work in? State a rationale for your selection. What if you were an associate-degree-diploma prepared nurse?

4. Which care delivery strategy would your chief financial officer favor? Why?

CHAPTER **23** WORKBOOK

Patient Classification, Staffing, and Scheduling

▌ INTRODUCTION

Staffing a patient unit is a complex task. There are many things that must be considered when calculating the staffing needs of the unit you are managing. These include the average census of the unit, length of stay, patient classification, and staff mix. It is important to have a good understanding of the needs of the unit before attempting to determine the number and type of staff needed. Also consider the staff's needs and the personnel policies and contracts with the staff when planning the schedule.

▌ ACTIVITY 23-1

You are the manager of a medical-surgical unit. The unit has 32 beds and has an occupancy rate of 75%. A decision was made that there should be four RNs, two LPNs/LVNs, and two nursing assistants on the day shift each day. There should be three RNs, one LPN/LVN, and two nursing assistants on the afternoon shift, and three RNs, one LPN/LVN, and one nursing assistant on the night shift. Using the formulas from your textbook (pages 448–449, determine how many FTEs of each category employee will be necessary to cover the staffing requirements. (Remember, your unit is operating 24 hours per day and all weekends and holidays.)

Your staff has the following allowed per contract:
>   7 holidays per year
>   10 sick days per year (funeral leaves deducted from sick time)
>   15 vacation days per year
All employees work every other weekend.

Determine:
>   Number of RN FTEs needed
>   Number of LPN/LVN FTEs needed
>   Number of nursing assistant FTEs needed

Using this same staffing pattern determine what percentage of staff is allowed for each shift.
_____ % allocated to 7 AM to 7 PM
_____ % allocated to 7 PM to 7 AM
100% Total

Now that your staffing pattern is determined, develop a priority-of-care guideline for one specific patient unit.

ACTIVITY 23-2

Scheduling

Using the same type of grid as represented on page 394 of your textbook (Figure 23-1), complete a unit staffing schedule for the 7 AM to 7 PM shift for a unit as described in Activity 23-1. (Suggest doing 2 weeks at least to establish weekend coverage.) Now consider the following revisions and constraints to your original planning.

1. What happens to the schedule if the second Monday is a holiday?

2. Include in the schedule one RN having a week of vacation time that includes her weekend to work.

3. Now assume you must suddenly include a funeral leave (3 consecutive days) for one LPN/LVN during the same time as the RN has vacation.

ACTIVITY 23-3

Self-Scheduling

You have called a staff meeting and have encouraged the staff to bring concerns regarding staff satisfaction. The meeting starts off with everyone wanting to start a self-scheduling program. Complete the following chart to illustrate and clarify the dilemmas, issues, and problems inherent in self-scheduling.

(+) Self-Scheduling	(+) Managerial Scheduling
1. Staff control over schedule	1. More efficient
2.	2.
3.	3.
4.	4.
5.	5.

(−) Self-Scheduling	(−) Managerial Scheduling
1. Negotiating with peers about schedule	1. Complaints from staff
2.	2.
3.	3.
4.	4.
5.	5.

Before starting self-scheduling you would need to write some guidelines. Identify four more guidelines that you believe are necessary to incorporate as you develop the new schedule. Review the chart above.

1. May only schedule Friday off with your weekend one time per month.

2.

3.

4.

5.

ACTIVITY 23-4

Patient Classification

1. Identify the patient classification instrument used at two different institutions.

2. Cite two similarities and differences between each form.
   Similarities:

   a)

   b)

   Differences:

   a)

   b)

3. Compare the use of a patient classification instrument with at least two patients. Identify how the use of it differs for each patient.

   a)

   b)

Role Transition

◼ INTRODUCTION

Roles in healthcare are changing rapidly. Are you in the midst of a role transition or are you anticipating the transition from nursing student to "real nurse"? No matter which situation you are in, Activities 24-1 and 24-2 can provide valuable insight. Thoughtful responses to the questions will help you clarify the roles of a nurse manager, your strengths, and areas for improvement.

◼ ACTIVITY 24-1

1. Read Chapter 24 and complete the "Roles Assessment" on pages 405–406. In that assessment you are asked to analyze job responsibilities, opportunities to contribute and grow professionally, lines of communication, and expectations of others around the nurse manager. Talk to two staff nurses and ask each of them, "What are the two most important roles that a nurse manager must fulfill?"
   a1)
   a2)
   b1)
   b2)
   Ask a nurse manager, "What are the two most important roles that you must fulfill?"
   a)
   b)
   Compare the responses:
   Similarities:

   Differences:

   Conflicts:

   Share your responses with two or three others in your class. Now what do all of you conclude about:
   Similarities:

   Differences:

   Conflicts:

Discuss responses with your classmates and others (managers, staff) and have them assist in clarifying the multiple roles and expectations.

2. What roles and responsibilities excite you? Why?

Which ones seem to demand a "risk and stretch" for you? Why?

Which roles and responsibilities would you rather not have? Why?

■ ACTIVITY 24-2

Complete the self-assessment on page 412. As it asks, talk with a mentor of yours and compare your perspective on yourself with the mentor's perspective. You also could use some of the sentence completions below as additional items on which to focus.

1. One recent example of my success in providing leadership is:

2. I'm especially proud of my ability to:

3. The part of my work I especially like is:

4. I believe in my capability to manage difficult:

5. I'm very responsible in relation to:

6. A goal I've met in the past year of which I'm most proud is:

7. I think my supervisor would evaluate my effectiveness as:

8. My colleagues would describe me as:

9. I accomplish the most when I:

10. One thing I'm more successful with this year is:

Power, Politics, and Influence

▎INTRODUCTION

Who would you say is the most important person at your hospital? Give it some thought before you respond! Is it the president or chief executive officer? Is it the person who makes the most money? Is it the person who supervises the most employees? Is it the person who has the authority to fire or demote you? Is it the physician with the most influence? Is it the patient who threatens to sue you? This chapter examines the nature, impact, and uses of power in nursing management.

▎ACTIVITY 25-1

1. Review the definitions of power in the box on page ??? (Types of Social Power). Write a short personal example fitting each definition:

   a. Expert:

   b. Information:

   c. Legitimate:

   d. Coercive:

   e. Reward:

   f. Referent:

   g. Connection:

2. Now reread the above introduction. Who is the most powerful person at your hospital? Explain why the most powerful person could be you, the nurse.

▎ACTIVITY 25-2

Read the case below, considering the different types of power. Reflect on the behaviors listed for Debbie, the emergency department charge nurse in the case.

Clinical Case Study

Debbie Starr (R.N., B.S.N., C.E.N.), the charge nurse in a very busy emergency department, was exhausted at the end of her 12-hour shift. Sixty-six patients had been triaged, assessed, cared for, counseled, educated, admitted, transferred, and/or discharged. One patient died. Some of the nursing responsibilities/behaviors carried out by Debbie on this shift included:

a) took/gave shift report every 4 hours.

b) assigned staff to patient care responsibilities.

c) assigned staff to nonnursing responsibilities such as ordering supplies, room checks, and testing emergency equipment.

d) oriented two new medical students to department protocols and expectations.

e) requested assistance from the nursing supervisor to obtain ICU beds for two critical patients.

f) called the children's protective agency to request emergency placement for three abandoned children brought in by the police.

g) yelled over the phone at a newspaper reporter who insisted on obtaining details of a recent accident.

h) assisted a staff nurse to support very distressed family members whose elderly parent had just died.

i) talked to the coroner for 10 minutes by phone.

j) cared for five patients whose nurse left for his dinner break.

k) assisted three staff members who were restraining an out-of-control inebriated patient.

l) intervened between a staff nurse and physician who disagreed about a patient care issue.

m) promised to talk privately to an angry unit secretary later in the shift if there was time.

n) gathered all staff together at 11 PM to thank them for their hard work and good care.

Write out short responses to the following questions about the case.

1. Cite all of the bases of power that Debbie exhibited. (Place the number of the power base that she used at the left side of each statement above.) Label each one according to the chapter definition: 1, expert; 2, information; 3, legitimate; 4, coercive; 5, reward; 6, referent; and 7, connection.

2. How did this nurse empower the staff? Cite two ways.

a)

b)

3. Cite two missed opportunities for empowerment that you saw.

a)

b)

4. Visualize this nurse and write a description of her. What does she look like?

How does she speak to people?

What values does she embody?

What influential person in your life does she remind you of?

ACTIVITY 25-3

Empowerment as defined in Chapter 25 is the "process by which we facilitate the participation of others in decision making and taking action in an environment where there is an equitable distribution of power." Empowerment is power sharing and a form of feminine leadership. All of the following can be powerful attributes of a professional nurse. Rank them in order of importance to you by numbering them in the blanks provided (1 being most important).

_____ a) professional knowledge, specialized knowledge
_____ b) technological competence
_____ c) professional experience
_____ d) problem-solving skills
_____ e) comfort with conflict resolution
_____ f) ability to communicate clearly with colleagues
_____ g) a commitment to organizational philosophy and mission
_____ h) above-average financial compensation
_____ i) a sense of humor
_____ j) positive feelings of work satisfaction

Give this same list to a nursing colleague and to a nonnursing colleague and ask them to rank these items. Compare all three rankings. What similarities and differences exist?

Similarities:

Differences:

ACTIVITY 25-4

1. Meet in groups of three or four. Discuss the responses you wrote for the questions about the case in Activity 25-2 featuring Debbie Starr, RN.

2. What "power tools" were most effective in this example?

   a)

   b)

   c)

   d)

3. Describe the "coalition building" behaviors Debbie demonstrated.

   a)

   b)

   c)

4. Discuss the following assertion and its implication for your future in nursing and in nursing management: "Collegiality demands mutual respect, not friendship!" (Chapter 25, page 426). Are friendship and being a respected manager mutually exclusive? Why or why not? Is friendship with colleagues essential to you for effective working relationships? Why or why not?

ACTIVITY 25-5

Meet in groups of five or six. Combine your group rankings from Activity 25-3 (or make arrangements to combine the entire class's rankings).

1. What conclusions can you draw from this exercise? Identify, describe, and explain differences that exist among the rankings by nurses.
   a)

   b)

   c)

2. What can you conclude?
   a)

   b)

   c)

3. Do differences exist between the nurse rankings and the nonnurse rankings? Discuss specific similarities, differences, and conclusions.
   Similarities:
   a)

   b)

   Differences:
   a)

   b)

   Conclusions:
   a)

   b)

Career Management

▌ INTRODUCTION

Managing a career takes time and energy. The alternative to managing your own career is to experience whatever happens and hope for the best. Managing a career isn't only related to finding a "good" position. It is about advancing in the profession in the way that you define you wish to proceed. It requires being proactive. This chapter identified specific strategies to launch a career and to keep it on a positive trajectory. The following activities are designed to use a data management system to create two commonly used documents to sell yourself and to experience an interview that focuses on positive outcomes.

▌ ACTIVITY 26-1

1. Using Chapter 26's Appendix, create a curriculum vitae. Then create a résumé reflective of your *best* abilities and accomplishments.

2. Give your CV or résumé to a classmate and ask that person to interview you. Consider Questions To Ask/ To Be Asked (p. 449) as a basis for the interview. That person can use the checklist for interviewing (such as items 7 to 14) to evaluate your performance.

Photo Credits*

Cover Photos, courtesy Chuck Dresner and Patrick Watson, photographers.

Chapter 1 [opener], p. 2, courtesy Chuck Dresner, photographer; [internal], p. 4, from Potter and Perry: *Fundamentals of Nursing*, ed 4, St. Louis, 1997, Mosby.

Chapter 2 [opener], p. 21, courtesy Chuck Dresner, photographer.

Chapter 3 [opener], p. 35, from Potter and Perry: *Fundamentals of Nursing*, ed 4, St. Louis, 1997, Mosby.

Chapter 5 [opener], p. 73, from Potter and Perry: *Fundamentals of Nursing*, ed 4, St. Louis, 1997, Mosby.

Chapter 7 [opener], p. 130, (top) © Patrick Watson, photographer; [bottom], courtesy of Gretchen Halstead, The Baptist Home, Rhinebeck, NY; [internal], p. 137, © Patrick Watson, photographer.

Chapter 8 [opener], p. 123, © Patrick Watson, photographer.

Chapter 11 [opener], p. 168, courtesy Chuck Dresner, photographer; [internal], p. 175, © Patrick Watson, photographer.

Chapter 12 [opener], p. 185, courtesy Chuck Dresner, photographer.

Chapter 13 [opener], p. 205, courtesy Corometrics Medical Systems, Wallingford, CT.

Chapter 16 [opener], p. 265, courtesy Chuck Dresner, photographer.

Chapter 17 [internal], p. 287, © Linda Bartlett, 1994.

Chapter 18 [opener], p. 300, from Elkin, Perry, and Potter: *Nursing Interventions and Clinical Skills*, St. Louis, 1996, Mosby; [internal], p. 307, from Potter and Perry: *Fundamentals of Nursing*, ed 4, St. Louis, 1997, Mosby.

Chapter 19 [opener], p. 318, courtesy Chuck Dresner, photographer.

Chapter 24 [opener], p. 400, and [internal], p. 411, courtesy Chuck Dresner, photographer.

* All other photos not listed specifically above are courtesy of Patrick Watson, photographer.

Index

Absenteeism, 337–339

Abuse, substance, in staff, 342–343

Accommodation in conflict resolution, 325

Accountability, 303
   collective action and, 154–155

Acknowledgment of strengths in team/group, 286

Acquisitions of healthcare organizations, 112

Action
   in conflict process, 321
   conversations for, 252–255

Active complaining, 255

Active listening
   in creating synergistic team, 289
   principles in, 290t

Activities, sharing, in delegation, 303

Advocacy, 355–357
   work place, 157–158

Affirmative action (AA), 48

Age Discrimination in Employment Act of 1967, 46t, 47

Agency
   apparent, temporary personnel and, 42
   consumer relationships with, 352

"Agency" personnel as issue for nurse manager, malpractice
      and, 42–43

Agenda for meeting, 200–201

Aggressors, individualistic behaviors of, uses of, 262

Agreements, group, in team, 287, 288

Alliances of healthcare organizations, 112

Ambulatory-based healthcare organization, 113–116

American Nurses' Association (ANA), human rights and, 124

American with Disabilities Act (ADA) of 1990, 46t, 47–48

Anecdotal notes in performance appraisal, 271–272

Apathetics in political activism, 418

Apparent agency, temporary personnel and, 42

Appraisals, performance, 270–276; see also Performance
      appraisals

Arrhythmia monitors, continuous, 208

Assertions, action caused by, 254–255

Assignment(s)
   delegation versus, 305
   in effective and ineffective teams, 283t

Associate nurse in primary nursing, 372

Attitude, empowering, power in work place and, 426–427

Authority
   appropriate, delegation and, 303–304
   collective action and, 154
   legal, to delegate, 306–307

Autocratic leadership, 98t, 99

Autonomy
   collective action and, 154
   as ethical principle, 51

Avoidance
   in conflict resolution, 324–325
   of sensitive/controversial issues, 133

Avoiders, individualistic behaviors of, uses of, 262

Bar chart in data analysis, 176, 179

Bargaining, collective, 49, 160–165
   agent for, selection criteria for, 163

Barriers to change, 76

BARS (behaviorally anchored rating scales) in performance
      appraisals, 275

Bedside computer terminals, 215–216

Behavior(s)
   individualistic, observing and using, 261–262
   maintenance, observing and using, 260–261
   task, observing and using, 259–260

Behavioral decision, 98

Behaviorally anchored rating scales (BARS) in performance
      appraisals, 275

Beletran v. Downey Community Hospital, 43

Beneficence as ethical principle, 51

Benefit packages, 117

Biofeedback in stress reduction, 191

Biomedical technology, 207–210

Bishop v. United States, 36

Blockers, individualistic behaviors of, uses of, 262

Blood gas analyzers, 208

Brainstorming for group problem solving and decision
      making, 101

Breach of duty of care to patient in malpractice, 38

Breakdowns, resolving, 255

Breakthroughs, 255

Budget(s), 235–240
   capital expenditure, 237
   cash, 237–238
      development of, in budgeting process, 239
      negotiating, in budgeting process, 239–240
   operating, 236–238
   resource management and, 30–31
   revenue, 237
   supply and expense, 237
   types of, 236–239
   unit
      development of, in budgeting process, 239
      managing, 240

Budgeting process, 239–240

Building shared vision in learning organization theory, 78

Bureaucracy, 144–145

Bureaucratic organizational structure, democratic structure
      differentiated from, 172, 173

Burnout; see also Stress
   characteristics of, 192–193
   definition of, 192
   as sign of organizational dysfunction, 189

Canadian Nurses' Association (CNA), 32

Capital expenditure budget, 237

Capitation as payment basis, 230

Care
   complexity of, in delegation decision making, 308

*Underlined page numbers indicate illustration or box;
t following page number indicates a table.

Care—*cont'd*
  delivery of
    strategies for, 365–383
      case management as, 374–376
      case method as, 366–367
      differentiated nursing practice as, 379–381
      functional method as, 367–369
      primary nursing as, 371–374
      team nursing as, 369–371
    systems for, 365–383
  integrated, 311
Care MAPS, 376, 377–378, 379
Care unit, patient-focused, 380
Career functions of mentors, 410–411
Career(s)
  definition of, 432
  management of, 431–450
    certification in, 438–439
    continuing learning in, 437–438
    marketing strategies in, 433, 435–437
    professional expectations in, 439–441
  potential, 441
  styles of, 433, 434
Caregiver information, satisfaction with, questionnaire on, 360
Caring
  team leadership and, 294
  Watson's theory of, 52
Case management, 374–376
  resource management and, 30
Case manager, nurse, 375–376
Case method of nursing care delivery, 366–367
Case mix in revenue budget, 237
Cash budget, 237–238
  development of, in budgeting process, 239
Causation in malpractice, 39
CDC (Centers for Disease Control and Prevention), 158
Centers for Disease Control and Prevention (CDC), 158
Centralization of organizational structure, 144
Certainty as defensive communication, 256
Certification, 438–439
Challenging assignments by mentor, 411
Change
  barriers to, 76
  chaos theory of, 76, 78
  conflict and, 318–334; *see also* Conflict
  definition of, 73
  environmental influences on, 86
  facilitators of, 76
  high-complexity, 75
  human side of, 80–81
  leading, 73–88
    strategies for, 81–82
  low-complexity, 75
  organizational development and, 141
  planned
    linear approaches to, 75–76

Change—*cont'd*
  planned—*cont'd*
    sequential stages of, 86–87
    seven-stage model of, 76, 77
    six-stage model of, 76, 77
  principles in guiding, 85
  receptiveness to, self-assessment of, 85
  responses to, 80–81
  as source of stress, 187
  systems side of, 81
  technology side of, 81
Change agent, 76
Change complexity continuum, 82
Change environment, context of, 75
Change leader(s)
  manager as, 73
  roles and functions of, 82–85
Change management
  definition of, 74
  functions of, 79–80
Change models, 75–76
Change outcome, 79
Change process, 80
Change situations, 75
Chaos theory, 76, 78
Character development in leadership and followership, 294, 295
Charge nurse, 368
Charges, 229
  capturing all, in timely fashion, 233
Charts, bar, in data analysis, 176, 179
Chemical dependency, 342–343
CHINs (community health information networks), 220
Civil Rights Act
  1991, 46–47
  1964, amended, 46
Clarifying questions, 258
Client; *see* Consumer(s); Patient(s)
Clinical incompetence, 340, 341
Coaching
  by mentor, 411
  in staff development, 272
Coalition, development of, power in work place and, 427–428
Coercion
  in conflict resolution, 325–326
  in leading change, 82, 83t
  in response to sensitive/controversial issues, 133–134
Coercive power, 418, 419, 420
Collaboration
  in conflict resolution, 327–328
  leaders in, 23
  in management, 29
  power in work place and, 426
Collaborative method for performance appraisal, 274–275
Collective action, 151–165
  nursing and, 152–155

Collective bargaining, 49, 159–164
  agent for, selection criteria for, 162
Collegiality, power in work place and, 426
Commitment
  exploring, 285
  to resolution in creating synergistic team, 290–291
  in team concept, 284
Committees, ethics, 53
Common law, 36–37
Communication(s), 246–264
  cultural diversity and, 127–128
  defensive, 256–257
  in leading change, 81, 83t
  lines of, in role transition, 403
    assessment of, 406
  management component of, 207
  skills in, as power strategy, 423
  supportive, 256
  in team concept, 283–284
Community health information networks (CHINs), 220
Community services, 113
Compassion in creating synergistic team, 289
Competition
  in conflict resolution, 325–326
  organizational development and, 141
Complaining as time waster, 197
Complaints, action caused by, 255
Complexity of organizational structures, 142–144
Compliments for action, 255
Comprehension in informed consent, 44
Compromise in conflict resolution, 326–327
Computer(s); see also Technology(ies)
  bedside, 215–216
  in information technology, 206
  mainframe, in integrated information system, 212
  nurse attitudes towards, 218
Computerized patient record (CPR), 219–220
Conceptualization in conflict process, 321
Confidence in team leadership, 294
Confidentiality
  computers and, 218–219
  privacy and, 44–45
Conflict(s), 318–334
  ability to handle, in effective and ineffective teams, 283t
  aspects of, 291t
  definition of, 319
  interpersonal, 320
  intrapersonal, 320
  organizational, 320
  process of, 320–324
    action in, 321
    conceptualization in, 321
    frustration in, 321
    outcomes in, 321–322
  productive vs. unproductive, 322
  resolution of
    accommodating in, 325

Conflict(s)—cont'd
  resolution of—cont'd
    assessing degree of, 322
    avoiding in, 324–325
    coercing in, 325–326
    collaborating in, 327–328
    competing in, 325–326
    compromising in, 326–327
    modes of, 324–328
    negotiating in, 326–327
    principles of, 12
    smoothing in, 325
  self-assessment of, 323
  types of, 320
  unresolvable
    identifying, 329
    managing, 328–332
Conflict managers, maintenance behaviors of, uses of, 261
Confrontation, constructive, 284
Connection power, 419, 420
Consensus decisions, 100
Consent, informed, 43–44
Consolidated systems, 112
Constructive confrontation, 284
Consultive leadership, 98t, 99
Consumer(s); see also Patient(s)
  attitudes of, healthcare costs and, 228
  focus on, 352
    services in, 353
  healthcare, 352
  needs of, identifying, in quality improvement
      process, 175
  in quality management/quality improvement, 173–174
  relationships with, 350–364
    advocacy in, 355–357
    of agency, 352
    leadership in, 360–361
    of nurses, 352–353
    of physicians, 352
    service in, 353–355
    teaching in, 357–360
Consumerism, organizational development and, 141
Contingency theory, 141
Continuing education in career management, 437–438
Continuous quality improvement, 170
Contractors, independent, temporary personnel as, 42
Contractual allowance, 229
Control
  as defensive communication, 256
  team leadership and, 294
  in teams, 285
Controversy, definition of, 319
Conversation(s)
  for action, 252–255
  life occurring in, 247–248
  for possibility, 251–252
  for relatedness, 249–251

Conversation(s)—cont'd
  for structure, 252
  types of, 249–255
Co-optation in leading change, 81, 83t
Coordinators, task behaviors of, uses of, 260
Coping, 188
Co-primary nursing model of patient care, 374
Corporate health alliance, 112
Corporate liability, 40
Cost(s)
  of care, discussing, with patient, 233
  fixed, 234
  healthcare, escalating, causes of, 228–229
  knowing, 232–233
  managing, 226–243
  nursing practices related to, 232–235
  variable, 234
    staffing as, 391–393
Cost center, 236
Cost-based reimbursement, 229
Cost-effectiveness of new technologies, evaluating, 234
Counseling
  by mentor, 411
  in resolving stress, 194
Counteroffer to request, 253
Cover letter, 448–449
CPR (computerized patient record), 219–220
Creativity in problem solving and decision making, 93
Critical Challenges: Revitalizing the Health Professions for the
    Twenty-First Century, 28
Critical paths, 376, 379
Critical thinking, 91–93
  definition of, 92
Criticism in effective and ineffective teams, 283t
Cross-culturalism, 129
Cross-training issues for nurse managers, malpractice and, 42
Cultural care, theory of, 128
Cultural diversity
  dealing effectively with, 131–134
  definition of, 125
  effects of, on staff performance, 130
  in healthcare, 123–135
  learning through role modeling and, 129–130
  in organization, meaning of, 125
  in work force, management techniques for, 126
Cultural sensitivity, definition of, 125–126
Culture(s)
  of area, governance structure and, 155
  Black, 126
  definition of, 125
  differences among, 356
  Hispanic, 126
  richness of, 130–131
Culture broker, 356
Curriculum vitae (CV), 435
  checklist for constructing, 445
  sample, 446

Curriculum vitae (CV)—cont'd
  writing of, 443–444
Customers; see Consumers
CV (curriculum vitae), 435; see also Curriculum vitae (CV)
Cybernetic theories of change, 86

Damages in malpractice, 39
Data
  analysis of, in problem-solving process, 95
  assembly of
    for curriculum vitae, 443–444
    for résumé, 444–446
  collection of
    for curriculum vitae and résumé, 443, 444
    in quality improvement process, 176–178
  gathering of, in problem-solving process, 95
  in information science, 207
Data processing, 210
Database, 210
Day, patient, 390
Decentralization in flat structures, 146
Decision(s)
  behavioral, 98
  consensus, 100
  descriptive, 98
  majority rule, 100
  making and implementing, providing support for,
    158–159
  normative, 98
  optimizing, 98
  prescriptive, 98
  in quality management/quality improvement, 174
  quality of, variables influencing, 99
  satisficing, 96–97, 98
Decision grids in decision making, 102, 103
Decision making, 91–93, 96–99
  on delegation, 307–309
  in effective and ineffective teams, 283t
  ethical
    framework for, 52–53
    research perspective on, 54
  factors affecting, 99
  group, 99–102
  styles of, 97–99
  tools for, 102–103
Decision models, 96–97, 98
Decisional participation, outcomes of, 157
Declarations, action caused by, 254
Defensive and supportive cycles, 257
Defensive communication, 256–257
Defining problem in problem-solving process, 95
Delegatee, 302
  ability and willingness of, 304–305
  selection of, 307
  supervising, 307
Delegation, 300–317
  in achieving performance outcomes, 302–303

Delegation—*cont'd*
  assignment versus, 305
  best of, 312–314
  decision making on, 307–309
  definition of, 302–304
  framework for, 304–305
  historical perspective on, 301–302
  importance of, 305–306
  integrated care and, 311
  legal authority for, 306–307
  by nurse managers, malpractice and, 40
  practicalities of, 311
  process of, 309, 310t
  in self-management, 201
  tips for, 311–312, 315–317
  worst of, 314–315
Delegator, 302
  behavior styles of, 304–305
Delphi technique for group problem solving and decision
      making, 102
Demand, induced, for healthcare services, 228
Deming's fourteen points of quality management, 170, 171
Democratic organizational structure, bureaucratic structure
      differentiated from, 172, 173
Demographic factors influencing healthcare organization
      development, 117–118
Deontological ethical theories, 50
Dependency, chemical, 342–343
Depersonalization in burnout, 193
Description in communicating support, 256
Descriptive decision, 98
Diagnosis-related groups (DRGs)
  hospital stays and, 373
  as payment basis, 230
  in prototype patient classification system, 385
Dialogue in learning organization theory, 78
Differentiated nursing practice, 379–381
Dignity, human, 253
Disability(ies)
  accommodation for, 48
  eligible, defining, 48
Discharge, wrongful, 49
Discipline
  nonpunitive, for absenteeism, 338–339
  progressive, for personal problems, 344
Discussion in effective and ineffective teams, 283t
Disorganization as time waster, 197–198
Distress; *see also* Stress
  definition of, 187
Diversity
  advocacy programs and, 356–357
  cultural, in healthcare, 123–135; *see also* Cultural diversity
"Do nothing" approach to problem solving, 93–95
Documentation of personnel problems, 343, 344
Doers, task behaviors of, uses of, 260
Dominant logic, guidelines for altering, 75
Dominators, individualistic behaviors of, uses of, 262

DRGs (diagnosis-related groups)
  hospital stays and, 373
  as payment basis, 230
  in prototype patient classification system, 385
Drug administration systems, 209
Dualism, team synergy and, 290–291
Duty
  of care to patient
    breach of, in malpractice, 38
    in malpractice, 37–38
  to educate by nurse managers, malpractice and, 40–41
  to evaluate, by nurse managers, malpractice and, 40–41
  to orient by nurse managers, malpractice and, 40–41

EAPs (employee assistance programs)
  in resolving stress, 194
  for substance abuse, 343
ECGs (electrocardiograms), 208
Economic environment, healthcare, changing, 230–231
Economic factors influencing healthcare organization
      development, 117
Educate, duty to, by nurse managers, malpractice and,
      40–41
Education
  consumer, 357–360
  continuing, in career management, 437–438
  graduate, 437–438
  in leading change, 81, 83t
  management, 411
  nursing, valuing, 422–423
Effectiveness, decreased, in burnout, 193
Elaborators, task behaviors of, uses of, 260
Electrocardiograms (ECGs), 208
Emancipated minors, informed consent and, 44
Emotional exhaustion in burnout, 193
Emotional problems of staff, 340, 342
Emotions, managing, in teams, 292–293
Empathy in communicating support, 256
Employee; *see* Personnel; Staff
Employee assistance programs (EAPs)
  in resolving stress, 194
  for substance abuse, 343
Employment laws, 45–49
  affirmative action as, 48
  Age Discrimination in Employment Act of 1967 as, 47
  Americans with Disabilities Act of 1990 as, 47–48
  collective bargaining as, 49
  employment-at-will as, 49
  equal employment opportunity, 46–47
  Equal Pay Act of 1963 as, 48–49
  Occupational Safety and Health Act as, 49
  wrongful discharge as, 49
Employment-at-will, 49
Empowering attitude, power in work place and, 426–427
Empowerment, 420–421
  Kanter's theory of, 25, 26t
  in leading change, 81

Empowerment—*cont'd*
    shared governance and, 156
    in staff development, 268, 270
Encouragers, maintenance behaviors of, uses of, 261
Energizers, task behaviors of, uses of, 260
Environment
    appraisal interview, 275–276
    change, context of, 75
    economic, healthcare, changing, 230–231
    external, assessment of, in strategic planning, 61
    healthcare, forces of unrest and insecurity in, 355
    internal, assessment of, in strategic planning, 61
    working, in effective and ineffective teams, 283t
Environmental influences on change, 86
Equal Employment Opportunity Commission (EEOC),
        46–47
Equal employment opportunity laws, 46–47
Equal Pay Act of 1963, 46t, 48–49
Equality in communicating support, 256
Ethical decision-making
    framework for, 52–53
    research perspective on, 54
Ethical issues, 35–56, 49–55
    future, 55
Ethical principles, 51–52
Ethical theories, 49–51
Ethics
    definition of, 49
    deontological theories of, 50
    law distinguished from, 50t
    principlism and, 51
    technology and, 219
    teleological theories of, 50–51
    values and, 50
Ethics committees, 53
Ethnocentrism, 129–130
Evaluate, duty to, by nurse managers, malpractice and, 40–41
Evaluation
    as defensive communication, 256
    in marketing, 66
    in problem-solving process, 96
    in quality improvement process, 180–181
    in strategic marketing planning process, 68
Evaluators, task behaviors of, uses of, 260
Executive Order 10988, 46t
Exercise in stress reduction, 191
Exhaustion, emotional, in burnout, 193
Expectancy theory of motivation, 9
Expectations
    in role transition, 403
        assessment of, 406
    as source of stress, 187
Expected outcomes in case method of care delivery, 367
Experimentation in problem solving, 93
Expert power, 418, 419
Expert systems in knowledge technology, 217–218
Expert witness, nurse as, 38–39

Expertise, development of, as power strategy, 425
Explaining as leadership task, 12–13

Facilitation
    in leading change, 81, 83t
    in management, 29
Facilitators of change, 76
Factor evaluation system of patient classification, 385–386
Failure to warn by nurse managers, malpractice and, 41
Family and Medical Leave Act, 46t
Federal labor legislation, 46t
Feedback
    in communication, 248
    delegation and, 309
    in performance appraisal, 271
Fee-for-service basis of payment, 113
Feelings in effective and ineffective teams, 283t
Feminine strengths related to androgynous management
        style, 17
Fidelity as ethical principle, 52
Financial soundness, understanding requirements for, 232
Financing of healthcare, 229
    healthcare costs and, 228–229
Fishbone diagram in data analysis, 176, 179
Fit between organizational structure and technologies, 141
"Five-why" technique of risk evaluation, 182
Fixed costs, 234
Flat structures, 146–147
Flexibility
    in communicating support, 256
    in creating synergistic team, 290
Flexible method for performance appraisal, 274–275
Flexible staffing, 393, 395
Floating staff issues for nurse managers, malpractice and, 42
Flow charts in data analysis, 176, 177
Focus in quality management/quality improvement, 174
Follower(s)
    maintenance behaviors of, uses of, 261
    role of, for nurse manager, 402
    roles of, 24
    traits of, compared with leader and manager trait, 25
Followership
    character development in, 294, 295
    in collective action, 153
    definition of, 4
Forced distribution scale in performance appraisal, 273
Foreseeability in malpractice, 39
Formal performance appraisal, 271, 272
Formalization of organizational structure, 144
Fortune v. National Cash Register Company, 49
Frustration in conflict process, 321
FTEs (full-time equivalents)
    in budgeting, 237–238
    in staffing budget, 390–391
Full-time equivalents (FTEs)
    in budgeting, 237–238
    in staffing budget, 390–391

Functional leadership, 258–259
Functional nursing, 367–369

GAS (general adaptation syndrome), 188, <u>189</u>
Gatekeepers
 maintenance behaviors of, uses of, 260
 nurses as, 352–353
Gender, cultural differences related to, 129
General adaptation syndrome (GAS), 188, <u>189</u>
Geographic dispersion of organization, 143–144
Gladiators in political activism, 418
Goals
 determining, in strategic marketing planning, 64
 envisioning, as leadership task, 7–8, 14t
 marketing, setting, 65
 in quality management/quality improvement, 173
 setting of
  as power strategy, 425
  in strategic planning, 62
  in time management, 198
Governance
 nursing, definition of, 155
 shared, 24, 156–157
Government in financing healthcare, 115–116
Graduate education, 437–438
Graphic rating scales in performance appraisal, 273–274
Graphs, line, in data analysis, 176, <u>178</u>
Group(s)
 "in" and "out," 285
 representing, as leadership task, 13, 15t
 teams and, 281
Group agreements in team, 287, <u>288</u>
Group leadership, 98t, 99
Group problem solving and decision making, 99–102
 strategies for, 101–102

Halo effect in graphic rating scales, 273
Hansen v. Caring Professionals, Inc., 42
Harm, potential for, in delegation decision making, 308
Harmonizers, maintenance behaviors of, uses of, 261
Health maintenance organizations (HMOs), 113
 in changing economic environment, 230–231
Healthcare, quality management in, 169–170
Healthcare consumers, 352
Healthcare providers, 352
Healthcare settings
 changes in, 28
 managing, 27–29
Hierarchy
 of needs as motivational theory, <u>9</u>
 in organizations, 143
High tech concept of nursing, 354
High touch concept of nursing, 354
High-complexity change, 75, 82
Histogram in data analysis, 176, <u>178</u>
HMOs (health maintenance organizations), 113
 in changing economic environment, 230–231

Home health agencies, 114
Home health organizations, 114
Honesty in creating synergistic team, 289–290
Horton v. Carolina Medicorp, Inc., 41
Hospices, 115
Hospital information system, 212–213
Hospital stay, average length of, 390
Howard v. North Mississippi Medical Center, 48
Hybrid organizational structure, 144, 147

ICP (intracranial pressure monitoring) systems, 209
Image, powerful, developing, strategies for, 422–423
Implementation
 in marketing, 66
 in problem-solving process, 96
 in strategic marketing planning process, 68
Incompetence, clinical, 340, 341
Indemnification, liability and, 40
Independent contractors, temporary personnel as, 42
Independent practice associations (IPAs), 113
Indicators, quality, development of, 31
Individualistic behaviors, observing and using, 261–262
Induced demand for healthcare services, 228
Influence, 420
 exercising, in work place and organizations, 426–428
Informal performance appraisal, 271
Informatics, 217
 resource management and, 30
Information
 caregiver satisfaction with, questionnaire on, <u>360</u>
 dealing with, in time management, 199–200
 definition of, 206
 gathering of, in budgeting process, 239
 in information science, 207
 management of, 205–224
  in leading change, 82, 83t
 relevant, ensuring, for participation in decision making, 158
 selection of, enabling, for participation in decision making, 158
Information givers, task behaviors of, uses of, 259
Information overload as time waster, 198
Information power, 418, <u>419</u>
Information science, 206–207
Information seekers, task behaviors of, uses of, 259
Information systems, 211–217
 integrated, 212–213
 nursing, 213–217
Information technology, 210–217
 definition of, 206, 208
 information systems in, 211–217
 information theory and, 210–211
 nurse-users of, characteristics of, <u>209</u>
Information theory, 210–211
Information triad, using, <u>207</u>
Informed consent, 43–44
Initiators, task behaviors of, uses of, 259

Injury, resultant, in malpractice, 39
Innovation
definition of, 73
need for, in delegation decision making, 308
Innovation-decision process of change, 76, 77
Innovator(s)
manager as, 73
response of, to change, 80
Institutional providers, 110–112
Insurance, health, private carriers of, in financing health-care, 116
Integrated care, 311
Integrated information systems, 212–213
Integrating factors in delegation decision making, 308
Interaction, level of, in delegation decision making, 308
Interactive Decision Model, 132–133
Internal resources in promoting role transition, 409
Internet, 220–221
health information path to, 222
Interpersonal conflict, 320
Interpersonal relations as source of stress, 187–188
Interruptions as time wasters, 197
Interview, 449–450
for performance appraisal, environment for, 275–276
to secure position, 436
checklist for, 448
in staff selection, 267
successful thank you for, 450
topics/questions of concern for, 450
Intracranial pressure monitoring (ICP) systems, 209
Intrapersonal conflict, 320
Involvement in quality management/quality improvement, 172–173
IPAs (independent practice associations), 113

JCAHO (Joint Commission on Accreditation of Healthcare Organizations), staffing regulations of, 389
Job satisfaction, management style and, 156
Joint Commission on Accreditation of Healthcare Organizations (JCAHO), staffing regulations of, 389
Justice as ethical principle, 51

Kanter's theory of structural power in organizations, 25, 26t
Knowledge base, 217
Knowledge in information science, 207
Knowledge technology, 217–218
definition of, 208
Knowledge workers, nurses as, 161–164
L
Labor acts, 160
Labor legislation, federal, 46t
Labor Management Reporting and Disclosure Act of 1959, 161
Labor relations, 49
Labor unions, 46
Landrum-Griffin Act, 160
Larrabee's theoretical model of quality for healthcare, 171, 171–172

Law(s)
common, 36–37
employment, 45–49
equal employment opportunity, 46–47
ethics distinguished from, 50t
protective, 43
reporting, 32
Leader(s)
change
manager as, 73
roles and functions of, 82–85
collaboration and, 23
personal attributes of, 4–5
role of, for nurse manager, 402
traits of, compared with manager and follower traits, 25
Leadership
androgynous style of, feminine and masculine strengths related to, 17
autocratic, 98t, 99
character development in, 294, 295
consultive, 98t, 99
in consumer relationships, 360–361
definition of, 4
diversity in, 13–16
in effective and ineffective teams, 283t
functional, 258–259
group, 98t, 99
methods of, Vroom and Yetton's, 98t
roles of, management roles versus, 23–27
situational, 304, 305
in stress management, 194–195
style of, 27
tasks of
achieving workable unity as, 11–12
affirming values as, 8
envisioning goals as, 7–8
explaining as, 12–13
managing as, 9–11
motivating as, 8, 9–10
renewing as, 13
representing groups as, 13
serving as symbol as, 13
of team, role of, 293–294
theories of, 304
traits of, 26
transformational, 16
Leadership theory development, 5, 6–7
Leading, tasks of, 7–13
Leading change, 73–88
strategies for, 81–82
Learning
about cultures through role modeling, 129–130
continuing, 437–438
team, in learning organization theory, 78
Learning organization theory, 78t
Legal authority to delegate, 306–307
Legal capacity in informed consent, 43–44

Legal issues, 35–57
    confidentiality as, 44–45
    employment laws as, 45–49; *see also* Employment laws
    informed consent as, 43–44
    liability as, 39–40; *see also* Liability
    malpractice as, 37–39, 40–43; *see also* Malpractice
    privacy as, 44–45
    protective laws as, 43
    reporting laws as, 43
Legislation, labor, federal, 46t
Legitimate power, 418, 419
Letter
    cover, 448–449
    thank you, successful, 450
Levelers, maintenance behaviors of, uses of, 261
Liability, 39–40
    confidentiality and, 44–45
    corporate, 40
    personal, 39
    privacy and, 44–45
    product, strict, 43
    vicarious, 39–40
Licensing standards for staff, 388–389
Licensure, 438
Line graphs in data analysis, 176, 178
Lines of communication in role transition, 403
    assessment of, 406
Listening
    active
        in creating synergistic team, 289
        principles in, 290t
    in effective and ineffective teams, 283t
    for meaning, 257–258
Logic, dominant, guidelines for altering, 75
Low-complexity change, 75, 82

Mainframe computer in integrated information system, 212
Maintenance behaviors, observing and using, 260–261
Maintenance situations, 250
Majority rule decisions, 100
Malpractice
    elements of, 37–39
    for nurse managers
        causes of, 40–43
        delegation and, 40
        duty to educate and, 40–41
        duty to evaluation and, 40–41
        duty to orient and, 40–41
        failure to warn and, 41
        staffing issues and, 41–43
        supervision and, 40
    professional, 37–39
Managed care, 230–231
    quality improvement programs and, 31
    resource management and, 30
    systems of, 113
Management theory, development of, 55

Management/managing
    androgynous style of, feminine and masculine strengths
        related to, 17
    of biases in patient classification, 387–388
    career, 431–450
    case, 374–376
    change
        definition of, 74
        functions of, 79–80
    collaboration in, 29
    of costs, 226–243
    education for, 411
    facilitating in, 29
    of healthcare settings, 27–29
    information, in leading change, 82, 83t
    as leadership task, 9–11, 14t
    of meetings, 200–201
    by objectives (MBO), 274
    of personal resources, 399–450
        role transition in, 400–413
    of personal/personnel problems, 335–346; *see also*
        Personal/personnel problems
    of polarities, 332
    quality, 168–181; *see also* Quality management
    of resources, 29–31, 151–243; *see also* Resources, managing
    risk, 181–182
    roles of, leadership roles versus, 23–27
    self, 185–203; *see also* Self-management
    of stress, 185–195; *see also* Stress, management of
    style of, job satisfaction and, 156
    tasks of, 7–13
    of time, 195–200; *see also* Time, management of
    of unit level budget, 240
    of unresolvable conflicts, 328–332
Manager(s)
    basic functions of, 23t
    conflict, maintenance behaviors of, uses of, 261
    functions of, 23
    nurse; *see* Nurse manager(s)
    personal attributes of, 4–5
    role of, for nurse manager, 402
    traits of, compared with leader and follower traits, 25
Managing by Values, 29
Manipulation in leading change, 82, 83t
MAPs (multidisciplinary action plans), care, 376, 377–378, 379
Marginalized populations, culturally competent
        care for, 132
Marketing, 63–69
    definition of, 63
    evaluation in, 66
    external threat analysis in, 65
    implementation in, 66
    opportunity analysis, 65
    planning in, 66
    strategic planning process for, 63–65
Marketing plan in strategic marketing planning process, 68
Marketing strategies in career management, 433, 435–437

Masculine strengths related to androgynous management style, 17
Matrix organization, 145–146
Mauro v. Borgess Medical Center, 48
MBO (management by objectives), 274
McIntosh v. Brookdale Hospital Medical Center, 48
Meaning, listening for, 257–258
Medical equipment supply systems, 116
Medical records
    confidentiality of, 44–45
    patient access to, 45
Meditation in stress reduction, 191
Mele v. St. Mary's Hospital of Rochester, Minnesota, and Mayo Foundations, 43
Mental models in learning organization theory, 78
Mentor(s), 158–159
    attracting, 424
    career functions of, 410–411
    in promoting role transition, 410–411
    psychosocial functions of, 411
Mentoring as power strategy, 424–425
Mentoring programs, cultural diversity and, 132
Mergers of healthcare organizations, 112
Metropolitan-based healthcare systems, 112
Minors, emancipated, informed consent and, 44
Mission(s)
    marketing, setting, 65
    of organization, 139, 140
    organizational-level, determining, in strategic marketing planning, 64
    in team concept, 284
Mission statement in strategic planning, 61–62
Modular method in team nursing, 371
MORAL model for ethical decision making, 53
Motivation
    as leadership task, 8, 9–10, 14t
    theories of, 9–10
Motivational theories, development of, 5
Motives
    individual and group, suggestions for unlocking, 8
    personal, self-awareness of, for leading/managing, 4–5
Multiculturalism, 128–129
Multidisciplinary action plans (MAPs), care, 376, 377–378, 379

National hospital companies, 112
National Labor Act, 46t
National Labor Relations Act, 161
National Labor Relations Board (NLRB), 49, 161
Needs, hierarchy of, as motivational theory, 9
Negligence, 40
Negotiation
    of budget in budgeting process, 239–240
    in conflict resolution, 326–327
    in leading change, 81, 83t
    power in work place and, 428
Networked information systems, 212
Networking as power strategy, 423–424

Networks
    community health information, 220
    healthcare, 112–113
Neutrality as defensive communication, 256
NISs (nursing information systems), 213–217
NLRB (National Labor Relations Board), 161
NMDS (nursing minimum data set), 210–211
No, inability to say, as time waster, 196
Nominal group technique for group problem solving and decision making, 101–102
Nonmaleficence as ethical principle, 51
Nonproductive hours in budgeting, 237
Nonproductive time in staffing budget, 390
Nonpunitive discipline for absenteeism, 338–339
Normative decision, 98
Norms as conversations for relatedness, 251
North American Free Trade Agreement (NAFTA), professional practice and, 32
Not-for-profit healthcare organizations, 111
Nurse(s)
    associate, in primary nursing, 372
    attitudes of, towards computers, 218
    in case method of nursing care delivery, 367
    charge, 368
    competencies of, descriptive, 26t
    consumer relationships with, 352–353
    in critical pathways/care MAPs, 379
    in differentiated nursing practice, 380–381
    as expert witness, 38–39
    in functional nursing, 368–369
    as gatekeepers, 352–353
    as knowledge workers, 162–165
    primary, in primary nursing, 371–372, 373–374
    in primary nursing, 373–374
    in team nursing, 371
    transition of, to nurse manager, 401
Nurse case manager, 375–376
Nurse manager(s)
    in case method of nursing care delivery, 367
    as change leader, 73
    in critical pathways/care MAPs, 379
    in differentiated nursing practice, 380
    in functional nursing, 368–369
    functions of, 23t
    key abilities/skills for, 27
    malpractice for, causes of, 40–43
    management style of, job satisfaction and, 156
    in primary nursing, 373
    role(s) of, 401–402
        perceptions of, 22
        tips for implementing, 33
    in team nursing, 371
    transition from staff nurse to, 401
Nurse practice acts, 36–37
Nursing
    co-primary, 374
    functional, 367–369

Nursing—*cont'd*
    future projections for, 453
    primary, 371–374
    reintegrated, 440
    team, 369–371
Nursing administration information systems, 213–214
Nursing centers, 114
Nursing information systems (NISs), 213–217
Nursing Leadership in the 21st Century, ARISTA II, 28
Nursing minimum data set (NMDS), 210–211
Nursing practice(s)
    changing healthcare economic environment and, 231
    cost-conscious, 232–235
    differentiated, 379–381
    professional, 36–39
    standard, using research to evaluate, 235
Nursing role and function changes in healthcare
        organizations, 119–120

Objectives
    determining, in strategic marketing planning, 64
    marketing, setting, 65
    in strategic planning, 62
Observers, maintenance behaviors of, uses of, 261
Occupancy, percentage of, staffing an, 389–390
Occupational Safety and Health Act of 1970, 49, 158
ODS (organized delivery systems), 231
On-line interactive information systems, 212
Operating budget, 236–238
Opinion givers, task behaviors of, uses of, 260
Opinion seekers, task behaviors of, uses of, 259
Opportunities
    provided by mentor, 410
    in role transition, 403
        assessment of, 405
Optimizing decision, 98
Organization(s)
    ancillary, 115
    bureaucratic, 144–145
    characteristics of, 110–112
    commitment of, to patient classification system, 386–387
    cultural diversity in, meaning of, 125
    definition of, 138
    development of, factors influencing, 141–142
    diversity in, 13–16
    exercising power and influence in, 426–428
    healthcare, 108–121
        acquisitions and, 112
        alliances of, 112
        ambulatory-based, 113–116
        in consolidated systems, 112
        development of, forces influencing, 116–118
        financial provisions of, 111–112
        mergers and, 112
        networks of, 112–113
        ownership of, 110–111
        service characteristics of, 110

Organization(s)—*cont'd*
    healthcare—*cont'd*
        systems theoretical perspective on, 118–119
        teaching status of, 112
    healthcare continuum of, 110t
    medical equipment supply, 116
    mission of, 139, 140
    nursing role and function changes in, 119–120
    pharmaceutical supply, 116
    philosophy of, 139–141
    planning, 15
    policies of, in managing absenteeism, 338
    professional, 116
    regulatory, 115
    structural power in, 25, 26t
    supportive, 115
    third-party financing, 115–116
    in time management, 199
    types of, 110–112
    vision statements for, 139
Organizational behavior modification as motivational
        theory, 10
Organizational charts, 143
Organizational conflict, 320
Organizational strengths, analyzing, in strategic marketing
        planning, 64–65
Organizational structure(s), 137–150
    characteristics of, 142–144
    democratic, bureaucratic structure differentiated from,
        172, 173
    fit between technologies and, 141
    flat, 146–147
    hybrid, 144, 147
    matrix, 145–146
    types of, 144–148
Organizational weakness, analyzing, in strategic marketing
        planning, 64–65
Organized delivery systems (ODS), 231
Orient, duty to, by nurse managers, malpractice and, 40–41
Orientation in staff development, 267
Orienters, task behaviors of, uses of, 260
Outcome(s)
    accountability for, in primary nursing, 371–372
    in conflict process, 321
    establishing, in quality improvement process, 178–180
    expected, in case method of care delivery, 367
    performance, achieving, delegation in, 302–303
    unpredictability of, in delegation decision making, 308
Outcome criteria for primary nurse, 372
Overstress, signs of, 190t
Overwork as source of stress, 188
Oximetry, 208

Paid time in staffing budget, 390
Paraphrasing, 257–258
Pareto chart in data analysis, 176, 179
Pareto's law, 189

Participation in leading change, 82, 83t
Partnership, foundation for, 248
Partnership models of patient care, 374
Paternalism as ethical principle, 52
Patient(s); *see also* Consumers
    classification of, 385–388
        factor evaluation system of, 385–386
        managing biases in, 387–388
        organizational commitment to, 386–387
        prospective system of, 386
        prototype system of, 385
        retrospective systems of, 386
        selecting/developinig systems for, 386
    discussing cost of care with, 233
    level of interaction with, in delegation decision making, 308
    needs of, meeting, 233–234
    outcomes for; *see* Outcome(s)
    satisfaction of, with care, in consumer relations, 361
Patient care standard in full-time equivalent calculation, 392
Patient day, 390
Patient-centered care, primary dimensions of, 353
Patient-focused care unit, 380
Payer mix in revenue budget, 237
Payers, third-party, 111
    healthcare costs and, 228–229
Payoff tables in decision making, 102–103
Peer review organizations (PROs), 115
People as source of stress, 187–188
Percentage
    of allocation in staffing matrix development, 392
    of occupancy, staffing and, 389–390
Perfectionism as time waster, 197
Performance appraisals, 270–276
    anecdotal notes in, 271–272
    collaborative method for, 274–275
    flexible method for, 274–275
    formal, 271, 272
    informal, 271
    interview environment for, 275–276
    scoring of, 272–273
    structured methods for, 273–274
    tools for, 272, 273–275
Performance outcomes, achieving, delegation in, 302–303
Personal liability, 39
Personal mastery in learning organization theory, 78
Personal motives, self-awareness of, for leading/
        managing, 4–5
Personal values, helping determine, 159
Personal view, disclosing, for participation in decision
        making, 158
Personal/personnel problems
    absenteeism as, 337–339
    chemical dependency as, 342–343
    clinical incompetence as, 340, 341
    documentation of, 343, 344
    emotional, 340, 342
    managing, 335–346

Personal/personnel problems—*cont'd*
    progressive discipline for, 344
    termination for, 344–345
    uncooperative employees as, 339–340
    unproductive employees as, 339–340
Personnel; *see also* Staff; Staffing
    problems of, managing, 335–346; *see also* Personal/
        personnel problems
    temporary, as issue for nurse manager,
        malpractice and, 42–43
    unlicensed assistive, in case method of delivery, 367
Pew Health Professions Commission, 28
Pharmaceutical supply systems, 116
Philosophy of organization, 139–141
Physical activity in stress reduction, 191
Physicians
    consumer relationships with, 352
    highly specialized, surplus of, healthcare costs and, 228
Physiological monitoring systems, 208
Planned change
    linear approaches to, 75–76
    sequential stages of, 86–87
    seven-stage model of, 76, 77
    six-stage model of, 76, 77
Planning, 58–72
    in budgeting process, 239
    in marketing, 66
    marketing in, 63–69; *see also* Marketing
    for quality improvement, 170
    requirements for, 10
    strategic, 60–63; *see also* Strategic planning
Planning organizations, 115
Plans, discussion of, in quality improvement process, 180
Polarity(ies)
    diagram of, 330, 331
    dynamics of, 330–331
    management of, 332
    structure of, 328–329, 330
    as unresolvable conflicts, 328–332
Policies in risk management, 45
Politics, 417
Position
    description of
        excerpts from, 271
        roles and, 270
    selection of, in career management, 433
    as source of stress, 188
Possibility, conversations for, 251–252
Power
    bases of, 418, 419
    coercive, 418, 419, 420
    connection, 419, 420
    definition of, 418
    exercising, in work place and organizations, 426–428
    expert, 418, 419
    focus on, 418–420
    history of, 416–418

Power—*cont'd*
  imbalance of, advocacy and, 356
  information, 418, <u>419</u>
  Kanter's theories on, 26t
  legitimate, 418, <u>419</u>
  personal, strategies for, 423–426
  referent, <u>419</u>, 420
  reward, 418, <u>419</u>, 420
  structural, in organizations, 25, 26t
  in teams, 285
Powerful image, developing, strategies for, 422–423
PPOs (preferred provider organizations), 113
Preferred provider organizations (PPOs), 113
Prescriptive decision, <u>98</u>
Prices, healthcare costs and, 228
Primary care healthcare organizations, 110t
Primary nurse in primary nursing, 371–372, 373–374
Primary nursing, 371–374
Principlism, 51
Priorities, setting of, in time management, 198–199
Prioritization in time management, 196
Privacy, liability and, 44–45
Private health insurance carriers in financing healthcare, 116
Private healthcare organizations, 110
Proactive, 59
Problem, defining, in problem-solving process, 95
Problem orientation in communicating support, 256
Problem solving, 90–105
  group, 99–102
  methods of, 93–95
  need for, in delegation decision making, 308
  process of, 95–96
Procedural facilitators, task behaviors of, uses of, 260
Procedures in risk management, 45
Procrastination, 196
Product, service differentiated from, <u>354</u>
Productive conflict vs. unproductive conflict, <u>322</u>
Productive hours in budgeting, 237
Productive time in staffing budget, 390
Productivity, monitoring of, by nurse managers, 240
Professional association in career management, 440
Professional expectations, 439–441
Professional malpractice, 37–39
Professional nursing practice, 36–39
  ethics in, 49–56
Professional organizations, 116
Professionalism, 32
Profit, need for, 231
Progressive discipline for personal problems, 344
Promises, action caused by, 252–253
Proprietary healthcare organizations, 111
PROs (peer review organizations), 115
Prospective patient classification system, 386
Prospective reimbursement, 229–230
Protection by mentor, 410
Protective laws, 43
Prototype system of patient classification, 385

Providers
  consumers and, 228
  healthcare, 352
  needs of, meeting patient needs rather than, 233–234
Psychosocial functions of mentors, 411
Public healthcare organizations, 110–111
Pulmonary function systems, 209
Purpose, clear, establishing, in creating synergistic team, 289
Purposeful inaction in problem solving, 93–95

QA (quality assurance), 181
QI; *see* Quality improvement (QI)
QM; *see* Quality management (QM)
Quality assurance (QA), 181
Quality care, 32
Quality improvement programs, managed care and, 31
Quality improvement (QI)
  definition of, 170
  planning for, 170
  process of, 174–181
    quality assurance compared with, 181t
  quality management and, 171–174
Quality indicators, development of, 31
Quality management (QM), 168–181
  benefits of, 170
  definition of, 170
  evolution of, 170–171
  in healthcare, 169–170
  quality improvement and, 171–174
  total, 32, 171
Questions, clarifying, 258

Racial differences, <u>356</u>
Recency effect in graphic rating scales, 273–274
Recognition seekers, individualistic behaviors of, uses of, 262
Recorders, task behaviors of, uses of, 260
Records, medical
  confidentiality of, 44–45
  patient access to, 45
Reengineering nursing care delivery system, 141
  philosophy and, 141
Referent power, <u>419</u>, 420
Reforming Health Care Workforce Regulation, 28
Regional healthcare systems, 112
Regulatory organizations, 115
Reimbursement
  cost-based, 229
  methods of, 229–230
  prospective, 229–230
Reimbursement practices, knowing, 232–233
Reintegration, 440
Relatedness, conversations for, 249–251
Relations, interpersonal, as source of stress, 187–188
Relationships
  building, as leadership task, 7–8
  consumer, 350–364; *see also* Consumers, relationships with
  in leading change, 82, 83t

Relationships—*cont'd*
  role transition and, 407, 408t
  work, supportive, in stress reduction, 192
Relaxation techniques in stress reduction, 191, 192
Renewing as leadership task, 13, 15t
Reporting laws, 43
Requests
  action caused by, 253
  possible responses to, 253–254
Research, use of, to evaluate standard nursing
          practices, 235
Resilience, 78–79
Resolution
  committment to, in creating synergistic team, 290–291
  conflict, 324–328; *see also* Conflict, resolution of
Resources
  division of, in staffing matrix development, 392
  internal, in promoting role transition, 409
  managing, 29–31, 151–243
    collective action in, 152–166
  nursing, predicting and using efficiently, 234
  personal, managing, 399–450
    role transition in, 400–413
Respect for others as ethical principle, 52
Respondeat superior, vicarious liability and, 39–40
Responses to change, 80–81
Responsibility(ies)
  collective action and, 154
  delegation and, 303
  in role transition, 403
    assessment of, 405
Resultant injury in malpractice, 39
Résumé, 435
  conventional approach to, 445
    sample, 447
  functional approach to, 446
Retrospective patient classification system, 386
Revenue budget, 237
Revenues, 231
Reward power, 418, 419, 420
Right-to-work states, 155
Risk(s)
  evaluating, 182
  management of, 181–182
Role(s)
  definition of, 404
  development of, 21–33, 407
  nurse manager, 401–402
  theory of, 404
  types of, 401–402
  understanding, 402–403
Role ambiguity, 266
Role conflict, 266
  as source of stress, 187
Role discrepancy, 407
Role expectations, definition of, 404
Role internalization, 407–408

Role modeling
  learning about cultures through, 129–130
  by mentor, 411
Role models, 158–159
Role negotiation in promoting role transition, 409–410
Role strain
  absenteeism and, 337
  definition of, 404
Role stress
  absenteeism and, 337
  definition of, 404
Role theory, 22, 270, 271
  absenteeism and, 337–339
Role transition, 400–413
  promoting
    internal resources in, 409
    management education in, 411
    mentors in, 410–411
    role negotiation in, 409–410
    strategies for, 409–413
  relationships and, 407, 408t
  role triumph after, 412
  unexpected, 408–409

Sabol v. Richard Heights General Hospital, 38–39
Safety in work place, 158
Satisficing decision, 96–97, 98
Scales in performance appraisals, 273–275
Schedule, 394, 395–396
Scheduling, 393–397
  self, 396–397
School health programs, 113
Scientific experimentation in problem solving, 93
Secondary care healthcare organization, 110t
Self-governance organizational structure, 147–148
Self-management, 185–203
  definition of, 186
  delegation in, 201
  of stress, 185–195; *see also* Stress, management of
  of time, 195–200; *see also* Time, management of
Self-regulation in effective and ineffective teams, 283t
Self-scheduling, 396–397
Service
  in consumer relationships, 353–355
  product differentiated from, 354
Service lines, 353
Sexual orientation, culture and, 129
Shared governance, 24, 156–157
Shared governance organizational structure, 147–148
Shared visions, 452
  building, in learning organization theory, 78
Sharing activities in delegation, 303
"Short-staffing" issues of nurse managers, malpractice and,
          41–42
Sigma Theta Tau International, 28
Situational assessment in strategic marketing planning
          process, 67–68

Situational leadership, 304, 305
Situational-contingency theories of leadership, 6
Skills checklist, 340, 341
Slang terms, meanings of, 127
Smart cards, 220
Smoothing in conflict resolution, 325
Social factors influencing healthcare organization
        development, 117
Social support in resolving stress, 193–194
Solutions, developing and selecting, in problem-solving
        process, 96
Special interest pleader, individualistic behaviors of,
        uses of, 262
Spectators in political activism, 418
Sponsorship by mentor, 410
Spontaneity in communicating support, 256
Staff
    assessment tool for, 361, 362
    development of, 267–270
    participation of, in patient classification, 387
    performance of, diversity and, 130
    problems of, managing, 335–346; see also Personal/
        personnel problems
    selection of, 267
    uncooperative, 339–340
    unproductive, 339–340
Staff mix, budget and, 369
Staffing, 388–391
    average length of stay and, 390
    budget for, 390–391
    flexible, 393, 395
    percentage of occupancy and, 389–390
    regulations on, 388–389
    resource use indicator and, 390
    schedules for, 393–397
    unit work load and, 389
    as variable cost, 391–393
Staffing issues of nurse managers, malpractice and, 41–43
Staffing matrix/pattern, 391–393
Stand-alone information systems, 212
Standard of care, determination of, 38
Standard setter, maintenance behaviors of, uses of, 261
Statute in defining legal age, 43–44
Stereotypes, cultural, 132
Strain, role
    absenteeism and, 337
    definition of, 404
Strategic marketing planning process, 63–65
    for breast screening program delivery, 67–68
    case studies on, 70–72
Strategic planning, 60–63
    definition of, 60
    evaluation in, 63
    external environmental assessment in, 61
    goal-setting in, 62
    implementation in, 63
    internal environmental assessment in, 61

Strategic planning—cont'd
    objectives in, 62
    process of, phases of, 61–63
    reasons for, 60–61
    review of mission statement in, 61–62
    steps in, 60
    strategy identification in, 62–63
Strategies
    for group problem solving and decision making, 101–102
    for leading change, 81–82
Strategizing as defensive communication, 256
Strengths, organizational, analyzing, in strategic marketing
        planning, 64–65
Stress
    definition of, 187
    dynamics of, 188
    excessive, signs of, 190t
    high levels of, resolving, 193–194
    management of, 185–195
        primary prevention in, 188–191
        secondary prevention in, 191–192
        strategies for, 191t
        tertiary prevention in, 192–193
    role
        absenteeism and, 337
        definition of, 404
    sources of, 187–188
Stress diagram, 189
Structural functional perspective in role theory, 22
Structure, conversations for, 252
Style theories of leadership, 6
Subacute facilities, 114–115
Substance abuse in staff, 342–343
Substituted liability, 39–40
Superiority as defensive communication, 256
Supervision
    of delegatee, 307
    by nurse managers, malpractice and, 40
Supply and expense budget, 237
Support
    in leading change, 81, 83t
    in role transition, 403
        assessment of, 406
Supportive and defensive cycles, 257
Supportive communication, 256
Supportive work relationships in stress reduction, 192
Symbol, serving as, as leadership task, 13, 15t
Symbolic interaction in role theory, 22
Synergy in team, creating, 289–291
Systems perspective in stress prevention, 189
Systems theory model of healthcare organization
        evolution, 118–119
Systems thinking in learning organization theory, 78

Taft-Hartley Act, 46t, 161
Task behaviors, observing and using, 259–260
Teaching in consumer relationships, 357–360

Teaching institutions, 112
Team(s)
    appreciation for individual skills in, 286–287
    assembly of, in quality improvement process, 175–176
    assessment questionnaire for, 282
    building of, 279–298
        value of, 291–292
    concepts of, 281, 283–285
    control in, 285
    creating synergy in, 289–291
    effective vs. ineffective, 281, 283t
    groups and, 281
    "in" groups and "out" groups in, 285
    leadership role in, 293–294
    managing emotions in, 292–293
    power in, 285
    tools and issues supporting, 285–289
    trust in, 287, 289
Team learning in learning organization theory, 78
Team nursing, 369–371
Technology(ies)
    biomedical, 207–210
    confidentiality and, 218–219
    ethics and, 219
    fit between organizational structure and, 141
    for future, 220–222
    future trends in, 219–220
    hospital mission and, 139
    information, 210–217; see also Information technology
        definition of, 206, 208
    knowledge, 217–218
        definition of, 208
    management of, 205–224
    new, evaluating cost-effectiveness of, 234
    professional issues involving, 218–219
    types of, 207–218
    voice, 217
Telehealth, 221
Teleological ethical theories, 50–51
Temporary personnel as issue for nurse manager,
        malpractice and, 42–43
Termination for personal problems, 344–345
Tertiary care healthcare organizations, 110t
Therapeutic systems, 209
Thinking
    critical, 91–93
        definition of, 92
    systems, in learning organization theory, 78
Third-party financing organizations, 115–116
Third-party payers, 111
    healthcare costs and, 228–229
Time
    effective use of, in cost-conscious nursing, 233
    management of, 195–200
        concepts in, 198
        prioritization in, 196
        strategies in, 198–200

Time—cont'd
    nonproductive, in staffing budget, 390
    paid, in staffing budget, 390
    productive, in staffing budget, 390
    wasting, 196–198
    worked, in staffing budget, 390
Time tools, 199
Total patient care method of nursing care
        delivery, 366–367
Total quality management (TQM), 32, 171
Trait theories of leadership, 6
Traits, leadership, 26
Transactional/tranformational theories of leadership, 7
Transculturalism, 127, 129
Transformational leadership, 16
    characteristics of, 24–25
    evolution of, 24
Transitionals in political activism, 418
Trial and error approach to problem solving, 93
Triangulation in risk evaluation, 182
Trust in team, 287, 289
Truth, telling, in creating synergistic team, 289–290
Two-factor theory of motivation, 9

Uncooperative employees, 339–340
Unionization, 159–164
Unions, labor, 46
Unit(s)
    of service, 236
    troubled/conflicted, 421
    work load of, staffing and, 389
Unit budget development in budgeting process, 239
Unit level budget, managing, 240
Unity, achieving workable, as leadership task, 11–12, 15t
Unlicensed assistive personnel in case method of
        delivery, 367
Unproductive conflict vs. productive conflict, 322
Unproductive employees, 339–340
Utilization rates, healthcare costs and, 228

Values
    affirming, as leadership task, 8, 14t
    ethics and, 50
    personal, helping determine, 160
Variable cost(s), 234
    staffing as, 391–393
Variables affecting staffing schedules, 393
Variance, 240
    in critical path/MAP, 376
Variance analysis in budgeting process, 240
Ventilators, 209
Veracity as ethical principle, 51
Vicarious liability, 39–40
View, personal, disclosing, for participation in decision
        making, 159
Violence, people and work place, 31
Visibility, high, as power strategy, 425–426

Vision(s)
  creating, in leading change, 82, 83t
  establishing, as leadership task, 8
  shared, 452
    building, in learning organization theory, 78
Vision statements of organizations, 139
Visioning, 452
Visiting nurse associations, 113, 114
Voice technology, 217
Voluntary action in informed consent, 44
Voluntary affiliated healthcare systems, 112

Wagner Act, 46t, 160
Wagner Amendments, 46t
Warn, failure to, by nurse managers, malpractice and, 41
Watkins v. Unemployment Compensation Board of Review, 49
Watson's theory of caring, 52
Weakness, organizational, analyzing, in strategic marketing
    planning, 64–65
Welcomers, maintenance behaviors of, uses of, 261

Wellness programs, 117
Whistle-blower protection, 163
Willingness to cooperate in team concept, 284
Wireless messaging (WL), 216–217
Witness, expert, nurse as, 38–39
WL (wireless messaging), 216–217
Work groups, troubled/conflicted, 421
Work load of unit, staffing and, 389
Work place
  exercising power and influence in, 426–428
  safety in, 158
  violence in, 31
Work place advocacy, 158–159
Worked time in staffing budget, 390
Working environment in effective and ineffective
    teams, 283t
World Wide Web, 221
Wrongful discharge, 49

Zamudio v. Patia, 48

Key Abilities and Skills for New Nurse Leaders/Managers and Effective Followers

- Critically analyze nursing care requirements
- Influence others in their enactment of nursing
- Create a desire in others to continue self-development; continue your own
- Synthesize data from multiple sources
- Develop staff, considering their abilities and the organization's needs; develop yourself
- Translate the organization's vision into work reality; live the mission
- Make informed decisions readily
- Solve problems fairly and effectively, using staff input; provide your own input
- Mentor, coach, acknowledge, empower, and challenge staff; accept the same from others
- Communicate clearly and accurately
- Exhibit flexibility, creativity, commitment, enthusiasm, caring, and cultural sensitivity
- Demonstrate clinical competence
- Evaluate others and their work in light of standards; do the same for yourself
- Predict, control, and evaluate needed resources
- Have "long-short" vision (balance today's demands without losing sight of tomorrow's needs); think about the future
- Build teams and their commitment; be a productive team member
- Choose your own leadership, followership, and management style